Managing Infectious Diseases

Managing Infectious Diseases

Edited by Jasmine Frost

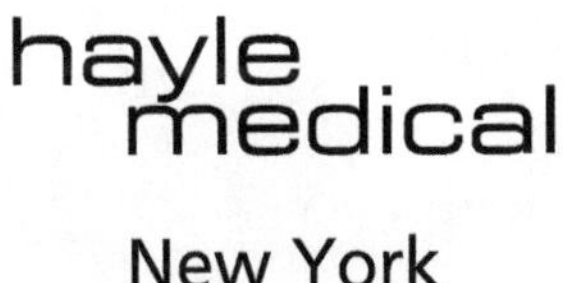

New York

Hayle Medical,
750 Third Avenue, 9th Floor,
New York, NY 10017, USA

Visit us on the World Wide Web at:
www.haylemedical.com

ISBN: 978-1-63241-650-6

Cataloging-in-Publication Data

Managing infectious diseases / edited by Jasmine Frost.
p. cm.
Includes bibliographical references and index.
ISBN 978-1-63241-650-6
1. Communicable diseases. 2. Infection. 3. Communicable diseases--Prevention.
4. Infection--Prevention. I. Frost, Jasmine.

RA643 .M36 2019
616.9 --dc23

Table of Contents

Preface

Illnesses resulting from an infection are called infectious diseases. Infection is caused by the invasion of the tissues of an organism's body by disease-causing agents. Virus, bacteria, nematode, viroid, prion, etc. are some of the agents that cause infections. An infectious disease is caused when the host's protective immune mechanisms are weak. Microorganisms damage tissues by releasing several toxins or destructive enzymes. Persistent infection is a severe form of infection. It occurs when the body is unable to clear the organism after the initial infection. Use of anti-infective drugs is the most common way to treat infections. The topics included in this book on infectious diseases are of utmost significance and bound to provide incredible insights to readers. It explores all the important aspects of infectious diseases in the present day scenario. Those in search of information to further their knowledge will be greatly assisted by this book.

The researches compiled throughout the book are authentic and of high quality, combining several disciplines and from very diverse regions from around the world. Drawing on the contributions of many researchers from diverse countries, the book's objective is to provide the readers with the latest achievements in the area of research. This book will surely be a source of knowledge to all interested and researching the field.

In the end, I would like to express my deep sense of gratitude to all the authors for meeting the set deadlines in completing and submitting their research chapters. I would also like to thank the publisher for the support offered to us throughout the course of the book. Finally, I extend my sincere thanks to my family for being a constant source of inspiration and encouragement.

Editor

1

Integrating HIV care and treatment into tuberculosis clinics in Lusaka, Zambia: results from a before-after quasi-experimental study

Michael E Herce[1,2*†], Jill Morse[1†], Dora Luhanga[1], Jennifer Harris[1,3], Helene J Smith[1], Stable Besa[1], Graham Samungole[4], Nzali Kancheya[1], Monde Muyoyeta[1] and Stewart E Reid[1,3]

Abstract

Background: Patients with HIV-associated tuberculosis (TB) often have their TB and HIV managed in separate vertical programs that offer care for each disease with little coordination. Such "siloed" approaches are associated with diagnostic and treatment delays, which contribute to unnecessary morbidity and mortality. To improve TB/HIV care coordination and early ART initiation, we integrated HIV care and treatment into two busy TB clinics in Zambia. We report here the effects of our intervention on outcomes of linkage to HIV care, early ART uptake, and TB treatment success for patients with HIV-associated TB in Lusaka, Zambia.

Methods: We provided integrated HIV treatment and care using a "one-stop shop" model intervention. All new or relapse HIV-positive TB patients were offered immediate HIV program enrolment and ART within 8 weeks of anti-TB therapy (ATT) initiation. We used a quasi-experimental design, review of routine program data, and survival analysis and logistic regression methods to estimate study outcomes before (June 1, 2010—January 31, 2011) and after (August 1, 2011—March 31, 2012) our intervention among 473 patients with HIV-associated TB categorized into pre- ($n = 248$) and post-intervention ($n = 225$) cohorts.

Results: Patients in the pre- and post-intervention cohorts were mostly male (60.1% and 52.9%, respectively) and young (median age: 33 years). In time-to-event analyses, a significantly higher proportion of patients in the post-intervention cohort linked to HIV care by 4 weeks post-ATT initiation (53.9% vs. 43.4%, $p = 0.03$), with median time to care linkage being 59 and 25 days in the pre- and post-intervention cohorts, respectively. In Cox proportional hazard modelling, patients receiving the integration intervention started ART by 8 weeks post-ATT at 1.33 times the rate (HR = 1.33, 95% CI: 1.00–1.77) as patients pre-intervention. In logistic regression modelling, patients receiving the intervention were 2.02 times (95% CI: 1.11–3.67) as likely to have a successful TB treatment outcome as patients not receiving the intervention.

Conclusions: Integrating HIV treatment and care services into routine TB clinics using a one-stop shop model increased linkage to HIV care, rates of early ART initiation, and TB treatment success among patients with HIV-associated TB in Lusaka, Zambia.

Keywords: TB-HIV integration, Tuberculosis, HIV/AIDS, Zambia, Linkage to care, Antiretroviral therapy, Sub-Saharan Africa

* Correspondence: michael.herce@cidrz.org
†Michael E Herce and Jill Morse contributed equally to this work.
[1]Centre for Infectious Disease Research in Zambia (CIDRZ), Lusaka, Zambia
[2]Division of Infectious Diseases, Department of Medicine, University of North Carolina School of Medicine, Chapel Hill, North Carolina, USA
Full list of author information is available at the end of the article

Background

Dual tuberculosis (TB) and HIV epidemics have disproportionately affected sub-Saharan Africa (SSA). In 2016, an estimated 30% of all incident TB in the World Health Organization (WHO) African region, or approximately 764,000 total TB cases, were HIV-associated [1]. In Zambia, one of the 30 WHO high TB burden countries, 58% of patients with new or relapse tuberculosis have HIV infection [1]. In Zambia and throughout SSA, patients with HIV-associated TB often have their TB and HIV managed independently, typically in disease-specific vertical care programs [2, 3].

Historically, these vertical programs have provided care for each disease with little to no coordination, relying instead upon separate clinics and different health workers [4]. As a result, these "siloed" programs are associated with diagnostic and treatment delays for both diseases, poor HIV counselling and testing (HCT) uptake, delays in, and low rates of, linkage to HIV care and antiretroviral therapy (ART) initiation, and increased patient morbidity and mortality [5–8] These non-integrated approaches have also been hampered by several operational challenges, including: a lack of resource sharing between TB and HIV programs; uncoordinated visit scheduling, which increases patient costs and work absenteeism; and poor communication between TB and HIV clinics about prescribed drug regimens, treatment-related side effects, and drug-drug interactions for shared patients [3, 9–11]. Importantly, the vertical approach also threatens TB infection control efforts when co-infected patients with newly diagnosed or undiagnosed TB congregate with other HIV-positive patients in ART clinics [12].

In response to these challenges, several models of coordinated TB/HIV care have emerged, reflecting a spectrum of service integration. These models range from referral-based approaches in which co-infected patients are directed from the TB clinic to a separate ART clinic, and vice versa, for TB/HIV services to a more integrated "one-stop shop" model where one healthcare team provides fully integrated TB/HIV services under one roof [3, 11]. Integrated TB/HIV care, in which the same healthcare team provides services to patients with HIV-associated TB, offers potential advantages over standard approaches. First, it allows clinicians to better co-manage TB/HIV co-infection and attendant complications, such as drug-drug interactions, side effects, and toxicities. Second, integrated care helps counsellors and treatment supporters provide psychosocial support and adherence counselling to co-infected patients in the same location. Finally, integrated TB/HIV services helps patients better access treatment and care, including ART, in a timely fashion, without having to wait in multiple clinics within one or more health facilities [3].

For ART provision, clinical trial evidence clearly demonstrates the importance of starting ART early, within 8 to 12 weeks, to reduce HIV-associated TB mortality, particularly for patients with advanced immunosuppression [13–16]. Despite the known benefits, however, several barriers to early ART initiation in patients with HIV-associated TB have hampered uptake of this evidence-based intervention in routine care settings. These barriers include poor coordination between vertical TB and HIV programs, patient and provider reluctance, delays in laboratory testing and result reporting, and the excessive number of steps patients must navigate along the HIV and TB care cascades [5, 9, 17, 18].

In Zambia, while recent progress has been made in improving the proportion of HIV-positive TB patients on ART reported to WHO, from 60% in 2012 to 83% in 2016 [1, 19], challenges remain. For example, in 2016, ART coverage as a percentage of the estimated number of new HIV-associated TB cases nationally stood at just under 60%, suggesting a need for continued work to improve access to ART for HIV-positive TB patients [1]. For HIV-positive TB patients accessing ART, little is known about the average time to ART initiation in routine care settings in SSA. Furthermore, there is limited data from Zambia and the region evaluating integrated TB/HIV care models in real-world clinical settings, and, in particular, few reports examining models that provide comprehensive HIV services, including ART initiation and follow-up, *within* TB clinics.

To increase the proportion of patients with HIV-associated TB who link to HIV care and initiate ART early in routine TB clinical settings, we piloted integration of HIV care and treatment—including HIV care enrolment and ART initiation and follow-up—into two busy TB clinics in Lusaka using a one-stop shop model. The Centre for Infectious Disease Research in Zambia (CIDRZ) implemented the pilot in partnership with the Lusaka District Health Office (DHO) of the Zambian Ministry of Health (MOH). We aim here to assess the feasibility of our pilot intervention and to evaluate its effects on timely linkage to HIV care, early ART uptake, and TB treatment outcomes among HIV-associated TB patients in Lusaka, Zambia.

Methods

Study design, population, and setting

We conducted a quasi-experimental before-after study from June 1, 2010 through March 31, 2012 to assess whether our TB/HIV treatment and care integration intervention had an effect on two primary outcomes: linkage to HIV care and early ART initiation. We defined "linkage to HIV care" as documented evidence of having enrolled in the national HIV program. We defined "early" ART initiation as a patient receiving ART within 8 to 12 weeks of anti-TB therapy (ATT) start. Patients were eligible for study inclusion if they had a recorded ATT start date documented in the TB register, and had documented HIV infection. We excluded patients who: were already on ART at the time of TB diagnosis; transferred into a study site TB clinic from a non-study site; were receiving HIV care through a private clinic or non-governmental organization; started ATT outside the defined pre- and post-intervention time periods; or were concurrently enrolled in another study. No patients with documented multi-drug resistant TB received treatment at primary health centre level during the study period.

We observed outcomes of interest among patients meeting study eligibility criteria at two TB clinics situated within two CIDRZ-supported primary health centres in Lusaka, Zambia—"Clinic A" and "Clinic B". Observations occurred during an 8-month pre-intervention period (June 1, 2010 through January 31, 2011) and an 8-month post-intervention period (August 1, 2011 to March 31, 2012). Patients who started ATT during the pre-intervention period were considered part of a "pre-intervention cohort"; those who initiated ATT during the post-intervention period were part of the "post-intervention cohort". The pre- and post-intervention periods were exactly the same duration, and were specified to enable an intervening 1-month "wash-out" window between when the last patient joining the pre-intervention cohort completed their 6-month ATT course and the start of our intervention during the post-intervention period.

Standard of care

Patients in the pre-intervention cohort received the standard of care. Under the standard of care, patients with TB/HIV co-infection are provided TB and HIV care separately in two distinct clinics using a referral-driven model. Typically, the standard of care follows one of two clinical pathways (detailed below) depending on whether HIV or TB is diagnosed first: 1) a newly diagnosed or established HIV-positive patient undergoes evaluation and treatment for TB; or 2) a new TB patient tests positive for HIV.

Newly diagnosed HIV-positive patients may be referred to the ART clinic from any of a number of locations in the facility, including the HCT room, the maternal & child health department, the out-patient department, or other department. At the ART clinic, the patient is enrolled in the national HIV program (requiring registration in the SmartCare electronic medical record system), and undergoes baseline clinical and laboratory evaluation in preparation for ART initiation. Those newly establishing HIV care also receive co-trimoxazole preventive therapy (CPT). All newly diagnosed HIV-positive patients undergo TB screening at the time of their first clinical evaluation by sputum smear microscopy, or, less commonly, by Xpert MTB/RIF (Cepheid, Sunnyvale, CA, USA) where available. Chest x-ray is not routinely available in all health facilities, and where available often requires that a user fee be paid. Patients found to be smear-negative are assessed by a clinician and may be treated empirically based on clinical findings suggestive of TB disease. After establishing HIV care, HIV-positive patients are screened for TB-compatible symptoms at every ART clinic visit per national guidelines [20, 21]. HIV-positive patients diagnosed with TB clinically (i.e. based on symptoms, physical exam, and/or chest x-ray) or microbiologically (i.e. by smear microscopy or Xpert MTB/RIF) are referred to the TB clinic to initiate ATT.

All newly diagnosed TB patients are offered HCT at enrolment into TB care, typically within the TB Clinic itself. To that end, the TB clinic usually houses one or more HCT counselling rooms, and is staffed by one to two nurses and peer health educators. Patients testing HIV-positive are referred to the ART Clinic to establish HIV care and undergo further evaluation for ART initiation as detailed above.

All patients with drug-susceptible TB, irrespective of HIV status, receive first-line ATT with a WHO-recommended, 6-month rifampicin-based fixed-dose combination regimen. ATT is initiated in the TB clinic according to national guidelines from the National Tuberculosis & Leprosy Control Programme (NTP). In Zambia, TB treatment is supported by a lay cadre of peer health educators who provide psychosocial support and adherence counselling to patients.

HIV care and treatment integration intervention

We implemented the same model of TB/HIV service integration in two routine TB clinics—Clinic A and Clinic B. The integration intervention was introduced first at Clinic A in August 2011, and then at Clinic B in October 2011. The intervention had five core components: 1) health worker training and mentorship; 2) timely provider-initiated HIV testing and counselling (PITC); 3) on-site HIV care enrolment; 4) dedicated ART clinic days; and 5) synchronized TB and HIV patient follow-up. We further describe these components below.

We trained all nurses and clinical officers from both the TB clinic and ART clinic on TB/HIV co-management. Training emphasized proper ATT and ART prescribing practices, and recognition and management of drug-related side effects and toxicity. Importantly, clinicians were trained to begin ART for all co-infected patients as soon as possible, and preferably within 8 to 12 weeks of ATT initiation, regardless of CD4 count. CIDRZ clinician mentors worked intensively with facility staff for approximately 6 months at the start of the intervention to reinforce training concepts. CIDRZ peer educators were trained to provide health education talks to patients on the relationship between TB and HIV and the need for early and sustained co-treatment.

All newly diagnosed TB patients were offered PITC at enrolment into TB care (Fig. 1). TB patients newly identified as HIV-positive who had not previously enrolled in HIV care were informed about the importance of linking to HIV care and starting ART, and were offered immediate enrolment into HIV care on site. MOH nursing staff conducted initial HIV care enrolment procedures in line with national guidelines in place at the time of the study, including: completion of the MOH HIV care enrolment form and blood draws for baseline laboratory tests (including complete blood count, CD4, creatinine, and liver function tests). Following HIV care enrolment, patients were scheduled for an on-site ART initiation visit with a clinical officer to undergo a thorough clinical evaluation, including history, physical exam, and laboratory test result review, and to start ART. HIV-positive TB patients already on ART at the time of ATT initiation were given the option to continue their HIV care at the ART clinic or to transfer their HIV care to the TB clinic for the duration of ATT.

To ensure adequate patient follow-up and efficient use of limited human resources for clinician staffing, each TB clinic scheduled a weekly 'ART clinic day' when the same MOH clinical officer was posted to provide "one-stop shop" TB/HIV services, including ART initiation. On the scheduled day, the MOH clinical officer evaluated patients, conducted a physical exam, and reviewed lab results and ART eligibility. Once patients enrolled in HIV care, and initiated ART, they attended the TB clinic according to their directly observed therapy (DOT) schedule (daily, weekly or monthly) for TB treatment. ART and TB follow-up was synchronized to harmonize clinical care and drug collection, and to maximize patient convenience. Specifically, the same clinical officer provided follow-up clinical evaluation for both TB and HIV and attendant co-morbidities and drug-related toxicities, and patients collected both their antiretrovirals (ARVs) and TB medications from the same open-air drug dispensary at the TB clinic. Eligible patients who declined to initiate ART continued to receive TB care in the TB clinic and were

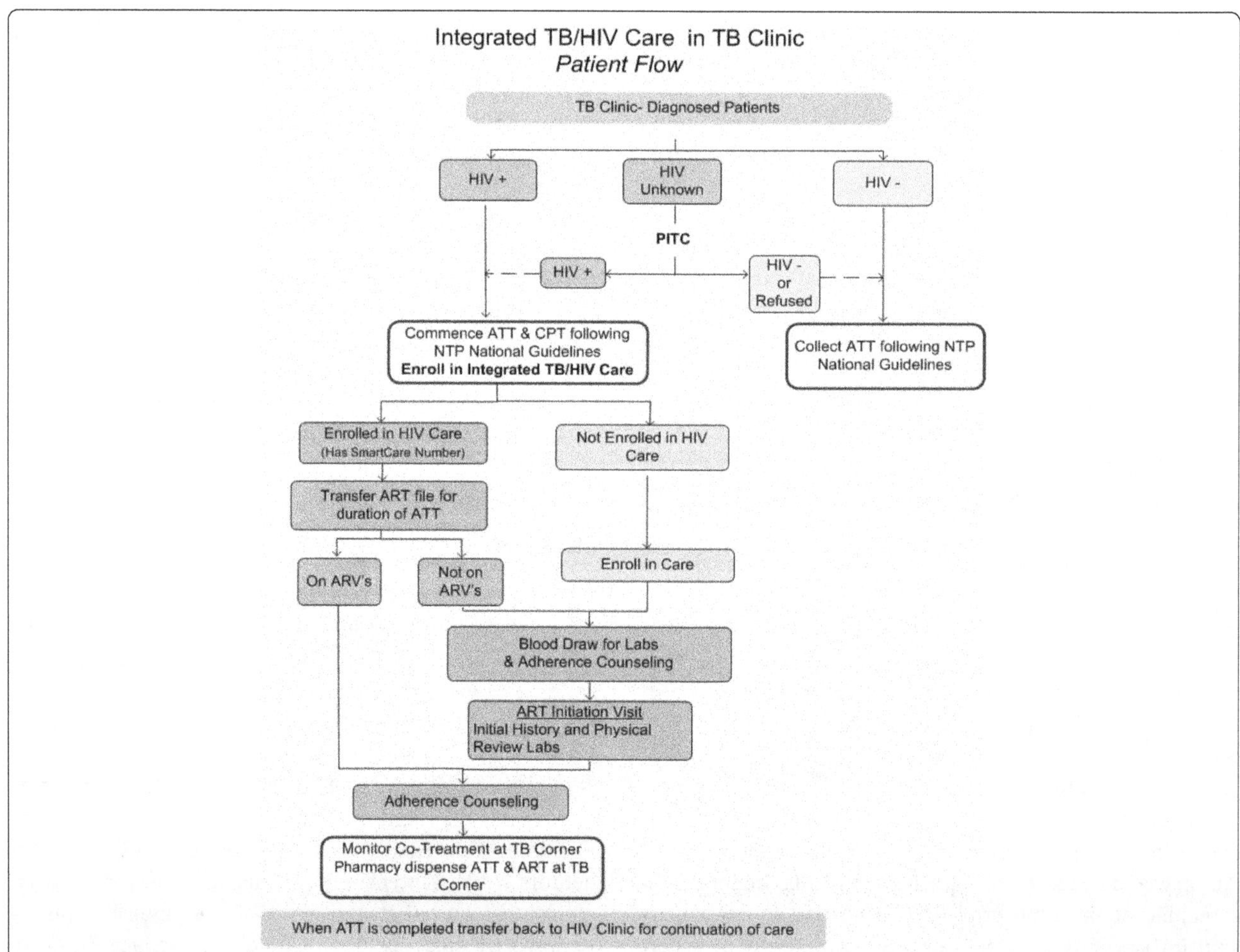

Fig. 1 Integrated TB/HIV care patient flow. HIV, human immunodeficiency virus; TB, tuberculosis; PITC, provider-initiated testing and counselling; ATT, anti-tuberculosis therapy; CPT, co-trimoxazole therapy; ART, anti-retroviral therapy; ARVs, antiretrovirals; NTP, National Tuberculosis and Leprosy Programme

encouraged to start ART at each visit. Upon ATT completion, patients were referred to the ART clinic in each facility for continuing their HIV care.

Data collection

For both the pre- and post-intervention periods, data were collected prospectively during routine clinical care, and recorded onto the following primary data sources: national TB registers, patient TB treatment cards, paper-based HIV care files, and the national SmartCare HIV electronic medical record system. From these data sources, we subsequently abstracted patient data fields of interest, including: age, sex, TB clinic serial number, TB registration date, TB case identification number, TB registration type (i.e. new, relapse, transferred in, treatment after default, or failure), TB anatomical site (i.e. pulmonary TB [PTB] or extra-pulmonary TB [EPTB]), TB treatment start date, recorded HIV status, SmartCare registration number, date of HIV care enrolment, date of initial history and physical exam, date of first CPT dispensation, date of first ART dispensation, and WHO TB treatment outcome [22, 23]. Blank data fields were coded as "missing." Per routine medical record keeping practice, any patient without a documented HIV care enrolment date is considered not to have linked to care, and any patient without a first ART dispensation date is thought not to have started ART. All data were de-identified at the time of abstraction to protect patient confidentiality. For the pre-intervention cohort, we administratively censored HIV care enrolment and ART initiation 6 months after the end of the pre-intervention period, on July 31, 2011. Similarly, for the post-intervention cohort, we censored HIV care enrolment and ART initiation 6 months after the end of the post-intervention period, on September 30, 2012.

Data analysis

Patient characteristics at the time of ATT initiation (i.e. at "baseline") were compared between pre- and post-intervention cohorts using the Chi-square test for categorical variables and the Student's t-test for continuous variables. Simple proportions were used to describe the primary outcomes: 1) the percentage of HIV-associated TB patients newly enrolled in HIV care by 4, 8, and 12 weeks of ATT initiation; and 2) the percentage of HIV-associated TB patients who newly initiated ART by 4, 8, and 12 weeks of starting ATT. We compared the proportion of patients with a primary outcome between the pre- and post-intervention cohorts, stratified by study clinic, using the Cochran-Mantel-Haenszel test. We estimated time to HIV care enrolment and ART initiation using Kaplan-Meier methods with follow-up time measured from ATT initiation. Cumulative failure functions were compared using the Log rank test. Cox proportional hazard modelling was employed to estimate the association between exposure to our TB/HIV integration intervention and ART start by 8 weeks post-ATT initiation. We selected 8 weeks post-ATT initiation as our threshold of interest as this is the WHO-recommended time frame by which ART should be initiated in patients with HIV-associated TB [24]. To estimate the effect of the intervention on successful TB treatment (i.e. TB cure or treatment completion), multi-variable logistic regression modelling was used to determine the odds ratio and associated 95% confidence interval (CI). For both our Cox proportional hazard and logistic regression models, we adjusted for potential confounders that were selected on the basis of clinical and programmatic plausibility, including age, sex, intervention clinic, TB anatomical site, and TB registration type (i.e. new case or cases of relapse, default, or treatment after failure). Patients who transferred out or had missing outcomes data were excluded from the models. We considered two-sided p-values ≤ 0.05 statistically significant. All statistical analyses were performed using STATA version 12.1 (College Station, TX, USA).

Ethics statement

Ethical approval for this study was granted by the University of Zambia Biomedical Research Ethics Committee and the Institutional Review Board at the University of North Carolina at Chapel Hill, without requiring patient consent given the use of de-identified, routinely collected data.

Results

Overview

Over the 22-month study period, Clinic A and B registered 578 and 983 total HIV-positive and HIV-negative TB patients, respectively; HIV prevalence among TB patients at Clinic A and B was 68.3% and 55.5%, respectively. A total of 473 patients met study eligibility criteria, including 248 patients in the pre-intervention cohort and 225 patients in the post-intervention cohort.

Baseline patient characteristics

Patient age and sex distribution did not differ significantly between the pre- and post-intervention cohorts, with a majority of patients being male with a mean age of 33 years (Table 1). Eighty-five percent of patients in both the pre- and post-intervention cohorts were classified as having new TB. A similar majority of patients in both cohorts had pulmonary tuberculosis, with the remaining patients in both cohorts having extra-pulmonary tuberculosis. While 52.8% of patients in the pre-intervention cohort hailed from Clinic A, 65.8% of patients in the post-intervention cohort were from Clinic B—a statistically significant difference (Table 1). The proportion of HIV-positive TB patients *not* linked to care at baseline as measured by enrolment in the HIV program at the time of ATT initiation was

Table 1 Baseline Characteristics of Pre- and Post-Intervention Cohorts

Characteristic	Pre-intervention $N = 248$ n (%)	Post-intervention $N = 225$ n (%)	*p*-value
Sex			
Male	149 (60.1)	119 (52.9)	0.12
Female	99 (39.9)	106 (47.1)	
Age, mean (se)	33.7 (0.7)	33.3 (0.7)	0.74
TB Registration Type			
New	211 (85.1)	192 (85.3)	0.40
Relapse	35 (14.1)	33 (14.7)	
Treatment after Default or Failure	2 (0.8)	0 (0)	
TB Anatomical Site			
Pulmonary TB	207 (83.5)	184 (81.8)	0.63
Extra-Pulmonary TB	41 (16.5)	41 (18.2)	
Clinic			
Clinic A	131 (52.8)	77 (34.2)	< 0.01
Clinic B	117 (47.2)	148 (65.8)	
Linkage to care Status			
Not Linked *(Not Enrolled in HIV Care, not receiving ART)*	159 (64.1)	167 (74.2)	0.02
Linked *(Enrolled in HIV Care, not receiving ART)*	89 (35.9)	58 (25.8)	

se Standard error, *TB* Tuberculosis, *ART* Antiretroviral therapy

significantly higher in the post-intervention cohort at 74.2%, compared to 64.1% in the pre-intervention cohort ($p = 0.02$) (Table 1).

Linkage to HIV care

A total of 147 patients had documented evidence of HIV program enrolment at the time of ATT initiation, and thus were excluded from the linkage to care analysis. Among patients who were not linked at baseline, a significantly higher proportion of patients in the post-intervention cohort linked to HIV care by 4, 8, and 12 weeks after ATT initiation, compared to patients in the pre-intervention cohort at the same time points (Table 2). By 12 weeks after ATT initiation, 62.9% of patients in the post-intervention cohort had linked to HIV care, compared to 54.7% in the pre-intervention cohort ($p = 0.03$). Stratified by clinic, we observed a significantly higher proportion of patients in the post-intervention cohort at Clinic A linking to care by 4, 8, and 12 weeks. For Clinic B, we did not observe a statistically significant difference in the proportion of patients in the pre- and post-intervention cohorts linking to HIV care by the time points of interest (Table 2).

In time-to-event analyses, a significantly higher proportion of patients in the post-intervention cohort

Table 2 Linkage to HIV care outcomes for patients not already in HIV care at baseline ($N = 326$)

Outcome	Pre-intervention	Post-intervention	*p*-value
Linked to HIV care within 4 weeks of ATT initiation			
All patients	69/159 (43.4%)	90/167 (53.9%)	0.01
Clinic A	40/81 (49.4%)	41/55 (74.6%)	< 0.01
Clinic B	29/78 (37.2%)	49/112 (43.8%)	0.37
Linked to HIV care within 8 weeks of ATT initiation			
All patients	82/159 (51.6%)	99/167 (59.3%)	0.04
Clinic A	46/81 (56.8%)	45/55 (81.8%)	< 0.01
Clinic B	36/78 (46.2%)	54/112 (48.2%)	0.78
Linked to HIV care within 12 weeks of ATT initiation			
All patients	87/159 (54.7%)	105/167 (62.9%)	0.03
Clinic A	48/81 (59.3%)	47/55 (85.5%)	< 0.01
Clinic B	39/78 (50.0%)	58/112 (51.8%)	0.81

ATT Anti-TB therapy

compared to the pre-intervention cohort linked to care by 4 weeks (53.9% vs. 43.4%, $p = 0.03$), but not by 8 weeks (59.3% vs. 51.6%, $p = 0.07$) or 12 weeks (62.9% vs. 54.7%, $p = 0.06$) (Fig. 2). The median time to HIV care linkage was 59 days in the pre-intervention cohort versus 25 days in the post-intervention cohort.

ART initiation

We evaluated ART initiation in both patients who were linked and not linked to HIV care at baseline (Table 3). The proportion of all patients at Clinics A and B initiating ART in the post-intervention cohort by 4 weeks after ATT initiation was higher in the post-intervention cohort (29.3%) than the pre-intervention cohort (25.0%), however, this difference was not statistically significant ($p = 0.18$) (Table 3). A significantly higher proportion of patients initiated ART by 8 weeks in the post-intervention (45.3%) versus pre-intervention cohort (38.3%) ($p = 0.04$). Similarly, by 12 weeks after ATT, significantly more HIV-positive TB patients receiving the intervention had started ART (52.0%) than those who had not been exposed to the intervention (41.5%) ($p < 0.01$). The proportion of patients starting ART within 4, 8, and 12 weeks of ATT initiation was observed to be consistently higher in Clinic A than Clinic B for both the pre- and post-intervention cohorts.

In time-to-event analyses, a significantly higher proportion of patients in the post-intervention versus pre-intervention cohort had initiated ART early, by 12 weeks (52.0% vs. 41.5%, $p = 0.03$) after TB treatment initiation (Fig. 3), but not by 8 weeks (45.3% vs. 38.3%, $p = 0.11$) or 4 weeks (29.3% vs. 25.0%, $p = 0.28$). Overall, median time to ART was 264 days in the pre-intervention cohort and 78 days in the post-intervention cohort.

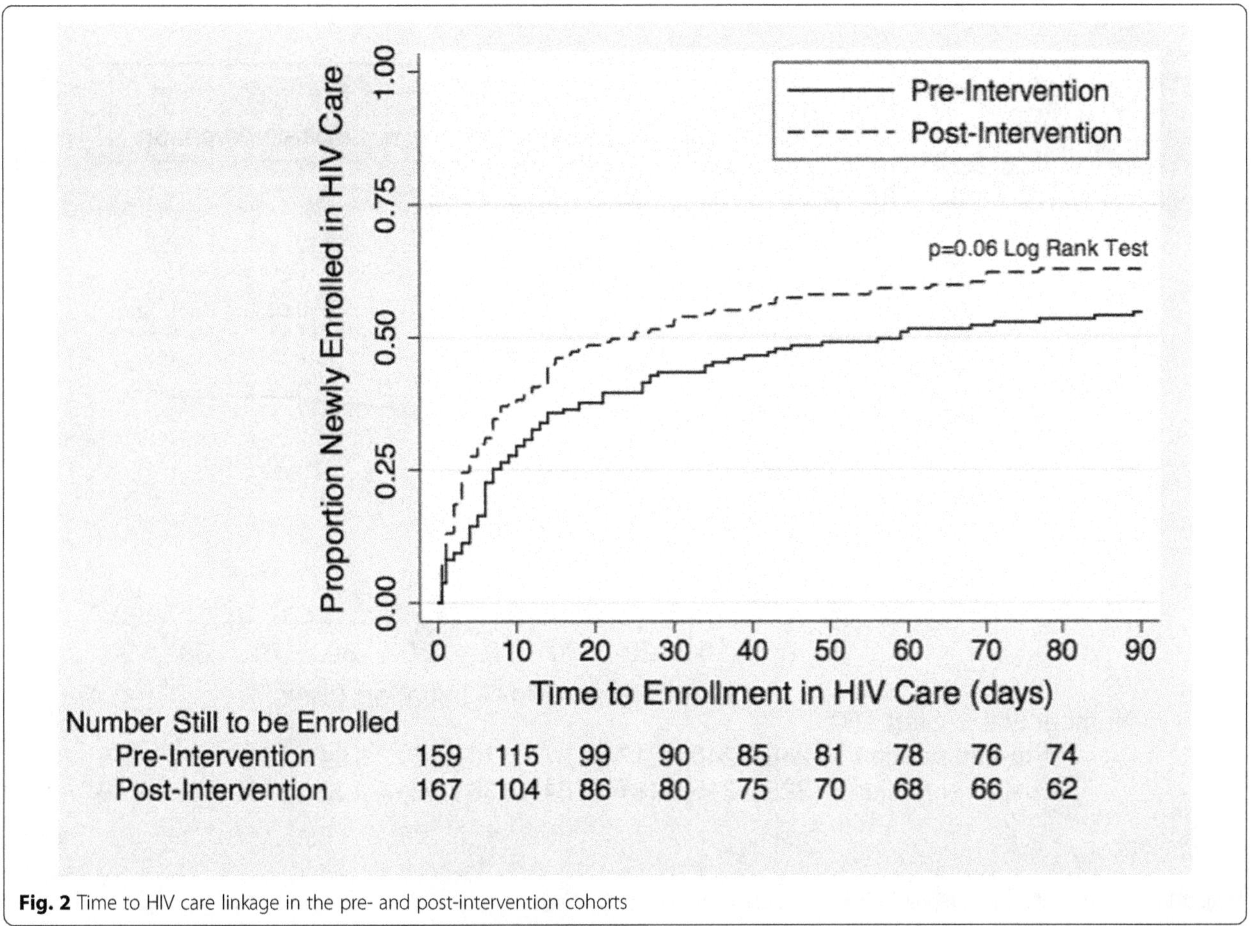

Fig. 2 Time to HIV care linkage in the pre- and post-intervention cohorts

In our adjusted multi-variable Cox proportional hazard model controlling for age, sex, clinic, TB anatomical site, and TB registration type, TB patients who received the integration intervention started ART by 8 weeks post-ATT at 1.33 times the rate (HR = 1.33, 95% CI: 1.00–1.77) as patients who were not exposed to the intervention, and this observation was statistically significant (Table 4).

Table 3 ART initiation outcomes for patients not yet on ART at the time of TB treatment initiation ($N = 473$)

Outcome	Pre-intervention	Post-intervention	*p*-value
Initiating ART within 0 to 4 weeks			
All patients	62/248 (25.0%)	66/225 (29.3%)	0.18
Clinic A	40/131 (30.5%)	23/77 (29.9%)	0.92
Clinic B	22/117 (18.8%)	43/148 (29.1%)	0.05
Initiating ART within 0 to 8 weeks			
All patients	95/248 (38.3%)	102/225 (45.3%)	0.04
Clinic A	58/131 (44.3%)	41/77 (53.3%)	0.21
Clinic B	37/117 (31.6%)	61/148 (41.2%)	0.11
Initiating ART within 0 to 12 weeks			
All patients	103/248 (41.5%)	117/225 (52.0%)	< 0.01
Clinic A	61/131 (46.6%)	51/77 (66.2%)	< 0.01
Clinic B	42/117 (35.9%)	66/148 (44.6%)	0.15

ART Antiretroviral therapy

TB treatment outcomes

Among the 473 total patients with HIV-associated TB in the pre- and post-intervention cohorts, 284 (60.0%) had a documented TB treatment outcome. Of these, a higher proportion had a successful outcome (i.e. either microbiological cure or documented treatment completion) in the post-intervention cohort (83.3%) compared to the pre-intervention cohort (73.9%), although the difference was of borderline statistical significance ($p = 0.051$) and the effect was less pronounced in Clinic B than Clinic A (Table 5).

In adjusted multivariable logistic regression modelling, patients receiving the TB/HIV integration intervention were 2.02 times (95% CI: 1.11–3.67) as likely to have a successful TB treatment outcome (i.e. achieving cure or completing treatment) as patients not receiving the intervention (Table 6).

Discussion

We demonstrate that implementing a one-stop shop model of TB/HIV service integration significantly

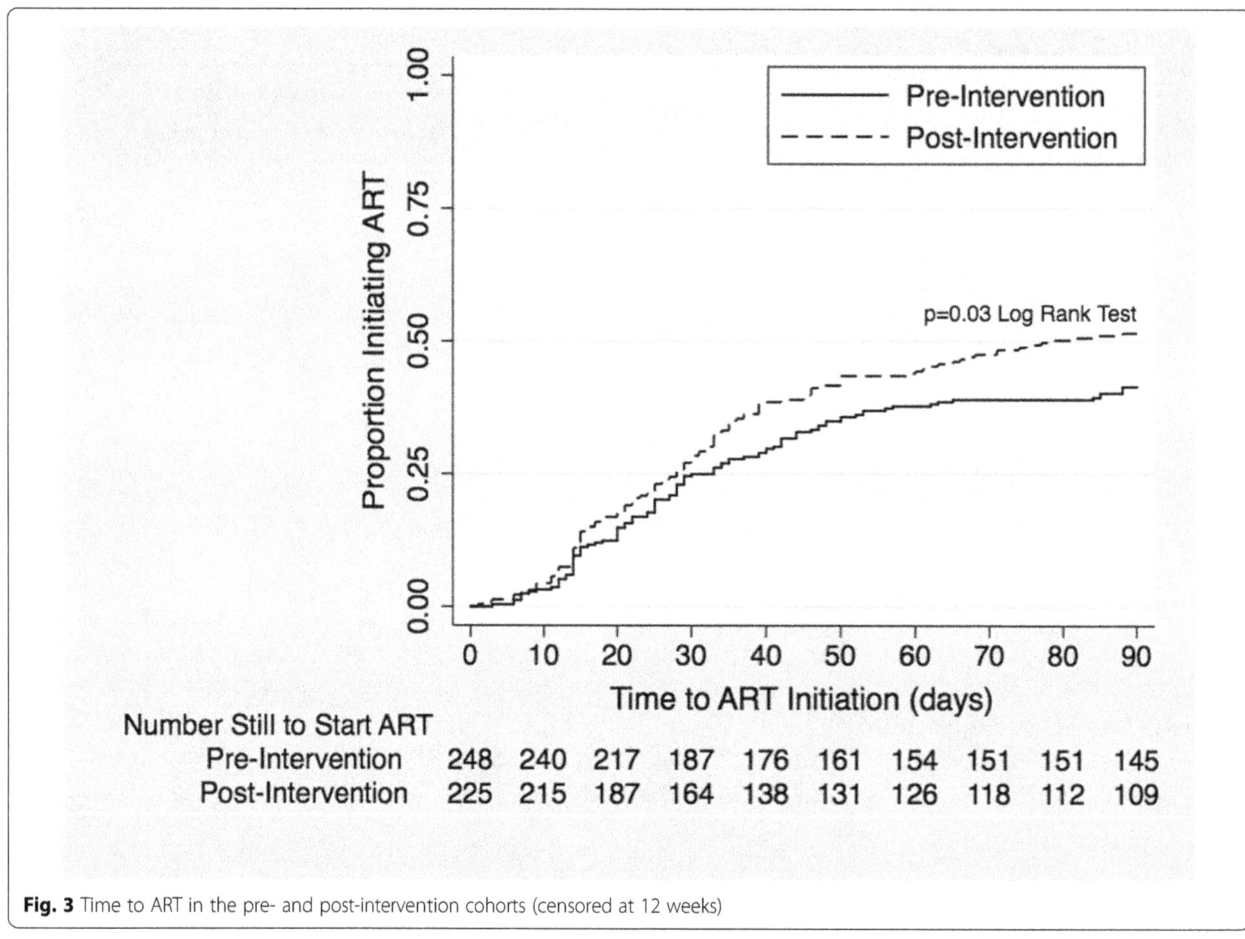

Fig. 3 Time to ART in the pre- and post-intervention cohorts (censored at 12 weeks)

increases linkage to HIV care and rates of early ART initiation among patients with HIV-associated TB. Providing this integrated model in TB clinics does not detract from TB services, but rather appears to increase the odds of TB cure or treatment completion. Taken together, our findings suggest the feasibility of integrating HIV care and treatment within routine TB clinical settings in Lusaka, Zambia.

Despite increasing access and coverage of ART in Zambia [25], there is an on-going need to implement and evaluate integrated TB/HIV service delivery models to ensure universal access to ART for patients with HIV-associated TB. Challenges with linkage to HIV care and ART initiation for HIV-positive TB patients persist despite clear national guidelines calling for prompt ART initiation and compelling clinical trial data documenting the clear benefits of early ART [13, 26–28]. Reasons for sub-optimal linkage to HIV care and ART uptake among patients with HIV-associated TB are thought to be multifactorial, and include: increased patient transport and opportunity costs related to the multiple visits generated by referral-based services; fear among patients and clinicians about the co-management of side effects and toxicities; the greater pill burden resulting from co-treatment; and stigma associated with establishing HIV care and initiating ART [6, 9, 11, 29–31].

WHO guidelines strongly recommend that ART be started within 8 weeks of ATT initiation [24]. Zambian national TB and HIV guidelines reinforce this guidance, calling for early ART initiation as soon as ATT is tolerated, ideally within 2 to 3 weeks of commencing TB treatment [20]. Yet, no published reports from Zambia describe the extent to which ART is started early, or the average time to ART initiation from ATT initiation, for patients with HIV-associated TB in routine care settings. In our post-intervention cohort, we observed an average time to ART from ATT initiation of 78 days, a marked reduction from the 264 days observed in the pre-intervention cohort. Similarly, patients who received our intervention had an increased rate of early ART initiation (by 8 weeks), although ART uptake remained below 50%. While these findings suggest our intervention improved access to early ART, the relatively low absolute proportion of patients who received ART by 8 weeks argues for greater investments in HIV services and health system strengthening to improve integrated TB/HIV care for patients with HIV-associated TB. In our Lusaka study clinics, we postulate that the relatively

Table 4 Estimated effect of the integrated TB/HIV treatment and care intervention, and other covariates, on ART initiation by 8 weeks (N = 473)

Characteristic	Unadjusted		*p*-value	Adjusted[a]		*p*-value
	HR	95% CI		HR	95% CI	
Integration Intervention						
After	1.25	(0.95, 1.66)	0.12	1.33	(1.00, 1.77)	0.05
Before	1.00					
Sex						
Female	0.82	(0.62, 1.09)	0.18	0.84	(0.63, 1.12)	0.23
Male	1.00					
Age						
≥ 35 years	1.21	(0.91, 1.60)	0.19	1.17	(0.89, 1.56)	0.26
< 35 years	1.00					
Clinic						
Clinic B	0.73	(0.55, 0.97)	0.03	0.71	(0.53, 0.94)	0.02
Clinic A	1.00					
TB Site						
Extra-pulmonary	0.79	(0.53, 1.17)	0.24	0.81	(0.55, 1.20)	0.29
Pulmonary	1.00					
TB Registration Type[b]						
Treatment after Default, Failure, OR Relapse	0.89	(0.60, 1.33)	0.57	0.84	(0.56, 1.26)	0.40
New	1.00					

HR Hazard ratio, *TB* Tuberculosis
[a]HR estimated by Cox proportional hazard modelling, adjusting for remaining variables presented in the table
[b]Relapse, treatment after default, and failure were collapsed into one category due to collinearity in the model

Table 6 Estimated effect of the integrated TB/HIV treatment and care intervention, and other covariates, on successful TB treatment (cure or completion) (N = 284)

Characteristic	Unadjusted		*p*-value	Adjusted[a]		*p*-value
	OR	95% CI		OR	95% CI	
Integration Intervention						
After	1.77	(0.99, 3.15)	0.05	2.02	(1.11, 3.67)	0.02
Before	1.00					
Sex						
Female	1.10	(0.61, 1.98)	0.75	1.16	(0.64, 2.13)	0.62
Male	1.00					
Age						
≥ 35 years	1.05	(0.59, 1.87)	0.87	1.08	(0.60, 1.95)	0.81
< 35 years	1.00					
Clinic						
Clinic B	0.57	(0.32, 1.02)	0.06	0.50	(0.27, 0.92)	0.03
Clinic A	1.00					
TB Site						
Extra-pulmonary	0.77	(0.35, 1.69)	0.52	0.82	(0.37, 1.82)	0.62
Pulmonary	1.00					
TB Registration Type[b]						
Treatment after Default, Failure OR Relapse	0.94	(0.42, 2.10)	0.89	0.99	(0.43, 2.28)	0.98
New	1.00					
ART started within 8 weeks of TB treatment						
Yes	1.30	(0.72, 2.32)	0.38	1.16	(0.63, 2.13)	0.63
No	1.00					

OR Odds ratio
[a]OR estimated by logistic regression modelling, adjusting for remaining variables presented in the table
[b]Relapse, treatment after default, and failure were collapsed into one category due to collinearity in the model

low ART uptake observed by 8 and 12 weeks was due to persistent gaps in human resources for health, clinical infrastructure in TB practice settings, and other service delivery barriers.

Our intervention featured a one-stop shop model characterized by complete integration of HIV treatment and care within existing TB clinics. Using this model, HIV-infected TB patients received PITC, CPT, ART and TB services in one clinic space under the care of the same providers who managed both TB and HIV at the same visit. Opt-out PITC may have been particularly important for linking co-infected patients to HIV care as it has been shown previously to result in higher testing uptake than traditional opt-in approaches across a variety of settings [32, 33]. In addition, offering on-site HIV care enrolment and co-localized treatment in the TB clinics minimized patient referral within and between facilities, which we postulate helped reduce the kind of pre-ART loss to follow-up associated with more traditional service integration models [6, 11, 34]. Despite the availability of these services, however, we observed only modest linkage to HIV care by 12 weeks post-ATT initiation, which suggests the influence of other patient-, health system-, and structural-level factors that likely went unaddressed by our intervention.

Table 5 Proportion of patients who either were cured or completed TB treatment during the pre- and post-intervention periods (*N* = 284)

Population	Pre-intervention *N* = 134 n (%)	Post-intervention *N* = 151 n (%)	*p*-value
All patients	99/134 (73.9%)	125/150 (83.3%)	0.05
Clinic A	60/77 (77.9%)	53/58 (91.4%)	0.04
Clinic B	39/57 (68.4%)	72/92 (78.3%)	0.18

Although single-facility integration models have been described previously, few reports characterize one-stop shop approaches to integrate ART provision and HIV care *within* TB clinics, and even fewer compare the effects of such approaches using data from historical or experimental controls [11, 29, 35, 36]. In Kenya, integrating HIV treatment and care into a rural TB clinic resulted in an increase in ART initiation (by the end of ATT), from 13% to between 29 and 36% [37]. In South Africa, integrated TB/HIV care was associated with significantly fewer unfavourable ART outcomes, which included death, default, and stopped treatment, than a vertical care approach [38].

We observed that integrated TB/HIV treatment and care was associated with increased odds of successful TB treatment. However, only 83.3% of patients achieved cure or completed treatment in the post-intervention period. While this proportion compares favourably with national figures reported to WHO for the study period, and TB outcomes for other integrated approaches documented in the region [38], it nonetheless falls below the Global Plan to End TB target of at least 90% of patients experiencing treatment success [19, 39]. Of note, TB treatment success at Clinic A exceeded 90%, but failed to surpass 80% in Clinic B, suggesting differences in the implementation context and barriers to introducing our intervention between TB clinics.

In both TB clinics, we encountered several noteworthy barriers to introducing integrated treatment and care. Limited clinic capacity and human resources, in particular, presented barriers to integrated service delivery, as reported elsewhere [11, 40]. At one study clinic, we encountered human resource challenges of frequent staff shortages, scheduling issues, and turnover, and addressed these directly through training, re-training, and mentorship. While it is possible that we could have strengthened our model by placing long-term project staff in the TB clinics, given our resource limitations we opted for a more sustainable approach focused on building the capacity of existing MOH staff to deliver integrated services. Similar to other settings, clinicians reported concerns over managing co-infected patients and co-administering ART and ATT, fearing the development of adverse events, such as immune reconstitution inflammatory syndrome [41, 42]. Some staff were not motivated to support integrated activities, especially if the activities were perceived as extra work. Indeed, overburdened staff has been cited as an important barrier to implementing integrated TB/HIV activities [43]. Anecdotally, we perceived this to be a clinic-specific issue: in Clinic B, reluctance among some staff to adopt the intervention may have contributed to poorer ART initiation outcomes; while in Clinic A, staff more uniformly welcomed TB/HIV integration and acknowledged it as a more efficient way to provide care. Results from other pilot projects suggest that TB/HIV integration may be a means to improve health worker knowledge, motivation, and retention [3]. Lastly, issues with supply chain management in the TB clinic resulted in intermittent sputum container and TB diagnostic reagent stock outs. In Malawi, similar supply chain challenges affected uptake of integrated HIV services among co-infected patients [9].

In responding to these challenges, several "key lessons learned" emerged. First, involving policy makers, facility in-charges, health workers, and other leadership in program planning from the outset was essential for obtaining local buy-in, and highlight the importance of obtaining visible MOH support and sensitizing staff pre-implementation to achieve adequate integration. Second, weekly clinic team meetings provided a forum to discuss challenges and identify and disseminate clinic-level best practices. Third, site-based mentoring enabled clinical officers to develop practical clinical skills and confidence in TB/HIV co-management. Fourth, longitudinal technical support for organizational and logistical problem solving led to improvements in patient flow and supply chain management for TB and HIV commodities. Fifth, adequate clinical space was essential for ensuring ART integration [40]. We found that clinics with at least 3 rooms worked best: one room allowed new patient enrolments and daily medication dispensing; a second room enabled patient examination on ART/TB clinic days; and a third room facilitated health commodity storage and private counselling space for HCT. Sixth, we found that integrated care functioned best when a dedicated, ART-trained clinical officer was assigned to staff the TB clinic. In Zambia, this clinical officer provided necessary clinical support to two nurses overseeing TB clinic operations. These nurses functioned daily to enrol into HIV care any TB patient newly diagnosed with HIV and to schedule appointments for clinician review and ART initiation.

From the client perspective, several patients anecdotally expressed a preference for our integrated care model. Similar patient preference has been reported previously in South Africa, especially for patients from lower socioeconomic strata [44]. Patients expressed an appreciation for the shorter waiting times and reduced stigma in the integrated TB clinic compared to the ART clinic, as well as the added convenience of our one-stop shop approach. In some cases, patients were reluctant to return to their general ART clinic after completion of TB treatment [11]. Qualitative research is required to further examine patient preferences regarding, and the patient-specific challenges surrounding, integrated TB/HIV care [31].

While the absence of qualitative data limited our ability to formally explore patient preferences regarding integrating HIV treatment and care into TB clinics, such an analysis was beyond the scope of this study. Our study was also limited by missing TB treatment outcome data for approximately 40% of the patients in our study. Missing data resulted from the inability to ascertain paper-based TB treatment outcomes for patients who did not return for a final TB clinic visit and could not be traced, and those who transferred out from our study sites during the course of their anti-TB therapy. These issues, along with our study having been conducted in only two urban Zambian clinics, limit the generalizability of our findings. Our study was also not designed to ascertain retention in HIV care, including retention after patient completion of ATT when they were referred to the ART clinic for continued HIV management. Similarly, we did not assess the effects of other important clinical, behavioural, and structural factors on linkage to care and ART uptake for patients with HIV-associated TB, including baseline CD4 count, perceived HIV- and TB-related stigma, co-morbid mental illness and substance use, and distance from patients' homes to the health facility. Lastly, the use of existing, de-identified program data precluded our ability to corroborate observational findings from elsewhere in SSA suggesting that integrated TB/HIV care reduces mortality among co-infected patients [45, 46].

Conclusions

We demonstrate that it is feasible to integrate HIV treatment and care, including ART, within public TB clinics in urban Zambia, while concurrently improving TB treatment outcomes. We describe an integrated model of TB/HIV treatment and care characterized by: the same health workers providing both TB and HIV services with the help of longitudinal training and mentorship; dedicated staffing, space, and clinic days for delivering all integrated services in the same clinic; and synchronized TB and HIV follow-up to ensure one-stop shopping for patients seeking care at a single TB clinic. Using this model, we achieved increases in linkage to care and early ART uptake for patients with HIV-associated TB. Additional studies are needed to identify new strategies to further improve integrated care and ART uptake, retention, and viral suppression among patients with HIV-associated TB in Zambia, in line with national and international targets. Further research is also needed to elucidate the patient-, health system-, and structural-level factors that enable or impede integrated care and the impact these factors have on joint, longitudinal TB/HIV clinical outcomes. Finally, additional investments are needed to ensure adequate human resources for health and health systems sufficiently robust to deliver high-quality, integrated services along the entire TB/HIV care continuum for patients with HIV-associated TB in SSA.

Abbreviations

ART: Antiretroviral Therapy; ARV: Antiretroviral; ATT: Anti-TB therapy; CIDRZ: Centre for Infectious Disease Research in Zambia; CPT: Co-trimoxazole Preventive Therapy; DOT: Directly observed therapy; EPTB: Extra-pulmonary Tuberculosis; HCT: HIV Counselling and Testing; HIV: Human Immunodeficiency Virus; HR: Hazard Ratio; MOH: Ministry of Health; OR: Odds Ratio; PLHIV: People Living with HIV; PTB: Pulmonary Tuberculosis; SSA: Sub-Saharan Africa; TB: Tuberculosis; WHO: World Health Organization

Acknowledgements

The authors thank the patients and staff of the study health facilities in Lusaka, Zambia. We acknowledge the important leadership of the National Tuberculosis and Leprosy Control Programme, the Lusaka Provincial Health Office, and the Lusaka District Health Office of the Zambia Ministry of Health that made this work possible.

Funding

This work was supported by funding from the U.S. Centers for Disease Control and Prevention (CDC) under grant U2GPS001421. The contents of this manuscript are the sole responsibility of the study authors and do not necessarily reflect the views of CDC or the United States government. The funding agencies had no role in the study design, data collection or analysis, manuscript writing, or the decision to submit for publication.

Authors' contributions

MEH helped conceive of the study, analysed the data, and led the manuscript writing. JM, JH, GS, NK, and SER contributed to developing the study concept and design. JM, DL, HJS, and SB contributed to data collection. MEH, JH, HJS, MM, and SER assisted with data analysis and results interpretation. MEH, JM, HJS, and SER contributed to drafting the manuscript. MEH, JM, DL, JH, HJS, SB, NK, MM, and SER reviewed the manuscript critically for intellectual content. All authors read and approved the final manuscript.

Competing interests

The authors declare that they have no competing interests.

Author details

[1]Centre for Infectious Disease Research in Zambia (CIDRZ), Lusaka, Zambia. [2]Division of Infectious Diseases, Department of Medicine, University of North Carolina School of Medicine, Chapel Hill, North Carolina, USA. [3]Division of Infectious Diseases, Department of Medicine, University of Alabama at Birmingham School of Medicine, Birmingham, AL, USA. [4]Lusaka District Health Office, Ministry of Health, Government of the Republic of Zambia, Lusaka, Zambia.

References

1. WHO. Global Tuberculosis Report. Geneva: World Health Organization; 2017. p. 249.
2. Friedland G, Harries A, Coetzee D. Implementation issues in tuberculosis/HIV program collaboration and integration: 3 case studies. J Infect Dis. 2007; 196(Suppl 1):S114–23.
3. Uyei J, Coetzee D, Macinko J, Guttmacher S. Integrated delivery of HIV and tuberculosis services in sub-Saharan Africa: a systematic review. Lancet Infect Dis. 2011;11(11):855–67.
4. Tsiouris SJ, Gandhi NR, El-Sadr WM, Gerald F. Tuberculosis and HIV-needed: a new paradigm for the control and Management of Linked Epidemics. J Int AIDS Soc. 2007;9(3):62.
5. Lawn SD, Campbell L, Kaplan R, Little F, Morrow C, Wood R. le DEASA: delays in starting antiretroviral therapy in patients with HIV-associated tuberculosis accessing non-integrated clinical services in a south African township. BMC Infect Dis. 2011;11:258.
6. Zachariah R, Harries AD, Manzi M, Gomani P, Teck R, Phillips M, Firmenich P. Acceptance of anti-retroviral therapy among patients infected with HIV and tuberculosis in rural Malawi is low and associated with cost of transport. PLoS One. 2006;1:e121.
7. Mukadi YD, Maher D, Harries A. Tuberculosis case fatality rates in high HIV prevalence populations in sub-Saharan Africa. AIDS (London, England). 2001; 15(2):143–52.
8. Zachariah R, Spielmann MP, Chinji C, Gomani P, Arendt V, Hargreaves NJ, Salaniponi FM, Harries AD. Voluntary counselling, HIV testing and adjunctive cotrimoxazole reduces mortality in tuberculosis patients in Thyolo, Malawi. AIDS (London, England). 2003;17(7):1053–61.
9. Kumwenda M, Tom S, Chan AK, Mwinjiwa E, Sodhi S, Joshua M, van Lettow M. Reasons for accepting or refusing HIV services among tuberculosis patients at a TB-HIV integration clinic in Malawi. Int J Tuberc Lung Dis. 2011;15(12):1663–9.
10. Chileshe M, Bond VA. Barriers and outcomes: TB patients co-infected with HIV accessing antiretroviral therapy in rural Zambia. AIDS Care. 2010;22(Suppl 1):51–9.
11. Legido-Quigley H, Montgomery CM, Khan P, Atun R, Fakoya A, Getahun H, Grant AD. Integrating tuberculosis and HIV services in low- and middle-income countries: a systematic review. Trop Med Int Health. 2013;18(2):199–211.
12. Maher D. Re-thinking global health sector efforts for HIV and tuberculosis epidemic control: promoting integration of programme activities within a strengthened health system. BMC Public Health. 2010;10:394.
13. Abdool Karim SS, Naidoo K, Grobler A, Padayatchi N, Baxter C, Gray AL, Gengiah T, Gengiah S, Naidoo A, Jithoo N, et al. Integration of antiretroviral therapy with tuberculosis treatment. N Engl J Med. 2011;365(16):1492–501.

14. Havlir DV, Kendall MA, Ive P, Kumwenda J, Swindells S, Qasba SS, Luetkemeyer AF, Hogg E, Rooney JF, Wu X, et al. Timing of antiretroviral therapy for HIV-1 infection and tuberculosis. N Engl J Med. 2011;365(16):1482–91.
15. Grinsztejn B, Hosseinipour MC, Ribaudo HJ, Swindells S, Eron J, Chen YQ, Wang L, Ou S-S, Anderson M, McCauley M, et al. Effects of early versus delayed initiation of antiretroviral treatment on clinical outcomes of HIV-1 infection: results from the phase 3 HPTN 052 randomised controlled trial. Lancet Infect Dis. 2014;14(4):281–90.
16. Nahid P, Dorman SE, Alipanah N, Barry PM, Brozek JL, Cattamanchi A, Chaisson LH, Chaisson RE, Daley CL, Grzemska M, et al. Official American Thoracic Society/Centers for Disease Control and Prevention/Infectious Diseases Society of America clinical practice guidelines: treatment of drug-susceptible tuberculosis. Clin Infect Dis. 2016;63(7):e147–95.
17. Harris JB, Hatwiinda SM, Randels KM, Chi BH, Kancheya NG, Jham MA, Samungole KV, Tambatamba BC, Cantrell RA, Levy JW, et al. Early lessons from the integration of tuberculosis and HIV services in primary care centers in Lusaka, Zambia. Int J Tuberc Lung Dis. 2008;12(7):773–9.
18. Howard AA, El-Sadr WM. Integration of tuberculosis and HIV services in sub-Saharan Africa: lessons learned. Clin Infect Dis. 2010;50(Suppl 3):S238–44.
19. WHO. Global Tuberculosis Report. Geneva: World Health Organization; 2013. p. 289.
20. Ministry of Health. Zambia Consolidated Guidelines for Treatment & Prevention of HIV Infection. Lusaka: Republic of Zambia, Ministry of Health; 2016. p. 75.
21. Ministry of Health. Managing Tuberculosis in the HIV setting in Zambia. Lusaka: Ministry of Health, Republic of Zambia; 2014. p. 52.
22. World Health Organization. Guidelines for treatment of drug-susceptible tuberculosis and patient care: 2017 update. Geneva: World Health Organization; 2017. p. 73.
23. WHO. Treatment of tuberculosis guidelines, 4th Edition, vol. 2010. Geneva: World Health Organization; 2010. p. 147.
24. WHO. Consolidated Guidelines on the Use of Antiretroviral Drugs for Treating and Preventing HIV Infection: Recommendations for a Public Health Approach. Second ed. Geneva: World Health Organization; 2016. p. 429.
25. Ministry of Health. Zambia Population-Based HIV Impact Assessment (ZAMPHIA 2015–2016): Summary Sheet. Lusaka: Ministry of Health, Republic of Zambia; 2016.
26. Cain LE, Logan R, Robins JM, Sterne JA, Sabin C, Bansi L, Justice A, Goulet J, van Sighem A, de Wolf F, et al. When to initiate combined antiretroviral therapy to reduce mortality and AIDS-defining illness in HIV-infected persons in developed countries: an observational study. Ann Intern Med. 2011;154(8):509–15.
27. Kitahata MM, Gange SJ, Abraham AG, Merriman B, Saag MS, Justice AC, Hogg RS, Deeks SG, Eron JJ, Brooks JT, et al. Effect of early versus deferred antiretroviral therapy for HIV on survival. N Engl J Med. 2009;360(18):1815–26.
28. Sterne JA, May M, Costagliola D, de Wolf F, Phillips AN, Harris R, Funk MJ, Geskus RB, Gill J, Dabis F, et al. Timing of initiation of antiretroviral therapy in AIDS-free HIV-1-infected patients: a collaborative analysis of 18 HIV cohort studies. Lancet. 2009;373(9672):1352–63.
29. Ferroussier O, Dlodlo RA, Capo-Chichi D, Boillot F, Gninafon M, Trébucq A, Fujiwara PI. Integrating HIV testing and care into tuberculosis services in Benin: programmatic aspects [short communication]. Int J Tuberc Lung Dis. 2013;17(11):1402–4.
30. Topp SM, Chipukuma JM, Giganti M, Mwango LK, Chiko LM, Tambatamba-Chapula B, Wamulume CS, Reid S. Strengthening health systems at facility-level: feasibility of integrating antiretroviral therapy into primary health care services in Lusaka, Zambia. PLoS One. 2010;5(7):e11522.
31. Daftary A, Padayatchi N. Social constraints to TB/HIV healthcare: accounts from coinfected patients in South Africa. AIDS Care. 2012;24(12):1480–6.
32. Van Rie A, Sabue M, Jarrett N, Westreich D, Behets F, Kokolomani J, Bahati ER. Counseling and testing TB patients for HIV: evaluation of three implementation models in Kinshasa, Congo. Int J Tuberc Lung Dis. 2008;12(3 Suppl 1):73–8.
33. Pope DS, Deluca AN, Kali P, Hausler H, Sheard C, Hoosain E, Chaudhary MA, Celentano DD, Chaisson RE. A cluster-randomized trial of provider-initiated (opt-out) HIV counseling and testing of tuberculosis patients in South Africa. J Acquir Immune Defic Syndr. 2008;48(2):190–5.
34. Wandwalo E, Kapalata N, Tarimo E, Corrigan CB, Morkve O. Collaboration between the national tuberculosis programme and a non governmental organisation in TB/HIV care at a district level: experience from Tanzania. Afr Health Sci. 2004;4(2):109–14.
35. Phiri S, Khan PY, Grant AD, Gareta D, Tweya H, Kalulu M, Chaweza T, Mbetewa L, Kanyerere H, Weigel R, et al. Integrated tuberculosis and HIV care in a resource-limited setting: experience from the Martin Preuss Centre, Malawi. Trop Med Int Health. 2011;16(11):1397–403.
36. Schwartz AB, Tamuhla N, Steenhoff AP, Nkakana K, Letlhogile R, Chadborn TR, Kestler M, Zetola NM, Ravimohan S, Bisson GP. Outcomes in HIV-infected adults with tuberculosis at clinics with and without co-located HIV clinics in Botswana. Int J Tuberc Lung Dis. 2013;17(10):1298–303.
37. Huerga H, Spillane H, Guerrero W, Odongo A, Varaine F. Impact of introducing human immunodeficiency virus testing, treatment and care in a tuberculosis clinic in rural Kenya. Int J Tuberc Lung Dis. 2010;14(5): 611–5.
38. Schulz SA, Draper HR, Naidoo P. A comparative study of tuberculosis patients initiated on ART and receiving different models of TB-HIV care. Int J Tuberc Lung Dis. 2013;17(12):1558–63.
39. Stop TB Partnership. The Paradigm Shift, 2016-2020: Global plan to end TB. Geneva: Stop TB Partnership; 2015. p. 122.
40. Martinot A, Van Rie A, Mulangu S, Mbulula M, Jarrett N, Behets F, Bola V, Bahati E. Baseline assessment of collaborative tuberculosis/HIV activities in Kinshasa, the Democratic Republic of Congo. Trop Dr. 2008;38(3):137–41.
41. Gandhi NR, Moll AP, Lalloo U, Pawinski R, Zeller K, Moodley P, Meyer E, Friedland G. Successful integration of tuberculosis and HIV treatment in rural South Africa: the Sizonq'oba study. J Acquir Immune Defic Syndr. 2009;50(1): 37–43.
42. McIlleron H, Meintjes G, Burman WJ, Maartens G. Complications of antiretroviral therapy in patients with tuberculosis: drug interactions, toxicity, and immune reconstitution inflammatory syndrome. J Infect Dis. 2007;196(Suppl 1):S63–75.
43. Pope DS, Atkins S, DeLuca AN, Hausler H, Hoosain E, Celentano DD, Chaisson RE. South African TB nurses' experiences of provider-initiated HIV counseling and testing in the eastern Cape Province: a qualitative study. AIDS Care. 2010;22(2):238–45.
44. Levin L, Irving K, Dikgang M, Punwasi J, Isaacs M, Myer L. TB patients' perspectives on integrated TB/HIV services in South Africa. Trop Dr. 2006; 36(3):173–5.
45. Van Rie A, Patel MR, Nana M, Vanden Driessche K, Tabala M, Yotebieng M, Behets F. Integration and task shifting for TB/HIV care and treatment in highly resource-scarce settings: one size may not fit all. J Acquir Immune Defic Syndr. 2014;65(3):e110–7.
46. Kerschberger B, Hilderbrand K, Boulle AM, Coetzee D, Goemaere E, De Azevedo V, Van Cutsem G. The effect of complete integration of HIV and TB services on time to initiation of antiretroviral therapy: a before-after study. PLoS One. 2012;7(10):e46988.

2

Retention of HIV infected pregnant and breastfeeding women on option B+ in Gomba District, Uganda: a retrospective cohort study

George Kiwanuka[1*], Noah Kiwanuka[2], Fiston Muneza[2], Juliet Nabirye[1], Frederick Oporia[3], Magdalene A. Odikro[2], Barbara Castelnuovo[4] and Rhoda K. Wanyenze[3]

Abstract

Background: Lifelong antiretroviral therapy for HIV infected pregnant and lactating women (Option B+) has been rapidly scaled up but there are concerns about poor retention of women initiating treatment. However, facility-based data could underestimate retention in the absence of measures to account for self-transfers to other facilities. We assessed retention-in-care among women on Option B+ in Uganda, using facility data and follow-up to ascertain transfers to other facilities.

Methods: In a 25-month retrospective cohort analysis of routine program data, women who initiated Option B+ between March 2013 and March 2015 were tracked and interviewed quantitatively and qualitatively (in-depth interviews). Kaplan Meier survival analysis was used to estimate time to loss-to-follow-up (LTFU) while multivariable Cox proportional hazards regression was applied to estimate the adjusted predictors of LTFU, based on facility data. Thematic analysis was done for qualitative data, using MAXQDA 12. Quantitative data were analyzed with STATA® 13.

Results: A total of 518 records were reviewed. The mean (SD) age was 26.4 (5.5) years, 289 women (55.6%) attended primary school, and 53% (276/518) had not disclosed their HIV status to their partners. At 25 months post-ART initiation, 278 (53.7%) were LTFU based on routine facility data, with mean time to LTFU of 15.6 months. Retention was 60.2 per 1000 months of observation (pmo) (95% CI: 55.9–64.3) at 12, and 46.3/1000pmo (95% CI: 42.0–50.5) at 25 months. Overall, 237 (55%) women were successfully tracked and interviewed and 43/118 (36.4%) of those who were classified as LTFU at facility level had self-transferred to another facility. The true 25 months post-ART initiation retention after tracking was 71.3% (169/237). Women < 25 years, aHR = 1.71 (95% CI: 1.28–2.30); those with no education, aHR = 5.55 (95% CI: 3.11–9.92), and those who had not disclosed their status to their partners, aHR = 1.59 (95% CI: 1.16–2.19) were more likely to be LTFU. Facilitators for Option B+ retention based on qualitative findings were adequate counselling, disclosure, and the desire to stay alive and raise HIV-free children. Drug side effects, inadequate counselling, stigma, and unsupportive spouses, were barriers to retention in care.

Conclusions: Retention under Option B+ is suboptimal and is under-estimated at health facility level. There is need to institute mechanisms for tracking of women across facilities. Retention could be enhanced through strategies to enhance disclosure to partners, targeting the uneducated, and those < 25 years.

Keywords: EMTCT, PMTCT, Retention, LTFU, HIV, Option B+

* Correspondence: georgekiwa@gmail.com
[1]Department of Health Policy Planning and Management, Makerere University School of Public Health, P.O Box 7072, Kampala, Uganda
Full list of author information is available at the end of the article

Background

Progress against HIV/AIDS over the last 15 years has inspired the global commitment to eliminate mother-to-child transmission of HIV (eMTCT) by 2020 [1], and the HIV epidemic by 2030 [2]. Since 1995, an estimated 1.6 million new HIV infections amongst children have been prevented due to the provision of antiretroviral medicines to women living with HIV during pregnancy or breastfeeding. Despite this achievement, many children are still being infected, and dying from AIDS-related illnesses [2].

Mother to child transmission (MTCT) of HIV is defined as the transmission of HIV from an HIV positive mother to her child during pregnancy, labor, delivery or breastfeeding [3]. In June 2013, the World Health Organization (WHO) recommended initiation of antiretroviral therapy (ART) for all pregnant and breastfeeding women with HIV, and continuation of ART for life (Option B+) [4]. Uganda started Option B+ rollout in December 2012. Gomba district was among the first districts to implement Option B+ [5] and had scaled up services to all levels of health facilities by the time this study was conducted. At District level, the Uganda Primary Health care system has four levels of care, including Health Center II, III, IV, and District Hospital. Health center II represents the first level of interface between the formal health sector and the communities and provides only ambulatory services. HC III offers continuous basic preventive, promotive and curative services, with provisions for laboratory services for diagnosis, and maternity care. HC IV provides all the above services including laboratory and comprehensive emergency obstetric services. The district hospital is the referral facility at district level offering specialized services [6].

Retention-in-care along the PMTCT cascade is an important indicator for quality of PMTCT services and a determinant of PMTCT outcomes [7, 8]. Retention-in-care is defined by the WHO as continuous engagement from diagnosis in a package of prevention, treatment, support and care services [9]. Poor retention-in-care is one of the leading causes of virologic failure, drug resistance, and MTCT [10].

It is therefore important that PMTCT retention-in-care is clearly defined, accurately estimated,, and its causes identified and addressed. However, many studies and evaluations that are based on facility data do not accurately estimate retention as they may not account for women who self-transfer to another health facility [11–14]. Without accounting for women who transfer to other facilities, retention-in-care may be under-estimated [15], and the extent of this under-estimation may vary based on the functionality of the referral mechanisms and tracking of patients across facilities. Studies that have attempted to address these gaps have had a short follow-up period and may not show the potential variations in retention during pregnancy, breastfeeding and after cessation of breastfeeding [16]. Further, the underlying barriers to retention have not been well-documented [17].

This study assessed retention-in-care in a 25-month cohort of pregnant and breastfeeding women on Option B+ in Uganda, using facility based data and integrated follow-up to ascertain transfers to other facilities to fully account for retention of women in care. The study also integrated in-depth interviews to explain the outcomes for the women.

Methods

Study setting and population

We conducted this study in Gomba district, in central Uganda between May 01st and June 30th, 2017. Gomba is a rural district with 92% of the population rural [18]. The HIV seroprevalence in Gomba is at eight 8.0%, higher than the national prevalence of 6.5% [19] Almost all women in Gomba attend at least one antenatal care visit [20]. The study was a retrospective cohort analysis of routine program data, combined with a mixed methods cross-sectional study. The study population was pregnant and breastfeeding women who started Option B+ between March 2013 and March 2015. We included women who were residents of Gomba for over 6 months and excluded all those who were visitors.

Data collection methods

Four research assistants were trained to extract the data using a structured abstraction tool. Client charts were reviewed for 1,3,6,12,18 and 25 months attendance, along the eMTCT cascade. The eMTCT cascade is a series of important stepwise events that constitute a vital roadmap to successful eMTCT. The cascade begins with identification of HIV positive pregnant women and ends with the detection of a final HIV status in HIV-exposed infants at 18 months [21].

An attempt to track all the women from the cohort was made, using the telephone contacts and physical addresses of the women which were retrieved from their records. The research assistants called the women for either phone or face-to-face cross-sectional interviews.

A total of 12 in-depth interviews were conducted, with clients purposively selected, including six women that were retained in care at health facility level and six women who were categorized as LTFU. These were deemed sufficient for data saturation given the recurrent themes with no new emerging leads [22]. Two trained research assistants with experience in qualitative inquiry were employed. Potential participants were called 1 week prior to the interview date to schedule the interview. The in-depth interview guide was structured around predefined broad themes, with preset open ended questions focusing on lived experiences of women on Option B+.

The dependent variable was retention in care and LTFU. A mother was defined as retained in care if she returned to the health facility for care, within 60 days of her last scheduled clinic visit. From clinic ART dispensing records, this was the period estimated for a mother to have run out of drugs. Women who were out of care at the time of conducting the interviews (whether or not they had returned into care at any time during the follow-up period) were categorized as LTFU.

Prior to the data collection, the research assistants were trained, and the data collection tools, including the data abstraction tool and the interview questionnaire pilot tested. Daily feedback during the data collection period was received through meetings of the research assistants and the principal investigator, to review challenges and identify solutions.

Sample size estimations and data analysis

Sample size estimation

The sample size was estimated using the online Stats-To-Do sample size calculator for survival analysis [23]. With a type one error (α) of 0.05, power (1 - β) of 0.84, survival rate in group 1 (SR1), which was the proportion of retention in care in adults receiving ART for health reasons (control group) of 0.87 [24], survival rate in group 2 (SR2), which is the anticipated proportion of retention under Option B+ (exposed group) of 0.69 [14], r = ratio of sample size in group 1 / sample size in group 2 (ssiz1/ssiz2) = (0.2), the total sample size was 232 women. However, we reviewed the records for all the women from all Health center II, III, and IV in the district that were enrolled in the 2-year period ($n = 518$), due to anticipated challenges of missing data.

Statistical analysis

Data were analyzed with STATA® 13. During univariate analysis, a descriptive analysis was conducted to calculate the proportions of Option B+ patients who died, stopped ART, were retained in care within the same health facility, and who self-transferred or were formally transferred to other facilities. Because our primary outcome is influenced by time along the Option B+ cascade, survival analysis method was used [14, 25]. The retention based on health facility records at 1, 3, 6, 12, 18 and 25 months after ART initiation was assessed using the Kaplan-Meir methods and survival functions were assessed over the 25-month period. The analysis was up to 25 months, because in our operational definition of retention, a mother was retained if she returned for care within 60 days of her scheduled visit, all those who were scheduled for 24 months reviews had until the end of 25 months to return for their visit. Bivariate analysis: Log-rank test of equality was used, for categorical variables to examine the relationships of individual and facility related independent variables with retention. Cox proportional hazards regression analysis was used to analyze all the variables associated with retention, with a p-value of 0.05.

For the qualitative data, audio tape recordings were simultaneously transcribed and translated verbatim from Luganda into English. Transcripts were then uploaded into the qualitative analysis software MAXQDA version 12 and data were analyzed following the six steps of thematic approach developed by Braun and Clarke [26].

Results

The study was conducted between 1st May and 30th June 2017. All the records of the 518 pregnant and breastfeeding women who were enrolled in care between March 2013 and March 2015 were included in the 25-month retrospective cohort analysis. Of the 518 women, 237 (46%) were successfully tracked for cross-sectional interviews and ascertainment of retention status; 12 were selected for in-depth interviews (Fig. 1). Of the 518 women, 281 (54%) were excluded because 234 (45%) had no phone or residential contacts to enable tracking, 27(10.1%) refused to speak to the interviewers on the phone or physically, and 20 had died.

Nearly half of the women, 234 (45%) were enrolled into Option B+ in 2014, 209 (40.2%) in 2013 and only 77 (14.8%) in 2015. Most of the women (346; 67.2%) started ART during pregnancy while 95 (18.3%) initiated ART before pregnancy, 7 (1.4%) during labor and 68 (13.1%) during breastfeeding. The women were aged between 16 and 48 years, with a mean age of 26.4 (SD: ±5. 5). All the women delivered live babies, and (379; 72.9%) had a DNA PCR test at 6 weeks (Table 1). Most of the women were enrolled at Health Center III, 353 (67.9%) against 167 (32.1) that were enrolled at the Health Center IV. About half of the women 289 (55.6%) had attended primary school, 141 (27.1%) had post-primary education while 90 (17.3%) had no formal education.

Of the 257 women who were tracked, 20 (7.8%) had died. Among the remaining 237 who agreed to be interviewed, 161 (62.7%) were in care, and 76 (29.6%) not in care. Of the 237 women tracked, 131 (51%) had been classified as LTFU and 126 (49%) as retained, as per facility records. Following analysis of tracking data, true retention was found to be 71.3% (169/237). It was found that 36.4% (43/131) of those initially categorized as LTFU at facility level had not dropped out of care, but had simply self-transferred to another facility,

Using the log-rank test, prespecified subgroups were assessed to determine whether differences in retention at 25 weeks were dependent on participants' baseline clinical characteristics (Table 2). The overall rate of

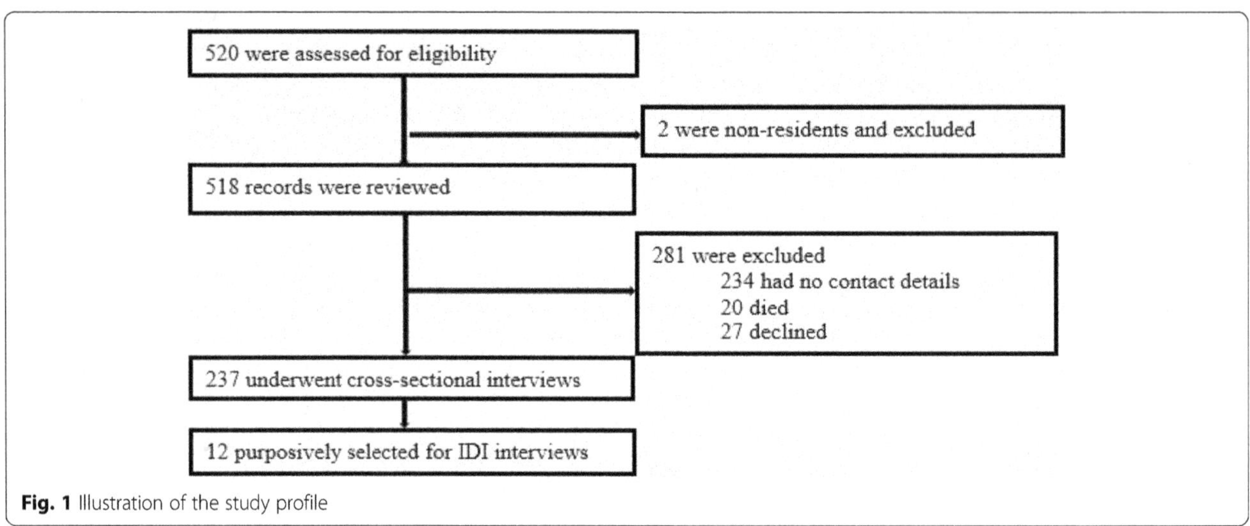

Fig. 1 Illustration of the study profile

health facility retention was 60.2/1000 pmo (95% CI: 55.9–64.3) at 12 months and 46.3/1000 pmo (95% CI: 42.0–50.5) at 25 months.

As shown in Table 3, there were 518 observations at the start with total time at risk of 8080 months. The overall number of women LTFU by 25 months based on the facility data was 278 (53.7%) translating into an overall incidence rate of LTFU of 30/1000 pmo. The mean time to LTFU was 15.6 months, with a minimum exit time of 1 month and a maximum exit time of 25 months. The 25th percentile of the survival time was 3 months while the 50th percentile was 25 months.

The Kaplan–Meier method was used to estimate the retention curve from the observed times, using facility data. Overall, retention along the whole Option B+ cascade was poor, with the highest risk in the first 6 months (Fig. 2). Between 18 and 24 months, the critical period of transfer from Option B+ care point to General ART clinic, a considerable proportion of mothers were still lost.

Figure 3 shows a significant difference between the retention curve for those who disclosed from those who had not disclosed their HIV status. By 25 months post ART-initiation, about 65% of those who had disclosed their status to their partners were retained in care while only 35% of those who had not disclosed were retained ($p = < 0.001$). Overall, non-disclosure of HIV status to spouse was associated with a risk of LTFU of about 35 percentage points higher than that associated with disclosure ($p = < 0.001$).

At multivariable analysis, women who were less than 25 years were more likely to be LTFU with adj.HR = 1.71; 95% CI: 1.28, 2.30. Those with no education had highest chance of LTFU, aHR 5.55 (95% CI: 3.11, 9.92), primary level of education had aHR 3.83 (95% CI: 2.31, 6.33) in comparison with those who had attained post-primary education (Table 4). Non-disclosure of HIV status was also significantly associated with LTFU, aHR 1.59 (95% CI: 1.16, 2.19). Starting ART during pregnancy, and while breastfeeding was associated with higher chances of LTFU compared to for women who started ART before pregnancy 2.66 (95% CI: 1.60, 4.44).

Analysis of personal behavioral practices revealed that, difficulty in travelling to health facility, aHR 2.30 (95% CI: 1.07, 4.92), and not receiving sufficient counselling, aHR 2.92 (95% CI: 1.49, 5.72) before initiation of ART were the negative predictors of retention under attitudes and perceptions, while presence of peer mothers was a positive predictor (Table 5). Women who had difficulty in obtaining support from the spouse were nearly four times more likely to be LTFU, compared to those who obtained support from their spouses aHR 3.59 (95% CI:2.21,5.81). Those who had difficulty in developing strategies to keep appointments were about two times more likely to be LTFU, aHR 1.89 (95% CI: 1.17,3.05).

Facilitators and barriers to retention in care for women on option B+

In-depth interviews for the women who were retained and those who were lost showed related issues, therefore, the arrangement of the results incorporates responses for both categories. The unique differences between the two categories are clearly emphasized during the description. Two major themes emerged from the analysis including initiation on Option B+ and adherence to clinic visits/retention in care.

Facilitators of option B+ initiation

All the women who were retained noted that disclosure, adequate partner counselling and support made their ART initiation ART very comfortable.

Table 1 Baseline characteristics of the women from abstracted cohort data

Characteristic	$N = 518$ (%)
Age	
16–24	220 (42.3)
25–48	298 (57.7)
Education Level	
None	90 (17.3)
Primary	287 (55.6)
Post-primary	141 (27.1)
Marital Status	
Single	94 (18.1)
Married/Cohabiting	404 (78.1)
Separated/Divorced	20 (3.8)
Number of children	
0–3	297 (57.5)
4–5	163 (31.4)
5+	58 (11.0)
Health Facility Level	
Health Center II/III	351 (67.9)
Health Center IV	167 (32.1)
Pregnancy Status at Enrollment	
Pregnancy	429 (82.8)
Breastfeeding	89 (17.2)
Disclosure Status	
No	273 (52.6)
Yes	245 (47.4)
Period of starting ART	
Before pregnancy	95 (18.3)
During Pregnancy	348 (67.2)
Labor	7 (1.4)
Breastfeeding	68 (13.1)
Place of Delivery	
Home/TBA[¶]	119 (23.0)
Health Center level II/III[†]	202 (39.0)
Health Center level IV/Hospital	157 (30.3)
Private Clinic	40 (7.7)
DNA-PCR at 6 weeks	
Yes	377 (72.9)
No	141 (27.1)
Final Status of Child†	
Negative	498 (95.8)
Positive	20 (4.2)

[†]The final status of the child at 18 months is done using a rapid antibody test
[†]The Health center II/III are facilities that conduct deliveries but do not provide EMOC services
[¶]Traditional birth attendants provide delivery services in the community, their services

Table 2 Showing demographic characteristics, perceptions and behavioral practices of women and the sub-group analysis for LTFU following cross-sectional interviews

Characteristic	Retained, $N = 119$ (%)	LTFU, $N = 118$ (%)	P-value
Income/Monthly (Uganda Shilling)			
< 50,000	74 (62.2)	92 (77.3)	0.0036
50,001-100,000	27 (22.7)	21 (17.6)	
> 100,000	18 (15.1)	6 (5.1)	
Distance from Health Facility			
< 1 km	19 (16.0)	7 (5.9)	< 0.001
1-5 km	80 (67.2)	60 (50.8)	
> 5 km	20 (16.8)	51 (43.3)	
Health Facility too far[a]			
Disagree	70 (58.8)	29 (24.6)	< 0.001
Agree	49 (41.2)	89 (75.4)	
Difficulty in travelling to Health Facility[a]			
Disagree	70 (58.8)	29 (24.6)	< 0.001
Agree	49 (41.2)	89 (75.4)	
Medicines available*			
Disagree	74 (62.2)	24 (20.3)	0.8214
Agree	45 (37.8)	94 (79.7)	
Counselling is sufficient[a]			
Disagree	0 (0)	34 (28.8)	< 0.001
Agree	119 (100)	84 (71.2)	
Peer Mothers help at Option B+ initiation[a]			
Disagree	6 (5)	32 (27.1)	< 0.001
Agree	113 (95)	86 (72.9)	
Difficulty in handling daily hassles[b]			
Disagree	85 (71.4)	51 (43.2)	< 0.001
Agree	34 (28.6)	67 (56.8)	
Difficulty in developing strategies to manage appointments[b]			
Disagree	100 (84)	44 (37.3)	< 0.001
Agree	19 (16)	74 (62.7)	
Difficulty in obtaining support from spouse[b]			
Disagree	80 (67.2)	24 (20.3)	< 0.001
Agree	39 (32.8)	94 (79.7)	
I have confidence in the available HIV care system[b]			
Disagree	0 (0)	6 (5.1)	0.6129
Agree	119 (100)	112 (94.9)	
Disclosed status to spouse?			
No	37 (31.1)	83 (70.3)	< 0.001
Yes	82 (68.9)	35 (29.7)	

[a]Individual attitudes and perceptions about health care services
[b]Personal behavioral practices that influence health services utilization

"I really did not face many challenges when starting ARVs because I came to test with my husband, we had talked about the possible outcomes and we were ready

Table 3 Probabilities of retention in Option B+ over a 24 months period

Time (Months)	No. of women	LTFU	Net[c] Lost	Retention probability[b]	SE[a]	95% CI[a]	
1	518	94	0	0.82	0.02	0.78	0.84
3	424	42	0	0.74	0.02	0.69	0.77
6	382	40	0	0.66	0.02	0.62	0.70
12	342	30	0	0.60	0.02	0.56	0.64
18	312	38	0	0.53	0.02	0.49	0.57
25	274	34	240	0.46	0.02	0.42	0.51

[a]SE stands for Standard error, CI, for Confidence intervals
[b]The probability of retention is 0.6 by 12 months and 0.46 by 25 months in care
[c]Right censoring was done, with all those who completed the duration of the study censored

> *for any of them. So, we both came here, and we were both found to be HIV positive. This made it very easy for me because we were counselled together as a couple"* 32-year-old, retained woman.

Other facilitators reported included desire to stay alive and raise HIV-negative babies.

Barriers of option B+ initiation

Patient unreadiness, inadequate counselling, HIV-related stigma and unsupportive partners and drug side-effects were the issues highlighted mostly by the women, especially those that were LTFU.

> *"I was not ready, as soon I tested positive, I was given medicines and was told to swallow them. I asked the health worker for time to think about it, but they said I had to start the medicines immediately. Other people I had heard about started with Septrin but for me I was started on ARVs immediately."* 23-year-old, LTFU.

HIV related stigma was another barrier. Some women feared discrimination and labeling of their children if their HIV status was known and thus felt the need to protect their children.

> *"I had the fear of coming to the health facility because I feared meeting my friends here. I would wonder how to fit in society where people knew that I was HIV positive. I feared that they would segregate against my other children, though they were HIV negative"* 26-year-old, LTFU.

Facilitators of adherence to clinic visits

One mother reported overcoming her daily hassles by better planning and keeping appointments by setting reminders in her phone and memorizing the upcoming appointment date.

> *"I have daily work such as farming, cooking would stand in the way of my appointments, but I would just overcome them by better planning such as waking up very early in the morning at 5am and take the cows to the bush for feeding, cook food early before I leave such that by 8am, I am done with all the home chores and I would be in time for my health facility appointment.*

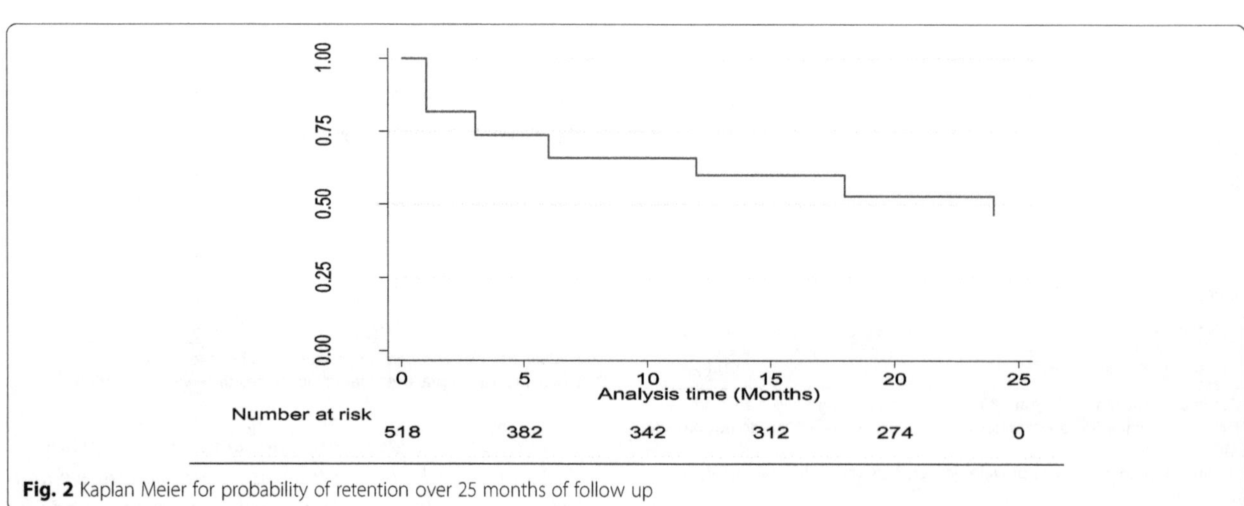

Fig. 2 Kaplan Meier for probability of retention over 25 months of follow up

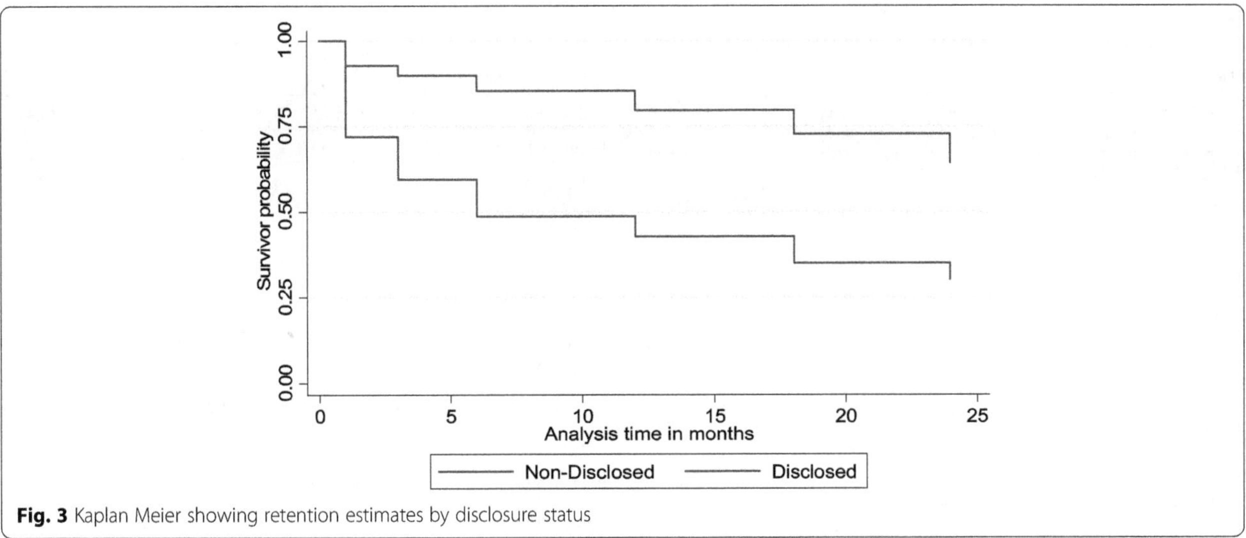

Fig. 3 Kaplan Meier showing retention estimates by disclosure status

> *On the day of appointment, I don't go for digging. I would remind myself by memorizing and checking my appointment book"* 27-year-old, retained.

Another mother who was retained in care reported that the only reason she managed to stay in care was because she overcame the fear of the negative consequences of disclosure, and she told her spouse about her status and noted that his positive attitude and support helped her adhere to her clinic visits. She however reports that despite his support, he refused to test for HIV, claiming to be immune to the virus.

> *"At delivery of the baby, I made up my mind to disclose, and I braced myself for being chased away from home after disclosure. I told him and to my surprise, he said that it was okay and started supporting me. Today he is the one who reminds me to take my ARVs, though for him he says he is immune to the HIV virus and refused to come for testing. Many women are hiding their status from the partners, I encourage them to disclose their status because the experience of living with a supportive partner is needed if one is to have successful care in Option B+"* 28-year-old, retained.

The desire to stay alive was also a strong motivation for mothers to adhere to their care and clinic visits. For most, this was because they wanted to raise their children and see them become independent.

> *"I was looking for a healthy life, so that I can live and raise my children. If I don't take my medicine, I will fall ill and die, and no one will take care of my children"* 27-year-old, retained.

Barriers of adherence to clinic visits

Side effects were mentioned by all the women who were retained and those who were LTFU. One mother reported that she felt like the side effects of the medicines were going to kill her, so she opted to drop out of care to live a better-quality life.

> *"The medicines used to give me a lot of side effects and when I talked to the health workers to change my medicines, they said that I would eventually get used to it, I tried but it became too much, and I stopped. I couldn't get out of bed, I was sleepless at night and I felt like it was going to kill me even before the HIV/AIDS, so I decided to stop"* 20-year-old, LTFU.

Failure to develop coping strategies was mentioned by about 75% percent of the women who were LTFU. A young mother reported that she had to choose between her employment, her studies and keeping her appointments. She chose the job because she needed the money, and she dropped both out of Option B+ care and school.

> *"I was trying to complete my Senior 4 at the time, and I also had to start working to get some money to keep me going. At the salon where I was working, the boss wanted me to work 7 days a week and if I did not work, I would not be paid. I failed to get around this because of the needs I had. My school and work were overwhelming, eventually I had to drop out of school as well, and I did not sit for my O-level exams."* 20-year-old, LTFU.

Lack of spousal support, coupled with violence and abandonment was another main reason for LTFU. One mother reported that her boyfriend, who had promised to stay with her for life abandoned her when she told

Table 4 Crude and adjusted hazard ratios (HRs) of LTFU in HIV care for Option B+ by socio-demographic characteristics and enabling resources

Characteristic	Crude HR (95% CI)	Adjusted HR (95% CI)	P-value
Age(years)			
≤ 24	1.8 (1.43,2,29)	1.71 (1.28,2.30)	< 0.001[a]
≥ 25	1.0	1.0	
Education level			
Post Primary	1.0	1.0	
Primary	3.479 (2.35,5.13)	3.83 (2.31,6.33)	< 0.001[a]
No Formal Education	6.92 (4.51,10.62)	5.55 (3.11,9.92)	< 0.001[a]
Marital status			
Single	1.0		
Married/Cohabiting	0.97 (0.53,1.78)		
Divorced/Separated	1.50 (0.79,2.85)		
Disclosure status			
Yes	1.0	1.0	
No	2.87 (2.21,3.71)	1.59 (1.16,2.19)	0.004[a]
Period of starting ART			
Before Pregnancy	1.0	1.0	
During Pregnancy	3.81 (2.41,6.03)	2.66 (1.60,4.44)	< 0.001[a]
Breastfeeding	3.17 (1.85,5.42)	1.88 (1.02,3.44)	0.042
Place of Delivery			
Home	1.0		
Health Center II/III	0.50 (0.35,0.70)	0.79 (0.54,1.14)	0.209
Health Center IV	0.31 (0.21,0.44)	0.61 (0.41,0.93)	0.021[a]
Private Clinic	1.81 (1.21,2.70)	1.73 (1.08,2.77)	0.021
Baby DNA-PCR at 6 weeks done			
Yes	1.0	1.0	
No	6.77 (5.52,8.76)	4.57 (3.17,6.57)	< 0.001[a]
Results for 6 weeks DNA-PCR received			
Yes	1.0	1.0	
No	2.41 (1.43,4.09)	1.57 (0.79,3.10)	0.192
Final Status of child			
Positive	1.0	1.0	
Negative	1.88 (1.17,3.04)	1.18 (0.63,2.20)	0.602
Income/Monthly (Uganda Shilling)			
< 50,000	3.32 (1.35,8.19)		
50,001-100,000	2.29 (0.86,6.12)		
> 100,000	1.00		
Distance from health facility			
< 1 km	1.00		
1-5 km	1.67 (0.77,3.67)		
> 5 km	3.48 (1.57,7.69)		

[a]Socio-demographic predictors of retention in care for women under Option B+

Table 5 Crude and adjusted hazard ratios (HRs) of LTFU in HIV care for Option B+ by attitudes, perceptions and personal behavioral practices

Characteristic	Crude HR (95% CI)	Adjusted HR (95% CI)	P-value
Health Facility too far			
Disagree	1.00		
Agree	2.54 (1.73,4.02)		
Difficulty in travelling to Health facility			
Disagree	1.00	1.00	
Agree	3.58 (2.28,5.62)	2.30 (1.07,4.92)	0.032
Counselling is sufficient			
Disagree	5.12 (3.32,7.87)	2.92 (1.49,5.72)	0.002
Agree	1.00	1.00	
Peer mothers help at Option B+ initiation			
Disagree	2.75 (1.81,4.16)		
Agree	1.00		
Difficulty in handling daily hassles			
Disagree	1.00		
Agree	2.05 (1.42,2.95)		
Difficulty in developing strategies to manage appointments			
Disagree	1.00	1.00	
Agree	3.69 (2.52,5.39)	1.89 (1.17,3.05)	0.009
Difficulty in obtaining support from spouse			
Disagree	1.00	1.00	
Agree	4.53 (2.88,7.13)	3.59 (2.21,5.81)	< 0.001
It's important to register into HIV care for Option B+			
Disagree	4.29 (2.54,7.23)		
Agree	1.00		
I have confidence in the available HIV care system			
Disagree	3.90 (1.42,10.67)		
Agree	1.00		

him about her HIV positive status. She felt purposeless and dropped out of care.

> *"I think I would have tried to stay in care if I had some form of support from my boyfriend. He had promised me that we would be together all our lives, the moment he got to know about my status, he changed. This made me very sad and I couldn't keep on coming for my appointments because I felt it was purposeless"* 20-year-old, LTFU.

Discussion

We conducted a study that was a combination of a retrospective cohort analysis and cross-sectional study, investigating retention in care for pregnant and breastfeeding women on Option B+ that were enrolled in care between March 2013 and March 2015, in Gomba district. We found that health facility retention was 60.2% at 12 months and 46.3% at 25 months. However, retention after contact tracing was 10% higher with many women found to have simply transferred to other health facilities. Nearly 50% of women were not traceable, mainly due to lack of contact details. There is a need to establishment a tracking system with reliable contact information and unique identifiers for example through the use of the recently introduced National Identity cards [27, 28]. The main predictors of retention were maternal age, level of education, counselling, disclosure status, timely DNA/PCR testing at 6 weeks and ability to develop strategies to keep appointments. The major facilitators for Option B+ initiation were adequate counselling, disclosure and spousal support, and the desire to stay alive and raise HIV-free children. Drug side effects, inadequate counselling and patient non-readiness, stigma, and un-supportive spouse were among the major barriers to the initiation of lifelong ART. Among the facilitators of adherence to clinic visits, ability to develop strategies to address daily hassles, ability to obtain spousal/family support, and disclosure were the most prominent. The barriers to adherence that were mentioned mostly by both retained and LTFU mothers included, drug side effects, failure to develop strategies to overcome daily hassles, lack of spousal support, and non-disclosure. Several of these barriers are modifiable and could be minimized through adequate counseling and support to enhance preparedness and planning to improve retention.

Retention in care for pregnant and breastfeeding women

The overall facility retention in care at 25 months, of 46.3% and all other time points was lower than that observed in a study done in northern Uganda [29] and in Malawi [12]. The true retention at 71.3% was similar to what was found in Malawi, in a setting that had electronic medical records system to track self-transfers [14]. High facility LTFU may be explained by poor follow up of women who are LTFU in rural, resource constrained facilities. In rural health facilities, health workers are not motivated enough to be vigilant about LTFU women, as it was found by Kallander [30–33]. It is also noteworthy that about half of the women had no phone or physical contact information, and some had incorrect contact details, which makes any attempt to follow them up virtually impossible. Ensuring complete and accurate contact information is a critical area for intervention [34].

We found that 32.8% of the women were misclassified as LTFU in routine data, underestimating the true level of retention at 25-months. A systematic review and meta-analysis of interventions to improve PMTCT service delivery and promote retention in Tanzania showed that up to 54.4% of LTFU clients had self-transferred to another facility [35]. The lack of a unified database with unique identifiers to help track the patients across facilities is a major challenge to HIV care in general and PMTCT specifically [36].

The rate of health facility LTFU was highest between initiation of ART and the 6-month visit. This may be explained by the failure to navigate the complexity of decisions a woman must make such as immediate initiation on ART [16]. In the second year, a large proportion of women were LTFU around the 18 months period, the critical period of transfer from Option B+ care point to adult care point. This could be explained by the poor health facility linkages between ART clinics and Option B+ care points, and the lack of desire by the mothers to stay on Option B+ once their baby is declared HIV negative [27, 37–40]. Studies have also highlighted the fear to be known as HIV positive and the stigma associated with HIV-only chronic care clinics. The integrated care within the ANC facilities masks the HIV status of the women, which is not possible once they transfer to the predominantly HIV chronic care clinics [41]. This highlights the need to explore integrated service and other models of chronic care for HIV infected pregnant and breast feeding women to minimize LTFU.

Women of a younger age of < 25 years with older spouses had more challenges with retention in care possibly because of their lack of independence from their spouses about decision making, and financial sustenance, which affects their ability to make decisions regarding their health [14, 42, 43]. Older women may have more settled lifestyles with less social pressures, which allow them to better cope with Option B+ care. Women with no or low formal education were also more likely to be LTFU in care possibly due to more challenges in appreciating HIV related information and schedules [43–47].

As documented in other studies, we found that adequate counselling was with a facilitator of retention in care [29, 43]. Pregnant HIV infected women face complex decisions that require major lifestyle and work related adjustments to cope with motherhood and HIV care and thus require counseling and other support to cope [48]. During this transition, support from family and especially their spouses is also crucial to their coping. It is thus not surprising that the women who disclosed their HIV status to the male partners did much better than their counterparts who had not done so [16, 29, 43]. Women are also inclined to provide false contact information because of fear of stigma and discrimination [43]. As documented elsewhere, ability to develop strategies to overcome daily hassles and keep appointments was associated with retention in care [30–32].

Mothers whose babies were not tested for HIV at 6 weeks were more likely to be LTFU. Women who do not adhere to their own care schedules will likely also miss those for their infants [29, 49]. A negative HIV test for the infant could also motivate the women to remain in care [37].

Drug side effects were a major barrier to adherence on Option B+. This may be due to the decreased morale caused by the side effects. These findings are consistent with recent studies in Uganda, Malawi and Ethiopia [16, 40, 42].

Study strengths and limitations

. The use of qualitative methods allowed for explanatory depth to the quantitative methods. However, there were some limitations. About half of the women were not reached due to lack of contact information—as ably demonstrated through the tracking of women, there is gross underestimation of retention which most likely equally applies to those who were not tracked. Further, the data used was from routine care program records not designed for research purposes, and several desired variables, such as occupation, religion, income, perceptions about eMTCT services were missed during the cohort data abstraction. This was mitigated by tracking and interviewing the women for additional data. Some mothers who were interviewed had to give information on events as far back as 2013, with possibility of recall bias.

Conclusions

Generally, LTFU was high especially in the first 6 months and during the 12–18-month period (at the time of transfer to chronic care) and was especially more pronounced among the young women with low educational status and those who had not disclosed their HIV status to their partners. Retention in care was also under-estimated at health facility level. Interventions to enhance PMTCT should focus on improving tracking of women across facilities, such as the use of an online electronic medical records system to automatically track self-transfers, and improving counseling and support for disclosure especially among young women and those with low education status.

Abbreviations

ANC: Antenatal Care; ART: Antiretroviral Therapy; EMOC: Emergency Obstetric care services; EMTCT: Elimination of Mother to Child Transmission; HIV: Human Immunodeficiency Virus; LTFU: Loss-to-follow-up; PMTCT: Prevention of Mother to Child Transmission; WHO: World Health Organization

Acknowledgements

The authors thank the Gomba district EMTCT cohort participants and study staff whose contributions made this work possible.

Funding

This study was partly funded by the Makerere University School of Public Health, the Supporting Policy Engagements for Evidence-based Decisions (SPEED) for Universal Health Coverage Project, and The Ugandan Academy for Health Innovation and Impact. The Ugandan Academy is initially funded by Janssen, the Pharmaceutical Companies of Johnson & Johnson as part of its commitment to global public health through collaboration with the Johnson & Johnson Corporate Citizenship Trust.

Authors' contributions

GK participated in designing the study, data collection, and statistical analyses and served as the lead author of the manuscript. FM, FO, MO, and BC participated in study conception and interpretation of results. RW and NK played active roles as supervisors during all stages of the study as well as manuscript writing. JN participated in qualitative data analysis and interpretation of results. All the authors read and approved the final manuscript.

Competing interests

The authors declare that they have no competing interests.

Author details

[1]Department of Health Policy Planning and Management, Makerere University School of Public Health, P.O Box 7072, Kampala, Uganda. [2]Department of Epidemiology and Biostatistics, School of Public Health, Makerere University College of Health Sciences, Kampala, Uganda. [3]Department of Disease Control and Environmental Health, Makerere University School of Public Health, Kampala, Uganda. [4]Department of Research, Infectious Diseases Institute, Makerere University College of Health Sciences, Kampala, Uganda.

References

1. UNAIDS, "Start Free, Stay Free, AIDS Free — A super-fast-track framework for ending AIDS among children, adolescents and young women by 2020," 2016. [Online]. Available: http://www.unaids.org/sites/default/files/media_asset/Stay_free_vision_mission_En.pdf. Accessed 02 Oct 2017.
2. UNAIDS, "Fact sheet 2016 | UNAIDS," *UNAIDS*, 2016. [Online]. Available: http://www.unaids.org/en/resources/fact-sheet. Accessed 02 Oct 2017.
3. WHO, "Progress Report 2016, prevent HIV, test and treat all," 2016.
4. IATT, "Monitoring & evaluation framework for antiretroviral treatment for pregnant and breastfeeding women living with HIV and their infants," 2015.
5. Hassinger R. Uganda Adopts New PMTCT Strategy, Option B +. 2015. Retrieved October 22, 2018 from https://www.msh.org/comment/8467.
6. MoH, "National Health Care Waste Management Plan 2009/10–2011/12." [Online]. Available: http://webcache.googleusercontent.com/search?q=cache:yl_5Jgg6YFUJ:library.health.go.ug/download/file/fid/1095+&cd=4&hl=en&ct=clnk&gl=ug. [Accessed: 16 Aug 2018].
7. Rollins NC, et al. Defining and analyzing retention-in-care among pregnant and breastfeeding HIV-infected women: unpacking the data to interpret and improve PMTCT outcomes. J Acquir Immune Defic Syndr. 2014;67: S150–6.
8. Sam-Agudu NA, et al. The impact of mentor mother programs on PMTCT service uptake and retention-in-care at primary health care facilities in Nigeria: a prospective cohort study (MoMent Nigeria). J Acquir Immune Defic Syndr. 2014;67(Suppl 2):S132Á8.
9. WHO, "Retention in HIV programmes. Defining the challenges and identifying solutions," 2012.
10. Nachega JB, et al. Adherence to antiretroviral therapy during and after pregnancy in low-income, middle-income, and high-income countries: a systematic review and meta-analysis. Aids. 2012;26(16):2039–52.
11. Kohler PK, et al. Community-based evaluation of PMTCT uptake in Nyanza Province, Kenya. PLoS One. 2014;9(10):e110110.
12. Tenthani L, et al. Retention in care under universal antiretroviral therapy for HIV infected pregnant and breastfeeding women ('Option B+') in Malawi. AIDS. 2014;28(4):589.
13. ElizabethGlazerFoundation, "Treatment for Life, Part 1: Option B+ Gives Mothers and Children Options," 2016. [Online]. Available: http://www.pedaids.org/blog/entry/treatment-for-life-part-1-option-b-gives-mothers-and-children-options. Accessed 22 Sept 2018.
14. Haas AD, et al. Retention in care during the first 3 years of antiretroviral therapy for women in Malawi's option B+ programme: an observational cohort study. Lancet HIV. 2014;3(4):e175–82.

15. Sibanda EL, Cowan FM. Good news for retention of women on option B+ in Malawi. Lancet HIV. 2016;3(4):e151–2.
16. Buregyeya E, et al. Facilitators and barriers to uptake and adherence to lifelong antiretroviral therapy among HIV infected pregnant women in Uganda: a qualitative study. BMC Pregnancy Childbirth. 2017;17(1):94.
17. Nabukeera-Barungi N, et al. Adherence to antiretroviral therapy and retention in care for adolescents living with HIV from 10 districts in Uganda. BMC Infect. Dis. 2015;15(1):520.
18. UBOS. National Population and Housing Census 2014. In: Uganda Bur. Stat. 2016, Natl. Popul. Hous. Census 2014 – Main Rep. , Kampala, Uganda; 2014. p. 1–209.
19. WHO, "Fact sheet on the Uganda Population HIV Impact Assessment | WHO | Regional Office for Africa," 2017. [Online]. Available: https://www.afro.who.int/publications/fact-sheet-uganda-population-hiv-impact-assessment. [Accessed: 16 Aug 2018].
20. MoH, "Uganda Demographic and Health Survey Report 2016 | Knowledge Management Portal," 2017. [Online]. Available: http://library.health.go.ug/publications/leadership-and-governance-monitoring-and-evaluation/statistics/uganda-demographic-and. [Accessed: 16 Aug 2018].
21. Hamilton E, et al. Using the PMTCT Cascade to accelerate achievement of the global plan goals. JAIDS J. Acquir. Immune Defic. Syndr. 2017;75:S27–35.
22. M. Mason, "Sample size and saturation in PhD studies using qualitative interviews," in Forum qualitative Sozialforschung/Forum: qualitative social research, 2010, vol. 11, 3.
23. StatsToDo, "StatsToDo : Sample Size for Survival (Kaplan Meier Log Rank Test) Program." [Online]. Available: https://www.statstodo.com/SSizSurvival_Pgm.php. Accessed 22 Sept 2018.
24. Kieffer MP, et al. Lessons learned from early implementation of option B+: the Elizabeth Glaser Pediatric AIDS Foundation experience in 11 African countries. JAIDS J Acquir Immune Defic Syndr. 2014;67:S188–94.
25. Clouse K, et al. Patient retention from HIV diagnosis through one year on antiretroviral therapy at a primary healthcare clinic in Johannesburg, South Africa. J. Acquir. Immune Defic. Syndr. 2013;62(2):e39.
26. Braun V, Clarke V, Terry G. Thematic analysis. Qual Res Clin Heal Psychol. 2014:95–114.
27. Helova A, et al. Health facility challenges to the provision of Option B+ in western Kenya: a qualitative study. Health Policy Plan. 2016;32(2):czw122.
28. F. Cataldo, et al. She knows that she will not come back: tracing patients and new thresholds of collective surveillance in PMTCT Option B. BMC Health Serv. Res. 2018;18(1):76.
29. Obai G, Mubeezi R, Makumbi F. Rate and associated factors of non-retention of mother-baby pairs in HIV care in the elimination of mother-to-child transmission programme, Gulu-Uganda: a cohort study. BMC Heal. Serv Res. 2017;17(1):48.
30. Kallander K, et al. Inscale cluster randomized trial evaluating the effect of innovative motivation and supervision approaches on community health worker performance and retention in uganda and mozambique: Intervention design. Am. J. Trop. Med. Hyg. 2012;1:243.
31. Bonenberger M, Aikins M, Akweongo P, Wyss K. The effects of health worker motivation and job satisfaction on turnover intention in Ghana: a cross-sectional study. Hum Resour Health. 2014;12:43.
32. Mathauer I, Imhoff I. Health worker motivation in Africa: the role of non-financial incentives and human resource management tools. Hum Resour Health. Aug. 2006;4:24.
33. Thi Hoai Thu N, Wilson A, McDonald F. Motivation or demotivation of health workers providing maternal health services in rural areas in Vietnam: findings from a mixed-methods study. Hum. Resour. Health. 2015;13(1):91.
34. McMahon JH, Elliott JH, Hong SY, Bertagnolio S, Jordan MR. Effects of Physical Tracing on Estimates of Loss to Follow-Up, Mortality and Retention in Low and Middle Income Country Antiretroviral Therapy Programs: A Systematic Review. PLoS One. 2013;8(2):e56047.
35. Ngarina M, et al. Women's preferences regarding infant or maternal antiretroviral prophylaxis for prevention of mother-to-child transmission of HIV during breastfeeding and their views on Option B+ in Dar es Salaam, Tanzania. PLoS One. 2014;9(1):e85310.
36. Rawizza HE, et al. "Loss to Follow-Up within the Prevention of Mother-to-Child Transmission Care Cascade in a Large ART Program in Nigeria." 2015;13(3):201–09.
37. Kalembo FW, Zgambo M. Loss to Followup: a major challenge to successful implementation of prevention of mother-to-child transmission of HIV-1 programs in sub-Saharan Africa. ISRN AIDS. 2012;2012:1–10.
38. Herce ME, et al. Supporting Option B+ scale up and strengthening the prevention of mother-to-child transmission cascade in central Malawi: results from a serial cross-sectional study. BMC Infect. Dis. 2015;15(1):328.
39. Gamell A, et al. Prevention of mother-to-child transmission of HIV Option B + cascade in rural Tanzania: The One Stop Clinic model. PLoS One. 2017; 12(7):e0181096.
40. Flax VL, Hamela G, Mofolo I, Hosseinipour MC, Hoffman IF, Maman S. Factors influencing postnatal Option B+ participation and breastfeeding duration among HIV-positive women in Lilongwe District, Malawi: A qualitative study. PLoS One. 2017;12(4):e0175590.
41. Valenzuela C, et al. HIV stigma as a barrier to retention in HIV care at a general hospital in Lima, Peru: a case-control study. AIDS Behav. 2015;19(2):235–45.
42. Mitiku I, Arefayne M, Mesfin Y, Gizaw M. Factors associated with loss to follow-up among women in Option B+ PMTCT programme in northeast Ethiopia: a retrospective cohort study. J. Int. AIDS Soc. 2016;19(1).
43. Tweya H, et al. Understanding factors, outcomes and reasons for loss to follow-up among women in option B+ PMTCT programme in Lilongwe, Malawi. Trop Med Int Heal. 2014;19(11):1360–6.
44. Rachlis B, et al. Facility-level factors influencing retention of patients in HIV care in East Africa. PLoS One. 2016;11(8):e0159994.
45. Ebuy H, Yebyo H, Alemayehu M. Level of adherence and predictors of adherence to the option B+ PMTCT programme in Tigray, northern Ethiopia. Int J Infect Dis. 2015;33:e123–9.
46. Gugsa S, et al. Exploring factors associated with ART adherence and retention in care under Option B+ strategy in Malawi: A qualitative study. PLoS One. 2017;12(6):e0179838.
47. Hoffman RM, et al. Factors associated with retention in Option B+ in Malawi: a case control study. J. Int. AIDS Soc. 2017;20(1):21464.
48. Stinson K, Myer L. Barriers to initiating antiretroviral therapy during pregnancy: a qualitative study of women attending services in Cape Town, South Africa. African J AIDS Res. 2012;11(1):65–73.
49. Ambia J, Mandala J. A systematic review of interventions to improve prevention of mother-to-child HIV transmission service delivery and promote retention. J Int AIDS Soc. 2016;19(1):20309.

3

Epidemiology of hepatitis B, C and D in Malawi

Alexander J Stockdale[1,2*], Collins Mitambo[3], Dean Everett[1,4], Anna Maria Geretti[2] and Melita A Gordon[1,2]

Abstract

Background: Viral hepatitis is an important public health issue in sub-Saharan Africa. Due to rising mortality from cirrhosis and hepatocellular carcinoma and limited implementation of screening and treatment programmes, it has been characterised as a neglected tropical disease. Synthesis of the existing evidence on the epidemiology of viral hepatitis B, C and D in Malawi is required to inform policy and identify research gaps.

Methods: We searched Pubmed, EMBASE and Scopus for studies reporting the epidemiology of viral hepatitis B, C and D in Malawi from 1990 to 2018. Articles reporting prevalence estimates were included provided they described details of participant selection, inclusion criteria and laboratory methods (detection of HBsAg, anti-HCV or anti-HDV antibody, HCV antigen or HCV RNA or HDV RNA). We assessed study quality using a prevalence assessment tool. Where appropriate, a pooled prevalence was calculated using a DerSimonian Laird random effects model.

Results: Searches identified 199 studies, 95 full text articles were reviewed and 19 articles were included. Hepatitis B surface antigen (HBsAg) seroprevalence was assessed in 14 general population cohorts. The pooled prevalence among adults was 8.1% (95% CI 6.1, 10.3). In 3 studies where HBsAg was stratified by HIV status, no effect of HIV on HBsAg prevalence was observed (OR 1.2 (95% CI: 0.8, 1.6, $p = 0.80$)). In a single study of HIV/HBV infected individuals, anti-hepatitis D antibody (anti-HDV) prevalence was low (1.5%). HCV antibody prevalence (anti-HCV) ranged from 0.7 to 18.0% among 12 cohorts in general populations. Among three studies which used PCR to confirm current infection, the pooled rate of HCV RNA confirmation among anti-HCV positive individuals was only 7.3% (95% CI: 0.0, 24.3).

Conclusions: Hepatitis B is highly prevalent in Malawi. There is a paucity of epidemiological data from rural areas where 85% of the population reside, and the Northern region. Priority research needs include large-scale representative community studies of HBV, HDV and HCV seroprevalence, assessment of children following introduction of the HBV vaccine in 2002, prevalence estimates of viral hepatitis among individuals with cirrhosis and HCC and data on HCV prevalence using PCR confirmation, to support a viral hepatitis strategy for Malawi.

Keywords: Epidemiology, Viral hepatitis, Hepatitis B, Hepatitis C, Hepatitis D, Malawi, Sub-Saharan Africa

Background

Viral hepatitis is the principal cause of liver cirrhosis and hepatocellular carcinoma (HCC) in sub-Saharan Africa [1]. Due to limited availability of screening and treatment programmes, it has been characterised as a neglected tropical disease [2]. In contrast with HIV, malaria and tuberculosis, where public health interventions have resulted in substantial reductions in mortality, viral hepatitis-associated mortality is rising: cirrhosis and HCC were the cause of an estimated 3.2% of adult deaths in 2005, rising to 4% in 2016 [3, 4]. In Malawi, the cirrhosis-associated mortality rate has been ranked in the top global decile [5]. Across Southern Africa, an estimated 50–64% of cases of HCC are attributable to viral hepatitis, and with limited treatment options outcomes are poor with an estimated annual mortality to incidence ratio of 96% [6–8]. HCC has been shown to occur in a younger age group among individuals in sub-Saharan Africa and in HBV-associated cases (relative to HCV-associated cases), contributing to increased disease impact [9, 10].

* Correspondence: a.stockdale@liverpool.ac.uk
[1]Malawi Liverpool Wellcome Trust Clinical Research Programme, Chichiri 3, PO Box 30096, Blantyre, Malawi
[2]Institute of Infection and Global Health, University of Liverpool, Ronald Ross Building, 8 West Derby Street, Liverpool L69 7BE, UK
Full list of author information is available at the end of the article

Data on the epidemiology of viral hepatitis are required to inform an effective public health response. In the Global Health Sector Strategy on Viral Hepatitis 2016–2021, the World Health Organisation (WHO) has identified the need to define the national disease burden and strategically target limited resources to counter the local epidemic. There is a WHO call for data on transmission and risk factors, to identify specific populations at risk and to quantify the health burden in terms of cirrhosis and hepatocellular carcinoma [11].

The Malawi Ministry of Health (MoH) has resolved to respond to viral hepatitis in a concerted and strategic manner. As part of the response, a National Viral Hepatitis Unit has been created in the MoH to guide the direction of policy and practice. In order to consolidate the current available evidence on epidemiology of viral hepatitis, identify the gaps in knowledge, practice and policy, we aimed to conduct a systematic review of all published epidemiological data on the prevalence of chronic hepatitis B, C and D in Malawi and identify further research needs.

Methods

Searches were performed in Pubmed, Scopus and EMBASE using the search terms Malawi AND (hepatitis or hepatitis B or HBV or HBsAg or hepatitis C or HCV or anti-HCV or HCV antibody or core HCV antigen or HCVcAg or HCV RNA or hepatitis D or HDV or anti-HD or anti-HDV or HDV IgG or HDV RNA or viral hepatitis). (Additional file 1: Table S1) Medical subject headings [MeSH] in Pubmed and EMBASE thesaurus tools were employed. Searches were restricted to publications between 1 Jan 1990 and 1 February 2018 with a search update on 22 June 18, to identify published data from the past 28 years (Fig. 1).

Data were grouped into two categories: "general populations" which provided data from potentially representative community samples, pregnant women, or blood donors; "HIV positive populations" adults or women, or children receiving routine HIV care, and "special groups", comprising populations likely to be unrepresentative of the general population such as medical inpatients, prisoners or medical students.

Studies reporting detection of hepatitis B surface antigen (HBsAg), or total or IgG anti-hepatitis delta antibody (anti-HDV) or HDV RNA among HBsAg positive people, or anti-hepatitis C antibody (anti-HCV), hepatitis C core antigen (HCVcAg) or HCV RNA were included, provided they presented details of selection and inclusion criteria and described the laboratory methods used.

Data extraction and quality assessment

We conducted this review in accordance with PRISMA guidelines [12]. We extracted details of study design, participant characteristics (age and gender distribution, population group), sampling method, dates, study locations, laboratory test used and prevalence estimates. A quality assessment tool for prevalence estimates was used and study quality was independently evaluated by two authors (AS, CM) with discordance resolved by discussion [13].

Statistical analysis

Confidence intervals for prevalence were calculated using the Wilson method. Pooled seroprevalence for hepatitis B was calculated with the DerSimonian-Laird random-effects model with Freeman-Tukey double arcsine transformation [14, 15]. A random effects model was applied due to anticipated heterogeneity. Study heterogeneity was assessed using the I^2 statistic. Analyses were performed in Stata release 14.2 (College Station, TX, USA) using the metaprop package [16].

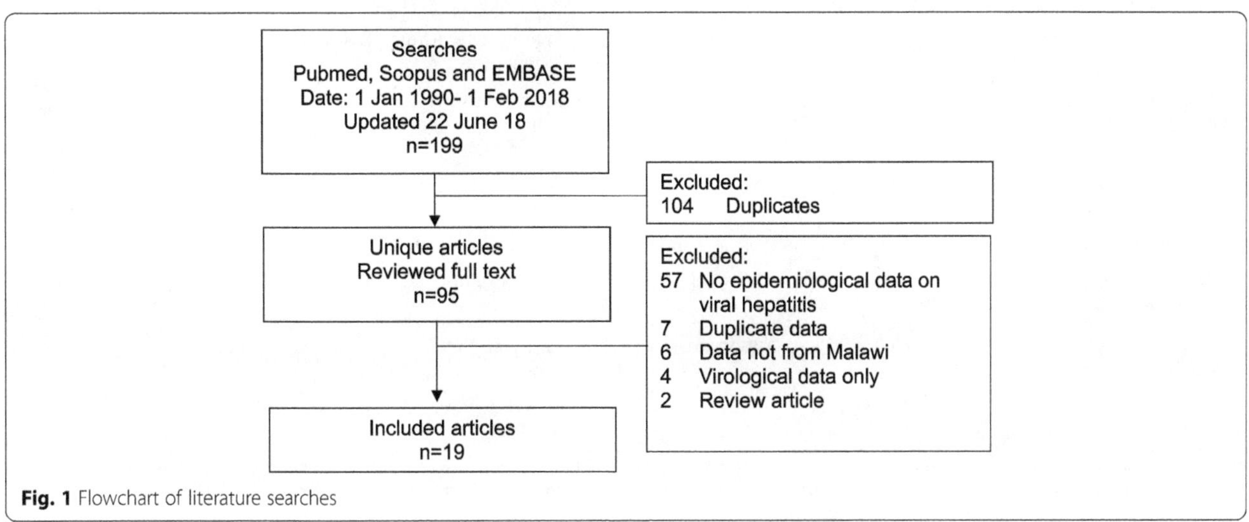

Fig. 1 Flowchart of literature searches

Results

The literature search identified 199 studies. Following removal of duplicates, 95 full-text articles were reviewed and 19 studies that reported epidemiological data on hepatitis B, C and D in diverse populations in Malawi were included (Fig. 1).

Description of included studies

The 19 included studies described a total of HBsAg seroprevalence data from 16 different cohorts that were general or HIV-positive populations (Table 1; Fig. 2) and three cohorts from specific unrepresentative subgroups (Table 2); hepatitis D antibody (anti-HDV) data was available from a single study (Table 3) and hepatitis C antibody (anti-HCV) data was available from 15 general or HIV-positive cohorts (Table 4; Fig. 4) and from four cohorts describing specific subgroups (Table 5). Fourteen of 18 studies were from urban centres.

Hepatitis B prevalence

HBsAg seroprevalence estimates ranged from 0.0 to 14.3% in general populations and 3.8 to 16.0% in

Table 1 Hepatitis B surface antigen (HBsAg) seroprevalence in Malawi: published data from 1990 to 2018

Population	Ref	Year	Location	Laboratory method	Prevalence (n/total)	Prevalence (%), (95% CI)
General Populations						
Pregnant women	[20]	1989–1994	QECH, Blantyre	MONOLISA HBsAg ULTRA (Biorad)	0/70	0.0 (0.0, 5.2)
Pregnant women, at delivery	[18]	1993–1995	Shire Valley	Bioelisa HBsAg (Biokit, S.A.)	12/100	12.0 (7.0, 19.8)
Pregnant women	[20]	2004–2008	QECH, Health Centres Blantyre	MONOLISA HBsAg ULTRA (Biorad)	16/134	11.9 (7.5, 18.5)
Male workers at sugar estate	[17]	1998	Nchalo	Auszyme monoclonal EIA (Abbott)	40/280	14.3 (10.7, 18.9)
Community, rural adults	[20]	2001	Mwanza District	MONOLISA HBsAg ULTRA (Biorad)	7/98	7.1 (3.5, 14.0)
Non-pregnant women (intravaginal MTZ gel RCT)	[20]	2003–2005	QECH, Blantyre	MONOLISA HBsAg ULTRA (Biorad)	8/137	5.8 (3.0, 11.1)
HIV-negative partners in a serodiscordant couple	[19]	2007–2010	Blantyre Lilongwe	HBsAg ELISA NS	26/433	6.0 (4.1, 8.7)
Blood donors	[21]	2001	Ntechu	HBsAg ELISA NS	13/159	8.2 (4.8, 13.5)
HIV-positive populations						
HIV-positive pregnant women, at delivery	[18]	1993–1995	Shire Valley	Bioelisa HBsAg (Biokit, S.A.)	8/50	16.0 (8.3, 28.5)
HIV-positive pregnant women	[20]	2000–2004	QECH, Blantyre	MONOLISA HBsAg ULTRA (Biorad)	6/156	3.8 (1.8, 8.1)
HIV-positive pregnant women	[22]	2004–2009	Lilongwe	Vitros Chemiluminescence Immunoassay (Ortho Clinical Diagnostics)	103/2049	5.0 (4.2, 6.1)
HIV-positive pregnant women	[23]	2008–2009	Blantyre	Murex HBsAg Version 3 with Confirmatory Assay (Murex Biotech)	27/309	8.7 (6.1, 12.4)
HIV positive: male workers at sugar estate	[17]	1998	Nchalo	Auszyme monoclonal EIA (Abbott)	32/189	16.9 (12.3, 22.9)
HIV-positive adults	[24]	2005	QECH, Blantyre	Bioelisa HBsAg (Biokit, S.A.)	20/300	6.7 (4.4, 10.1)
HIV positive adults, ART starters	[25]	2007–2009	QECH, Blantyre	Bioelisa HBsAg (Biokit, S.A.)	133/1117	11.9 (10.1, 13.9)
HIV-positive adults in sero-discordant couple	[19]	2007–2010	Blantyre Lilongwe	HBsAg ELISA NS	26/432	6.0 (4.1, 8.7)
HIV-infected children	[26]	2008–2010	Lilongwe	Genetic Systems HBsAg 3.0 (Bio-Rad)	2/91	2.2 (0.6, 7.7)

Abbreviations: *QECH* Queen Elizabeth Central Hospital, Blantyre. This is a tertiary referral hospital, *MTZ* metronidazole, *RCT* randomised controlled trial. Biorad: HBsAg ELISA, Biorad, Hercules, CA, USA; Bioelisa: HBsAg 3.0 Biokit SA Barcelona, Spain; Ortho Clinical Diagnositics: Raritan, New Jersey, United States: Siemens: ADVIA Centaur, Siemens, Munich, Germany; Abbott: Murex HBsAg, Abbott, Illinois, USA; HBsAg ELISA NS- manufacturer not specified

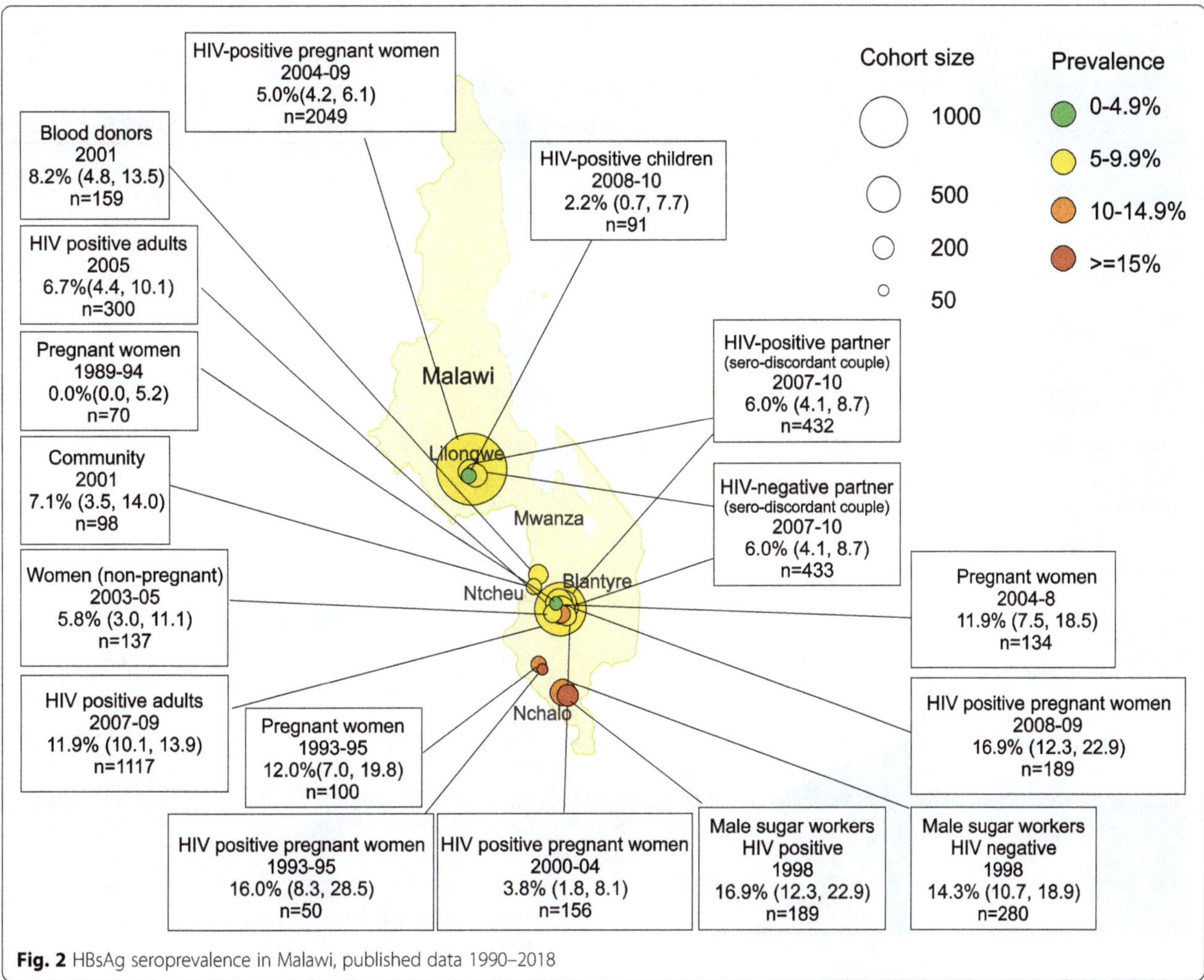

Fig. 2 HBsAg seroprevalence in Malawi, published data 1990–2018

HIV positive populations (Table 1). One small study reporting from HIV positive children aged 3 months - 15 years (median 36 months) reported seroprevalence of 2.2% [95% confidence interval (CI) 0.6, 7.7]. This study did not estimate HBV vaccine efficacy as the vaccine was introduced in Malawi in 2002 and both vaccinated and non-vaccinated cohorts were combined. Pooled estimates of HBsAg seroprevalence among adult general populations was 7.6% (95% CI 4.6, 11.2) and 8.5 (95% CI 5.7, 11.7) in HIV positive populations (Fig. 3). The overall pooled estimate of HBsAg seroprevalence in adults was 8.1% (95% CI 6.1, 10.3).

No significant difference in HBsAg prevalence was noted between HIV-positive and -negative populations ($p = 0.74$). The effect of HIV status on HBV seroprevalence was assessed directly in three studies, with a total of 1484 participants, that tested HBsAg prevalence, stratified by HIV status within the same population. These populations comprised male workers at a sugar factory ($n = 469$) [17], pregnant women recruited at delivery ($n = 150$) [18] and HIV positive and negative sero-discordant couples recruited for a randomised control trial of antiretroviral therapy for prevention of transmission ($n = 865$) [19]. Among the three groups, the odds ratio of HBsAg positivity among HIV positive compared

Table 2 HBsAg seroprevalence among special unrepresentative populations in Malawi: Published data from 1990 to 2018

Population	Ref	Year	Location	Laboratory method	Prevalence (n/total)	Prevalence (%, (95% CI))
Adult medical inpatients	[27]	2004	Medical ward, QECH, Blantyre	Determine HBsAg Rapid Test (Alere)	34/194	17.5 (12.8, 23.5)
Prisoners	[28]	2007	Chichiri Prison, Blantyre	HBsAg kit (Abbott)	5/164	3.0 (1.3, 6.9)
Medical students	[29]	2013	College of Medicine, Blantyre	SD Bioline Rapid Test (Alere)	0/89	0.0 (0.0, 4.9)

Abbreviations: *QECH* Queen Elizabeth Central Hospital, *ART* antiretroviral therapy

Table 3 Published data on hepatitis D seroprevalence in Malawi among HBsAg positive individuals

Population	Ref	Year	Location	Method	Prevalence (n/total)	Prevalence (%, (95% CI))
HIV-HBV infected adults	[30]	2007–2009	HIV clinic, QECH Blantyre	1. ETI-AB-DELTAK (Diasorin)	2/133	1.5 (0.4, 5.3)
				2. HDV RNA PCR (in-house)	0/133	0.0 (0.0, 2.8)

Table 4 Published data on hepatitis C seroprevalence in Malawi

Population	Ref	Year	Location	Method	Prevalence (n/total)	Prevalence (%, (95% CI))
General Populations						
Pregnant women	[20]	1989–1994	QECH, Blantyre	Anti-HCV (Biorad)	2/70	2.9 (0.8, 9.8)
Pregnant women, at delivery	[18]	1993–1995	Shire Valley	Ortho anti-HCV (Ortho Diagnostics)	18/100	18.0 (11.7, 26.7)
Pregnant women	[20]	2004–2008	QECH, Health Centres Blantyre	Anti-HCV (Biorad)	8/138	5.8 (3.0, 11.0)
Community, rural adults	[20]	2001	Mwanza District	Anti-HCV (Biorad)	9/99	9.0 (4.9, 16.4)
Non-pregnant women (intravaginal MTZ gel RCT)	[20]	2003–2005	QECH, Blantyre	Anti-HCV (Biorad)	9/146	6.1 (3.3, 11.3)
Male workers at sugar estate	[17]	1998	Nchalo	Ortho anti-HCV (Ortho Diagnostics)	35/279	10.0 (7.0, 14.1)
Blood donors	[32]	1996	KCH, Lilongwe	Anti-HCV EIA (Roche) Confirmed with Anti-HCV (Abbott)	4/100	4.0 (1.6, 9.8)
Blood donors	[21]	2001	Ntechu	1. Murex anti-HCV	10/148	6.8 (3.7, 12.0)
				2. HCV RNA by in-house PCR	1/140	0.7 (0.1, 3.9)
HIV positive populations						
HIV-positive pregnant women, at delivery	[18]	1993–1995	Shire Valley	Ortho anti-HCV (Ortho Diagnostics)	6/50	12.0 (5.6, 23.8)
HIV-positive pregnant women	[23]	2008–2009	Blantyre	1. Innotest HCV Ab IV (Innogenetics),	8/309	2.6 (1.3, 5.0)
				2. Versant HCV RNA 1.0 assay (Siemens)	1/309	0.3 (0.1, 1.8)
HIV positive patients	[24]	2005	QECH, Blantyre	Monolisa HCV Ag-Ab (Biorad) confirmed with ADVIA Centaur anti-HCV) and InnoLIA HCV immunoassay (Innogenetics)	17/300	5.7 (3.6, 8.9)
HIV-positive male workers at sugar estate	[17]	1998	Nchalo	Ortho anti-HCV Ab (Ortho Clinical Diagnostics)	28/280	10.0 (7.0, 14.1)
HIV-positive pregnant women	[20]	2000–2004	QECH, Blantyre	Anti-HCV (Biorad)	8/148	5.4 (2.8, 10.3)
HIV positive adults starting ART	[31]	2014–15	Lilongwe	1. HCV IgG Architect (Abbott)	5/227	2.2 (0.9, 5.1)
				2. RealTime HCV RNA (Abbott)	0/227	0.0 (0.0, 1.7)
HIV positive patients on ART for > 10 years	[33]	2014–16	Chiradzulu	OraQuick HCV Rapid antibody test (Orasure)	2/385	0.5 (0.1, 1.9)

Abbreviations: *QECH* Queen Elizabeth Central Hospital, *HCV* hepatitis C virus Biorad: Hercules, CA, USA; Ortho Clinical Diagnostics: Raritan, New Jersey, United States; Roche: Basel Switzerland; Abbott: Illinois, USA; Innogenetics: Ghent, Belgium; Siemens: Munich, Germany; Orasure: Bethlehem, Pennsylvania, United States

Table 5 Published data on hepatitis C seroprevalence among special unrepresentative populations in Malawi: Published data from 1990 to 2018

Population	Ref	Year	Location	Method	Prevalence (n/total)	Prevalence (%, (95% CI))
Prisoners	[28]	2007	Chichiri Prison, Blantyre	Anti-HCV (Biotec)	0/164	0.0 (0.0, 2.3)
Adult inpatients (Dermatology, Urology)	[32]	1996	KCH, Lilongwe	Anti-HCV EIA (Roche) Confirmed with Anti-HCV (Abbott)	13/333	3.9 (2.3, 6.6)
Adult medical inpatients	[27]	2004	Medical ward, QECH, Blantyre	HCV Ag/Ab (Monolisa, Biorad) confirmed with Immunoassay (Innogenetics)	9/202	4.5 (2.4, 8.2)
Malawian women and children with childhood malignancies	[34]	2006–10	QECH, Blantyre	HBV ELISA (MP Biomedicals)	Mothers: 2/418	0.5 (0.1, 1.7)
				Confirmed by HCV BLOT (MP Biomedicals)	Children: 1/418	0.2 (0.0, 1.3)

Abbreviations: Biotec: Dorset, United Kingdom; Roche: Basel, Switzerland; Abbott: Illinois, USA; Innogenetics: Ghent, Belgium; MP Biomedicals: California, USA*KCH* Kamuzu Central Hospital, *QECH* Queen Elizabeth Central Hospital, *HCV* hepatitis C virus

to HIV negative individuals from within the same population was 1.2 (95% CI 0.8, 1.6, $p = 0.80$), indicating no evidence of association between HBV infection and HIV infection status. (Fig. 4).

Studies among three unrepresentative groups deemed at altered risk of HBV infection: (adult medical inpatients, prisoners and medical students) found HBsAg prevalence rates of 17.5%, 3.0% and 0% respectively (Table 2).

Hepatitis D prevalence

A single study was available reporting HDV prevalence among HIV/HBV co-infected individuals commencing ART in Blantyre [30] (Table 3). This demonstrated

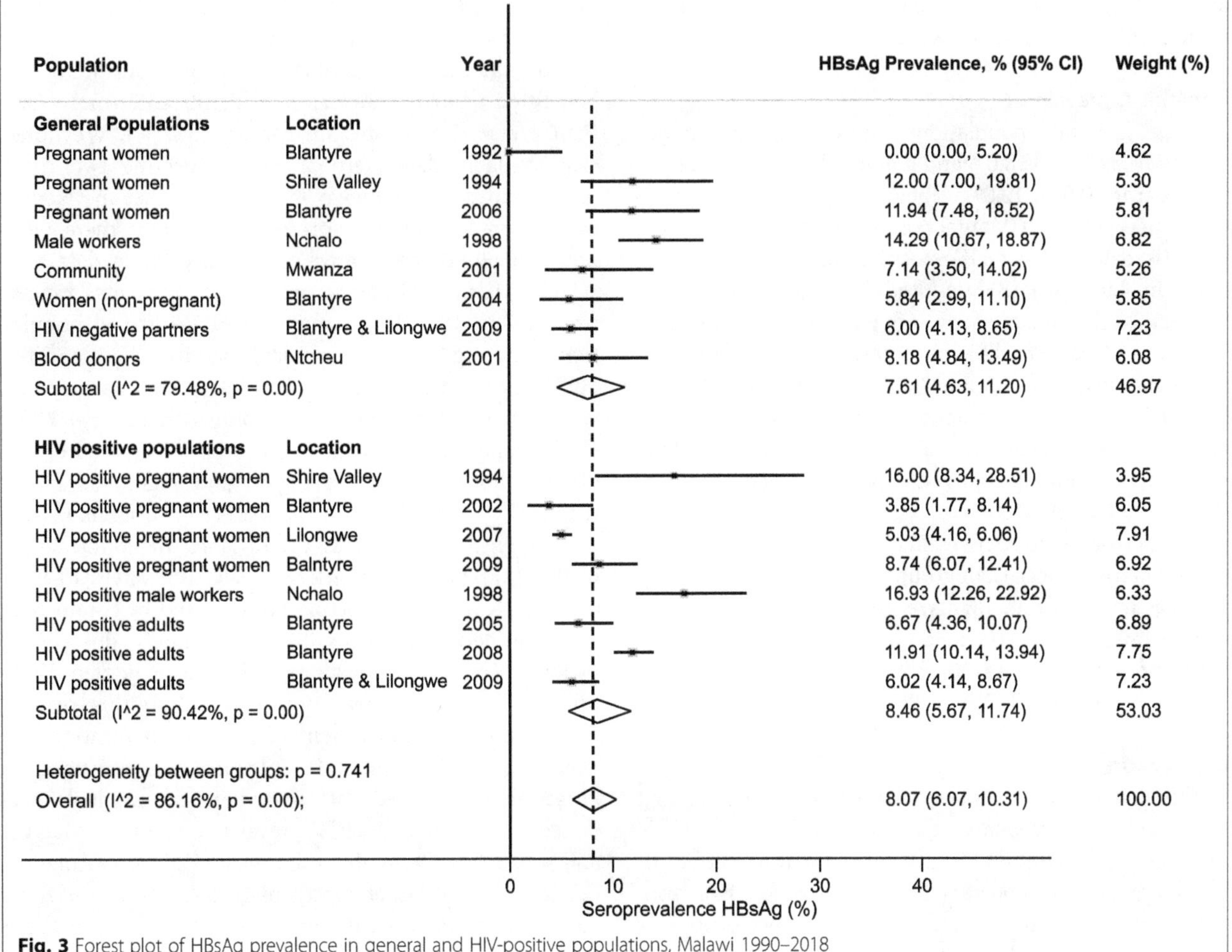

Fig. 3 Forest plot of HBsAg prevalence in general and HIV-positive populations, Malawi 1990–2018

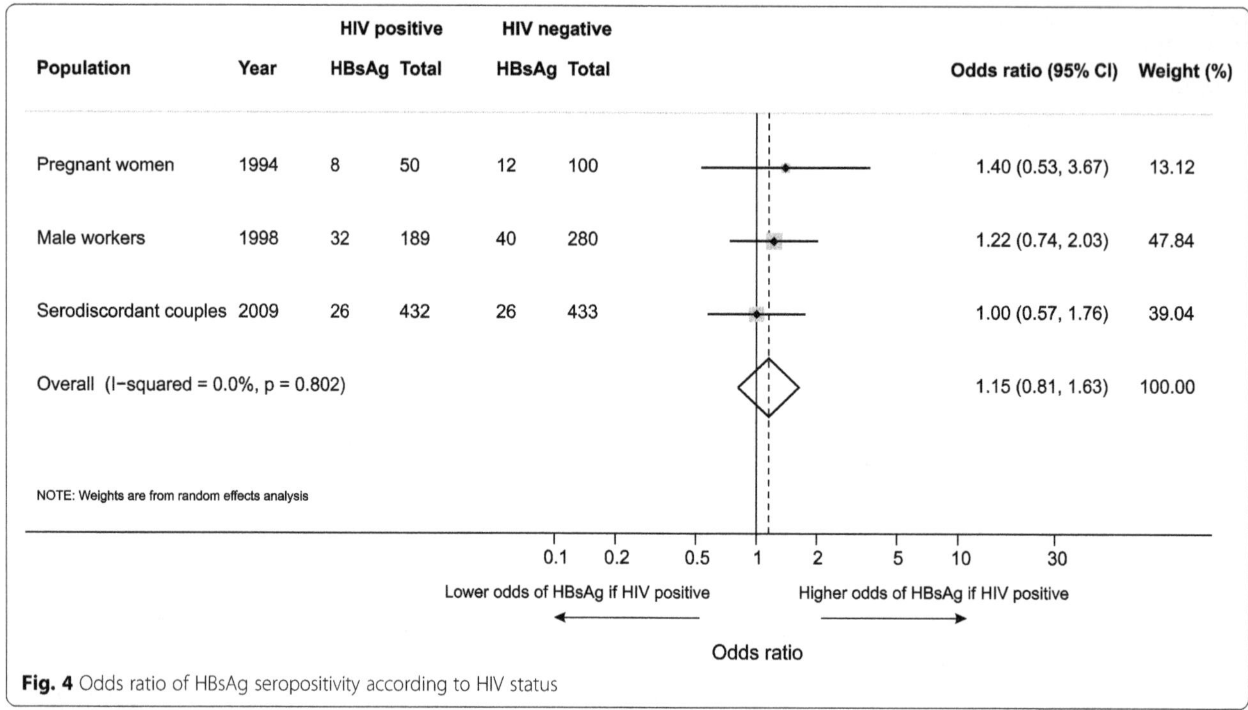

Fig. 4 Odds ratio of HBsAg seropositivity according to HIV status

anti-HDV prevalence of 2/133 (1.5%) but none of the participants were HDV RNA PCR positive.

Hepatitis C prevalence

Among general populations, anti-HCV prevalence ranged from 0.7 to 18.0% and among HIV-positive populations from 0.0 to 12.0%. (Table 4, Fig. 5) Three studies confirmed active HCV infection using RNA PCR. These comprised a study of HIV-positive adults commencing ART in Lilongwe [31], a study of blood donors in Ntcheu [21] and a study of HIV-positive pregnant women in Blantyre [23]. In these studies, anti-HCV prevalence was 2.2, 6.8 and 2.6% respectively but HCV RNA PCR demonstrated active HCV prevalence of 0, 0.7 and 0.3% respectively, with a pooled rate of HCV RNA confirmation among anti-HCV positive participants of 7.3% (95% CI 0.0–24.3).

Among four studies assessing HCV prevalence in unrepresentative special subgroups comprising: prisoners; medical inpatients in Blantyre and Lilongwe; and children with malignancies and their mothers, the prevalence of anti-HCV was 0; 3.9 and 4.5; 0.2 and 0.5% respectively (Table 5).

Discussion

In this systematic review, we have compiled the existing epidemiological evidence on HBV, HCV and HDV prevalence in Malawi and have highlighted a number of key findings and important knowledge gaps. Data from studies reporting from general and HIV-infected populations showed a pooled HBsAg seroprevalence estimate of 8.1% (95% CI 6.1, 10.3). This finding is in keeping with regional estimates from Mozambique (8.3%), Tanzania (7.2%) and Zambia (6.1%) [35]. Our study has benefitted from the inclusion of significantly more data than previous estimates for Malawi [35, 36]. We noted that available data were biased toward the two main urban centres of Lilongwe and Blantyre, that the Northern region was under-represented and that there were no nationally representative community survey data.

Hepatitis C antibody seroprevalence estimates ranged from 2.9 to 18% from general or HIV-infected populations. Among the three available studies that reported HCV RNA confirmation, only 7.3% of 676 participants with anti-HCV antibody were confirmed to have HCV RNA replication. This finding has been consistent with other cohorts across the region and highlights issues with using anti-HCV as the basis for obtaining epidemiological estimates in the absence of confirmatory testing [37]. Confirmation of anti-HCV results with PCR or core HCV antigen testing are required to obtain reliable prevalence estimates [38]. Accordingly, due to the paucity of studies reporting PCR data, a pooled HCV prevalence estimate was not provided in this review. Furthermore, an assessment of possible association between HCV, HBV and HIV infection was not possible based on the limited data. Based on the available evidence, it is likely that HCV prevalence is low in Malawi, and was below 1% in all studies using RNA confirmation [21, 23, 31], but larger representative samples employing confirmatory PCR testing are required to confirm these findings. Further work to establish whether false positive

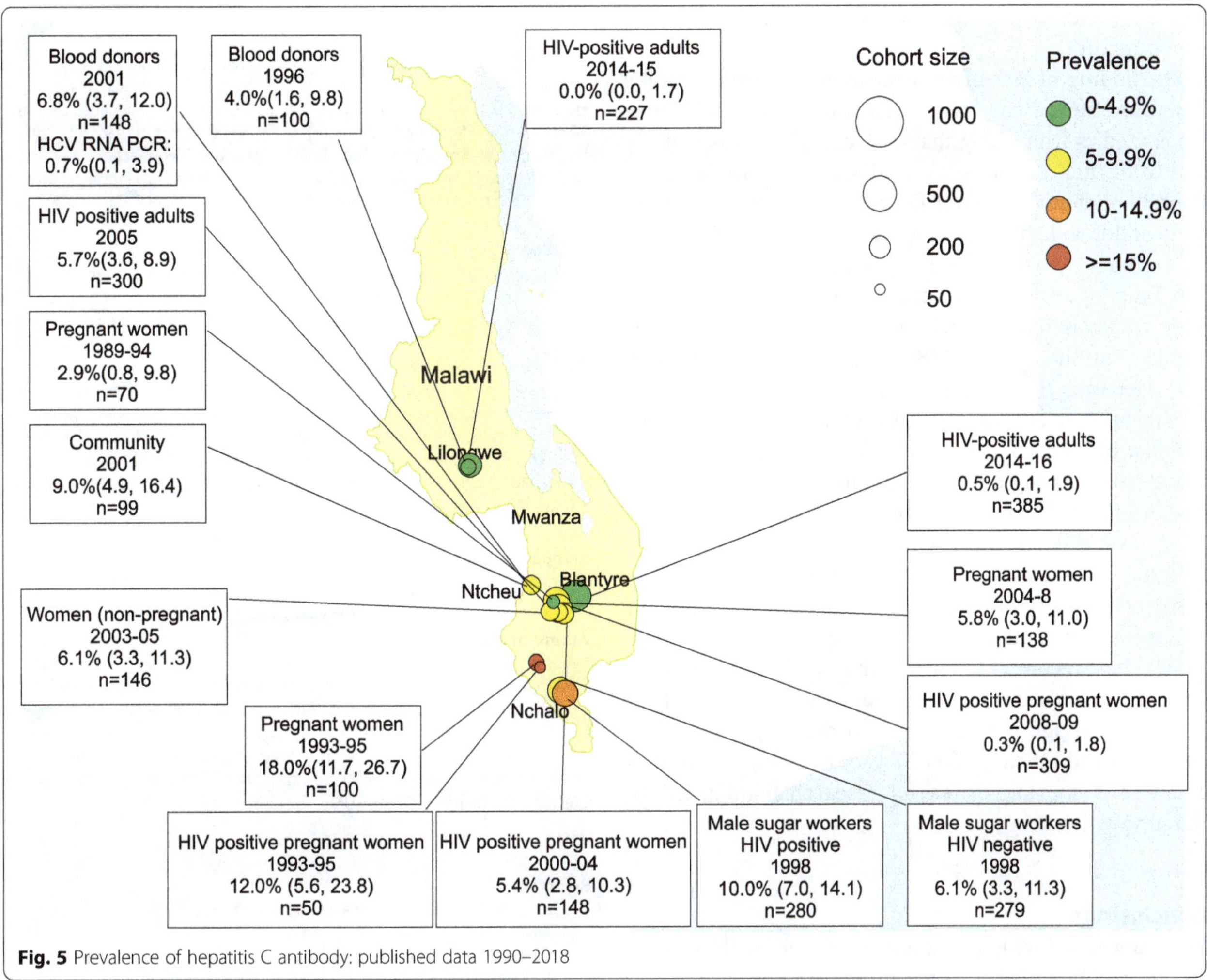

Fig. 5 Prevalence of hepatitis C antibody: published data 1990–2018

anti-HCV antibody tests or failure of HCV RNA assays to detect local HCV strains is required, particularly in view of the paucity of available genotypic HCV data from sub-Saharan Africa [39].

Only a single study reporting HDV prevalence was available, demonstrating a low rate of anti-HDV among HIV/HBV co-infected patients in Blantyre (1.5%), with none of the participants showing replication of HDV RNA by PCR. This finding is in keeping with available limited data demonstrating a low rate of HDV seroprevalence from Southern Africa relative to Central or West Africa, though the paucity of available data from the Southern Africa region should be noted [30]. Due to the rapid progression to fatal liver disease associated with HBV/HDV superinfection or co-infection, cross-sectional community estimates of HDV seroprevalence are unlikely to reliably estimate the true burden of disease caused by HDV. Studies of hospitalised patients with well-characterised liver disease are required and will facilitate the ascertainment of the attributable fraction of viral hepatitis to liver disease [40].

There are several limitations in this analysis, highlighted by our assessment of study quality (Additional file 2: Table S2). The epidemiological evidence presented in this study is drawn from predominantly small cohorts studies in diverse populations employing convenience sampling. A striking bias toward urban centres was observed with only four of 18 included studies drawn from rural areas, despite an estimated 85% of the Malawian population residing in rural areas [41]. There were no available data from the Northern region of Malawi, where 13% of the population live [41]. To overcome these issues of lack of nationally representative unbiased community data, the use of the demographic health survey using dried blood spot sampling represents a promising solution. Dried blood spots have excellent diagnostic performance relative to venous blood sampling for HBsAg and anti-HCV screening and this method has been recently recommended for large surveys by the WHO [38]. Use of dried blood spots for hepatitis D screening of the demographic health survey has recently been used in Burkina Faso [42], and represent an efficient method to obtain samples without requiring a cold chain or venepuncture.

The finding of lack of an association between hepatitis B seroprevalence and HIV status is in keeping with previous studies from sub-Saharan Africa [43]. This is likely due to distinct transmission epidemiology, with hepatitis B predominantly acquired perinatally or horizontally in early childhood, and HIV acquired predominantly during adolescence or adulthood by sexual transmission in sub-Saharan Africa. By contrast, recent evidence of incident transmission of HBV in HIV-infected adults has highlighted the risk of HBV acquisition in adulthood [44]. Hepatitis B vaccination is provided as a component of the pentavalent vaccine (also containing, diphtheria, tetanus, pertussis and *Haemophilis influenzae* type B) in the expanded programme of immunisation schedule for Malawian infants, provided at 6, 10 and 14 weeks since 2002. The Demographic Health Survey 2015–16 estimated 3-dose coverage of the vaccine of 93.0%, with consistently high coverage exceeding 90%, regardless of socioeconomic status or geographic location [45]. The WHO has recently proposed that gathering data on hepatitis B seroprevalence among a vaccinated cohort at 5 years of age is a priority in order to generate evidence on the efficacy of HBV vaccination programmes and this is a priority area for research highlighted by this review [46].

Conclusions

Hepatitis B is highly prevalent in Malawi with an estimated seroprevalence among the general population of 8.1%. HCV prevalence was below 1% in three general population cohorts that used nucleic amplification confirmatory testing. There is a need for representative unbiased community seroprevalence estimates of HBV, HDV and HCV prevalence. These should include confirmatory PCR testing to establish reliable HCV prevalence estimates. Future studies examining seroprevalence among community samples, with a particular focus on rural areas and the Northern region, are required. Assessment of the effectiveness of the hepatitis B vaccination programme introduced in 2002 and data on HDV prevalence among HBsAg positive individuals represent further research priorities. Prevalence estimates of viral hepatitis among people with well-characterised liver disease with cirrhosis and HCC are required to ascertain the attributable fraction and burden of disease. These data will help to support a viral hepatitis strategy for Malawi, facilitate the introduction of screening and treatment programmes for HBV and HCV and begin to reverse the current trend of increasing viral hepatitis-associated mortality.

Abbreviations

Anti-HCV: hepatitis C virus antibody; Anti-HDV: anti-hepatitis C virus antibody; ART: antiretroviral therapy; DNA: deoxyribonucleic acid; EIA: Enzyme immunoassay; HBsAg: hepatitis B surface antigen; HBV: hepatitis B virus; HCC: hepatocellular carcinoma; HCV: hepatitis C virus; HDV: hepatitis D virus; KCH: Kamuzu Central Hospital, Lilongwe, Malawi (National tertiary referral hospital); MoH: Ministry of Health; PCR: polymerase chain reaction; QECH: Queen Elizabeth Central Hospital, Blantyre, Malawi (National tertiary referral hospital); RNA: ribonucleic acid; WHO: World Health Organisation

Funding

AS is supported by a Wellcome Trust Clinical PhD Fellowship, grant 109130/Z/15/Z. The funder had no role in the design of the study and collection, analysis, and interpretation of data nor in writing the manuscript.

Authors' contributions

AS performed the literature searches, extracted the data, performed statistical analyses, wrote the manuscript, CM performed quality assessment of included articles, reviewed and revised the manuscript, DE, AMG and MG developed the concept and study design, reviewed and revised the manuscript and assisted in data analysis and interpretation. All authors read and approved the final manuscript.

Competing interests

The authors declare they have no competing interests.

Author details

[1]Malawi Liverpool Wellcome Trust Clinical Research Programme, Chichiri 3, PO Box 30096, Blantyre, Malawi. [2]Institute of Infection and Global Health, University of Liverpool, Ronald Ross Building, 8 West Derby Street, Liverpool L69 7BE, UK. [3]HIV and AIDS Department, Malawi Ministry of Health, PO Box 30377, Lilongwe, Malawi. [4]MRC Centre for Inflammation Research, The Queen's Medical Research Institute, University of Edinburgh, 47 Little France Crescent, Edinburgh EH16 4TJ, UK.

References

1. Lemoine M, Thursz MR. Battlefield against hepatitis B infection and HCC in Africa. J Hepatol. 2017;66(3):645–54.
2. O'Hara GA, McNaughton AL, Maponga T, Jooste P, Ocama P, Chilengi R, Mokaya J, Liyayi MI, Wachira T, Gikungi DM, et al. Hepatitis B virus infection as a neglected tropical disease. PLoS Negl Trop Dis. 2017;11(10):e0005842.
3. Global Burden of Disease Causes of Death Collaborators. Global, regional, and national age-sex specific mortality for 264 causes of death, 1980-2016: a systematic analysis for the global burden of disease study 2016. Lancet. 2017;390(10100):1151–210.
4. Global Burden of Disease Collaboratorative Network. Global Burden of Disease Study 2016 (GBD 2016) Results. Seattle: Institute for Health Metrics and Evaluation; 2017. http://ghdx.healthdata.org/gbd-results-tool Accessed 24 June 2018
5. Mokdad AA, Lopez AD, Shahraz S, Lozano R, Mokdad AH, Stanaway J, Murray CJL, Naghavi M. Liver cirrhosis mortality in 187 countries between 1980 and 2010: a systematic analysis. BMC Med. 2014;12:145.
6. Akinyemiju T, Abera S, Ahmed M, Alam N, Alemayohu MA, Allen C, Al-Raddadi R, Alvis-Guzman N, Amoako Y, Artaman A, et al. The burden of primary liver Cancer and underlying etiologies from 1990 to 2015 at the global, regional, and National Level: results from the global burden of disease study 2015. JAMA Oncol. 2017;3(12):1683–91.
7. Parkin DM, Bray F, Ferlay J, Jemal A. Cancer in Africa 2012. Cancer Epidemiol Biomark Prev. 2014;23(6):953–66.
8. Yang JD, Mohamed EA, Aziz AO, Shousha HI, Hashem MB, Nabeel MM, Abdelmaksoud AH, Elbaz TM, Afihene MY, Duduyemi BM, et al. Characteristics, management, and outcomes of patients with hepatocellular carcinoma in Africa: a multicountry observational study from the Africa liver Cancer consortium. Lancet Gastroenterol Hepatol. 2017;2(2):103–11.
9. de Martel C, Maucort-Boulch D, Plummer M, Franceschi S. World-wide relative contribution of hepatitis B and C viruses in hepatocellular carcinoma. Hepatology. 2015;62(4):1190–200.

10. Yang JD, Gyedu A, Afihene MY, Duduyemi BM, Micah E, Kingham TP, Nyirenda M, Nkansah AA, Bandoh S, Duguru MJ, et al. Hepatocellular carcinoma occurs at an earlier age in Africans, particularly in association with chronic hepatitis B. Am J Gastroenterol. 2015;110(11):1629–31.
11. World Health Organisation. Global health sector strategy on viral hepatitis 2016–2021. Geneva: WHO; 2016.
12. Moher D, Liberati A, Tetzlaff J, Altman DG. Preferred reporting items for systematic reviews and meta-analyses: the PRISMA statement. BMJ. 2009; 339:b2535.
13. Munn Z, Moola S, Lisy K, Riitano D, Tufanaru C. Methodological guidance for systematic reviews of observational epidemiological studies reporting prevalence and cumulative incidence data. Int J Evid Based Healthc. 2015; 13(3):147–53.
14. Freeman MF, Tukey JW. Transformations related to the angular and the square root. Ann Math Stat. 1950;21(4):607–11.
15. Barendregt JJ, Doi SA, Lee YY, Norman RE, Vos T. Meta-analysis of prevalence. J Epidemiol Community Health. 2013;67(11):974–8.
16. Nyaga VN, Arbyn M, Aerts M. Metaprop: a Stata command to perform meta-analysis of binomial data. Archives Public Health. 2014;72(1):39.
17. Sutcliffe S, Taha TE, Kumwenda NI, Taylor E, Liomba GN. HIV-1 prevalence and herpes simplex virus 2, hepatitis C virus, and hepatitis B virus infections among male workers at a sugar estate in Malawi. J Acquir Immune Defic Syndr. 2002;31(1):90–7.
18. Ahmed SD, Cuevas LE, Brabin BJ, Kazembe P, Broadhead R, Verhoeff FH, Hart CA. Seroprevalence of hepatitis B and C and HIV in Malawian pregnant women. J Inf Secur. 1998;37(3):248–51.
19. Greer AE, Ou SS, Wilson E, Piwowar-Manning E, Forman MS, McCauley M, Gamble T, Ruangyuttikarn C, Hosseinipour MC, Kumarasamy N, et al. Comparison of hepatitis B virus infection in HIV-infected and HIV-uninfected participants enrolled in a multinational clinical trial: HPTN 052. J Acquir Immune Defic Syndr. 2017;76(4):388–93.
20. Taha TE, Rusie LK, Labrique A, Nyirenda M, Soko D, Kamanga M, Kumwenda J, Farazadegan H, Nelson K, Kumwenda N. Seroprevalence for hepatitis E and other viral Hepatitides among diverse populations. Malawi Emerg Infect Dis. 2015;21(7):1174–82.
21. Candotti D, Mundy C, Kadewele G, Nkhoma W, Bates I, Allain JP. Serological and molecular screening for viruses in blood donors from Ntcheu, Malawi: high prevalence of HIV-1 subtype C and of markers of hepatitis B and C viruses. J Med Virol. 2001;65(1):1–5.
22. Chasela CS, Kourtis AP, Wall P, Drobeniuc J, King CC, Thai H, Teshale EH, Hosseinipour M, Ellington S, Codd MB, et al. Hepatitis B virus infection among HIV-infected pregnant women in Malawi and transmission to infants. J Hepatol. 2014;60(3):508–14.
23. Andreotti M, Pirillo MF, Liotta G, Jere H, Maulidi M, Sagno JB, Luhanga R, Amici R, Mancini MG, Gennaro E, et al. The impact of HBV or HCV infection in a cohort of HIV-infected pregnant women receiving a nevirapine-based antiretroviral regimen in Malawi. BMC Infect Dis. 2014;14:180.
24. Moore E, Beadsworth MB, Chaponda M, Mhango B, Faragher B, Njala J, Hofland HW, Davies J, Hart IJ, Beeching NJ, et al. Favourable one-year ART outcomes in adult Malawians with hepatitis B and C co-infection. J Inf Secur. 2010;61(2):155–63.
25. Aoudjane S, Chaponda M, Gonzalez Del Castillo AA, O'Connor J, Noguera M, Beloukas A, Hopkins M, Khoo S, van Oosterhout JJ, Geretti AM. Hepatitis B virus sub-genotype A1 infection is characterized by high replication levels and rapid emergence of drug resistance in HIV-positive adults receiving first-line antiretroviral therapy in Malawi. Clin Infect Dis. 2014;59(11):1618–26.
26. Varo R, Chris Buck W, Kazembe PN, Phiri S, Andrianarimanana D, Weigel R. Seroprevalence of CMV, HSV-2 and HBV among HIV-infected Malawian children: a cross-sectional survey. J Trop Pediatr. 2016;62(3):220–6.
27. Nyirenda M, Beadsworth MB, Stephany P, Hart CA, Hart IJ, Munthali C, Beeching NJ, Zijlstra EE. Prevalence of infection with hepatitis B and C virus and coinfection with HIV in medical inpatients in Malawi. J Inf Secur. 2008;57(1):72–7.
28. Chimphambano C, Komolafe I, Muula A. Prevalence of HIV, HepBsAg and Hep C antibodies among inmates in Chichiri prison, Blantyre. Malawi Malawi Med J. 2007;19(3):107–10.
29. Chipetah F, Chirambo A, Billiat E, Shawa IT. Hepatitis B virus seroprevalence among Malawian medical students: a cross-sectional study. Malawi Med J. 2017;29(1):29–31.
30. Stockdale AJ, Chaponda M, Beloukas A, Phillips RO, Matthews PC, Papadimitropoulos A, King S, Bonnett L, Geretti AM. Prevalence of hepatitis D virus infection in sub-Saharan Africa: a systematic review and meta-analysis. Lancet Glob Health. 2017;5(10):e992–e1003.
31. Demir M, Phiri S, Kaiser R, Chaweza T, Neuhann F, Tweya H, Fatkenheuer G, Steffen HM. HIV/hepatitis C virus co-infection among adults beginning antiretroviral therapy, Malawi. Emerg Infect Dis. 2016;22(11):2018–20.
32. Maida MJ, Daly CC, Hoffman I, Cohen MS, Kumwenda M, Vernazza PL. Prevalence of hepatitis C infection in Malawi and lack of association with sexually transmitted diseases. Eur J Epidemiol. 2000;16(12):1183–4.
33. Loarec A, Carnimeo V, Maman D, Molfino L, Walter K, Nzomukunda Y, Muyindike W, Andrieux-Meyer I, Balkan S, Mwanga-Amumpaire J, et al. Low hepatitis C virus prevalence among human immunodeficiency virus+ individuals in Sub-Saharan Africa. J Hepatol. 2017;66(1):S270–S271.
34. Fox JM, Newton R, Bedaj M, Keding A, Molyneux E, Carpenter LM, Martin F, Mutalima N. Prevalence of hepatitis C virus in mothers and their children in Malawi. Tropical Med Int Health. 2015;20(5):638–42.
35. Schweitzer A, Horn J, Mikolajczyk RT, Krause G, Ott JJ. Estimations of worldwide prevalence of chronic hepatitis B virus infection: a systematic review of data published between 1965 and 2013. Lancet. 2015;386(10003):1546–55.
36. Rao VB, Johari N, du Cros P, Messina J, Ford N, Cooke GS. Hepatitis C seroprevalence and HIV co-infection in sub-Saharan Africa: a systematic review and meta-analysis. Lancet Infect Dis. 2015;15(7):819–24.
37. Sonderup MW, Afihene M, Ally R, Apica B, Awuku Y, Cunha L, Dusheiko G, Gogela N, Lohouès-Kouacou M-J, Lam P, et al. Hepatitis C in sub-Saharan Africa: the current status and recommendations for achieving elimination by 2030. Lancet Gastroenterol Hepatol. 2017;2(12):910–9.
38. World Health Organisation. Guidelines of hepatitis B and C testing. Geneva: WHO; 2017. http://www.who.int/hepatitis/publications/guidelines-hepatitis-c-b-testing/en/ Accessed 26 June 18
39. Niebel M, Singer JB, Nickbakhsh S, Gifford RJ, Thomson EC. Hepatitis C and the absence of genomic data in low-income countries: a barrier on the road to elimination? Lancet Gastroenterol Hepatol. 2017;2(10):700–1.
40. Lempp FA, Ni Y, Urban S. Hepatitis delta virus: insights into a peculiar pathogen and novel treatment options. Nat Rev Gastroenterol Hepatol. 2016;13(10):580–9.
41. Government of Malawi. Population and housing census. Zomba: National Statistical Office; 2008.
42. Tuaillon E, Kania D, Gordien E, Van de Perre P, Dujols P. Epidemiological data for hepatitis D in Africa. Lancet Glob Health. 2018;6(1):e33.
43. Matthews PC, Geretti AM, Goulder PJ, Klenerman P. Epidemiology and impact of HIV coinfection with hepatitis B and hepatitis C viruses in sub-Saharan Africa. J Clin Virol. 2014;61(1):20–33.
44. Seremba E, Ssempijja V, Kalibbala S, Gray RH, Wawer MJ, Nalugoda F, Casper C, Phipps W, Ocama P, Serwadda D, et al. Hepatitis B incidence and prevention with antiretroviral therapy among HIV-positive individuals in Uganda. AIDS. 2017;31(6):781–6.
45. Government of Malawi. Malawi demographic and health survey 2015–16. Zomba: National Statistical Office; 2017.
46. World Health Organisation. World health statistics 2017: monitoring health for the sustainable development goals. Geneva: WHO; 2017.

4

Outcome of untreated lung nodules with histological but no microbiological evidence of tuberculosis

Che-Liang Chung[1], Yen-Fu Chen[2], Yen-Ting Lin[3], Jann-Yuan Wang[3*], Shuenn-Wen Kuo[4] and Jin-Shing Chen[4]

Abstract

Background: The outcome of lung nodule(s) with histopathological findings suggestive of tuberculosis (TB) but lack of microbiologic confirmation remains unclear. Whether these patients require anti-TB treatment remains unknown. The aim of the study was to compare the risk of active TB within 4 years in untreated patients with histological findings but no microbiological evidences suggestive of TB.

Methods: From January 2008 to June 2013, patients with either solitary or multiple lung nodules having histological findings but no microbiological evidences suggestive of TB were identified from a medical center in Taiwan and were followed for 4 years unless they died or developed active TB.

Results: A total of 107 patients were identified. Among them, 54 (51%) were clinical asymptomatic. Biopsy histology showed granulomatous inflammation in 106 (99%), and caseous necrosis was present in 55 (51%) cases. Forty (37%) patients received anti-TB treatment, and 21 (53%) of them had adverse events, including 13 initially asymptomatic patients. Anti-TB treatment was favored in patients with caseous necrosis, whereas observation was preferred in subjects whose nodules were surgically removed. Only 1 case in the untreated group developed culture-confirmed active pulmonary TB during 4-year follow-up (1 case per 251.2 patient-years). None of the 16 cases having co-existing histologic finding of malignancy became incident TB case within a follow-up of 56.7 patient-years.

Conclusions: In patients having lung nodules with only histologic features suggestive of TB, the incidence rate of developing active TB was low. Risk of adverse events and benefit from immediate treatment should be carefully considered.

Keywords: Caseous necrosis, Granulomatous inflammation, Pulmonary nodule, Surgery, Tuberculosis

Background

Tuberculosis (TB) is an infectious disease prevalent worldwide. Currently, its diagnosis, which is mainly based on medical history, clinical manifestation, radiographic features, microbiological evidence, and laboratory findings, remains challenging. The definite diagnosis of TB is made through a positive culture from infected sputum or tissue samples. In Taiwan, among all infectious diseases, TB is associated with the highest incidence and mortality rate, with 12,338 TB cases (53.0 per 100,000 individuals) recorded in 2012; of these, 19% had sputum smear-negative and culture-negative TB [1]. If noninvasive methods cannot provide a definite diagnosis, presumptive diagnosis can be made through tissue biopsy [2].

The histological features suggestive of TB include granulomatous inflammation, caseous necrosis, and positive acid-fast stain (AFS); however, these are not pathognomonic for active TB. For example, granulomatous inflammation and caseous necrosis may be caused by various pathogens other than *Mycobacterium tuberculosis*, such as nontuberculous mycobacteria (NTM) and fungi [3]. Moreover, granulomatous inflammation may sometimes be seen in noninfectious diseases. The characteristic morphological feature of hypersensitivity pneumonitis is

* Correspondence: jywang@ntu.edu.tw
[3]Department of Internal Medicine, National Taiwan University Hospital, #7, Chung-Shan South Road, Zhongzheng District, Taipei 10002, Taiwan
Full list of author information is available at the end of the article

bronchiolocentric granulomatous lymphocytic alveolitis [4]. Sarcoidosis is also characterized by noncaseating granulomas [5].

Solitary or multiple lung nodules are frequently encountered during health checkup and clinical examination. Histological examination of biopsy specimens is often required to establish a definite diagnosis and exclude the possibility of malignancy. However, even if the histological examination reveals findings suggestive of TB, differentiating an active disease from old tuberculoma is difficult without serial radiographic studies. Hence, whether all patients with such nodules should receive standard anti-TB treatment immediately remains unknown.

Therefore, in this study, we identified patients with lung nodules having histological findings but no microbiological evidence suggestive of TB and compared the clinical characteristics and incidence of active TB within the subsequent 2 years between patients receiving and not receiving anti-TB treatment.

Methods

Patients and setting

This was a retrospective cohort study conducted in National Taiwan University Hospital (NTUH). The Research Ethics Committee of NTUH approved this study (REC No.: 201205025RIC). Under Taiwan's National TB control policy, all cases of culture-confirmed and suspected TB should be reported to the Taiwan Centers for Disease Control (CDC), and all TB contacts should receive contact investigation and be reported to Taiwan CDC, as well. Permission is required to access the online reporting database of Taiwan CDC (https://tb.cdc.gov.tw/slow/ca/loginbycard.asp). Standard regimen used in Taiwan for treating new TB cases follows the guidelines of the World Health Organization (WHO), consisting isoniazid (5 mg/kg), rifampicin (10 mg/kg), pyrazinamide (25 mg/kg), and ethambutol (15 mg/kg) for 2 months, followed by isoniazid (5 mg/kg), rifampicin (10 mg/kg), plus ethambutol (15 mg/kg) if results of susceptibility test is not available, for 4 months [6, 7].

We searched the histopathology database of NTUH for findings of caseous necrosis or granulomatous inflammation from January 2008 to June 2013. Patients were excluded if (1) the *M. tuberculosis* complex or NTM were isolated within 60 days before or after biopsy, (2) biopsy samples were extrapulmonary, (3) biopsy was performed during anti-TB treatment, (4) computed tomography (CT) images of the chest were unavailable, (5) histological or microbiological evidence of fungal or parasitic infection was noted, (6) patients had pure or mixed with non-nodular radiographic patterns suggestive for active disease, such as tree-in-buds pattern, consolidation, and miliary lesions [8], and (7) a positive tissue AFS, since these cases were usually treated as TB until proven otherwise.

Follow-up and outcome

All included patients were followed up for 4 years after biopsy unless they died or received a diagnosis of active TB. Active TB was defined if either of the following two criteria was fulfilled [9, 10]: (1) mycobacterial cultures of sputum or other respiratory samples yielded the *M. tuberculosis* complex; and (2) chest radiography revealed new lesions without other proven etiology, which improved after standard anti-TB treatment, determined by serial chest radiography or by follow-up CT, if the pre-treat pulmonary lesion was not detectable by chest radiography.

Data collection

Medical records were reviewed to obtain demographic data, including age, sex, symptoms, comorbidity, history of TB, biopsy method, histology, AFS results, mycobacterial culture of sputum and tissue specimens, and adverse events of anti-TB treatment. At the beginning of tissue diagnosis, we obtained laboratory test results, including leukocyte and differential leukocyte counts and hemoglobin, albumin, and C-reactive protein levels. CT images were further reviewed by a pulmonologist. Furthermore, radiographic patterns; presence of solitary or multiple nodules, background fibrocalcified lesions, and bronchiectasis; maximum diameter and density of lesions; cavitation; and mediastinal lymphadenopathy were recorded.

Statistical analyses

Categorical variables were compared using the *chi*-square test or Fisher's exact test, as appropriate, whereas continuous variables were compared using independent sample t tests. Multivariate logistic regression analysis was performed in a backward manner to identify the predictors for prescribing anti-TB treatment. The analyzed variables included age, sex, history of TB, presence of respiratory or constitutional symptoms suggestive of TB, histological findings (caseous necrosis, granulomatous inflammation on biopsy histology, concomitant malignancy on biopsy histology), biopsy method, mycobacterial culture for respiratory specimens or biopsy specimens, comorbidity (diabetes mellitus, end-stage renal disease, malignancy, hepatitis B virus infection, human immunodeficiency virus infection, organ transplant recipient, alcoholism, and autoimmune disease), findings on chest computed tomography (multiple nodules, lesion size > 3 cm, cavitary lesions, ground-glass opacity, fibrocalcified lesions, mediastinal lymphadenopathy), and laboratory test results (leukocyte count and hypoalbuminemia [defined as serum albumin level < 3.5 g/dL]). Kaplan–Meier curves were generated to represent the time to subsequent development of active TB in different groups and were compared using the log-rank test. All analyses were performed using IBM SPSS statistics (version 23; IBM Corp., Armonk, NY, USA). Statistical significance was set at $p < 0.05$.

Results

Case identification

From January 2008 to June 2013, a total of 470 patients with histological findings suggestive of TB were identified; among them, 439 had granulomatous inflammation, 233 had caseous necrosis, and 143 had positive tissue AFS. In total, 363 patients were excluded because of various reasons shown in Fig. 1. The remaining 107 (22.8%) patients were analyzed further.

Among all 107 patients, 54 (51%) were clinically asymptomatic and were referred for further evaluation because of abnormal chest images noted during health examination or routine checkup for other medical problems. Among all 107 patients, 40 (37%) received anti-TB treatment (treated group); of them, 17 were clinically asymptomatic. The remaining 67 patients (63%) received follow-up without immediate treatment (untreated group). Among all 107 cases, 78 had multiple lung nodules or masses, while the remaining 29 patients had solitary nodule. Typical CT images of solitary and multiple lung nodules or masses are illustrated in Fig. 2.

Clinical characteristics and follow-up

The clinical characteristics of all 107 patients are presented in Table 1. The mean age was 56.3 ± 13.4 years, with a male predominance (60%). The most common underlying disease was malignancy (35%), followed by diabetes mellitus (10%). Tissue samples were collected through surgical resection in 65 patients (61%). In total, 91 patients (85%) were tested through sputum or tissue mycobacterial culture. The most common histological finding was granulomatous inflammation (99%), followed by caseous necrosis (51%); 18 patients (17%) had concomitant histological findings of malignancy.

The mean follow-up duration was similar between the treated and untreated groups. During the follow-up period, 3 treated and 8 untreated patients died. Of the 8 untreated patients, 3 received surgical resection of the lesion. Five died of malignancy, and the remaining 3 died of heart disease, upper gastrointestinal bleeding, and pneumonia, respectively. Half of the 8 untreated patients had the past history of treated pulmonary TB; seven of them (88%) had been tested through either sputum or tissue mycobacterium culture, or both. No evidence of active TB was noted during the entire clinical course of the 8 cases.

No significant difference was observed in age, sex, clinical symptoms, and history of TB between the treated and untreated groups. More patients in the untreated group had malignancy than did those in the treated group (46% vs. 15%, $p = 0.001$). More patients in the treated group had the histological features of caseous necrosis (78% vs. 36%, $p < 0.001$), but fewer patients had the histological features of concomitant malignancy (5% vs. 24%, $p = 0.012$). Anti-TB treatment was not administered to 24 of the 55 patients (44%) with biopsy histology showing caseous necrosis; none of these patients developed active TB in the subsequent 4 years.

The radiographic patterns and laboratory data of the patients are summarized in Table 1. In general, most patients had normal hemogram and serum albumin levels. The laboratory data were similar in the treated and untreated groups, except that the treated group had higher albumin levels. In both groups, the most common radiographic findings were multiple lung nodules and mediastinal lymphadenopathy. The associated findings, such as cavitary lesions and ground-glass opacity, did not differ significantly between the 2 groups. Fibrocalcified lesions, bronchiectasis, and mediastinal lymphadenopathy, implying inactive or chronic disease status, did not differ significantly between the 2 groups.

Predictors of anti-TB treatment initiation

The multivariate logistic regression analysis identified 2 independent factors for predicting whether physicians initiate anti-TB treatment: caseous necrosis on biopsy histology (OR = 9.60, 95% CI = 3.38–27.23), and surgical resection (OR = 0.25, 95% CI = 0.09–0.69; Table 2).

Development of active pulmonary TB

In the untreated group, during a total of 251.2 follow-up patient-years, only 1 patient developed pulmonary TB approximately 19 months after biopsy (Day 574). None of the 16 cases having co-existing histologic finding of malignancy became incident TB case within a follow-up of 56.7 patient-years.

The patient, aged between 50 and 60, had a history of left maxillary acinic cell carcinoma, which had been surgically resected 13 years ago and had recurred 2 months before the index biopsy. Chest CT for staging work-up revealed a 1.8-cm nodule in the right upper lobe (Fig. 3a). The case reported weight loss and a tendency to become easily fatigued, but denied any airway symptoms. CT-guided biopsy revealed granulomatous inflammation with lymphocyte aggregation and negative tissue AFS. Sputum AFS and mycobacterial cultures were also negative. Anticancer chemotherapy and target therapy were administered consequently. Although follow-up chest CT at 10 months after the index biopsy showed progression in bilateral alveolar infiltrates, sputum studies for a total of 6 specimens collected at 9 and 11 months after the index biopsy were all negative for the *M. tuberculosis* complex. Follow-up

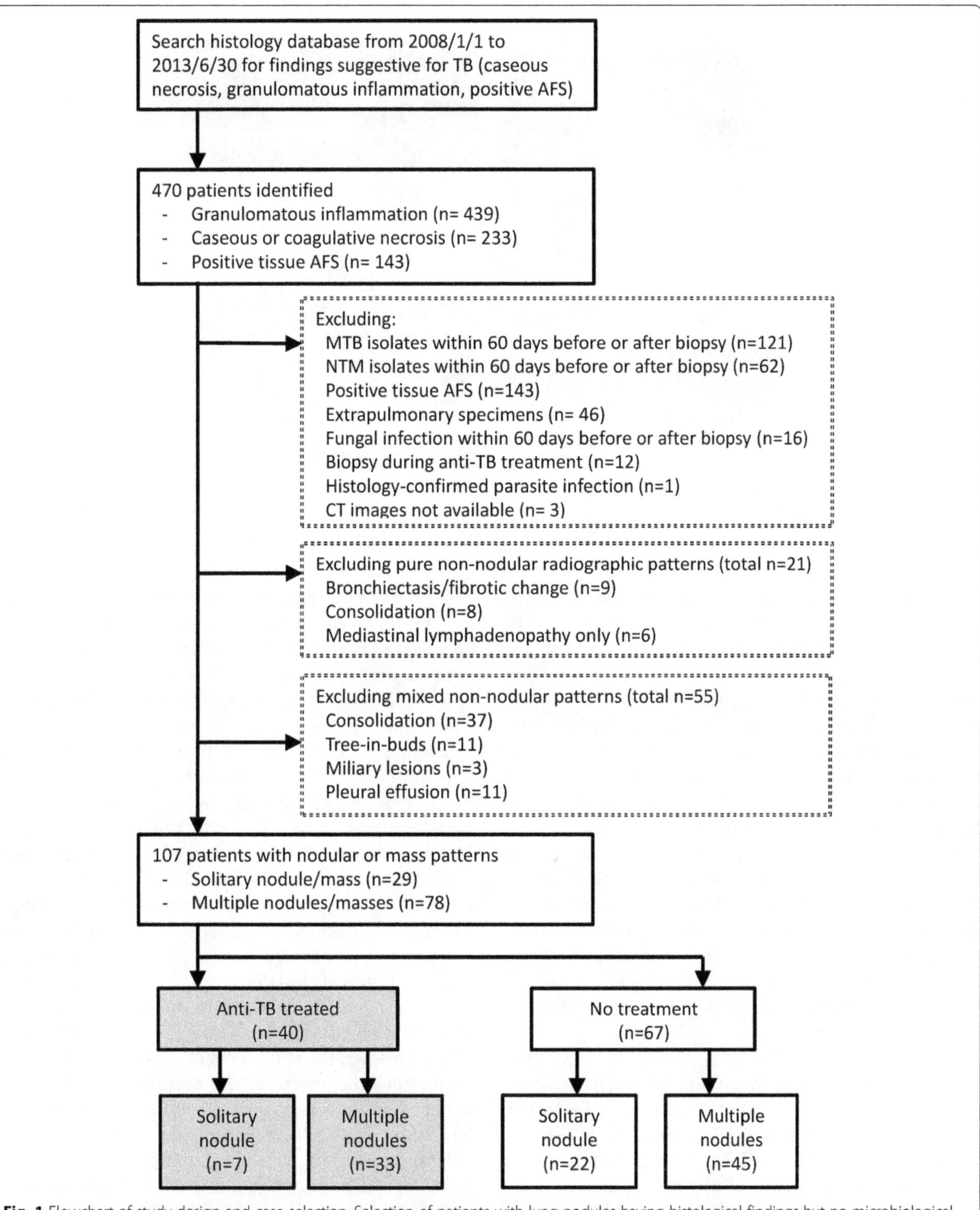

Fig. 1 Flowchart of study design and case selection. Selection of patients with lung nodules having histological findings but no microbiological evidence suggestive of tuberculosis

chest CT at 17 months after the index biopsy demonstrated multiple bilateral cavitary consolidations (Fig. 3b). Sputum culture at that time yielded the *M. tuberculosis* complex. No records of recent contact to active TB case were found in the online reporting database of Taiwan CDC.

Among the 40 treated patients, none fulfilled the criteria of active TB in the 4 years after the date of the

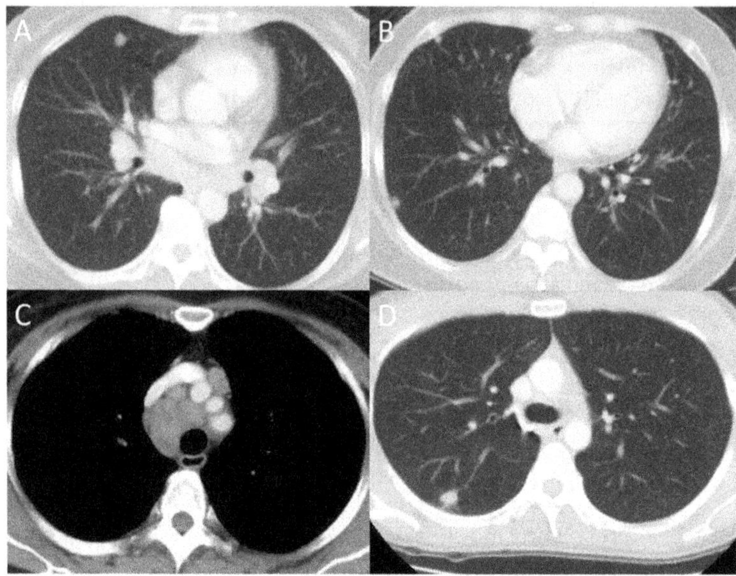

Fig. 2 Image presentation of chest computed tomography (CT) in 2 cases. Chest CT of a patient, aged between 50 and 60 (untreated group), revealed multiple round nodules in the bilateral lungs (**a**, **b**) and mediastinal lymphadenopathy (**c**). Chest CT of a patient, aged between 30 and 40 (treated group), revealed an ill-defined speculated, 1.2-cm nodule with pleural tagging at the posterior aspect of the right upper lobe (**d**)

index biopsy. The risk of active TB did not differ between the treated and untreated groups (p = 0.433; power = 0.118, Kaplan–Meier analysis).

Adverse events of anti-TB treatment

Among the 40 patients receiving anti-TB treatment after the index biopsy, adverse events occurred in 21 (53%). The most common adverse event was rash (20%), followed by hepatotoxicity (18%) and constitutional symptoms including fever, malaise, dizziness, and chest tightness (18%; Fig. 4). The development of adverse events led to treatment interruption in 8 patients (20%), including 6 patients who developed hepatotoxicity. Among the 17 clinically asymptomatic patients who received anti-TB treatment, 13 (76%) had adverse events, leading to therapeutic regimen modification in 3 patients (18%) and treatment interruption in 6 patients (35%).

Discussion

This is the first study to investigate the incidence of active TB within the subsequent 4 years in patients with histological findings but no microbiological evidence suggestive of TB. This study has 3 major findings. First, if untreated, the incidence of active TB was 1 in 251.2 patient-years, which represents an annual incidence of 398 cases per 100,000 individuals (approximately 7 times the incidence in Taiwan); immediately anti-TB treatment may not be necessary in most of these cases. Second, if treated, the risk of adverse events was 53%; one-fifth of the treated cases even demonstrated severe adverse events necessitating interruption of their anti-TB treatment. Third, primary physicians appeared to favor anti-TB treatment in patients with caseous necrosis but appeared to disfavor it in those whose lung nodules had been surgically resected.

The understanding of the natural course of pulmonary tuberculoma is mainly based on reports before the establishment of effective anti-TB treatment. Approximately 30–50% of the cases of pulmonary tuberculoma may demonstrate a stationary course [11–13]. In an early report recording 18 patients with 23 tuberculomas totally, 11 tuberculomas calcified or showed no interval changes during the follow-up period of 12–148 months, and the remaining 12 tuberculomas showed progressive changes within 5–90 months [12]. Currently, anti-TB treatment is typically administered postoperatively when tuberculoma is diagnosed [13–15].

The histological examination of tissue sections of mycobacterial lesions often shows few or no acid-fast bacilli, even when the culture result is positive. This might result from the effects of the fixation fluid or organic solvent [16]. In a report, the identification of mycobacteria through Ziehl–Neelsen staining was accurate in only approximately 60% of culture-positive cases [17]. Some reports have indicated that the nucleic acid amplification (NAA) test for *M. tuberculosis* complex is much more sensitive than the AFS histopathological test; however, the NAA test cannot differentiate between live and dead TB bacilli [16, 18].

The proportion of NTM recovered from AFS-positive respiratory specimens was highly variable among the geographic areas and populations, ranging from 7.3 to

Table 1 Clinical characteristics, radiographic patterns, and laboratory data of treated and untreated groups

	All patients (*n* = 107)	Treated group (*n* = 40)	Untreated group (*n* = 67)	*P* value
Age (year)	56.3 ± 13.4	55.5 ± 12.4	56.8 ± 14.0	0.629
Male gender	64 (60)	26 (65)	38 (57)	0.398
Clinically asymptomatic	54 (51)	17 (43)	37 (55)	0.203
Previous history of tuberculosis				0.272
No	95 (89)	38 (95)	57 (85)	
Yes, treatment status unknown	1 (1)	0	1 (2)	
Yes, treated	11 (10)	2 (5)	9 (13)	
Biopsy method				0.090
Bronchoscopy	6 (6)	1 (3)	5 (8)	
CT-guided	33 (31)	18 (45)	15 (22)	
Echo-guided	3 (3)	1 (3)	2 (3)	
Surgery	65 (61)	20 (50)	45 (67)	
Histology				
Granulomatous inflammation	106 (99)	40 (100)	66 (99)	> 0.999
Caseous necrosis	55 (51)	31 (78)	24 (36)	< 0.001
Lymph node sampling	32 (30)	3 (8)	29 (43)	< 0.001
Lymph node involvement	13 (12)	2 (5)	11 (16)	0.125
Concomitant malignancy	18 (17)	2 (5)	16 (24)	0.012
Mycobacterial culture				
Tissue culture performed	68 (64)	21 (53)	47 (70)	0.066
Sputum culture performed	81 (76)	33 (83)	48 (72)	0.205
Either one	91 (85)	34 (85)	57 (85)	0.992
Comorbidity				
Malignancy	37 (35)	6 (15)	31 (46)	0.001
Diabetes mellitus	11 (10)	2 (5)	9 (13)	0.204
ESRD under regular hemodialysis	2 (2)	1 (3)	1 (2)	> 0.999
Liver cirrhosis	2 (2)	2 (5)	0	0.138
Organ transplant recipient	2 (2)	1 (3)	1 (2)	> 0.999
Autoimmune disease	2 (2)	0	2 (3)	0.527
Hepatitis B virus infection	8 (8)	3 (8)	5 (8)	> 0.999
HIV infection	2 (2)	2 (5)	0	0.138
Alcoholism	1 (1)	1 (3)	0	0.374
Main findings on chest CT				
Multiple nodules	78 (73)	33 (83)	45 (67)	0.084
Solitary nodule	29 (27)	7 (18)	22 (33)	0.084
Lesion size > 3 cm	9 (8)	2 (5)	7 (10)	0.400
Associate findings[a]				
Cavitation	3 (3)	0	3 (5)	0.291
Ground glass opacity	20 (19)	9 (23)	11 (16)	0.435
Calcification	22 (21)	9 (23)	13 (19)	0.701
Fibrosis	36 (34)	15 (38)	21 (31)	0.514
Bronchiectasis	13 (12)	5 (13)	8 (12)	> 0.999
Mediastinal LAP	72 (67)	25 (63)	47 (70)	0.415
Lab data				

Table 1 Clinical characteristics, radiographic patterns, and laboratory data of treated and untreated groups *(Continued)*

	All patients (*n* = 107)	Treated group (*n* = 40)	Untreated group (*n* = 67)	*P* value
Albumin (g/dL)[b]	4.2 ± 0.6	4.4 ± 0.5	4.1 ± 0.6	0.005
Hemoglobin (mg/dL)	13.0 ± 1.8	13.4 ± 1.6	12.8 ± 1.9	0.091
Leukocyte count (K/uL)	7.2 ± 3.4	7.2 ± 4.1	7.2 ± 3.0	0.968
Segment (%)	62.4 ± 10.2	61.5 ± 9.9	62.9 ± 10.4	0.479
Band (%)	0.05 ± 0.30	0.10 ± 0.47	0.02 ± 0.12	0.293
Lymphocyte (%)	29.0 ± 9.2	30.8 ± 8.8	27.9 ± 9.2	0.120
CRP (mg/dL)[c]	3.1 ± 5.5	2.8 ± 3.2	3.2 ± 5.9	0.824
Death during follow up period	11 (10)	3 (8)	8 (12)	0.464
Mean follow-up duration (days)	1395.3 ± 217.0	1440.4 ± 85.5	1368.4 ± 263.4	0.097
Developing active tuberculosis	1 (1)	0	1 (2)	> 0.999

CRP C-reactive protein, *CT* Computed tomography, *ESRD* End-stage renal disease, *HIV* Human immunodeficiency virus, *LAP* Lymphadenopathy, Data are expressed as number (%) or mean ± standard deviation

[a]Each case might have more than one associate finding

[b]Data were missing for 2 cases of the treated group

[c]Data were available for 9 and 35 cases of the treated and untreated groups, respectively

50%, which reduced the positive predictive value of AFS for pulmonary TB [19–22]. In a study on 360 biopsy specimens, mycobacterial culture of 166 specimens was performed. Of them, the percentages of specimens that were culture-positive for mycobacteria with histological features of necrotizing granulomas, nonnecrotizing granulomas, and poorly formed granulomas were 38.2%, 32.4%, and 30.0%, respectively. Of the 39 specimens that were culture-positive for mycobacteria, 14 (36%) yielded the *M. tuberculosis* complex, whereas the remaining 25 (64%) yielded NTM [23]. In a retrospective study, the "TB-like" granulomatous reaction (epithelioid cell granuloma with central caseous necrosis) was the most common pathological feature in NTM infections [24].

In addition to *Mycobacteria*, granulomatous inflammation can be seen in infections caused by fungi, parasites, and *Actinomycetes* [17, 25]. However, the occurrence of active TB in all patients with histological features of caseous necrosis or granulomatous inflammation varies because of the differences in local prevalence. Thus, no histological finding has been identified to be pathognomonic for active TB. Therefore, whether immediately anti-TB treatment should be administered to patients with histological findings but no microbiological evidence suggestive of TB remains debatable [25, 26]. Our study demonstrated that primary care physicians favored anti-TB treatment for patients with histological findings of caseous necrosis. However, no untreated patient with similar histological features of caseous necrosis developed active TB within the subsequent 4 years.

Eighteen (17%) cases in this cohort had concomitant findings of malignancy in biopsy specimens. There were no incident TB cases in these patients, while one TB case was noted during a follow-up of 194.5 patient-years for those without co-existing malignancy in biopsy samples. The prevalence of coexistence of granulomatous inflammation and malignancy in lung biopsy is unknown. Previous reports showed coexisting malignancy in 3 of 616 lung specimens with granulomatous inflammation [27–29]. Because of retrospective design, the reasons for the primary care physicians not favoring anti-TB treatment in patients with underlying malignancy are unknown. These patients might be so weak that anti-TB drugs were considered too toxic as compared with close observation. On the contrary, some doctors might start treatment immediately because of the fear of disseminated TB during subsequent cancer chemotherapy.

Surgical procedures to reduce the bacterial load or to collapse the lung are the mainstay treatments during the

Table 2 Factors associated with prescribing anti-tuberculosis treatment in logistic regression analysis

	Adjusted Odds Ratio[a]	95% CI	*p* Value
Surgical resection	0.25	0.09–0.69	0.007
Caseous necrosis on biopsy histology	9.60	3.38–27.23	< 0.001

CI Confidence interval

[a]Adjusted variables included age, sex, history of TB, symptomatic, granulomatous inflammation on biopsy histology, concomitant malignancy on biopsy histology, mycobacterial culture for respiratory specimens or biopsy specimens, comorbidity (diabetes mellitus, end-stage renal disease, malignancy, hepatitis B virus infection, human immunodeficiency virus infection, organ transplant recipient, alcoholism, and autoimmune disease), findings on chest computed tomography (multiple nodules, lesion size > 3 cm, cavitary lesions, ground-glass opacity, fibrocalcified lesions, mediastinal lymphadenopathy), leukocyte count, and hypoalbuminemia

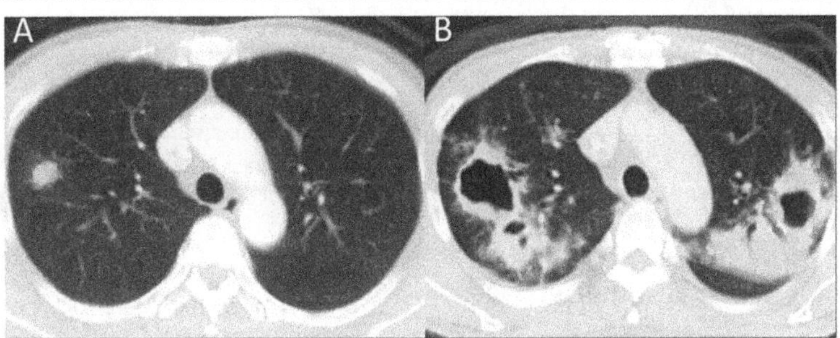

Fig. 3 Chest CT of an asymptomatic patient, aged between 50 and 60 (untreated group), revealed a 1.8-cm nodule in the right upper lobe (**a**). Follow-up chest CT at 17 months later showed multiple bilateral cavitary consolidations (**b**). Sputum culture yielded the *Mycobacterium tuberculosis* complex

preantibiotic period [13, 30, 31]. Because of the high surgical complication rate [14] and development of effective treatment, surgery is currently only indicated as a diagnostic procedure, an adjuvant for multidrug-resistant TB, and a therapeutic strategy for refractory lesions despite adequate anti-TB treatment [13, 32]. Theoretically, if pulmonary lesions are removed completely, the remaining tissues are macroscopically and microscopically normal. In this case, a patient can be considered to be either cured or having latent TB infection (LTBI), which carries the lifetime risk of subsequent active TB by 5–15% [33].

With the increasing use of chest CT for health checkups, the identification of lung nodules has increased [34]. Therefore, pulmonary lesions with histological findings but no microbiological evidence suggestive of TB have become frequently encountered clinical problems. However, guidelines for managing this special clinical entity have not been well established. Given that in our cohort study, none of the 45 untreated patients who received surgical resection developed active pulmonary TB during 4-year follow-up, and only 1 patient in the whole untreated group became incident case, the TB incidence rate in this special group maybe lower than that in LTBI cases [34]. Another concern for initiating empirical anti-TB treatment is the frequently encountered adverse events, particularly in patients with systemic comorbidity, such as malignancy, hypoalbuminemia, and anemia [35–37]. Considering the low risk of progression into active TB and the high risk of adverse events, the decision on either regular follow-up or immediate initiation of anti-TB treatment should be carefully judged based on risk and benefit assessment. A prospective study is required to confirm this finding and our speculation.

This study has some limitations. First, although demographic data and radiological findings were not significantly different between the treated and untreated groups, the physician's judgment on initiating anti-TB treatment may still bias the risk of subsequent active TB (confounded by indication). Second, while NAA test [38] and immunohistological staining [39] for *Mycobacterium tuberculosis* complex on biopsy specimens are promising for the diagnosis of active TB, they were not routinely

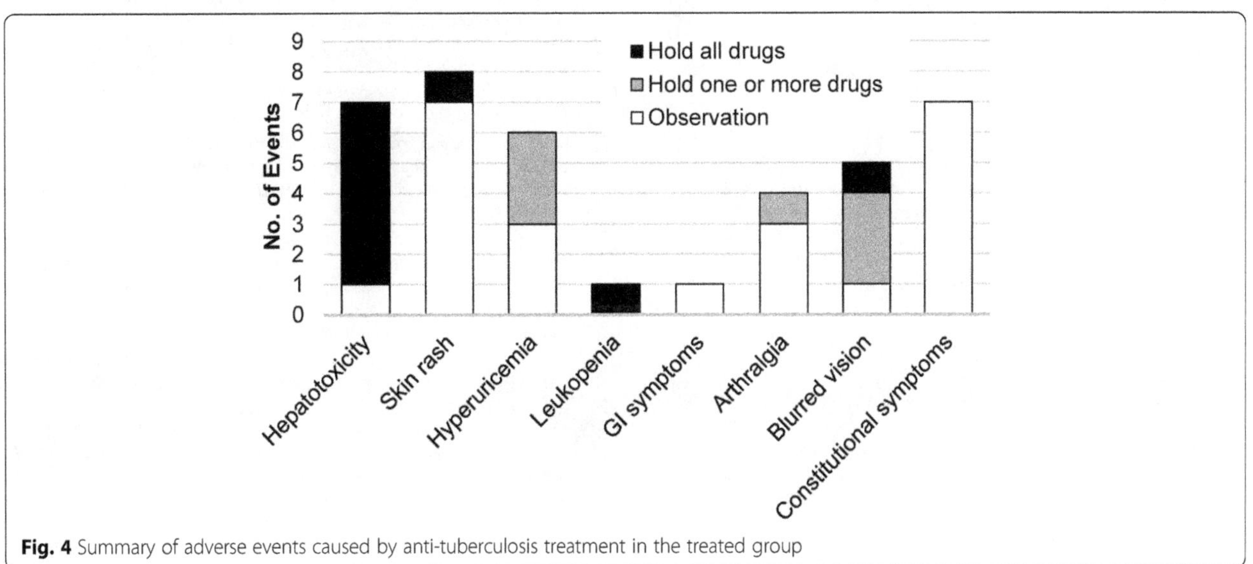

Fig. 4 Summary of adverse events caused by anti-tuberculosis treatment in the treated group

performed in all hospitals in Taiwan and most hospitals in the world. Finally, in some cases, respiratory specimens for AFS and mycobacterial culture were not collected because of the lack of sputum; however, this might not be a major concern and might indicate no active pulmonary disease.

Conclusion

In patients having lung nodules with histological findings but no microbiological evidence suggestive of TB, the incidence rate of active TB is 1 in 251.2 patient-years, lower than that in LTBI cases. Given the low risk of active TB and the high risk of adverse events, regular follow-up sputum and imaging studies, rather than immediate anti-TB treatment administration, may be considered. However, an additional prospective study is necessary to confirm our current findings.

Abbreviations

AFS: Acid-fast stain; CI: Confidence interval; CT: Computed tomography; LTBI: Latent tuberculosis infection; NAA: Nucleic acid amplification; NTM: Nontuberculous mycobacteria; NTUH: National Taiwan University Hospital; OR: Odds ratio; TB: Tuberculosis

Acknowledgements

The authors thank Dr. Meng-Rui Lee for his kindly help on statistical analysis. CLC was an attending physician at National Taiwan University Hospital Yunlin Branch, Yunlin, Taiwan, when this study was completed and submitted for publication.

Funding

This work was supported by the Centers for Disease Control, Taiwan [MOHW105-CDC-C-114-000103]. The funders had no role in the study design, data collection and analysis, decision to publish, or manuscript preparation.

Authors' contributions

CLC drafted the manuscript and designed the study with YFC and JYW. SWK, JSC, and JYW were involved in data processing. CLC, YTL, and JYW performed statistical analysis. All authors reviewed, provided input and approved the final manuscript. JYW is the guarantor of the study.

Competing interests

The authors declare that they have no competing interests.

Author details

[1]Department of Internal Medicine, Yuanlin Christian Hospital, Changhua, Taiwan. [2]Department of Internal Medicine, National Taiwan University Hospital Yunlin Branch, Douliu, Yunlin, Taiwan. [3]Department of Internal Medicine, National Taiwan University Hospital, #7, Chung-Shan South Road, Zhongzheng District, Taipei 10002, Taiwan. [4]Division of Thoracic Surgery, Department of Surgery, National Taiwan University Hospital and National Taiwan University College of Medicine, Taipei, Taiwan.

References

1. Centers for Disease Control, Minitry of Health and Welfare, Taiwan: Taiwan Tuberculosis Control Report 2013. 2014.
2. Sihoe A, Yew W. Role of surgery in the diagnosis and Management of Tuberculosis. In: Schlossberg D, editor. Tuberculosis and nontuberculous mycobacterial infections. 6th ed. Washington, DC: ASM Press; 2011. p. 141–61.
3. Zumla A, James DG. Granulomatous infections- etiology and classification. Clin Infect Dis. 1996;23(7):146–58.
4. Selman M, Pardo A, King TE Jr. Hypersensitivity pneumonitis: insights in diagnosis and pathobiology. Am J Respir Crit Care Med. 2012;186(4):314–24.
5. Ma Y, Gal A, Koss MN. The pathology of pulmonary sarcoidosis: update. Semin Diagn Pathol. 2007;24(3):150–61.
6. Centers for Disease Control, Minitry of Health and Welfare, Taiwan. Taiwan Guidelines for TB Diagnosis & Treatment (6E). 6th ed. Taiwan: Centers for Disease Control, Ministry of Health and Welfare, R.O.C.(Taiwan); 2017.
7. WHO. Treatment of tuberculosis: guidelines for national programmes. 4th ed; 2010.
8. Ko JM, Park HJ, Kim CH, Song SW. The relation between CT findings and sputum microbiology studies in active pulmonary tuberculosis. Eur J Radiol. 2015;84(11):2339–44.
9. Wang JY, Shu CC, Lee CH, Yu CJ, Lee LN, Yang PC. Interferon-gamma release assay and rifampicin therapy for household contacts of tuberculosis. J Inf Secur. 2012;64(3):291–8.
10. Nahid P, Dorman SE, Alipanah N, Barry PM, Brozek JL, Cattamanchi A, Chaisson LH, Chaisson RE, Daley CL, Grzemska M, et al. Official American Thoracic Society/Centers for Disease Control and Prevention/Infectious Diseases Society of America clinical practice guidelines: treatment of drug-susceptible tuberculosis. Clin Infect Dis. 2016;63(7):e147–95.
11. Lee HS, Oh JY, Lee JH, Yoo CG, Lee CT, Kim YW, Han SK, Shim YS, Yim JJ. Response of pulmonary tuberculomas to anti-tuberculous treatment. Eur Respir J. 2004;23(3):452–5.
12. Grenville-Mathers R. The Natural History of so-called tuberculoma. J Thorac Surg. 1952;23(3):251–2.
13. Subotic D, Yablonskiy P, Sulis G, Cordos I, Petrov D, Centis R, D'Ambrosio L, Sotgiu G, Migliori GB. Surgery and pleuro-pulmonary tuberculosis: a scientific literature review. J Thorac Dis. 2016;8(7):E474–85.
14. Prytz S, Hansen JL. Surgical treatment of "Tuberculoma". Scand J Thorac Cardiovasc Surg. 1976;10(2):179–82.
15. Evman S, Baysungur V, Alpay L, Uskul B, Misirlioglu AK, Kanbur S, Dogruyol T. Management and surgical outcomes of concurrent tuberculosis and lung Cancer. Thorac Cardiovasc Surg. 2016. https://doi.org/10.1055/s-0036-1583167.
16. Fukunaga H, Murakami T, Gondo T, Sugi K, Ishihara T. Sensitivity of acid-fast staining forMycobacterium tuberculosisin formalin-fixed tissue. Am J Respir Crit Care Med. 2002;166(7):994–7.
17. Kradin RL, Mark EJ. Pulmonary infections. In: Kradin R, editor. Diagnostic pathology of infectious disease. 1st ed; 2010. p. 125–88.
18. Hernández-Pando R, Jeyanathan M, Mengistu G, Aguilar D, Orozco H, Harboe M, Rook GAW, Bjune G. Persistence of DNA from Mycobacterium tuberculosis in superficially normal lung tissue during latent infection. Lancet. 2000;356(9248):2133–8.
19. Doucette K, Cooper R. Tuberculosis. In: Grippi MA, Elias JA, Fishman JA, Kotloff RM, Pack AI, Senior RM, Siegel MD, editors. Fishman's pulmonary diseases and disorders. 5th ed. New York: McGraw-Hill Education; 2015.
20. Kendall BA, Varley CD, Choi D, Cassidy PM, Hedberg K, Ware MA, Winthrop KL. Distinguishing tuberculosis from nontuberculous mycobacteria lung disease, Oregon, USA. Emerg Infect Dis. 2011;17(3):506–9.
21. Grubek-Jaworska H, Walkiewicz R, Safianowska A, Nowacka-Mazurek M, Krenke R, Przybylowski T, Chazan R. Nontuberculous mycobacterial infections among patients suspected of pulmonary tuberculosis. Eur J Clin Microbiol Infect Dis. 2009;28(7):739–44.
22. Koh WJ, Yu CM, Suh GY, Chung MP, Kim H, Kwon OJ, Lee NY, Chung MJ, Lee KS. Pulmonary TB and NTM lung disease- comparison of characteristics in patients with AFB smear-positive sputum. Int J Tuberc Lung Dis. 2006; 10(9):1001–7.
23. Tang YW, Procop GW, Zheng X, Myers JL, Roberts GD. Histologic parameters predictive of mycobacterial infection. Am J Clin Pathol. 1998;109(3):331.
24. Marchevsky A, Damsker B, Gribetz A, Tepper S, Geller SA. The Spectrum of pathology of nontuberculous mycobacterial infections in open-lung biopsy specimens. Am J Clin Pathol. 1982;78(5):695.
25. Aubry MC. Necrotizing granulomatous inflammation: what does it mean if your special stains are negative? Mod Pathol. 2012;25(Suppl 1):S31–8.
26. Ulbright TM, Katzenstein AL. Solitary necrotizing granulomas of the lung: differentiating features and etiology. Am J Surg Pathol. 1980;4(1):13–28.
27. Rui Y, Han M, Zhou W, He Q, Li H, Li P, Zhang F, Shi Y, Su X. Non-malignant pathological results on transthoracic CT guided core-needle biopsy: when is benign really benign? Clin Radiol. 2018;73(8):757.e751–7.

28. Kim JI, Park CM, Kim H, Lee JH, Goo JM. Non-specific benign pathological results on transthoracic core-needle biopsy: how to differentiate false-negatives? Eur Radiol. 2017;27(9):3888–95.
29. Mukhopadhyay S, Farver CF, Vaszar LT, Dempsey OJ, Popper HH, Mani H, Capelozzi VL, Fukuoka J, Kerr KM, Zeren EH, et al. Causes of pulmonary granulomas: a retrospective study of 500 cases from seven countries. J Clin Pathol. 2012;65(1):51–7.
30. Fox GJ, Mitnick CD, Benedetti A, Chan ED, Becerra M, Chiang CY, Keshavjee S, Koh WJ, Shiraishi Y, Viiklepp P, et al. Surgery as an adjunctive treatment for multidrug-resistant tuberculosis: an individual patient data Metaanalysis. Clin Infect Dis. 2016;62(7):887–95.
31. FurÁk J, TrojÁn I, Szöke T, Tiszlavicz L, Morvay Z, Csada E, Balogh Á. Surgical intervention for pulmonary tuberculosis: analysis of indications and perioperative data relating to diagnostic and therapeutic resections. Eur J Cardiothorac Surg. 2001;20(4):722–7.
32. WHO. The role of surgery in the treatment of pulmonary TB and multidrug-and extensively drug-resistant TB: WHO; 2014. http://www.euro.who.int/en/health-topics/communicable-diseases/tuberculosis/publications/2014/the-role-of-surgery-in-the-treatment-of-pulmonary-tb-and-multidrug-and-extensively-drug-resistant-tb. Accessed 3 Sept 2018
33. Getahun H, Matteelli A, Chaisson RE, Raviglione M. Latent Mycobacterium tuberculosis infection. N Engl J Med. 2015;372(22):2127–35.
34. Gould MK, Tang T, Liu IL, Lee J, Zheng C, Danforth KN, Kosco AE, Di Fiore JL, Suh DE. Recent trends in the identification of incidental pulmonary nodules. Am J Respir Crit Care Med. 2015;192(10):1208–14.
35. Yee D, Valiquette C, Pelletier M, Parisien I, Rocher I, Menzies D. Incidence of serious side effects from first-line Antituberculosis drugs among patients treated for active tuberculosis. Am J Respir Crit Care Med. 2003;167(11): 1472–7.
36. Singla R, Sharma S, Mohan A, Makharia G, Sreenivas V, Jha B, Kumar S, Sarda P, Singh S. Evaluation of risk factors for antituberculosis treatment induced hepatotoxicity. Indian J Med Res. 2010;132(1):81–6.
37. Yew WW, Leung CC. Antituberculosis drugs and hepatotoxicity. Respirology. 2006;11(6):699–707.
38. Raslan WF, Rabaan A, Al-Tawfiq JA. The predictive value of gen-Probe's amplified Mycobacterium tuberculosis direct test compared with culturing in paraffin-embedded lymph node tissue exhibiting granulomatous inflammation and negative acid fast stain. J Infect Public Health. 2014;7(4): 251–6.
39. Ulrichs T, Lefmann M, Reich M, Morawietz L, Roth A, Brinkmann V, Kosmiadi GA, Seiler P, Aichele P, Hahn H, et al. Modified immunohistological staining allows detection of Ziehl–Neelsen-negative Mycobacterium tuberculosis organisms and their precise localization in human tissue. J Pathol. 2005; 205(5):633–40.

5

Study of Healthcare Personnel with Influenza and other Respiratory Viruses in Israel (SHIRI): study protocol

Avital Hirsch[1*], Mark A. Katz[1,2,3], Alon Laufer Peretz[4], David Greenberg[5], Rachael Wendlandt[6], Yonat Shemer Avni[7], Gabriella Newes-Adeyi[6], Ilan Gofer[1], Maya Leventer-Roberts[1], Nadav Davidovitch[8], Anat Rosenthal[8], Rachel Gur-Arie[8], Tomer Hertz[9,10], Aharona Glatman-Freedman[11,14], Arnold S. Monto[3], Eduardo Azziz-Baumgartner[12], Jill Morris Ferdinands[12], Emily Toth Martin[3], Ryan E. Malosh[3], Joan Manuel Neyra Quijandría[13], Min Levine[12], William Campbell[6], Ran Balicer[1], Mark G. Thompson[12] and on behalf of the SHIRI workgroup

Abstract

Background: The Study of Healthcare Personnel with Influenza and other Respiratory Viruses in Israel (SHIRI) prospectively follows a cohort of healthcare personnel (HCP) in two hospitals in Israel. SHIRI will describe the frequency of influenza virus infections among HCP, identify predictors of vaccine acceptance, examine how repeated influenza vaccination may modify immunogenicity, and evaluate influenza vaccine effectiveness in preventing influenza illness and missed work.

Methods: Cohort enrollment began in October, 2016; a second year of the study and a second wave of cohort enrollment began in June 2017. The study will run for at least 3 years and will follow approximately 2000 HCP (who are both employees and members of Clalit Health Services [CHS]) with routine direct patient contact. Eligible HCP are recruited using a stratified sampling strategy. After informed consent, participants complete a brief enrollment survey with questions about occupational responsibilities and knowledge, attitudes, and practices about influenza vaccines. Blood samples are collected at enrollment and at the end of influenza season; HCP who choose to be vaccinated contribute additional blood one month after vaccination. During the influenza season, participants receive twice-weekly short message service (SMS) messages asking them if they have acute respiratory illness or febrile illness (ARFI) symptoms. Ill participants receive follow-up SMS messages to confirm illness symptoms and duration and are asked to self-collect a nasal swab. Information on socio-economic characteristics, current and past medical conditions, medical care utilization and vaccination history is extracted from the CHS database. Information about missed work due to illness is obtained by self-report and from employee records. Respiratory specimens from self-collected nasal swabs are tested for influenza A and B viruses, respiratory syncytial virus, human metapneumovirus, and coronaviruses using validated multiplex quantitative real-time reverse transcription polymerase chain reaction assays. The hemagglutination inhibition assay will be used to detect the presence of neutralizing influenza antibodies in serum.

Discussion: SHIRI will expand our knowledge of the burden of respiratory viral infections among HCP and the effectiveness of current and repeated annual influenza vaccination in preventing influenza illness, medical utilization, and missed workdays among HCP who are in direct contact with patients.

* Correspondence: avitalhi@clalit.org.il
[1]Chief Physician's Office, Clalit Health Services, Clalit Research Institute, Tel Aviv, Israel
Full list of author information is available at the end of the article

Background

Healthcare personnel (HCP) are believed to be at increased risk of respiratory viral infections, with one in five estimated to be infected with seasonal influenza each year [1]. These estimates vary widely, however, depending on the extent of active surveillance and the use of serologic vs. molecular diagnostics. Respiratory infections are of particular concern among HCP because of the close contact of HCP with patients [2], and the risk of HCP transmitting respiratory viruses to others [3]. Although recent research suggests that certain subgroups of HCP, such as those who perform aerosol-generating procedures, may be at heightened risk of infection with influenza and other respiratory pathogens [4], incidence of infections among HCP is not well characterized across different occupations and responsibilities. Furthermore, although HCP often work while ill [5–7], the extent to which infected HCP transmit respiratory pathogens to patients is not clear [8]. Further research is needed on the frequency and types of interactions HCP have with patients when they have symptomatic, atypical, or asymptomatic [1, 9] influenza virus infections.

Vaccination of HCP against influenza is an important component of infection control in healthcare settings [10], but persistently low rates of vaccine uptake among HCP in most countries remains an international concern [10–12]. Numerous studies on the knowledge, attitudes, and practices (KAP) associated with influenza vaccine acceptance and rejection have been conducted among HCP in high-income countries in North America and Europe [13–16]. However, much less is known about the barriers to vaccine acceptance among HCP in countries in the Middle East [12]. In Israel, a high-income country, less than half (49%) of HCP received influenza vaccine for the 2015–2016 influenza season; vaccine coverage was somewhat higher among hospital-based physicians (53%) than nurses (46%) [17]. More information is needed on the occupational, socio-demographic, and KAP factors that may explain variations in influenza vaccine acceptance in Israel, including how the personal KAP of HCP may impact on their promotion of influenza vaccination among their patients.

Although recent reviews confirm that the seasonal influenza vaccine is moderately effective in reducing the risk of influenza illness among adults [18], multiple gaps in knowledge remain about the preventive value of the vaccine among HCP [1]. To date, there has been only one randomized controlled trial of influenza vaccine efficacy among HCP, and this study measured serologic outcomes only [19]. Given that vaccinated individuals are less likely to seroconvert after an influenza virus infection and so can appear as not having been infected [20, 21], the use of serologic outcomes likely biases (and specifically, inflates) vaccine efficacy estimates.

Gaps are especially evident in our understanding of the value of influenza vaccine for reducing secondary adverse outcomes, including nosocomial infections among patients [22, 23] and missed work due to illness [24, 25]. Evidence is also needed to validate the potential of the vaccine in reducing the severity and duration of disease and diminish infectiousness among those who have breakthrough infections despite being vaccinated [24, 26]. Because HCP often receive influenza vaccine during multiple years, studies of HCP also provide an opportunity to examine how prior vaccinations may modify immunogenicity and vaccine effectiveness, and may provide answers to questions regarding the extent of residual protection and/or negative vaccine interference across seasons [27–29].

Here we provide an overview of the design and methods of a prospective study of influenza vaccine effectiveness in HCP named "Study of Healthcare Personnel with Influenza and other Respiratory Viruses in Israel" (SHIRI). The SHIRI cohort will follow approximately 600 HCP, all of whom have direct patient contact, during at least three influenza seasons, and an additional 1400 HCP during at least two influenza seasons.

Our study has four primary objectives: (1) to describe the frequency of respiratory, atypical (e.g., febrile only), and asymptomatic influenza virus infection among HCP; (2) to identify predictors of vaccine acceptance (and hesitancy) among HCP; (3) to examine how repeated influenza vaccination may modify immunogenicity; and (4) to evaluate influenza vaccine effectiveness in preventing influenza illness, associated missed work, and working while ill. Table 1 lists the knowledge gaps we identified within each of these aims and the study features intended to address these gaps.

The findings of this study will contribute to our knowledge about the burden of influenza and the vaccine effectiveness among HCP, and thus may influence a vaccination policy change in Israel and internationally.

Methods/design

Study design

This prospective cohort study of influenza vaccine effectiveness in HCP is funded by the United States Centers for Disease Control and Prevention (US CDC). A steering committee, consisting of principal investigators from the two hospitals, Clalit Health Services (CHS), the Israeli Center for Disease Control, Abt Associates, and the US CDC was established and charged with making critical decisions related to the study. Additional investigators from the University of Michigan School of Public Health and the Ben Gurion University School of Public Health will advise on laboratory methods and qualitative methods related to the study. Study activities are described in Fig. 1.

Table 1 Study Goals and Features Intended to Address Specific Knowledge Gaps

Knowledge Gap	Study Feature
1. Description of the frequency of influenza virus infection among healthcare personnel, including those manifesting as acute respiratory illness, atypical illness, or asymptomatic infection	
Studies of influenza illness among HCP using laboratory-confirmed outcomes are scarce.	Identification of symptomatic influenza virus infections with mqRT-PCR assay.
Typical surveillance strategies have focused on acute respiratory illness using highly specific case definitions which overlook non-respiratory and non-febrile manifestations of influenza disease.	Usage of a broad case definition: "illness with cough, runny nose, body aches, or feverishness in the past seven days."
Few studies have used both molecular and serologic diagnostics to assess the total burden of influenza virus infection among HCP.	In addition to mqRT-PCR, 4-fold increases in HI from pre- to post-season will also be used to identify possible influenza virus infection among unvaccinated HCP.
It is unclear how differences in sex, age, occupation, and underlying health may contribute to the frequency of influenza illness among HCP.	Usage of random stratified sampling to enroll a mixture of HCP by sex, age, and occupation. Assess underlying health status by self-report and medical record extraction.
Further research is needed on whether specific HCP roles and responsibilities increase the risk of infection with influenza and other respiratory pathogens.	Comparison of the frequency of ARFI (and infection with influenza and other respiratory viruses) by number of hours of direct patient care and by performance of aerosol-generating procedures (such as suction of fluids and tracheal intubation).
More information is needed on the impact of influenza illness on HCP's absence from work due to illness and working while ill.	Assessment of the duration of illness, missed, and rescheduled work due to illness, hours worked during illness, and ability to do usual activities.
2. Identification of predictors of vaccine acceptance (and hesitancy)	
Most studies of HCP have focused on influenza vaccine uptake in specific seasons and less on behavior over multiple years.	Description of how the frequency of influenza vaccination during the five years prior to enrollment and during the two to three years of participation in the cohort varies by sex, age, occupation, and socio-economic status.
Most studies of KAP associated with influenza vaccination among HCP have been conducted in the United States or Western European countries.	This study is conducted in Israel, and will examine KAP topics including association between frequency of vaccination and perceived susceptibility to influenza, perceived benefits and risks of influenza vaccination, readiness to be vaccinated, and anticipated worry and regret about influenza vaccination decisions.
3. Examination of how repeated influenza vaccination may modify immunogenicity	
Few studies have assessed the effects of repeated influenza vaccination across multiple seasons on immunogenicity.	Examination of how HI differs depending on the receipt of influenza vaccines up to ten years prior to the study for consistent health plans members.
Further research is needed on the mechanisms through which prior vaccination affects immunogenicity.	Examination of whether any link between repeated vaccination and HI can be explained by HCP's "antibody landscape".
Further research is needed on whether repeated prior vaccination impacts cell mediated immune response to influenza vaccines.	In a subset of participants who provide peripheral blood mononuclear cells before and after vaccination, examination of whether repeated prior vaccination is associated with suppression of B-cell and T-cell immunogenicity.
4. Evaluation of influenza vaccine effectiveness in preventing influenza illness and associated missed work and working while ill	
Prior study of IVE among HCP used serologic outcomes, which are likely biased among vaccinees.	Estimate the effectiveness of the influenza vaccine in preventing mqRT-PCR confirmed influenza illness among HCP.
It is unclear whether influenza vaccines may reduce missed work due to influenza illness or reduce time spent working while ill (i.e., presenteeism) with influenza.	Examine the hours of missed work and presenteeism between the dates of onset and resolution of influenza illness; apply these observations to estimate potential IVE in averting missed work or presenteeism.
More information is needed on the extent to which prior vaccination may offer residual protection and/or interfere with IVE in subsequent seasons.	Examination of IVE associated with combinations of current season vaccination and frequent vs. infrequent prior vaccinations.
Further research is needed on whether the influenza vaccination may modify influenza disease severity and duration among those who become infected despite vaccination.	Among HCP with influenza illness, examination of whether symptom severity and illness duration are lower among vaccinated vs. unvaccinated HCP.

Abbreviations: *HCP* healthcare personnel, *mqRT-PCR* multiplex quantitative real-time reverse transcription polymerase chain reaction, *HI* hemagglutination inhibition, *ARFI* acute respiratory illness or febrile illness, *KAP* knowledge, attitudes, and practices, *IVE* influenza vaccine effectiveness

Setting

The study is being conducted among HCP at two hospitals in Israel: (1) Soroka University Medical Center (located in Beer Sheva, a city in southern Israel), and (2) Beilinson Hospital (located in Petah Tivka, a city in central Israel) (Table 2). Both hospitals are managed and primarily staffed

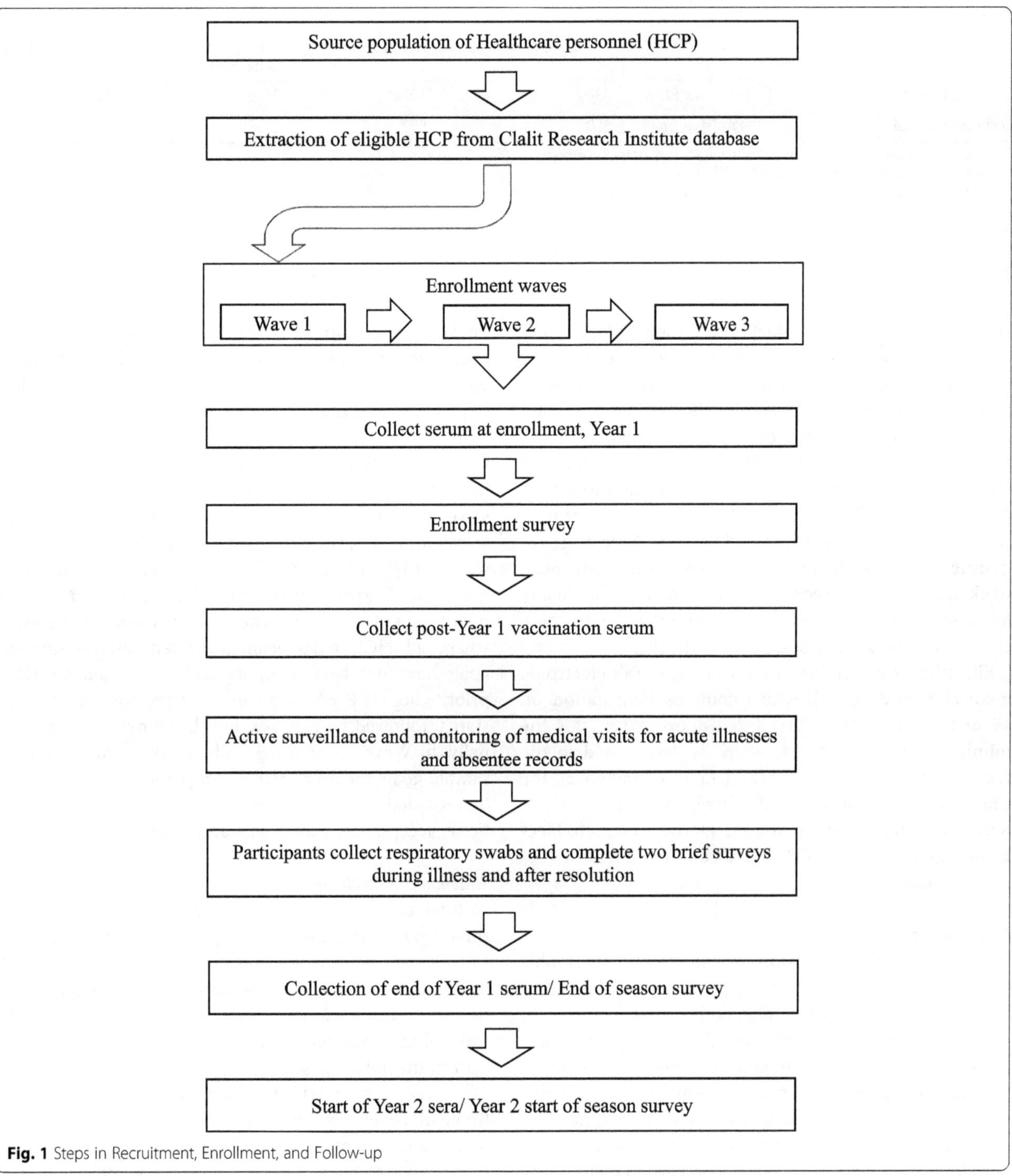

Fig. 1 Steps in Recruitment, Enrollment, and Follow-up

by CHS, the largest insurer and integrated care provider in Israel with over 4.4 million members in 2017, which constitute over 50% of the population.

Participants

Eligibility criteria

Eligible participants include HCP employed at a participating hospital who meet the following criteria: at least 18 years old; work full-time (≥30 h per week); and have routine direct hands-on or face-to-face contact with patients (within one meter) as part of a typical work shift. These eligibility criteria are similar to previous studies of HCP with direct patient contact [24, 30]. Participation is offered to physicians, nurses, respiratory therapists, physical therapists, unit clerks, radiograph technicians, medical assistants, transporters, and other

Table 2 Study Sites

Name of study site	Location	Number of employees	Number Of beds	Number of eligible participants, 2016[c]	Number of eligible participants, 2017[d]
Soroka University Medical Center	Beer Sheva, Israel	4300[b]	1074[a]	2436	2853
Beilinson Hospital	Petah Tikva, Israel	5500[b]	850[b]	1988	2260

[a]Data as of 2016; Data were extracted from Israeli Ministry of Health reports
[b]Data of 2017; Data were extracted from employee records from the CHS EHR and Israeli Ministry of Health reports
[c]Recruitment in 2016 began in October, when nationwide vaccination was already in progress. HCP who had already been vaccinated in the current season were not eligible for the study
[d]Excludes participants enrolled in 2016
Number of beds data was obtained from Israeli Ministry of Health reports
Abbreviations: *CHS* Clalit Health Services, *EMR* electronic medical record, *HCP* healthcare personnel

HCP who have direct contact with patients. All participants must also be members of CHS and have had continuous membership in CHS for at least 1 year prior to enrollment (in order to access medical and vaccination records). HCP are invited to join the study whether or not they intend to be vaccinated. HCP are excluded if they received the current season's flu vaccine more than 48 h before enrollment. If enrollment goals are not met, some enrollment restrictions can be eliminated (e.g., requiring prior year membership in the Clalit health plan, working, ≥30 h per week, or plans to stay at the facility for at least 2 years) and differences in outcomes by these characteristics can be examined analytically.

Eligibility is determined by reviewing CHS's electronic medical record (EMR), which contains information on all of the eligibility criteria listed above except for the number of working hours, which is determined in the recruitment phone call. EMR data is extracted at the Clalit Research Institute, the research arm of CHS. Screening information is logged in the Research Electronic Data Capture (REDCap), a common database (described below).

Recruitment

In order to recruit HCP with diverse socio-demographic characteristics, occupational responsibilities, and influenza vaccination histories, eligible HCP were invited to participate using a stratified sampling strategy that targeted eligible participants in groups (strata) categorized by sex, age, occupation, and previous year influenza vaccination status. This systematic approach was intended to minimize convenience sampling, which can introduce both known and unknown biases. Each group includes individuals with unique characteristics known to potentially affect influenza vaccine immunogenicity and effectiveness.

At CHS, a list of eligible HCP at each facility was generated and categorized into groups based on age (18–34, 35–49, ≥50 years old), sex, occupational categories (1- Physicians; 2 - Nurses, medical therapists, and professional technicians; and 3 - Medical assistants and support staff), and prior season influenza vaccination status (yes vs. no). Thus, prior to each year of the study, the sample is drawn from 36 unique strata (2 sexes * 3 age groups * 3 occupation groups * 2 prior season vaccination status groups). This stratified sampling strategy will be applied to potential new participants each year.

At each hospital, goals are set for the minimum and maximum number of enrollees per strata; then, recruitment is implemented in three waves. During the first wave of recruitment, HCP from the 36 strata are invited at random to participate in the study. Next, in Wave 2, we identify study strata where additional recruitment is needed and expand direct invitations to additional HCP who have not yet been invited to join the study. In strata where all HCP have been contacted but recruitment goals have not been met, we will recruit similar HCP, prioritizing HCP who are similar in previous vaccination status, followed by age, sex, and lastly by profession. Finally, in Wave 3, we accept volunteers to meet the total sample goals for each facility. All potential enrollees will be recorded in a recruitment log in order to track invitations, acceptance, and refusal and reasons for refusal.

Timeline of enrollment

A total cohort of 2000 HCP will be enrolled over a three-year period. Enrollment periods are targeted prior to influenza seasons. During Year 1 of the study, which targeted the 2016/2017 influenza season, enrollment could not begin until October 6, 2016 due to funding and institutional approval delays. Recruitment continued until the start of the influenza season (December 4, 2016) for a total of 8 weeks. This recruitment period included a month of frequent Israeli national holidays (October 2016), during which enrollment was challenging because many HCP were on vacation. In Year 1 of the study, 596 HCP were enrolled, and will contribute to Years 1, 2 and 3 of this 3-year cohort study. Enrollment in Year 2 began in June 2017. New enrollees in Year 2 will contribute to Years 2 and 3 of the study.

Active surveillance

During the influenza season, participants receive twice-weekly short message service (SMS) messages asking them to confirm whether they have acute illness symptoms, defined as one or more of the following symptoms within the past 7 days: cough, runny nose, body aches, or feverishness. In addition to these SMS messages, participants are asked to contact the study staff immediately when they experience symptoms of acute illness. If a participant reports an acute illness, he or she is asked follow-up questions about specific symptoms and date of onset. Participants are first contacted by SMS message. If they do not respond, they are contacted by telephone. If participants do not respond to phone calls, an attempt is made to contact them in-person. Ill participants receive follow-up SMS messages about whether the illness has resolved. Once an illness resolution is reported by a participant, he or she is sent five follow-up questions by SMS message about illness presentation, duration, and impact on work attendance. These surveillance activities are described in Fig. 2.

The start and end of active surveillance is determined by the study investigators and steering committee based on historical patterns for seasonal influenza circulation and available clinical and surveillance indicators of laboratory-confirmed influenza virus circulation in Israel. In the first year of the study, active surveillance started on December 4, 2016 and continued through March 23, 2017.

Data collection

We collect data for all participants from multiple sources. Key variables and their sources in the years prior to the study and during each study year are summarized in Table 3.

Electronic medical records

Information on socio-demographic characteristics, current medical conditions, medical history, medical care utilization, and influenza vaccination history are extracted from the CHS EMR at enrollment and at the end of each study year. For all participants, chronic medical conditions are identified using a combination of the International Classification of Diseases, Ninth Revision (ICD-9) codes from inpatient and outpatient records, International Classification of Primary Care Coding (ICPC), physician-entered free text diagnoses from outpatient medical records, and electronic chronic disease registries maintained by the Clalit Research Institute (details in Additional file 1: Annex 1 and Annex 2).

Routine influenza vaccine administration for CHS HCP members who receive the vaccine is recorded in the health fund's EMR. Because the vaccine is offered free of charge for members in CHS hospitals and clinics, nearly all of those who are vaccinated do so in such settings. Participants are considered vaccinated for a specific season if they received influenza vaccine from September 1 through March 31 of the relevant influenza season. To date, influenza vaccine has not been offered in Israel prior to September 1. We document prior vaccine history, according to EMR records, from the the 2006–2007 season, 10 years prior to the first year of our study.

In addition, we document medical visits for ARFI during weeks of active surveillance in every study year. We also document medically attended ARFI in the 10 years prior to enrollment, distinguishing between medical visits that occurred during the influenza season and those that occurred outside of the influenza season. Medically attended ARFI episodes during active surveillance and for years prior to enrollment are captured through evaluation of outpatient visits, emergency room visits, and hospital admissions. Criteria used for medically attended ARFI are described in Additional file 1: Annex 3.

Outpatient visits, emergency room visits, medications dispensed at CHS pharmacies, and hospital admissions are regularly updated in the CHS EMR, making it possible to document medical visits nearly in real-time by recording ICD-9 codes and free text entered by physicians. We also access the EMR to document influenza antiviral medications and antibiotics dispensed during acute illnesses.

Self-reported data

At enrollment and at the beginning of each subsequent season, all participants complete a brief survey with questions about socio-demographic characteristics that are not available in the EMR, occupational responsibilities, health status, and KAP regarding seasonal influenza vaccination.

At the end of each influenza season, participants are asked to complete another brief survey that includes questions about their overall health and to describe previously unreported illnesses ('End-of-season survey'). Surveys are designed to be self-administered electronically through the Internet using the REDCap system.

Work absenteeism

During active surveillance, we document days of missed work associated with respiratory illnesses. Missed workdays are identified by self-report (as part of acute illness and illness follow-up SMS messages) and by periodic reviews of human resource department employee absentee records. Illness days are identified as all days between self-reported illness onset and illness resolution dates (from SMS surveillance messages or by direct phone screening). Thus, missed work due to illness includes days that participants directly reported missing due to illness and days of absence (according to employee records) between the illness onset and resolution dates.

Laboratory methods

Nasal specimens

When participating HCP report being ill with a respiratory illness during the influenza season, they are instructed to self-collect a nasal swab using a self-swabbing kit [31] that includes illustrated instructions, a nasal mid-turbinate

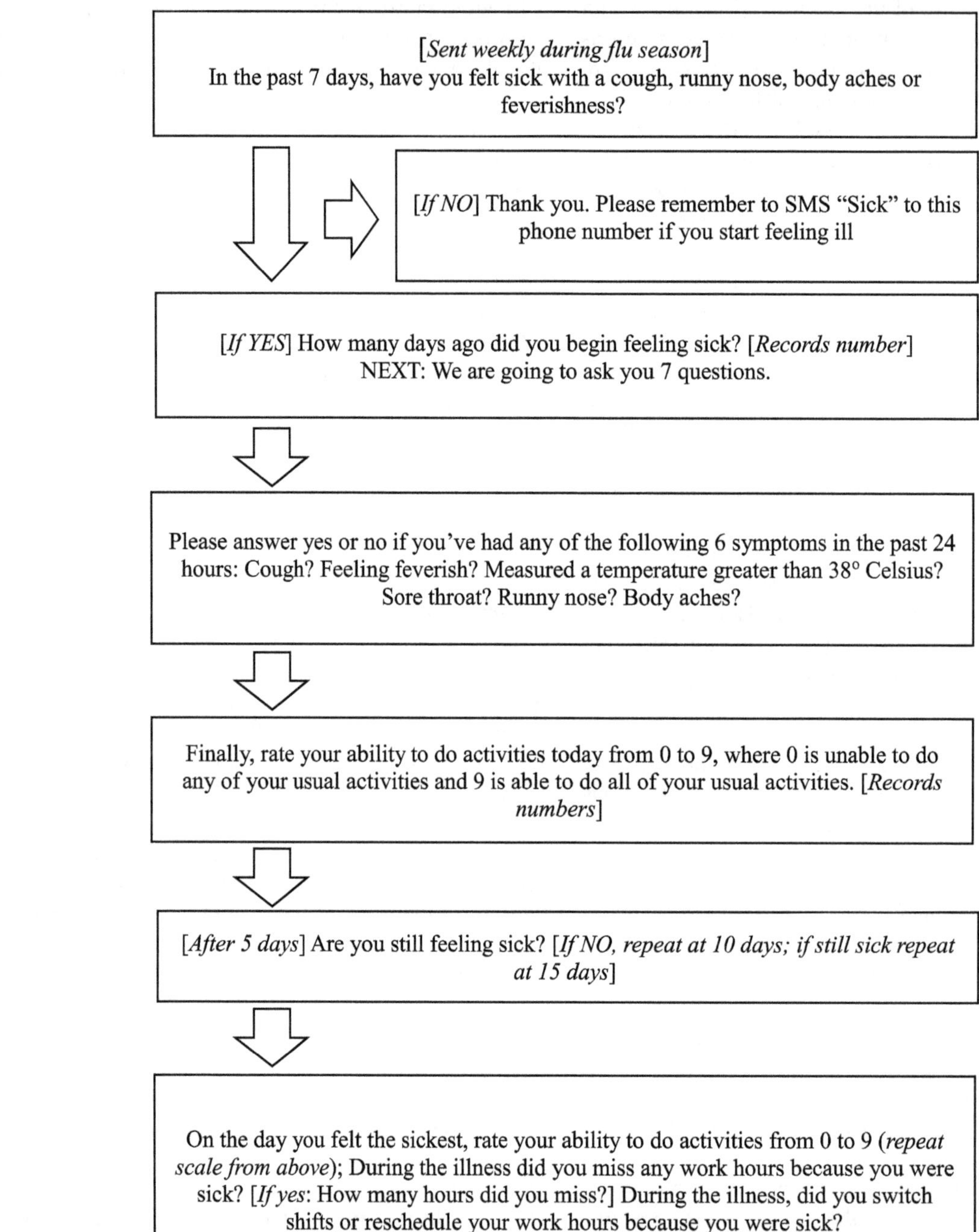

Fig. 2 Active Surveillance SMS Messaging Flow

swab, and a tube with room temperature transport medium. Respiratory specimens are placed in viral transport medium and delivered to the respective hospitals from HCP's residences by a courier service or are hand-carried by participants to study staff at their respective hospitals. If participants prefer not to collect the nasal swab themselves, study staff are able to collect it for them.

Molecular diagnostics

Specimens from Beilinson Hospital are stored at 4 °C and delivered by courier to the Clinical Virology Laboratory (CVL) at Soroka University Medical Center twice a week, where they are immediately aliquoted and frozen at – 80 °C. Specimens from participating Soroka University Medical Center HCP are brought to the laboratory daily, where they are aliquoted and frozen.

Table 3 Key Variables and Sources of Information for Participants

	Self-reported		Electronic Medical Records		Time Period	
	Enrollment survey	EOS survey	EMR	Employee Records	From year(s) prior to the study	Data from years enrolled in study
Demographic						
Sex					✓	
Date of birth					✓	
Marital status	✓		✓			✓
Country of birth			✓		✓	
Immigration date			✓		✓	
Ethnicity by country of birth of individual, the parents, or grandparents			✓		✓	
Socio-economic status by clinic address			✓		✓	✓
Supplementary insurance status			✓		✓	
Dates enrolled as CHS member			✓		✓	
Level of education	✓					✓
Household composition (number of rooms; number of family members in the house)	✓					✓
Occupation and work responsibilities	✓				✓	✓
Family income	✓					✓
Health Status and Risk Behaviors						
Health status and health behaviors	✓	✓			✓	
Smoking status, history			✓		✓	
Pack years			✓		✓	
Height			✓		✓	
Weight			✓		✓	
Body mass index			✓		✓	
Medication use for chronic conditions and immunosuppressants			✓		✓	
Attitudes						
Perceptions of illness, vaccines, missing work	✓					✓
Recollection of influenza vaccination (for vaccinated HCP)		✓				✓
Reasons for not receiving the influenza vaccine (for unvaccinated HCP)		✓				✓
Job satisfaction	✓					✓
Influenza Vaccination Documentation						
Vaccine administration date			✓		✓	✓
Vaccine type			✓		✓	✓
Vaccine manufacturer & lot			✓		✓	✓
Employee Records of Illness Absences				✓		✓
Acute Respiratory Illness						
Number of inpatient admissions associated with acute illness			✓		✓	✓
Chronic Medical Conditions and Pregnancy						
Number of ambulatory or inpatient medical encounters associated with chronic medical condition			✓		✓	✓
Chronic medical conditions			✓		✓	
Pregnancy					✓	✓

Abbreviations: *EOS* end of season, *EMR* electronic medical record, *CHS* Clalit health plan, *HCP* healthcare personnel

After one freeze-thaw cycle, specimens are tested for influenza A viruses [A(H1N1)pdm09 and A(H3N2)], influenza B viruses, respiratory syncytial virus (RSV), human metapneumovirus, and coronaviruses (NL63, 229E, OC43, HKU1) using validated multiplex quantitative real-time reverse transcription polymerase chain reaction (mqRT-PCR) assays [32], with protocols, primers, probes, and reagents supplied by Hy-labs (Israel) and Integrated DNA Technologies (USA). The CVL, in collaboration with the University of Michigan (Ann Arbor, Michigan, US), has completed the World Health Organization and US CDC influenza proficiency panels. Quality Control for Molecular Diagnostics (Glasgow, Scotland, UK) proficiency panels were also completed for influenza, RSV, human metapneumovirus (hMPV) and coronaviruses.

Some specimens will have molecular characterization with genetic sequencing and other assays to detect genetic markers to determine viral subclades and antiviral resistance at a reference laboratory approved by the study steering committee. Remaining aliquots of all study specimens may be sent to a US CDC-designated facility (also approved by the study steering committee) for additional virus characterization, banking, and storage. No specimens will contain personal identifiers.

Blood Specimens At enrollment, prior to each influenza season, 10 mL specimens of whole blood are collected from all participants. In addition, 5 mL specimens of whole blood are collected at the end of season 1 and the start and end of subsequent seasons. Participants who received the influenza vaccine during the study period will be asked to provide an additional sample of 5 mL of whole blood approximately 28 days (within a range of 21–42 days) after vaccination. Sera are extracted from whole blood and stored frozen until testing.

Participants who consent to providing additional blood at enrollment, as an optional part of the study, provide an additional 10 mL heparinized whole blood at enrollment and the end of season for extraction of peripheral blood mononuclear cells (PBMC). In addition, we collect 10 mL of heparinized whole blood approximately 7 days after vaccination from participants who agree to this optional part of the study. All PBMC samples are centrifuged, undergo cell count, diluted to 1-5 × 10^6 cells/ml and gradually frozen to − 80 °C, and placed in liquid nitrogen within 24 h. PBMC samples will be used for cell-mediated immunity assays.

Hemagglutination inhibition assay

The hemagglutination inhibition (HI) assay will be used to detect the presence of influenza antibodies in serum. HI to inactivated influenza vaccine components and influenza circulating strains will be performed at a reference laboratory using standard methods [33] as described previously [28, 34] (See Additional file 1: Annex 4). Egg-grown viruses will be supplied by the US CDC's International Reagent Resource. Preparation of serum samples will include (a) treatment with a receptor-destroying enzyme to remove nonspecific inhibitors, and (b) removal of nonspecific agglutinins by serum adsorption with packed red blood cells (RBC). Standard 0.5% turkey RBC will be prepared for influenza A (H1N1)pdm09 antigens and ether-treated B influenza antigens. Given indications that neuraminidase of circulating antigenic clusters of influenza A(H3N2) viruses (since 2014) have acquired the ability to bind to RBC, modified HI assays will be conducted for influenza A(H3N2) antigens using guinea pig red blood cells in the presence of the antiviral oseltamivir carboxylate, which inhibits influenza neuraminidase. Serum will be diluted 2-fold starting from 1:10. The HI titer will be the reciprocal of the serum dilution in the last well with complete HI. The geometric mean titer from duplicate results will be reported; HI < 10 will be considered 5 for the purposes of statistical analyses.

Additional immunological assays

Additional serologic testing may occur, including neuraminidase inhibition assay testing, antigen microarray testing [35] and other approaches. Neuraminidase-specific antibodies have been shown to play a role in protection against influenza infection [36, 37]. However, many questions remain about the role of neuraminidase in vaccine effectiveness [38].

Attitudes toward morbidity due to influenza and other respiratory illnesses

As a sub-study within this project, approximately 15–25 in-depth open-ended qualitative interviews are conducted each year with participants who recently had a wintertime respiratory illness and agree to participate in this sub-study.

Participants are contacted by phone approximately 1 week after confirmation of respiratory illness resolution and asked to participate in an interview. Interviews cover topics including illness experience, including symptoms, duration, perceived severity, and disruption to their daily activities and responsibilities, perceptions of how the illness impacted work responsibilities, perceptions of how the illness impacted life outside of work, and reasons for choosing to receive or not receive the influenza vaccine this season (see Additional file 1: Annex 5). Interviews will be recorded by audio recorder and later transcribed. After transcription, the data are translated from Hebrew to English and qualitatively analyzed using NVivo Software (QSR International, Melbourne, Australia) to identify themed code-words that may point to common patterns of comments across the interviews.

Data management

REDCap

Data collection and site-level management are conducted using REDCap, a browser-based metadata-driven software system (Vanderbilt University, Nashville, TN, USA) [39]. Most study instruments, including the recruitment log, online surveys, and laboratory results, allow for real-time data entry directly into REDCap. Surveys are designed to be self-administered electronically through the Internet using home computers, personal mobile telephones, or on computers or tablets provided at the workplace by study staff. In addition, study staff enter participants' responses directly into the REDCap database for interviews administered by telephone. Routine quality assurance monitoring is conducted locally by the project manager and centrally by the data coordinator (Abt Associates). Missing or unclear information is corrected through follow-up contact with participants.

TextIt

TextIt (TextIt, Kigali, Rwanda) is an online platform that uses logic flows to send tailored SMS messages to participants. Custom decision trees were developed in order to trigger exchanges with participants during active surveillance (described above). Specifically, TextIt documents answers to weekly illness inquiries, dates of illness onset and resolution, ratings of symptoms, and missed work. Study staff perform bi-weekly exports of TextIt data and import the data into an Excel macro-enabled workbook in order to track participant responses and illness events over time (see Additional file 1: Annex 6 for more details about TextIt).

Statistical considerations

Cohort size

The required number of participants depends on multiple factors, including expected influenza attack rate, vaccination coverage, and anticipated study attrition. We estimated that with 2340 participants contributing 5 months at-risk for influenza infection per season, 40% vaccine coverage, and 10% influenza illness attack rate, we would be powered to estimate a true vaccine effectiveness of 50% with confidence intervals that do not overlap with zero.

Sample size for incidence calculations

The full cohort provides the sample needs for estimating the frequency (or incidence within the study sample) of influenza illness. Given the larger sample demands for the vaccine effectiveness objectives, we expect to have ample statistical power for most objectives that involve estimating incidence or frequencies.

Sample size for immune response to vaccine and infection objectives

To assess the immune response to the vaccine, we plan to collect serum from the cohort members prior to vaccine availability, after vaccination, and at the end of each season. Our study design mirrors approaches used in previous studies that assessed the HI antibody titers among HCP analyzed sera from subgroups of 300–800 participants who provided sera at the same three time points [28]. See Additional file 1: Annex 7 for more details.

Data analysis of VE

Rates of acute illness associated with mqRT-PCR confirmed influenza virus infection (influenza illness) will be calculated as the number of influenza illnesses divided by person-time measured in weeks of active surveillance. Regression models will be used to estimate influenza vaccine effectiveness (1 – rate of influenza illness among vaccinated HCP/rate among unvaccinated HCP * 100) with 95% confidence intervals. Adjusted models of influenza vaccine effectiveness will include study year, calendar time (i.e., weeks between illness onset and week of peak of influenza season), and a propensity for vaccination score calculated using multivariable logistic regression [40]. Other potential confounders, including study site, will be examined and included in the adjusted model if they change IVE point estimates by > 5%.

Data analysis of immunogenicity

Since distributions of HI titer data are typically highly left-skewed, all statistical analyses will be conducted using log base-2 transformed titer data; results are then back-transformed to the original scale for ease of interpretation [28, 41]. Pre- and post-vaccine draws are assumed to be correlated within each person, thus repeated measures linear mixed models will be fitted to estimate geometric mean titers (GMT) and geometric mean ratios (GMR). Compound symmetric covariance error structures will be assumed for repeated measures within individuals. GMT will be calculated by back-transforming the least squares mean estimates of logged titer data. GMR will be calculated by back-transforming the difference of least squares means of post-vaccination and pre-vaccination logged titer estimates. GMR will be interpreted as the geometric mean fold ratio of post-vaccination titer to pre-vaccination titer. Multivariate estimates adjusted a priori for age and sex. Linear, quadractic, and cubic terms for age will be examined to consider possible nonlinear associations with age. Other covariates (e.g., education, household size, working in a hospital setting) may also be adjusted within multivariable models if they were associated with the number of prior vaccinations and either preseason GMT or post-vaccination GMR among vaccines.

Ethical considerations

The study protocol and procedures have been reviewed and approved by the Helsinki committees (institutional review board) at both of the study sites, and by Abt Associates (the coordinating institution on which US CDC relies). In addition, extraction of data from the CHS EMR was approved by the Data Use Committee of the Clalit Research Institute.

All participants complete written informed consent in Hebrew. Small gifts (such as a gift card) are given to participants at study milestones like completion of enrollment, blood draws, and completion of end-of-season survey. Influenza test results are given to those participants who ask to receive them. Given the research nature of the laboratory methods and time delays in batch testing, mqRT-PCR findings are not available to inform clinical decisions.

Discussion

We described the recruitment, enrollment, active surveillance, data collection, laboratory methods, and data management procedures for the SHIRI cohort – a US CDC-sponsored prospective study, overseen by CHS, of approximately 2300 HCP at two hospitals in Israel. In this study, we will describe the frequency of influenza virus infections among HCP in Israel. Using a broad case definition of respiratory illness, we aim to identify a wide range of ARFI in order to assess more accurately the burden of respiratory illness among HCP. Due to CHS's extensive EMR, we will have the ability to look at HCP influenza vaccination records up to 10 years prior to study enrollment in order to better understand how HI antibody titers differ depending on the number and specific combinations of prior influenza vaccinations. We will also be able to evaluate influenza vaccine effectiveness in preventing medically attended and non-medically attended influenza illness and associated missed work days.

The findings from the SHIRI cohort will increase our understanding of the burden of acute respiratory illnesses, and influenza virus illness specifically, among HCP in Israel. The unique design of the study, which includes comprehensive medical and vaccination data, active surveillance using a broad case definition, and both molecular and serologic diagnostics, will provide important data on influenza vaccine immunogenicity and effectiveness among HCP. The combination of insights about influenza burden and vaccine effectiveness may potentially inform influenza vaccine policy for HCP in Israel and internationally.

Strengths

Our study benefits from the fact that all enrolled HCP are members of CHS, and therefore extensive information is recorded in the EMR, which provides real-time data about ambulatory visits, hospitalizations, and medication use. In addition, the EMR provides reliable historic data about the participants, such as prior vaccination information, socio-economic variables, and data about health status and health behaviors. In our study, even if an ARFI is not reported through the SMS surveillance system, daily monitoring of the EMR for medical visits and medications will allow us to identify illnesses and contact participants directly in order to collect respiratory specimens and complete the illness survey. Combining our study with EMR data and data from the two hospitals' human resources departments will also allow us to reliably map the impact of illness on missed work and to evaluate days worked when ill (presenteeism).

In addition, the broad case definition of an ARFI promises to be more sensitive for influenza illness than case definitions used in previous HCP research [24] and should allow us to characterize a continuum of mild to moderately severe illnesses. Another strength is that the two study sites (Soroka University Medical Center and Beilinson Hospital) are among the largest hospitals in Israel, and the populations they serve and the HCP they employ vary in socio-demographic and economic characteristics. Soroka University Medical Center, the only general hospital in the Negev region in southern Israel, serves two main local populations: Jews, who mostly live in urban settings, and Bedouin Arabs, who live in a range of settlement types, from cities to unrecognized rural villages that lack electricity and running water [42, 43]. Beilinson Hospital, located in central Israel, serves a mostly urban population of a relatively higher socio-economic status compared to Soroka University Medical Center. Conducting our study in these two different settings may allow us to identify socio-demographic differences in KAP, vaccine uptake, and influenza illness attack rates. The use of mixed methods, including laboratory, clinical and epidemiological quantitative data, and in-depth qualitative interviews, creates a comprehensive approach, which is particularly important when trying to understand issues of influenza vaccine compliance and hesitancy. Finally, the study cohort includes several unique sub-studies.

Limitations

Our study has at least four limitations. First, our ability to generalize vaccine effectiveness findings from the study years to the potential preventive value of an influenza vaccine program may be limited. The effectiveness of the vaccine depends in part on the types of viruses circulating and the antigenic and genetic match between vaccine components and circulating strains in a given year. The precision of the estimates will also depend on the number of influenza cases.

Second, we will be cautious in interpreting self-reported information, given potential biases in recall and self-presentation. While some of the information collected through active surveillance can be verified with administrative data, other information, such as symptoms for non-medically attended illnesses, cannot be verified by another data source.

Third, although the random stratified sampling design intentionally includes HCP with a mixture of characteristics and work responsibilities, there are relatively few HCP in some of the strata. For example, few male medical assistants and support personnel are employed at the two hospitals, and therefore it is unlikely that we will be able to enroll large numbers from this category. This may limit our ability to examine the association between the frequency of influenza illness and specific combinations of age, sex, and occupation.

Fourth, during the third wave of recruitment we accept volunteers, regardless of age, profession, or vaccine status, which can present a sampling bias. However, characteristics of these volunteer participants will be compared with those of participants recruited during the first two waves in order to evaluate potential differences between the groups.

Abbreviations

ARFI: Acute respiratory illness or febrile illness; CHS: Clalit Health Services; CVL: Clinical Virology Laboratory; EMR: Electronic medical record; GMT: Geometric mean titer; GMR: Geometric mean ratios; HCP: Healthcare personnel; HI: Hemagglutination inhibition; hMPV: Human metapneumovirus; ICD-9: The international classification of diseases, ninth revision; ICPC: International Classification of Primary Care Coding; IVE: Influenza vaccine effectiveness; KAP: Knowledge, attitudes, and practices; mqRT-PCR: Multiplex quantitative real-time reverse transcription polymerase chain reaction; PBMC: Peripheral blood mononuclear cells; RBC: Red blood cells; REDCap: Research Electronic Data Capture; RSV: Respiratory syncytial virus; SHIRI: Study of Healthcare Personnel with Influenza and other Respiratory Viruses in Israel; SMS: Short message service; US CDC: United States Centers for Disease Control and Prevention

Acknowledgments

The authors would like to thank Becca Feldman (Clalit Research Institute) for epidemiological support, Nataliya Sokolski (Clalit Research Institute) for administrative support, Sydney Krispin (Clalit Research Institute) for assistance in editing and reviewing the manuscript, Orly Barashi Zamir (Soroka Universitty Medical Center) for on-site study coordination, and Jacob Dreiher (Soroka University Medical Center) for on-site study leadership. The authors would like to thank Sonja Olsen, Jerome Tokars, and Meredith McMorrow for feedback on an earlier version of this manuscript (US CDC). We would like to thank the study staff at all participating hospitals. Finally, we are extremely grateful to the study participants.

Funding

Contract HHSD2002013M53890B within CDC's Achieving Public Health Impact through Research and task 200–2014-F-60406 ("The Epidemiology and Prevention of Influenza Virus Infections in Low- and Middle-Income Countries") to Abt Associates from US CDC.

Authors' contributions

Study concept and design: MGT, RB, ASM, REM, ALP, DG, RW, GNA, MLR, and ND; Laboratory methods: YAS, ETM, MGT; Literature search: MGT, MAK, AH; Acquisition of data: IG, WC; Coordination of the study: AH, MAK; Wrote the manuscript: AH, MAK, MGT, RW; Drafting of the manuscript and critical revision of the manuscript for important intellectual content: ALP, DG, RW, YSA, GNA, IG, MLR, ND, AR, RGA, TH, AGF, ASM, EAB, JMF, ETM REM, JMNQ, ML, WC, RB; All authors read and approved the final manuscript.

Competing interests

No conflicts of interest were reported. The findings and conclusions in this report are those of the authors and do not necessarily represent the official position of the US CDC.

Author details

[1]Chief Physician's Office, Clalit Health Services, Clalit Research Institute, Tel Aviv, Israel. [2]School of Public Health, Medical School for International Health, Faculty of Health Sciences, Ben Gurion University of the Negev, Beer Sheva, Israel. [3]Department of Epidemiology, University of Michigan School of Public Health, Ann Arbor, MI, USA. [4]Rabin Medical Center, Occupational Medicine Department, Petah Tikva, Israel. [5]Pediatric Infectious Disease Unit, Soroka University Medical Center, Beer Sheva, Israel. [6]Abt Associates, Inc, Atlanta, GA, USA. [7]Clinical Virology, Soroka University Medical Center, Ben Gurion University of the Negev, Beer Sheva, Israel. [8]Department of Health Systems Management, School of Public Health, Faculty of Health Sciences, Ben Gurion University of the Negev, Beer Sheva, Israel. [9]Department of Microbiology Immunology and Genetics, Faculty of Health Sciences, Ben Gurion University of the Negev, Beer Sheva, Israel. [10]Vaccine and Infectious Disease Division, Fred Hutch Cancer Research Center, Seattle, WA, USA. [11]Israel Center for Disease Control, Ministry of Health, Tel Hashomer, Ramat Gan, Israel. [12]Influenza Division, Centers for Disease Control and Prevention (CDC), Atlanta, GA, USA. [13]U.S. Naval Medical Research Unit N° 6 – Lima, Lima, Peru. [14]Department of Epidemiology and Preventive Medicine, School of Public Health, Sackler Faculty of Medicine, Tel Aviv University, Tel Aviv, Israel.

References

1. Kuster SP, Shah PS, Coleman BL, Lam PP, Tong A, Wormsbecker A, et al. Incidence of influenza in healthy adults and healthcare workers: a systematic review and meta-analysis. PLoS One. 2011;6. https://doi.org/10.1371/journal.pone.0026239.
2. Brankston G, Gitterman L, Hirji Z, Lemieux C, Gardam M. Transmission of influenza a in human beings. Lancet Infect Dis. 2007;7:257–65. https://doi.org/10.1016/S1473-3099(07)70029-4.
3. Thomas RE. Do we have enough evidence how seasonal influenza is transmitted and can be prevented in hospitals to implement a comprehensive policy? Vaccine. 2016;34:3014–21. https://doi.org/10.1016/j.vaccine.2016.04.096.
4. Tran K, Cimon K, Severn M, Pessoa-Silva CL, Conly J. Aerosol generating procedures and risk of transmission of acute respiratory infections to healthcare workers: a systematic review. PLoS One. 2012;7. https://doi.org/10.1371/journal.pone.0035797.
5. Molinari NAM, Ortega-Sanchez IR, Messonnier ML, Thompson WW, Wortley PM, Weintraub E, et al. The annual impact of seasonal influenza in the US: measuring disease burden and costs. Vaccine. 2007;25:5086–96. https://doi.org/10.1016/j.vaccine.2007.03.046.
6. Pearson ML, Bridges CB, Harper S a. Influenza vaccination of health-care personnel: recommendations of the healthcare infection control practices advisory committee (HICPAC) and the advisory committee on immunization practices (ACIP). MMWR Recomm Rep. 2006;55:1–16.
7. Vanhems P, Voirin N, Roche S, Escuret V, Regis C, Gorain C, et al. Risk of influenza-like illness in an acute health care setting during community influenza epidemics in 2004-2005, 2005-2006, and 2006-2007: a prospective study. Arch Intern Med. 2011;171:151–7. https://doi.org/10.1001/archinternmed.2010.500.
8. De Serres G, Skowronski DM, Ward BJ, Gardam M, Lemieux C, Yassi A, et al. Influenza vaccination of healthcare workers: critical analysis of the evidence for patient benefit underpinning policies of enforcement. PLoS One. 2017;12. https://doi.org/10.1371/journal.pone.0163586.
9. Carrat F, Vergu E, Ferguson NM, Lemaitre M, Cauchemez S, Leach S, et al. Time lines of infection and disease in human influenza: a review of volunteer challenge studies. Am J Epidemiol. 2008;167:775–85. https://doi.org/10.1093/aje/kwm375

10. Poland GA, Tosh P, Jacobson RM. Requiring influenza vaccination for health care workers: seven truths we must accept. Vaccine. 2005;23:2251–5. https://doi.org/10.1016/j.vaccine.2005.01.043.
11. Rakita RM, Hagar B a, Crome P, Lammert JK. Mandatory influenza vaccination of healthcare workers: a 5-year study. Infect Control Hosp Epidemiol. 2010;31:881–8. https://doi.org/10.1086/656210.
12. Abu-Gharbieh E, Fahmy S, Rasool BA, Khan S. Influenza vaccination: healthcare workers attitude in three Middle East countries. Int J Med Sci. 2010;7:319–25.
13. Hollmeyer H, Hayden F, Mounts A, Buchholz U. Review: interventions to increase influenza vaccination among healthcare workers in hospitals. Influenza Other Respir Viruses. 2013;7:604–21. https://doi.org/10.1111/irv.12002.
14. Hollmeyer HG, Hayden F, Poland G, Buchholz U. Influenza vaccination of health care workers in hospitals-a review of studies on attitudes and predictors. Vaccine. 2009;27:3935–44. https://doi.org/10.1016/j.vaccine.2009.03.056.
15. Naleway AL, Henkle EM, Ball S, Bozeman S, Gaglani MJ, Kennedy ED, et al. Barriers and facilitators to influenza vaccination and vaccine coverage in a cohort of health care personnel. Am J Infect Control. 2014;42:371–5. https://doi.org/10.1016/j.ajic.2013.11.003.
16. Thompson MG, Gaglani MJ, Naleway A, Ball S, Henkle EM, Sokolow LZ, et al. The expected emotional benefits of influenza vaccination strongly affect pre-season intentions and subsequent vaccination among healthcare personnel. Vaccine. 2012;30:3557–65. https://doi.org/10.1016/j.vaccine.2012.03.062.
17. Influenza vaccination of Medical Teams n.d. https://www.health.gov.il/PublicationsFiles/Flu_stuff2015_2016.pdf.
18. Osterholm MT, Kelley NS, Sommer A, Belongia EA. Efficacy and effectiveness of influenza vaccines: a systematic review and meta-analysis. Lancet Infect Dis. 2012;12:36–44. https://doi.org/10.1016/S1473-3099(11)70295-X.
19. Wilde JA, McMillan JA, Serwint J, Butta J, O'Riordan MA, Steinhoff MC. Effectiveness of influenza vaccine in health care professionals: a randomized trial. JAMA. 1999;281:908–13. https://doi.org/10.1001/jama.281.10.908.
20. Petrie JG, Ohmit SE, Johnson E, Cross RT, Monto AS. Efficacy studies of influenza vaccines: effect of end points used and characteristics of vaccine failures. J Infect Dis. 2011;203:1309–15. https://doi.org/10.1093/infdis/jir015.
21. Thompson MG, Gaglani MJ, Naleway AL, Dowell SH, Spencer S, Ball S, et al. Reduced serologic sensitivity to influenza a virus illness among inactivated influenza vaccinees. Vaccine. 2016;34:3443–6. https://doi.org/10.1016/j.vaccine.2016.04.085.
22. Thomas RE, Jefferson T, Lasserson TJ. Influenza vaccination for healthcare workers who work with the elderly: systematic review. Vaccine. 2010;29:344–56. https://doi.org/10.1016/j.vaccine.2010.09.085.
23. Thomas RE, Jefferson T, Lasserson TJ. Influenza vaccination for healthcare workers who care for people aged 60 or older living in long-term care institutions. Cochrane Database Syst Rev. 2013;7:CD005187. https://doi.org/10.1002/14651858.CD005187.pub4.
24. Henkle E, Irving S a, Naleway AL, Gaglani MJ, Ball S, Spencer S, et al. Comparison of laboratory-confirmed influenza and noninfluenza acute respiratory illness in healthcare personnel during the 2010-2011 influenza season. Infect Control Hosp Epidemiol. 2014;35:538–46. https://doi.org/10.1086/675832.
25. Ng a NM, Lai CKY. Effectiveness of seasonal influenza vaccination in healthcare workers: a systematic review. J Hosp Infect. 2011;79:279–86. https://doi.org/10.1016/j.jhin.2011.08.004.
26. Kenah E, Chao DL, Matrajt L, Halloran ME, Longini IM. The global transmission and control of influenza. PLoS One. 2011;6. https://doi.org/10.1371/journal.pone.0019515.
27. McLean HQ, Thompson MG, Sundaram ME, Meece JK, McClure DL, Friedrich TC, et al. Impact of repeated vaccination on vaccine effectiveness against influenza A(H3N2) and B during 8 seasons. Clin Infect Dis. 2014;59:1375–85. https://doi.org/10.1093/cid/ciu680.
28. Gaglani M, Spencer S, Ball S, Song J, Naleway A, Henkle E, et al. Antibody response to influenza A(H1N1)pdm09 among healthcare personnel receiving trivalent inactivated vaccine: effect of prior monovalent inactivated vaccine. J Infect Dis. 2014;209:1705–14. https://doi.org/10.1093/infdis/jit825.
29. Belongia EA, Skowronski DM, McLean HQ, Chambers C, Sundaram ME, De Serres G. Repeated annual influenza vaccination and vaccine effectiveness: Review of evidence. Expert Rev Vaccines 2017:14760584.2017.1334554. doi: https://doi.org/10.1080/14760584.2017.1334554.
30. Melia M, O'Neill S, Calderon S, Hewitt S, Orlando K, Bithell-Taylor K, et al. Development of a flexible, computerized database to prioritize, record, and report influenza vaccination rates for healthcare personnel. Infect Control Hosp Epidemiol. 2009;30:361–9. https://doi.org/10.1086/596043.
31. Thompson MG, Ferber JR, Odouli R, David D, Shifflett P, Meece JK, et al. Results of a pilot study using self-collected mid-turbinate nasal swabs for detection of influenza virus infection among pregnant women. Influenza Other Respir Viruses. 2015;9:155–60. https://doi.org/10.1111/irv.12309.
32. Lieberman D, Lieberman D, Shimoni A, Keren-Naus A, Steinberg R, Shemer-Avni Y. Identification of respiratory viruses in adults: nasopharyngeal versus oropharyngeal sampling. J Clin Microbiol. 2009;47:3439–43. https://doi.org/10.1128/JCM.00886-09.
33. Who. Manual for the laboratory diagnosis and virological surveillance of influenza. World Heal Organ. 2011;2011:153.
34. Thompson MG, Naleway A, Fry AM, Ball S, Spencer SM, Reynolds S, et al. Effects of repeated annual inactivated influenza vaccination among healthcare personnel on serum hemagglutinin inhibition antibody response to a/Perth/16/2009 (H3N2)-like virus during 2010-11. Vaccine. 2016;34:981–8. https://doi.org/10.1016/j.vaccine.2015.10.119.
35. Hertz T, Shagal A, Ohmit S. Immune history to influenza infection and vaccination predicts antibody responses to the seasonal influenza vaccine. J Immunol. 2016;196(1 Supplement):146.24.
36. Couch RB, Atmar RL, Franco LM, Quarles JM, Wells J, Arden N, et al. Antibody correlates and predictors of immunity to naturally occurring influenza in humans and the importance of antibody to the neuraminidase. J Infect Dis. 2013;207:974–81. https://doi.org/10.1093/infdis/jis935.
37. Monto AS, Petrie JG, Cross RT, Johnson E, Liu M, Zhong W, et al. Antibody to influenza virus neuraminidase: an independent correlate of protection. J Infect Dis. 2015;212:1191–9. https://doi.org/10.1093/infdis/jiv195.
38. Laguio-Vila MR, Thompson MG, Reynolds S, Spencer SM, Gaglani M, Naleway A, et al. Comparison of serum hemagglutinin and neuraminidase inhibition antibodies after 2010-2011 trivalent inactivated influenza vaccination in healthcare personnel. Open Forum Infect Dis. 2015;2. https://doi.org/10.1093/ofid/ofu115.
39. Harris PA, Taylor R, Thielke R, Payne J, Gonzalez N, Conde JG. Research electronic data capture (REDCap)-A metadata-driven methodology and workflow process for providing translational research informatics support. J Biomed Inform. 2009;42:377–81. https://doi.org/10.1016/j.jbi.2008.08.010.
40. D'Agostino RB Jr, D'Agostino RBS. Estimating treatment effects using observational data. JAMA. 2007;297:314–6.
41. Coudeville L, Bailleux F, Riche B, Megas F, Andre P, Ecochard R. Relationship between haemagglutination-inhibiting antibody titres and clinical protection against influenza: development and application of a bayesian random-effects model. BMC Med Res Methodol. 2010;10. https://doi.org/10.1186/1471-2288-10-18.
42. Greenberg D, Givon-Lavi N, Newman N, Bar-Ziv J, Dagan R. Nasopharyngeal carriage of individual Streptococcus pneumoniae serotypes during pediatric pneumonia as a means to estimate serotype disease potential. Pediatr Infect Dis J. 2011;30:227–33. https://doi.org/10.1097/INF.0b013e3181f87802.
43. Abuhazira YS. The Bedouin population in IsraelPopulation register compared with population estimation as basis of demographic indexes. Jerusalem: CBS; 2010. http://cbs.gov.il/www/publications/pw50.pdf.

6

Efficacy and safety of cefazolin versus antistaphylococcal penicillins for the treatment of methicillin-susceptible *Staphylococcus aureus* bacteremia

Changcheng Shi[1,2†], Yubo Xiao[3†], Qi Zhang[2†], Qingyu Li[1], Fei Wang[1], Jing Wu[4] and Nengming Lin[1,2,5*]

Abstract

Background: Antistaphylococcal penicillins (ASPs) and cefazolin have become the most frequent choices for the treatment of methicillin-susceptible *Staphylococcus aureus* (MSSA) infections. However, the best therapeutic agent to treat MSSA bacteremia remains to be established.

Methods: We conducted a systematic review and meta-analysis to evaluate the efficacy and safety of these two regimens for the treatment of MSSA bacteremia. PubMed, EMBASE and the Cochrane Library from inception to February 2018 were searched. The primary outcome was mortality. The secondary outcomes included treatment failure, recurrence of bacteremia, adverse effects (AEs) and discontinuation due to AEs. Data were extracted and pooled odds ratios (ORs) and 95% confidence intervals (CIs) were calculated.

Results: A total of ten observational studies met the inclusion criteria. The results indicate that compared to ASPs, cefazolin was associated with significant reduction in mortality (OR, 0.69; 95% CI, 0.58 to 0.82; $I^2 = 3.4\%$) and clinical failure (OR, 0.56; 95% CI, 0.37 to 0.85; $I^2 = 44.9\%$) without increasing the recurrence of bacteremia (OR, 1.12; 95% CI, 0.94 to 1.34; $I^2 = 0\%$). There were no significant differences for the risk of anaphylaxis (OR, 0.91; 95% CI, 0.36 to 2.99; $I^2 = 0\%$) or hematotoxicity (OR, 0.56; 95% CI, 0.17 to 1.88; $I^2 = 0\%$). However, nephrotoxicity (OR, 0.36; 95% CI, 0.16 to 0.81; $I^2 = 0\%$) and hepatotoxicity (OR, 0.12; 95% CI, 0.04 to 0.41; $I^2 = 0\%$) were significantly lower in the cefazolin group. Moreover, cefazolin was associated with lower probability of discontinuation due to AEs compared with the ASPs (OR, 0.24; 95% CI, 0.12 to 0.48; $I^2 = 18\%$).

Conclusion: The results of present study favor the application of cefazolin and should be regarded as important evidence to help make clinical decisions in choosing a treatment option for treating MSSA bacteremia.

Keywords: Cefazolin, Antistaphylococcal penicillins, Methicillin-susceptible *Staphylococcus aureus*, Bacteremia, Meta-analysis

* Correspondence: lnm1013@163.com
†Changcheng Shi, Yubo Xiao and Qi Zhang contributed equally to this work.Changcheng Shi, Yubo Xiao and Qi Zhang co-first authors.
[1]Department of Clinical Pharmacy, Affiliated Hangzhou First People's Hospital, Zhejiang University School of Medicine, Hangzhou, China
[2]Department of Clinical Pharmacy, Hangzhou First People's Hospital, Nanjing Medical University, Hangzhou, China
Full list of author information is available at the end of the article

Background

Staphylococcus aureus is the principal cause of community-acquired and nosocomial infections. Although more clinical research has focused on the methicillin-resistant *Staphylococcus aureus* (MRSA), bloodstream infections due to methicillin-susceptible *Staphylococcus aureus* (MSSA) remain a significant healthcare burden worldwide with high morbidity and mortality [1, 2].

Prevailing evidence has established the use of β-lactam antibiotics in preference to vancomycin as optimum therapy for MSSA bacteremia [3, 4]. According to the relevant clinical practice guidelines, cefazolin and antistaphylococcal penicillins (ASPs) such as nafcillin, oxacillin, and cloxacillin are the most frequent choices [5–8]. However, the optimal choice of β-lactam antibiotic for MSSA bacteremia is still unclear. To our knowledge, randomized control trials (RCTs) directly comparing clinical outcomes between cefazolin and ASPs for MSSA bacteremia are lacking, but data are emerging to support the role of cefazolin as a first-line agent for MSSA bacteremia [9, 10]. The aim of this meta-analysis was to summarize all the available evidence and compare the efficacy and safety of cefazolin versus ASPs for the treatment of MSSA bacteremia.

Literature search strategy

We searched PubMed, EMBASE and the Cochrane Library from inception to February 2018. The search terms were "(oxacillin OR nafcillin OR methicillin OR cloxacillin OR floxacillin OR dicloxacillin OR flucloxacillin OR antistaphylococcal penicillin OR semisynthetic penicillin) AND (methicillin-susceptible *Staphylococcus aureus* OR methicillin susceptible *Staphylococcus aureus* OR MSSA) AND (bacteremia OR bacteraemia OR bloodstream infection OR sepsis) AND cefazolin)". Reference lists of the relevant publications were searched for additional literature. No language or publication restriction were imposed.

Inclusion criteria and study selection

Two review authors independently reviewed the results to screen relevant studies for further assessment. Any discrepancy was resolved through discussion. Original studies included in our meta-analysis were required to meet the following criteria: (i) RCTs or observational designs, including cohort and case-control studies; (ii) comparing the efficacy or safety of treatment between cefazolin and ASPs for MSSA bacteremia in two groups of patients; (iii) at least one of the following outcomes: mortality, treatment failure, recurrence of bacteremia, adverse effects (AEs) and discontinuation due to AEs. Exclusion criteria were as follows: (i) no outcome data were available; (ii) studies investigating only cefazolin or ASPs; (iii) presented solely as abstract at scientific conferences; (iv) duplicate publications.

Outcomes

The primary outcome assessed in this meta-analysis was mortality. The secondary outcomes included treatment failure, recurrence of bacteremia, AEs and discontinued treatment due to AEs. While extracting data, we found that for 'mortality', some studies reported 'all-cause mortality', 'all-cause in-hospital mortality', 'over mortality' or 'bacteremia-associated mortality'. In our meta-analysis, all of these terms were regarded as approximate 'mortality'. When data for more than one endpoint were available, mortality in the main analysis was recorded at the latest point in the study (e.g., 90-day mortality had precedence over 30-day mortality). Treatment failure and other secondary outcomes were defined according to descriptions provided by each study.

Data extraction and quality assessment

The variables that were abstracted from each study included the investigator, publication year, study design, location, enrolment period, number of participants, patient characteristics (age, sex, disease severity, the source of infection), intervention and comparison, dose and duration of administration, and outcome measures. Data were extracted independently by two authors. Discrepancies were resolved in meetings. Because only observational studies were available for inclusion, the quality of the included publications was appraised based on the Newcastle-Ottawa scale (NOS), as recommended by the Cochrane Collaboration [11]. Each study was scored from 0 to 9, based on eight items within the three following domains: selection, comparability and exposure (or outcome) [12].

Statistical analysis

Pooled odds ratios (ORs) and 95% confidence intervals (CIs) of all outcomes were used to determine whether there were significant differences between the compared data. Heterogeneity was evaluated using the I^2 statistic and a value of > 50% was defined to indicate significant heterogeneity. If no significant heterogeneity was found, a fixed-effects model was used. Otherwise, a random-effect model was selected. Sensitivity analyses were undertaken by excluding each publication. Subgroup analyses were performed based on the study design, location, study period, time of mortality reporting and control group.

Additionally, we presented separate subgroup analyses of adjusted or unadjusted estimates. Publication bias was assessed by generating funnel plots and tested used Begg's and Egger's asymmetry test. A *P*-value of < 0.05 was considered statistically significant. Meta-analysis statistical analyses were performed using STATA software (version 12.0, Stata Corporation, College Station, TX, USA).

Results

Search results

A total of 237 articles were identified in the initial search. After selection, ten studies involving 4779 patients met our inclusion criteria [13–22]. The details of the study selection process are shown in Fig. 1. Eight retrospective studies [13–18, 20, 21] and two prospective studies [19, 22] were included. No RCTs were identified. The studies were conducted in different countries as follows: the USA (5 trials) [16, 18–21], South Korea (2 trials) [13, 22], Canada (1 trial) [17], Singapore (1 trial) [15] and Israel (1 trial) [14]. The studies were published from 2011 to 2018. The mean or median patient age ranged between 50 and 69 years. Four studies compared cefazolin with nafcillin [13, 19, 20, 22], three compared cefazolin with cloxacillin [14, 15, 17], two compared cefazolin with oxacillin [16, 18], and one compared cefazolin with nafcillin or oxacillin [21]. Seven studies reported the dose or duration of administration [13, 15–20]. The detailed characteristics of included studies are represented in Table 1 and Additional file 1: Table S1. Most studies included were given five or more Newcastle-Ottawa Scale stars, indicating high quality (Additional file 1: Table S2).

Mortality

All included studies reported on mortality. Our meta-analysis indicated that mortality was significant decreased in MSSA bacteremia patients treated with cefazolin compared to those treated with ASPs (OR, 0.69; 95% CI, 0.58 to 0.82; $I^2 = 3.4\%$) (Fig. 2). Sensitivity analysis was used to evaluate the robustness of the findings after exclusion of each publication (Additional file 1: Table S3). We also performed subgroups analyses based on the study design, location, study period, time of mortality reporting, control group. Most of the subgroups analyses showed that cefazolin was associated with lower mortality than ASPs, except for the studies which the control group was cloxacillin. Six studies provided adjusted mortality data after controlling for potential confounders and similar results were obtained (OR, 0.69; 95% CI, 0.58 to 0.83; $I^2 = 23.6\%$) (Table 2).

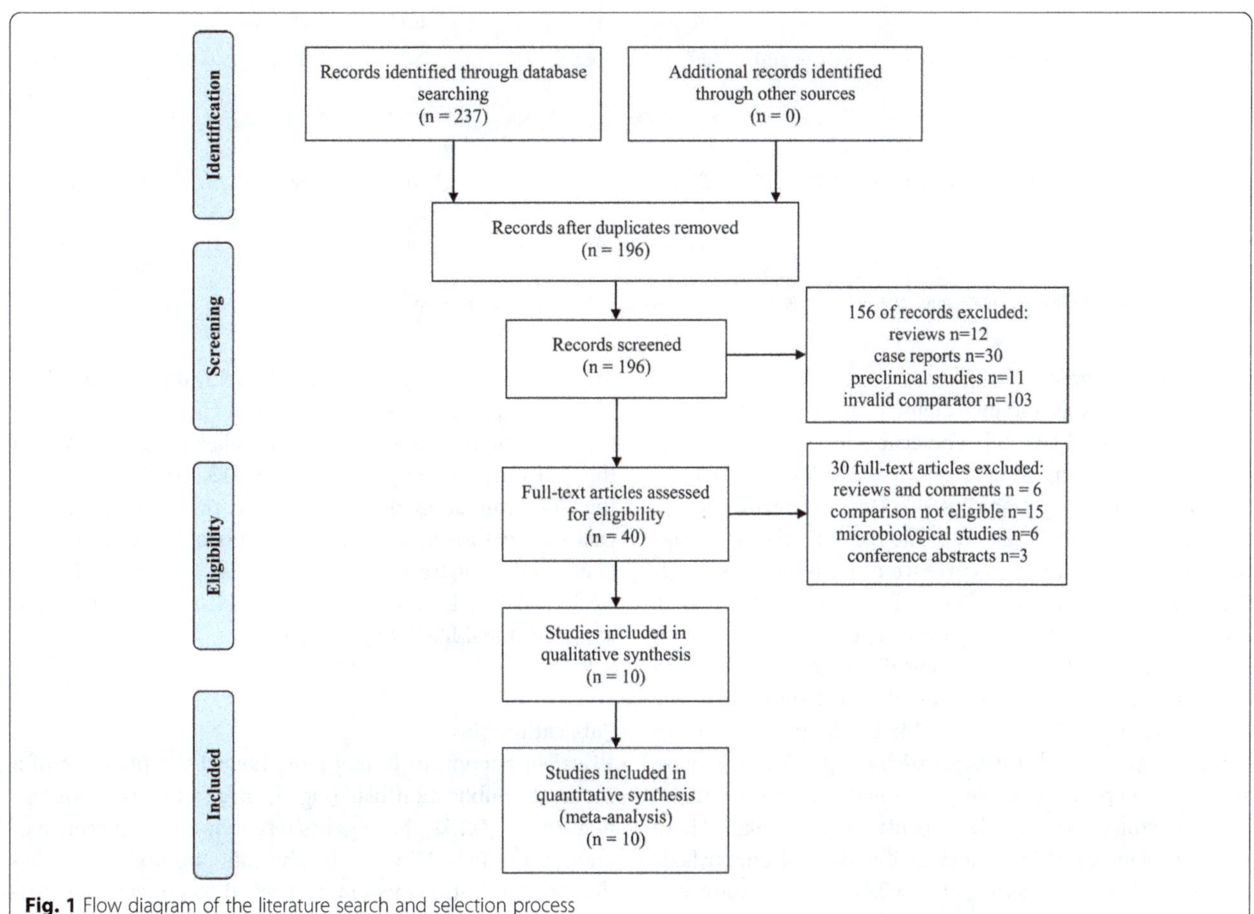

Fig. 1 Flow diagram of the literature search and selection process

Table 1 Characteristics of the studies included in the meta-analysis

Study	Design	Location	Study period	Treatment groups	No. of patients	Median dose (g/d)	Median duration (d)	ICU admission %	Definition of mortality
Lee 2011 [13]	SC retrospective PS-matched case- control study	South Korea	2004–2009	CFZ	49	NR	17	NR	30-day over mortality
				NAF	84	NR	15	NR	90-day SAB-related mortality
Paul 2011 [14]	SC retrospective cohort study	Israel	1988–1994 & 1999–2007	CFZ	72	NR	NR	5.2	30-day all-cause mortality
				CLX	281	NR	NR		90-day mortality
Renaud 2011 [15]	SC retrospective cohort study	Singapore	2009	CFZ	14	2	NR	NR	30-day mortality
				CLX	13	2–8	NR	NR	
Li 2014 [16]	MC retrospective cohort study	USA	2008–2012	CFZ	59	6	31	7	30-day all-cause mortality
				OXA	34	12	39	18	90-day all-cause mortality
Bai 2015 [17]	MC retrospective PS-matched cohort study	Canada	2007–2010	CFZ	105	3	NR	10	90-day mortality
				CLX	249	12	NR	18	
Rao 2015 [18]	MC retrospective cohort study	USA	2010–2013	CFZ	103	6	29	41.8	All-cause in-hospital mortality
				OXA	58	12	32.5	32.8	
Pollett 2016 [19]	SC prospective PS-matched cohort study	USA	2008–2013	CFZ	70	NR	20	13	90-day all-cause mortality
				NAF	30	NR	12	27	
Flynt 2017 [20]	MC retrospective cohort study	USA	2013–2015	CFZ	68	6	NR	NR	30-day all-cause mortality
				NAF	81	12	NR	NR	
McDanel 2017 [21]	MC retrospective cohort study	USA	2003–2010	CFZ	1163	NR	NR	15	30-day all-cause mortality
				NAF/ OXA	2004	NR	NR	19	90-day all-cause mortality
Lee 2018 [22]	MC prospective PS-matched cohort study	South Korea	2013–2015	CFZ	79	NR	NR	NR	90-day all-cause mortality
				NAF	163	NR	NR	NR	30-day all-cause mortality

CFZ cefazolin, *CLX* cloxacillin, *MC* multicenter, *NAF* nafcillin, *NR* not reported, *OXA* oxacillin, *PS* propensity score, *SC* single center

Secondary outcomes

Clinical failure was variably defined and reported in five studies [13, 16, 18, 20, 22]. The cefazolin group had a significantly lower clinical failure (OR, 0.56; 95% CI, 0.37 to 0.85; $I^2 = 44.9\%$). Eight studies reported the recurrence of bacteremia [13, 15–18, 20–22]. The results indicate no significant difference in the recurrence of bacteremia between the two groups (OR, 1.12; 95% CI, 0.94 to 1.34; $I^2 = 0\%$). Data on the number of AEs were reported in five studies [15, 16, 18, 20, 22]. No significant differences in AEs rates between the two group were found with high consistency (OR, 0.37; 95% CI, 0.10 to 10.14; $I^2 = 83.1\%$). The most common AEs included hepatotoxicity (e.g., elevated transaminases), nephrotoxicity (e.g., elevated serum creatinine), and hematotoxicity (e.g., leukopenia, neutropenia). There were no significant differences in the risks of anaphylaxis (OR, 0.91; 95% CI, 0.36 to 2.99; $I^2 = 0\%$) and hematotoxicity (OR, 0.56; 95% CI, 0.17 to 1.88; $I^2 = 0\%$). However, we found nephrotoxicity (OR, 0.36; 95% CI, 0.16 to 0.81; $I^2 = 0\%$) and hepatotoxicity (OR, 0.12; 95% CI, 0.04 to 0.41; $I^2 = 0\%$) were significantly lower in the cefazolin group than in the ASPs group. Only three studies [13, 16, 22] compared the discontinuation due to AE. The results indicate that cefazolin was associated with lower probability of being discontinuation of treatment due to AEs compared with the ASPs (OR, 0.24; 95% CI, 0.12 to 0.48; $I^2 = 18\%$) (Table 3 and Additional file 2: Figure S1-S8).

Publication bias

Visual inspection of funnel plot showed the presence of a moderate publication bias (Fig. 3). Begg's test was not significant ($P = 0.152$), but Egger's test showed the presence of publication bias ($P = 0.043$). Fail-safe methods indicated that 56 publications would be needed to convert our estimated result.

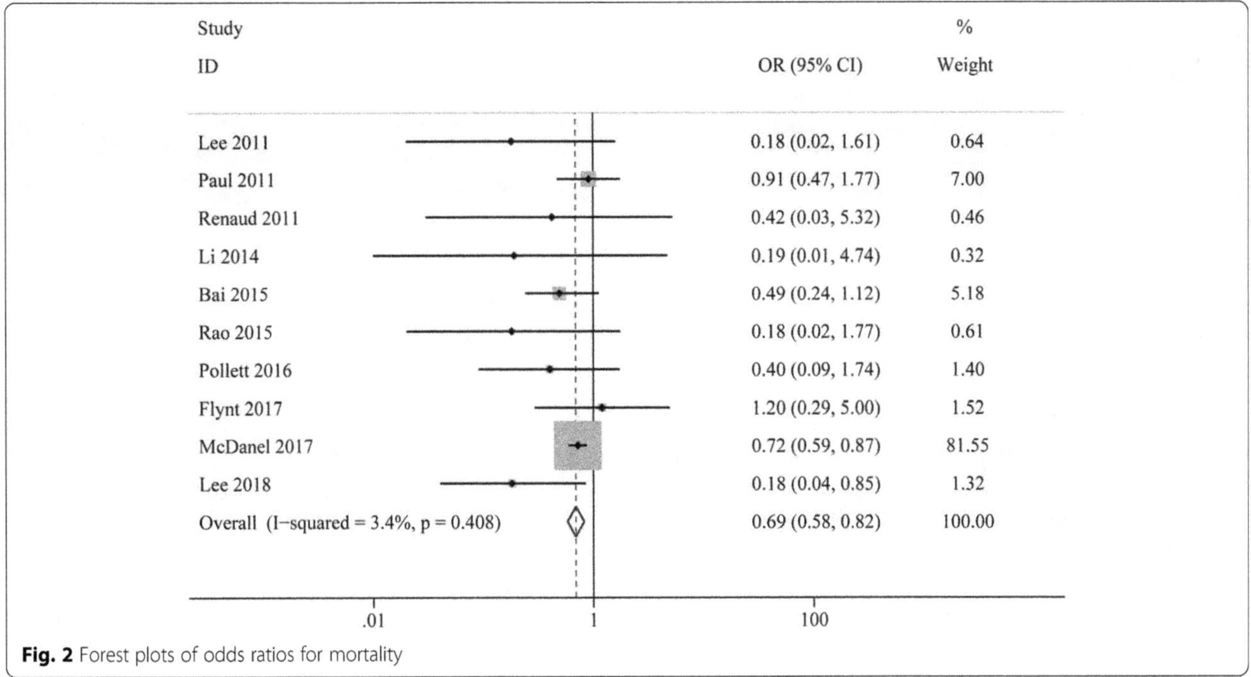

Fig. 2 Forest plots of odds ratios for mortality

Discussion

This meta-analysis systematically reviewed studies focusing on the efficacy and safety of cefazolin and ASPs in treating bacteremia caused by MSSA. The results of our meta-analysis demonstrated that cefazolin was associated with a significant reduction in mortality and clinical failure without increasing recurrence of bacteremia, when compared to ASPs. In addition, the safety of cefazolin was superior to ASPs, especially regarding the risk of hepatotoxicity and nephrotoxicity.

Table 2 Subgroup analysis of mortality with cefazolin versus ASPs for the treatment of MSSA bacteremia

Variable	No. of studies	No. of patients	OR (95% CI)	*P* Value	I^2%
Study design					
Retrospective	8	4212	0.71 (0.59–0.84)	0.57	0
Prospective	2	258	0.27 (0.09–0.79)	0.46	0
Location					
USA	5	3670	0.71 (0.59–0.86)	0.52	0
Other	5	800	0.57 (0.36–0.91)	0.25	25.4
Study period					
Initiated before 2008	4	3782	0.58 (0.36–0.92)	0.15	43.4
Initiated after 2008	6	688	0.71 (0.59–0.85)	0.64	0
Mortality recording time					
30-day mortality	6	3676	0.60 (0.48–0.75)	0.81	0
90-day mortality	7	4133	0.69 (0.58–0.82)	0.30	16.9
Adjustment					
Propensity score matched or multiple adjusted	6	4040	0.69 (0.58–0.83)	0.26	23.6
Unadjusted	10	4779	0.74 (0.64–0.87)	0.11	37.6
Control group					
NAF or OXA	7	3910	0.69 (0.57–0.83)	0.26	22.6
CLX	3	560	0.69 (0.42–1.12)	0.46	0

ASPs antistaphylococcal penicillins, *CFZ* cefazolin, *CI* confidence interval, *CLX* cloxacillin, *MSSA* methicillin-susceptible *Staphylococcus aureus*, *NAF* nafcillin, *OR* odds ratio, *OXA* oxacillin

Table 3 Meta-analysis of each secondary outcome

Outcome	No. of studies	No. of patients	OR (95% CI)	*P* Value	I^2%	Effects model
Clinical failure	5	778	0.56 (0.37–0.85)	0.12	44.9	Fixed
Recurrence of bacteremia	8	4017	1.12 (0.94–1.34)	0.80	0	Fixed
AEs	5	672	0.37 (0.10–1.41)	0	83.1	Random
Hepatotoxicity	4	645	0.12 (0.04–0.41)	0.51	0	Fixed
Nephrotoxicity	3	484	0.36 (0.16–0.81)	0.88	0	Fixed
Anaphylaxis	5	672	0.91 (0.36–2.99)	0.53	0	Fixed
Hematotoxicity	4	511	0.56 (0.17–1.88)	0.42	0	Fixed
Discontinuation due to AEs	3	468	0.24 (0.12–0.48)	0.30	18	Fixed

AEs adverse effects, *CI* confidence interval, *OR* odds ratio

The results of the primary outcome were robust and were not significantly altered during most of the subgroup and sensitivity analyses. A subgroup analysis based on the control group showed that the non-significant association in the analysis of the studies in which the control group was cloxacillin could be due to lack of power, as the trend towards lower mortality with cefazolin was evident. Although Egger's test showed significant publication bias, the fail-safe number was large enough ($n = 56$).

Regarding the safety profile, this present study supported the superior tolerability of cefazolin over ASPs. A recent meta-analysis (published after completion of our work) also reviewed the literature comparing the safety of cefazolin and ASPs for the treatment of MSSA infections [23]. Although the previous meta-analysis focused on MSSA infections but not MSSA bacteremia, these results are consistent with our findings. The results of this study showed that cefazolin was associated with lower rates of nephrotoxicity and hepatotoxicity compared with ASPs among hospitalized patients or outpatients treated for MSSA infections. Moreover, cefazolin was associated with lower probability of discontinuation due to AEs in hospitalized patients and hypersensitivity reactions in outpatients [23].

In clinical practice, the preference for ASPs over cefazolin for MSSA bacteremia is primarily due to concerns about the inoculum effect. The inoculum effect has been defined as a significant elevation in the cefazolin minimum inhibitory concentration with an inoculum higher than standard bacterial inoculum [24]. This is usually due to the production of a type A β-lactamase that can hydrolyze cefazolin [25]. Two recent review articles summarized clinical reports focused on cefazolin inoculum effect [9, 10]. However, most of these reports are case reports or case series and no study show any significant difference in outcomes when comparing isolates

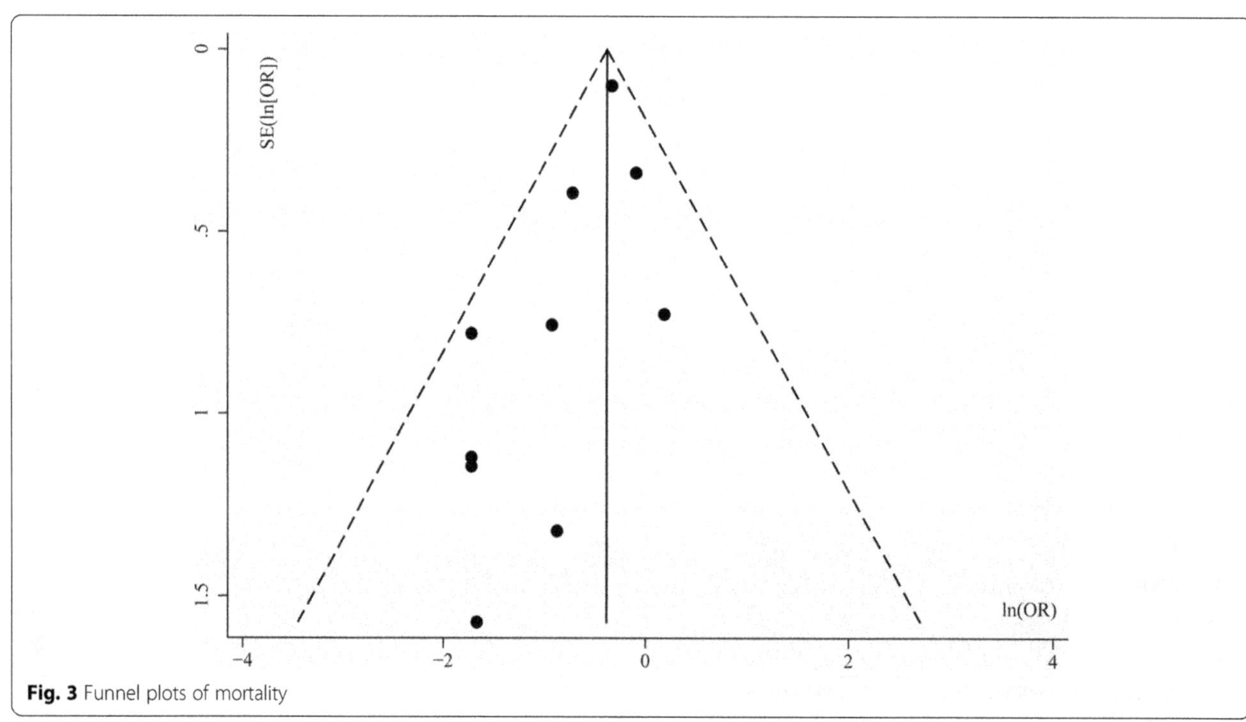

Fig. 3 Funnel plots of mortality

with or without the inoculum effect [26–28]. A recent study by Lee et al. found that treatment failure (61.5% vs. 28.9%) and mortality (15.4% vs. 0%) were significantly higher in the inoculum effect-positive arm than in the negative arm among patients who received cefazolin [22]. Therefore, the clinical relevance of the cefazolin inoculum effect is still unclear. More properly designed studies comparing cefazolin to ASPs for high-inoculum MSSA bacteremia, such as endocarditis, are required.

The selection of a regimen for the treatment of MSSA bacteremia is primarily based on efficacy, safety, costs and availability. In addition to the reduction in mortality, clinical failure, risks of hepatotoxicity and nephrotoxicity, and the probability of discontinuation due to AEs as noted above, cefazolin offers several additional advantages such as being less expensive and being more convenient to dose [15, 18]. Taken together, the evidence of supports a beneficial effect of cefazolin over ASPs for MSSA bacteremia in the absence of endocarditis or high-burden infection.

Two recent meta-analyses (both published after completion of our work) have compared the use of cefazolin and ASPs for the treatment of MSSA bacteremia [29, 30]. The conclusions of these two meta-analyses were similar and consistent: the survival rates and safety profiles of cefazolin were superior to ASPs. The meta-analysis conducted by Bidell et al. concluded that cefazolin was associated with a significant reduction in all-cause 90-day mortality (OR, 0.63; 95% CI, 0.41 to 0.99; $I^2 = 58\%$) and discontinuation due to AEs (OR, 0.25; 95% CI, 0.11 to 0.56; $I^2 = 13\%$), when compared to ASPs [29]. Another meta-analysis conducted by Rindone et al. demonstrated that the mortality (RR, 0.78; 95% CI, 0.69–0.88; $I^2 = 51\%$) and withdrawals from AEs (RR, 0.27; 95% CI, 0.16 to 0.47; $I^2 = 37\%$) were significantly lower in the cefazolin group than in the ASPs group [30]. These two meta-analyses had some differences compared with ours: (i) these two previous meta-analyses did not report the differences in AEs rates. Our study compared the differences in AEs (e.g., hepatotoxicity, nephrotoxicity, hematotoxicity, and anaphylaxis) between the cefazolin and ASPs and concluded the safety of cefazolin was superior to ASPs, especially regarding the risk of hepatotoxicity and nephrotoxicity; (ii) our meta-analysis demonstrated that the clinical failure was significantly lower in the cefazolin group than in the ASPs group. However, the meta-analysis by Bidell et al. found no significant differences in clinical failure rate between the two groups [29]. The difference may be due to the included studies. Of note, the meta-analysis conducted by Bidell et al. included only seven out of the ten observational studies analyzed in our meta-analysis. Moreover, two original studies [17, 21] included in the meta-analysis did not report the clinical failure rate. However, these two original studies were used in the analysis of clinical failure in the meta-analysis conducted by Bidell et al. [29]; (iii) all analyses were conducted unadjusted in these two previous meta-analyses. It is commonly believed that adjusted estimates are consistently closer to the true values than unadjusted estimates. The present meta-analysis used the adjusted estimates if appropriate and presented separate subgroup analyses of adjusted or unadjusted estimates.

There were several limitations that should be considered. First, all studies included in the present meta-analysis were observational studies, which have a high selection bias and may expose the analysis to confounders. For example, patients in the ASPs treatment arms had numerically higher rates of endocarditis [13, 17, 18, 20, 22] and ICU admission [16, 17, 19, 21]. The subgroup analysis of the adjusted odds ratios of primary outcome continued to favor cefazolin. Although these publications tried to adjust for the confounders, residual confounding factors remain. Second, despite the absence of statistical heterogeneity, the inherent heterogeneity across the studies analyzed (i.e., source of bacteremia, source control, dose and duration, etc.) should not be discounted. Third, as the source of bloodstream infection were diverse in the present study, we could not conclude that cefazolin was superior to ASPs for a specific type of bacteremia, especially in deep-seated infection, such as endocarditis.

Conclusion

The results of present study favor the application of cefazolin for the treatment of MSSA bacteremia. Therefore, we suggest that cefazolin be used as a first-line regimen for MMSA bacteremia in the absence of endocarditis or high-burden infection. Our study should be regarded as important evidence to help make clinical decisions in choosing a treatment option for MSSA bacteremia.

Abbreviations

AEs: Adverse effects; ASPs: Antistaphylococcal penicillins; CFZ: Cefazolin; CIs: Confidence intervals; CLX: Cloxacillin; MC: Multicenter; MRSA: Methicillin-resistant *Staphylococcus aureus*; MSSA: Methicillin-susceptible *Staphylococcus aureus*; NAF: Nafcillin; NOS: Newcastle-Ottawa scale; NR: Not reported; OR: Odds ratio; OXA: Oxacillin; PS: Propensity score; SC: Single center

Funding

This work was supported by Zhejiang Provincial Program for the Cultivation of High-level Innovative Health Talents (grant number: 2010-190-4), Clinical Pharmacy of Zhejiang Medical Key Discipline (grant number: 2018-2-3) and Clinical Pharmacy of Hangzhou Medical Key Discipline (grant number: 2017-68-7).

Authors' contributions

Conceived and designed the protocol: LNM and SCC. Execution of literature search: SCC and XYB. Execution of data extraction: SCC and WJ. Execution of quality assessment: XYB and ZQ. Data analysis and interpretation: SCC, ZQ, LQY and WF. All authors have read and approved the final manuscript.

Competing interests
The authors declare that they have no competing interests.

Author details
[1]Department of Clinical Pharmacy, Affiliated Hangzhou First People's Hospital, Zhejiang University School of Medicine, Hangzhou, China. [2]Department of Clinical Pharmacy, Hangzhou First People's Hospital, Nanjing Medical University, Hangzhou, China. [3]Department of Pharmacometrics, Mosim Co., Ltd, Shanghai, China. [4]Department of Pharmacy, Hangzhou Obstetrics & Gynecology Hospital, Hangzhou, China. [5]Department of Clinical Pharmacology, Translational Medicine Research Center, Affiliated Hangzhou First People's Hospital, Zhejiang University School of Medicine, Hangzhou, China.

References

1. Laupland KB, Lyytikäinen O, Søgaard M, Kennedy KJ, Knudsen JD, Ostergaard C, et al. The changing epidemiology of Staphylococcus aureus bloodstream infection: a multinational population-based surveillance study. Clin Microbiol Infect. 2013;19:465–71.
2. Cosgrove SE, Sakoulas G, Perencevich EN, Schwaber MJ, Karchmer AW, Carmeli Y. Comparison of mortality associated with methicillinresistant and methicillin-susceptible Staphylococcus aureus bacteremia: a meta-analysis. Clin Infect Dis. 2003;36:53–9.
3. McDanel JS, Perencevich EN, Diekema DJ, Herwaldt LA, Smith TC, Chrischilles EA, et al. Comparative effectiveness of beta-lactams versus vancomycin for treatment of methicillin-susceptible Staphylococcus aureus bloodstream infections among 122 hospitals. Clin Infect Dis. 2015;61:361–7.
4. Wong D, Wong T, Romney M, Leung V. Comparative effectiveness of β-lactam versus vancomycin empiric therapy in patients with methicillin-susceptible Staphylococcus aureus (MSSA) bacteremia. Ann Clin Microbiol Antimicrob. 2016;15:27.
5. Baddour LM, Wilson WR, Bayer AS, Fowler VG Jr, Tleyjeh IM, Rybak MJ, et al. Infective endocarditis in adults: diagnosis, antimicrobial therapy, and management of complications: a scientific statement for healthcare professionals from the american heart association. Circulation. 2015;132: 1435–86.
6. Gudiol F, Aguado JM, Almirante B, Bouza E, Cercenado E, Domínguez MÁ, et al. Diagnosis and treatment of bacteremia and endocarditis due to Staphylococcus aureus. A clinical guideline from the Spanish Society of Clinical Microbiology and Infectious Diseases (SEIMC). Enferm Infecc Microbiol Clin. 2015;33(625):e1–e23.
7. Liu C, Bayer A, Cosgrove SE, Daum RS, Fridkin SK, Gorwitz RJ, et al. Clinical practice guidelines by the infectious diseases society of america for the treatment of methicillin-resistant Staphylococcus aureus infections in adults and children. Clin Infect Dis. 2011;52:e18–55.
8. Mermel LA, Allon M, Bouza E, Craven DE, Flynn P, O'Grady NP, et al. Clinical practice guidelines for the diagnosis and management of intravascular catheter-related infection: 2009 update by the Infectious Diseases Society of America. Clin Infect Dis. 2009;49:1–45.
9. Li J, Echevarria KL, Traugott KA. β-Lactam therapy for methicillin-susceptible Staphylococcus aureus bacteremia: a comparative review of cefazolin versus antistaphylococcal penicillins. Pharmacotherapy. 2017;37: 346–60.
10. Loubet P, Burdet C, Vindrios W, Grall N, Wolff M, Yazdanpanah Y, et al. Cefazolin versus anti-staphylococcal penicillins for treatment of methicillin-susceptible Staphylococcus aureus bacteraemia: a narrative review. Clin Microbiol Infect. 2018;24:125–32.
11. Higgins JPT, Green S. Cochrane handbook for systematic reviews of interventions. Version 5.1.0. Cochrane Collaboration. 2011. https://handbook-5-1.cochrane.org.
12. Stang A. Critical evaluation of the Newcastle-Ottawa scale for the assessment of the quality of nonrandomized studies in meta-analyses. Eur J Epidemiol. 2010;25:603–5.
13. Lee S, Choe PG, Song KH, Park SW, Kim HB, Kim NJ, et al. Is cefazolin inferior to nafcillin for treatment of methicillin-susceptible Staphylococcus aureus bacteremia? Antimicrob Agents Chemother. 2011;55:5122–6.
14. Paul M, Zemer-Wassercug N, Talker O, Lishtzinsky Y, Lev B, Samra Z, et al. Are all beta-lactams similarly effective in the treatment of methicillin-sensitive Staphylococcus aureus bacteraemia? Clin Microbiol Infect. 2011;17:1581–6.
15. Renaud CJ, Lin X, Subramanian S, Fisher DA. High-dose cefazolin on consecutive hemodialysis in anuric patients with staphylococcal bacteremia. Hemodial Int. 2011;15:63–8.
16. Li J, Echevarria KL, Hughes DW, Cadena JA, Bowling JE, Lewis JS 2nd. Comparison of cefazolin versus oxacillin for treatment of complicated bacteremia caused by methicillin-susceptible Staphylococcus aureus. Antimicrob Agents Chemother. 2014;58:5117–24.
17. Bai AD, Showler A, Burry L, Steinberg M, Ricciuto DR, Fernandes T, et al. Comparative effectiveness of cefazolin versus cloxacillin as definitive antibiotic therapy for MSSA bacteraemia: results from a large multicentre cohort study. J Antimicrob Chemother. 2015;70:1539–46.
18. Rao SN, Rhodes NJ, Lee BJ, Scheetz MH, Hanson AP, Segreti J, et al. Treatment outcomes with cefazolin versus oxacillin for deep-seated methicillin-susceptible Staphylococcus aureus bloodstream infections. Antimicrob Agents Chemother. 2015;59:5232–8.
19. Pollett S, Baxi SM, Rutherford GW, Doernberg SB, Bacchetti P, Chambers HF. Cefazolin versus Nafcillin for methicillin-sensitive Staphylococcus aureus bloodstream infection in a California tertiary medical center. Antimicrob Agents Chemother. 2016;60:4684–9.
20. Flynt LK, Kenney RM, Zervos MJ, Davis SL. The safety and economic impact of cefazolin versus Nafcillin for the treatment of methicillin-susceptible Staphylococcus aureus bloodstream infections. Infect Dis Ther. 2017;6:225–31.
21. McDanel JS, Roghmann MC, Perencevich EN, Ohl ME, Goto M, Livorsi DJ, et al. Comparative effectiveness of cefazolin versus nafcillin or oxacillin for treatment of methicillin-susceptible Staphylococcus aureus infections complicated by bacteremia: a nationwide cohort study. Clin Infect Dis. 2017;65:100–6.
22. Lee S, Song KH, Jung SI, Park WB, Lee SH, Kim YS, et al. Comparative outcomes of cefazolin versus nafcillin for methicillin-susceptible Staphylococcus aureus bacteraemia: a prospective multicentre cohort study in Korea. Clin Microbiol Infect. 2018;24:152–8.
23. Eljaaly K, Alshehri S, Erstad BL. Systematic review and meta-analysis of the safety of Antistaphylococcal Penicillins compared to cefazolin. Antimicrob Agents Chemother. 2018. https://doi.org/10.1128/AAC.01816-17.
24. Soriano F, García-Corbeira P, Ponte C, Fernández-Roblas R, Gadea I. Correlation of pharmacodynamic parameters of five beta-lactam antibiotics with therapeutic efficacies in an animal model. Antimicrob Agents Chemother. 1996;40:2686–90.
25. Lee SH, Park WB, Lee S, Park S, Kim SW, Lee JM, et al. Association between type a blaZ gene polymorphism and cefazolin inoculum effect in methicillin-susceptible Staphylococcus aureus. Antimicrob Agents Chemother. 2016;60:6928–32.
26. Nannini EC, Stryjewski ME, Singh KV, Bourgogne A, Rude TH, Corey GR, et al. Inoculum effect with cefazolin among clinical isolates of methicillin-susceptible Staphylococcus aureus: frequency and possible cause of cefazolin treatment failure. Antimicrob Agents Chemother. 2009;53:3437–41.
27. Chong YP, Park SJ, Kim ES, Bang KM, Kim MN, Kim SH, et al. Prevalence of blaZ gene types and the cefazolin inoculum effect among methicillin-susceptible Staphylococcus aureus blood isolates and their association with multilocus sequence types and clinical outcome. Eur J Clin Microbiol Infect Dis. 2015;34:349–55.
28. Lee S, Kwon KT, Kim HI, Chang HH, Lee JM, Choe PG, et al. Clinical implications of cefazolin inoculum effect and β-lactamase type on methicillin-susceptible Staphylococcus aureus bacteremia. Microb Drug Resist. 2014;20:568–74.
29. Bidell MR, Patel N, O'Donnell JN. Optimal treatment of MSSA bacteraemias: a meta-analysis of cefazolin versus antistaphylococcal penicillins. J Antimicrob Chemother. 2018. https://doi.org/10.1093/jac/dky259.
30. Rindone JP, Mellen CK. Meta-analysis of trials comparing cefazolin to antistaphylococcal penicillins in the treatment of methicillin-sensitive Staphylococcus aureus bacteraemia. Br J Clin Pharmacol. 2018;84:1258–66.

7

No polymorphisms in K13-propeller gene associated with artemisinin resistance in *Plasmodium falciparum* isolated from Brazzaville, Republic of Congo

Pembe Issamou Mayengue[1,2*], Roch Fabien Niama[1,2], Dezi Kouhounina Batsimba[1], Alida Malonga-Massanga[1], Igor Louzolo[2], Nadia Claricelle Loukabou Bongolo[2], Lucette Macosso[2], Reyna Ibara Ottia[1], Ghyslain Kimbassa Ngoma[1], Louis Régis Dossou-Yovo[2,3], Brice Pembet Singana[1], Gabriel Ahombo[1], Géril Sekangue Obili[4], Simon Charles Kobawila[1] and Henri Joseph Parra[2]

Abstract

Background: In the Republic of Congo, artemisinin-based combinations have been recommended for the treatment of uncomplicated malaria since 2006. However, the emergence of resistant parasites again these combinations in Southeast Asia is a threat for the control of this disease, especially in sub-Saharan Africa where the weight of the disease is important. Indeed, polymorphisms in *Plasmodium falciparum* K13-propeller gene have been involved in variations of drug sensitivity of *Plasmodium falciparum* to artemisinin-based combinations. The aim of the current study is to determine the prevalence of mutations of this gene in isolates collected in three health centers in Brazzaville.

Methods: From May 2015 to May 2016, a total of 131, 259 and 416 samples from patients with suspected malaria were collected at the Laboratoire National de Santé Publique, Hôpital de Mfilou, and the CSI «Maman Mboualé» respectively. After DNA isolation, genotyping and sequencing of *Plasmodium falciparum* K13-propeller were performed in positive *Plasmodium falciparum* isolates identified after *msp-2* gene genotyping.

Results: All 806 samples collected were *msp-2* genotyped and *Plasmodium falciparum* infections were confirmed in 287 samples with 43, 85, 159 samples from Laboratoire National de Santé Publique, Hôpital de Mfilou, and the CSI «Maman Mboualé» respectively. Of these 287 *msp-2* positives samples, K13-propeller nested PCR products were successfully obtained from 145 (50.52%) isolates and sequences were generated from 127(87.58%) nested products. None of mutations that were associated with ACTs resistance in Southeast Asia were detected on the samples from three different study sites from Brazzaville. However, one mutation type was observed at position 578, where alanine was substituted by serine (A578S) in two isolates (1.57%, 2/127), those from the Hôpital de Mfilou. No mutation was found in isolates from the two other sites.

Conclusion: The current study shows a very limited polymorphism in the K13-propeller gene in isolates from the Republic of Congo and K13 polymorphisms associate with ACT resistance are not present in this country. However, permanent and large surveillance of resistant parasite population using K13-propeller gene is recommended.

Keywords: *Plasmodium falciparum*, K13-propeller gene, Resistance, ACTs, Brazzaville, Republic of Congo

* Correspondence: pmayengue@yahoo.fr
[1]Faculté des Sciences et Techniques, Université Marien Ngouabi, BP 69, Brazzaville, République du Congo
[2]Laboratoire National de Santé Publique, BP 120, Brazzaville, République du Congo
Full list of author information is available at the end of the article

Background

In the Republic of Congo, malaria remains one of the main causes of consultation in health centers, with children under 15 years old and pregnant women being the most vulnerable groups [1, 2]. Like in almost all sub-Saharan African countries, the high level of resistance of *Plasmodium falciparum* to chloroquine as well as the inefficacy of sulphadoxine-pyrimethamine and amodiaquine either singly or in combination for the treatment of uncomplicated malaria have led the Republic of Congo to change its anti-malarial drug policy for treating uncomplicated malaria to artemisinin-combination therapies (ACTs) in 2006 [3]. Previous studies have shown that ACTs remain highly efficacious in Sub-Saharan Africa, including the Republic of Congo [4–7]. However, the emergence of resistance to artemisinin derivatives, including ACTs in Southeast Asia is a serious public health concern. If resistance to ACTs may spread, particularly in sub-Saharan Africa, the public health implications could be disastrous, because no alternative drug is currently available with the same level of efficacy and tolerance than ACTs. In order to limit the development of *Plasmodium falciparum* resistance to current antimalarial, the World Health Organization (WHO) has recommended a vigilant surveillance of resistant parasites [8]. Recently, five principal mutations, namely the M476I, Y493H, I543T, R539T and C580Y in the *Plasmodium falciparum* Kelch propeller domain (K13-propeller) have been found to be associated with delayed parasite clearance after ACTs therapy in Cambodia [9]. Although no mutations associated with prolonged artemisinin clearance in Southeast Asia are found in sub-Saharan African regions, while diverse others mutations are identified even in isolates collected before or after the introduction of ACTs, regular surveillance is needed, taking into consideration the critical importance of ACTs in the control and elimination of malaria in these regions [10–14]. Thus, the current study aimed at measuring the prevalence of *Plasmodium falciparum* K13-propeller polymorphisms in clinical isolates collected from Brazzaville 10 years after the introduction of ACTs.

Methods

Study areas and site preparation

Brazzaville, the political capital hosts 38% (1,642,105 inhabitants) of the total population of the Republic of Congo, estimated at 4312715 inhabitants. With the population expansion due to urbanization, Brazzaville is now divided into nine districts: Bacongo, Makelekele, Poto-Poto, Moungali, Ouenze, Talangaï, Mfilou, Madibou and Djiri. The present study was conducted in three health centers: Centre de Santé Intégré (CSI) « Maman Mboualé» located in the district of Talangaï, in the north part of city (4°13'S, 15°17′E); Hôpital de Mfilou located in the district of Mfilou, in the south part of the city (4°15'S, 15°13′E) and the Laboratoire National de Santé Publique (LNSP), the national reference laboratory located in the center part of city, in the district of Poto-Poto (4°16'S, 15°15′E).

Malaria transmission in the study areas varies from low, moderate to intense with meso-, hyper- to perennial endemicity. Malaria infection is primarily due to *P. falciparum*. Two rainy seasons are observed each year with the main one during the months of February to May, and a short one from October to December [15].

In the early project stage, first, a meeting with the site actors including the head of each laboratory and microscopists was organized for the purpose of presenting the project objectives, methodology and expected results, as well as to obtain microscopists consent.

Study population, blood samples and data collection

From May 2015 to May 2016, patients with clinical signs of uncomplicated malaria, presenting at the laboratory of one of the three study sites were invited to participate in this study. Exclusion criteria comprised pregnancy, severe malaria or other severe illness as judged by the attending physician. A number of representative patients to be included each month, per week and per day has been estimated by the statistician taking into account the proportion of malaria reported in each health center, 1 year before starting the study. In sample size calculations, considering the proportion of malaria at 73.29% for the CSI « Maman Mbouale», 87.75% for Hôpital de Mfilou and 2.33% for LNSP, using a confidence level of 95% and a marge error of 5%, the SCHWARZ method [16] yielded a minimum number of 310, 200 and 100 patients to be recruited at the CSI « Maman Mbouale», Hôpital de Mfilou and the LNSP, respectively. Recruited patients were randomly selected from Monday to Friday. At the CSI « Maman Mbouale», a minimum of 7 patients were recruited per week, with at least one patient per day, whereas, at the Hôpital de Mfilou, the minimum number was 5 patients per week, with one per day. For the LNSP, 3 patients were enough, with one included on Monday, on Wednesday and on Friday. After informed consent was obtained, records were made on patient demographics, fever or history of fever in the last 48 h, other signs of malaria, provenance, previous antimalarial drugs intake used of bed net treated. The axillary temperature was taken for fever confirmation.

At each study site, blood sample from each patient was blotted on the Whatman filter paper (3MM CHR) while preparing the thick blood smears, dried and transferred to the "Laboratoire National de Santé Publique" in Brazzaville, where isolation of deoxyribonucleic acid (DNA), polymerase chain reaction (PCR) and sequencing were performed. Before reading, thick blood smears were dried and stained with 10% Giemsa solution (Sigma

Chemical, Sigma Aldrich ChemieGmbh, Taufkirchen, Germany) in pH 7.2, for approximately 10 min. The stain was gently washed away by adding drops of clean water and the slide was completely dried before examination. Thick blood smears were assessed by micrsocopists until 200 leucocytes had been counted. Parasite density was calculated for each patient assuming an average of 8000 leucocytes per μl of blood using the proposed method of the WHO [17]. Individual diagnostic result was given to each patient and advised to meet the prescribers for possible antimalarial chemotherapy.

Extraction of parasite DNA

Genomic DNA was extracted from samples collected on the Whatman filter paper by QIAamp DNA mini Kit (Qiagen, Hilden, Germany) according to the manufacturer's instruction. Briefly, 3 circles of approximately 3 mm diameter were punched out from a blood spot and placed into a 1.5 mL micro centrifuge tube in which 180 μL of ATL buffer was added. Successive washing steps with AW1 buffer and AW2 buffer were followed by DNA elution with 150 μL of AE buffer. Extracted DNA was stored at – 20 °C until use.

Genotyping

For multiple purposes, the highly polymorphic central region of *Merozoite Surface Protein-2* (*msp-2*) gene was firstly genotyped as described previously [18], and positive *Plasmodium falciparum* samples were used for K13-propeller genotyping. PCR amplification was performed following a 2-step amplification procedure in which the initial amplifications were followed by the nested PCR reactions using specific primers K13–1 and K13–4 for the first round and K13-inF2 and K13-inR2 for the nested PCR (Table 1), flanking the codons T474I, M476I, A481V, Y493H, T508 N, P527T, G533S, N537I, R539T, I543T, P553L, R561H, V568G, P574L, A578S, and C580Y; as described by Li et al. [12]. The amplification reactions were carried out as described by Ariey et al. [9]. For the first round, 1 μL of DNA was amplified with 200 μM of each deoxynucleotide triphosphate (dNTP), 1 μM of each primer, 3 mM $MgCl_2$, 1.5 units of Taq DNA polymerase and sterile ultrapure water to a final reaction of 25 μL. The mixtures were denatured at 95 °C for 5 min, followed by 40 amplification cycles (94 ° C for 30 min, 60 °C for 1 min 30 s, and 72 °C for 1 min 30 s), and final elongation at 72 °C for 10 min. For the second round PCR, similar procedure with specific primers was used and 5 μL of the first PCR product were used as template.

All PCR products were analyzed using 2% agar gel electrophoresis. Thereafter PCR products were purified using PureLink™ Quick PCR Purification Kit (Invitrogen, by Thermo Fischer Scientific) and directly used as templates for DNA sequencing using an ABI 3500xL automated sequencer (Applied Biosystems Genetic Analyzer, HITACHI). The data was analyzed using Geneious 10.2.3 [19]. Mutations were assessed by comparing each sequence with the 3D7 K13-propeller (PF3D7_1343700) used as the reference.

Data analysis

Data were entered and verified in Microsoft Excel (Microsoft Corp., Seattle, USA) and validated in EpiInfo for Windows version 3.5.1. Data were analyzed using the SPSS 16.0 for Windows (Inc., Chicago, USA).The mutant and wild-type alleles identified in the analyzed isolates were used to generate the prevalence of the alleles.

Results

Characteristics of febrile patients with symptoms of malaria

A total of 131, 259 and 416 patients with suspected malaria were enrolled at the LNSP, Hôpital de Mfilou and the CSI «Maman Mboualé» respectively.

Out of 259 patients enrolled at the Hôpital de Mfilou, gender and age were recorded for 257 of them, while with regards to the CSI « Maman Mboualé», out of the 416 recruited patients, 410 had records on gender (Table 2).

All 806 samples collected were *msp-2* genotyped and *Plasmodium falciparum* infections were confirmed in 287 samples with 43, 85, 159 samples from LNSP, Hôpital de Mfilou, and CSI «Maman Mboualé» respectively. These *msp-2* positive samples were then considered for K13-propeller genotyping and nested PCR products was successfully obtained from 145 (50.52%) isolates, with 5, 50 and 90 from LNSP, Hôpital de Mfilou, and CSI «Maman Mboualé» respectively (Table 3). K13-propeller sequences were generated from 127(87.58%) nested

Table 1 K13- propeller primers sequences

Primer name	Sequences 5'.....3'	Size (bp)
K13–1(forward)	CGGAGTGACCAAATCTGGGA	2097
K13–4 (reverse)	GGGAATCTGGTGGTAACAGC	
K13-inF2 (forward)	TCAACAATGCTGGCGTATGTG	501
K13-inR2 (reverse)	TGATTAAG GTAATTAAAAGCTGCTCC	

Table 2 Characteristics of patients

Characteristics	LNSP	Hôpital de Mfilou	CSI « Maman Mboualé»
Total numbers	131	259	416
Gender (F/M)	68/63	131/126	207/203
Median age (years)	42 (11–74)	26 (0.5–84)	10 (0.5–75)
Groups of age (%)			
< 5 years	0 (0.0)	38 (14.8)	99 (23.8)
≥ 5 years	131 (100)	219 (85.2)	317 (76.2)

products (17 isolates did not generate good quality sequences that could be analyzed). To analyze polymorphisms in the K13-propeller, sequences alignment was done by comparing with the 3D7 strain (PF3D7_1343700).

None of mutations that were associated with ACTs resistance in Southeast Asia were detected on the samples from three different study sites from Brazzaville. However, one mutation type was observed at position 578, where alanine was substituted by serine (A578S). Only two isolates (with the frequency of 1.57%, 2/127) had carried the A578S substitution, and those from the Hôpital de Mfilou. No mutation was found in isolates from CSI « Maman Mbouалé » and LNSP.

Discussion

The present study of which all steps were carried out in Brazzaville, including K13-propeller sequencing, allowed us to analyze the polymorphism related to ACTs resistance in 127 *Plasmodium falciparum* isolates from Brazzaville. In the Republic of Congo, ACTs are recommended as first- and second-line treatment for uncomplicated malaria since 2006, and the efficacy of these combinations remains high as reported by Ndounga et al. [5, 6]. However, it is important to monitor the eventual occurrence of the ACTs-resistant parasite population. The causes of the occurrence of resistance are multiple, including self-medication, which does increase drug pressure. Although the WHO recommendations require a preliminary parasitological test before taking any ACT, it is not surprising to notice the intake of these drugs without medical prescription in Brazzaville. Resistance to artemisinin and its derivatives is considered as major risk to public health, which would have a greater impact in sub-Saharan Africa where the burden remains high. The emergence of *Plasmodium falciparum* resistance to artemisinin and its derivatives, which appear as delayed parasite clearance after ACT treatment, has been reported in Southeast Asia [20]. At the molecular level, five major mutations in the *Plasmodium falciparum* K13-propeller gene, namely the M476I, Y493H, I543T, R539T, and C580Y mutations have been found to be associated with in vitro resistance to artemisinin and delayed parasite clearance following treatment with ACTs [9]. However, in the current study none of these mutations were found. Moreover, only a single limited A578S mutation has been found only in two isolates, all from Hôpital de Mfilou. A very low proportion of this A578S mutation has been also reported in Cambodia by Straimer et al. [21] and in many sub-Saharan countries such as Uganda, Mali, Equatorial Guinea, Kenya, Democratic Republic of Congo, and Ghana [10–12, 22–24].

The treatment outcomes and parasite clearance profiles for patients with A578S mutations in the current study were not evaluated. However, study conducted in Mali has shown that parasite clearance time was comparable between infections with non-synonymous K13-propeller mutations (including A578S mutation) and infections with the reference allele [11]. Thus, due to the common presence of this mutation in many countries, further characterization is needed as well as assessment of the role of this mutation in in vivo parasite clearance in others sub-Saharan Africa countries including the Republic of Congo is required.

Furthermore, the A557S mutation detected in the Republic of Congo by Taylor et al. [25] has not been detected in the current study. None of the 13 new mutations not associated with resistance to ACTs identified in the Republic of Congo by Koukouikila-Kousounda et al. [14] were also identified in the current study. Taking into account this large

Table 3 Identification of *Plasmodium falciparum* isolates and total number of K13-propeller sequence

Sites	Number of *Plasmodium falciparum* isolates	Number of K13 nested PCR	Number of K13-propeller sequence
LNSP	43	5 (11.62%)	3 (60%)
Hôpital de Mfilou	85	50 (58.82%)	48 (96%)
CSI « Maman Mbouалé »	159	90 (56.60%)	76 (84.4%)
Total	287	145 (50.52%)	127 (87.58%)

difference, repeated studies including different sites in all departments and increasing the number of isolates to be analyzed, are needed to better characterize the actual profile of polymorphisms in the K13- propeller gene in this country.

Although none of the mutations associated with artemisinin resistance in South-East Asia are present in sub-Saharan Africa including the Republic of Congo, new mutations are emerging on the African continent [26]. Thus, the impact of these mutations on resistance to ACTs is to be explored.

Conclusion

The current study shows very limited polymorphism in the K13-propeller gene in clinical isolates from the Republic of Congo and polymorphisms associate with ACTs resistance are not present in this country. Only one mutation type was observed at position 578, where alanine was substituted by serine (A578S) in two isolates, those from the Hôpital de Mfilou. However, permanent and large surveillance of resistant parasite population using K13-propeller gene is recommended.

Abbreviations

ACTs: artemisinin-combination therapies; CERSSA: Comité d'Ethique de la Recherche en Sciences de la Santé; CSI: Centre de Santé Intégré; DNA: deoxyribonucleic acid; dNTP: deoxynucleotide triphosphate; LNSP: Laboratoire National de Santé Publique; PCR: polymerase chain reaction; WHO: World Health Organization

Acknowledgements

We are grateful to all patients and all microscopists working in our three sites, who participated in this study. We thank also Professor Michael Ramharter for carefully reading of manuscript.

Funding

The study was supported by the "Laboratoire National de Santé Publique" and the World Academy of Sciences (RGA No.16–040 RG/BIO/AF/AC_I-FR3240293321).

The "Laboratoire National de Santé Publique" has contributed in the design of the study, the collection, the analysis and interpretation of data; the World Academy of Sciences has contributed in the collection and analysis of samples as well as in writing the manuscript.

Authors' contributions

PIM designed and coordinated field study, analyzed the data and wrote the draft of the article. RFN, DKB, IL, NCLB, LM, RIO, GKN, BPS, GA, GSO, SGK, HJP supervised field samples and data collection; LRDY participated in patients recruitment; AMM analyzed samples. All authors read and approved the final version and the final manuscript.

Competing interests

The authors declare that they have no competing interests.

Author details

[1]Faculté des Sciences et Techniques, Université Marien Ngouabi, BP 69, Brazzaville, République du Congo. [2]Laboratoire National de Santé Publique, BP 120, Brazzaville, République du Congo. [3]Ecole Normale Supérieure, Université Marien Ngouabi, BP 69, Brazzaville, République du Congo. [4]Centre Hospitalier Universitaire de Brazzaville, BP 1846, Brazzaville, République du Congo.

References

1. Ministry of Health and Population. Programme Biennal de Développement Sanitaire 2015-2016. Ministère de la Santé et de la Population, Brazzaville, République du Congo. 2014.
2. Mbongo JA, Ekouya BG, Koulimaya GC, Iloki L. Paludisme Congénital au Centre Hospitalier et Universitaire de Brazzaville : une Étude Épidémiologique de 90 Cas. Health Sci Dis. 2015;16:1–4.
3. Ministry of Health and Population. Politique nationale de lutte contre le paludisme. Ministère de la Santé et de la Population, Brazzaville, République du Congo. 2006. Accessed 4 May 2018.
4. Ndounga M, Tahar R, Casimiro PN, Loumouamou D, Basco LK. Clinical efficacy of artemether lumefantrine in Congolese children with acute uncomplicated falciparum malaria in Brazzaville. Malar Res Treat. 2012;2012:749479.
5. Ndounga M, Mayengue PI, Casimiro PN, Loumouamou D, Basco LK, Ntoumi F, Brasseur P. Artesunate-amodiaquine efficacy in Congolese children with acute uncomplicated falciparum malaria in Brazzaville. Malar J. 2013;12:53.
6. Ndounga M, Mayengue PI, Casimiro PN, Koukouikila-Koussounda F, Bitemo M, Matondo DB, Ndounga DLA, Basco LK, Ntoumi F. Artesunate–amodiaquine versus artemether-lumefantrine for the treatment of acute uncomplicated malaria in Congolese children under 10 years old living in suburban area: a randomized study. Malar J. 2015;14:423.
7. Singana BP, Bogreau H, Matondo BD, Dossou-Yovo LR, Casimiro PN, Mbouka R, Ha Nguyen KY, Pradines B, Basco LK, Ndounga M. Malaria burden and anti-malarial drug efficacy in Owando, northern Congo. Malar J. 2016;15:16.
8. World Health Organizaion. Malaria report. Geneva: World Health Organization; 2015.
9. Ariey F, Witkowski B, Amaratunga C, Beghain J, Langlois AC, Khim N, et al. A molecular marker of artemisinin-resistant *Plasmodium falciparum*. Nature. 2014;505:50–5.
10. Conrad MD, Bigira V, Kapisi J, Muhindo M, Kamya MR, Havlir DV, et al. Polymorphisms in K13 and falcipain-2 associated with artemisinin resistance are not prevalent in Plasmodium falciparum isolated from Ugandan children. PLoS One. 2014;9:e105690.
11. Ouattara A, Kone A, Adams M, Fofana B, Maiga AW, Hampton S, et al. Polymorphisms in the K13-propeller gene in artemisinin-susceptible *Plasmodium falciparum* parasites from Bougoula-Hameau and Bandiagara, Mali. Am J Trop Med Hyg. 2015;92:1202–6.
12. Li J, Chen J, Xie D, Eyi UM, Matesa RA, Ondo Obono MM, et al. Limited artemisinin resistance-associated polymorphisms in *Plasmodium falciparum* K13-propeller and PfATPase6 gene isolated from Bioko Island, Equatorial Guinea. Int J Parasitol Drugs Drug Resist. 2016;6:54–9.
13. Mita T, Culleton R, Takahashi N, Nakamura M, Tsukahara T, Hunja CW, et al. Little polymorphism at the K13 propeller locus in worldwide *Plasmodium falciparum* populations prior to the introduction of artemisinin combination therapies. Antimicrob Agents Chemother. 2016;60:3340–7.
14. Koukouikila-Koussounda F, Jeyaraj S, Nguetse CN, Nkonganyi CN, Kokou KC, Etoka-Beka MK, et al. Molecular surveillance of *Plasmodium falciparum* drug resistance in the republic of Congo: four and nine years after the introduction of artemisinin-based combination therapy. Malar J. 2017;16:155.
15. Ntoumi F, Vouvoungui JC, Ibara R, Landry M, Sidibé A. Malaria burden and case management in the republic of Congo: limited use and application of rapid diagnostic tests results. BMC Public Health. 2013;13:135.
16. Schwartz D. Méthodes statistiques à l'usage des médecins et des biologistes /Troisième édition. Paris: Flammarion Médecine-sciences. 1969; ISBN-2-257-30326-1; http://www.sudoc.fr/005623065.
17. World Health Organization. Bench aids for malaria Microscopy. Geneva. 2009; ISBN-13 9789241547864.
18. Mayengue PI, Ndounga M, Malonga FV, Bitemo M, Ntoumi F. Genetic polymorphism of mérozoïte surface protein-1 and merozoite surface protein-2 in *Plasmodium falciparum* isolates from Brazzaville, republic of Congo. Malar J. 2011;10:276.
19. Kearse M, Moir R, Wilson A, Stones-Havas S, Cheung M, Sturrock S, et al. Geneious basic: an integrated and extendable desktop software platform for the organization and analysis of sequence data. Bioinformatics. 2012;28:1647–9.
20. Dondorp AM, Nosten F, Yi P, Das D, Phyo AP, Tarning J, et al. Artemisinin resistance in *Plasmodium falciparum* malaria. J Trop Med. 2009;5:455–67.
21. Straimer J, Gnadig NF, Witkowski B, Amaratunga C, Duru V, Ramadani AP, et al. Drug resistance K13-propeller mutations confer artemisinin resistance in *Plasmodium alciparum* clinical isolates. Science. 2015;347:428–31.
22. Muwanguzi J, Henriques G, Sawa P, Bousema P, Colin J, Sutherland Beshir K. Lack of K13 mutations in *Plasmodium falciparum* persisting after artemisinin combination therapy treatment of Kenyan children. Malar J. 2016;15:36.

23. Makaba MD, Kayembe M, Situakibanza HT, Bobanga LC, Nsibu GN, Mvumbi P, et al. Falciparum malaria molecular drug resistance in the Democratic Republic of Congo: a systematic. Malar J. 2015;14:354.
24. Feng J, Li J, Yan H, Feng X, Xia Z. Evaluation of antimalarial resistance marker polymorphism in returned migrant workers in China. Antimicrob Agents Chemother. 2015;59:326–30.
25. Taylor SM, Parobek CM, DeConti DK, Kayentao K, Coulibaly SO, Greenwood BM, et al. Absence of putative artemisinin resistance mutations among plasmodium falciparum in sub-Saharan Africa: a molecular epidemiologic study. J Infect Dis. 2014;211:680–8.
26. Conrad MD, LeClair N, Arinaitwe E, Wanzira H, Kakuru A, Bigira V, et al. Comparative impacts over 5 years of artemisininbasedcombination therapies on *Plasmodium falciparum* polymorphismsthat modulate drug sensitivity in Ugandan children. J Infect Dis. 2014;210:344–53.

8

Zoonotic disease research in East Africa

Naomi Kemunto[1,2], Eddy Mogoa[3], Eric Osoro[1,2], Austin Bitek[4], M. Kariuki Njenga[1,2,5] and S. M. Thumbi[1,2,5*]

Abstract

Background: The East African region is endemic with multiple zoonotic diseases and is one of the hotspots for emerging infectious zoonotic diseases with reported multiple outbreaks of epidemic diseases such as Ebola, Marburg and Rift Valley Fever. Here we present a systematic assessment of published research on zoonotic diseases in the region and thesis research in Kenya to understand the regional research focus and trends in publications, and estimate proportion of theses research transitioning to peer-reviewed journal publications.

Methods: We searched PubMed, Google Scholar and African Journals Online databases for publications on 36 zoonotic diseases identified to have occurred in the East Africa countries of Burundi, Ethiopia, Kenya, Tanzania, Rwanda and Uganda, for the period between 1920 and 2017. We searched libraries and queried online repositories for masters and PhD theses on these diseases produced between 1970 and 2016 in five universities and two research institutions in Kenya.

Results: We identified 771 journal articles on 22, and 168 theses on 21 of the 36 zoonotic diseases investigated. Research on zoonotic diseases increased exponentially with the last 10 years of our study period contributing more than half of all publications 460 (60%) and theses 102 (61%) retrieved. Endemic diseases were the most studied accounting for 656 (85%) and 150 (89%) of the publication and theses studies respectively, with publications on epidemic diseases associated with outbreaks reported in the region or elsewhere. Epidemiological studies were the most common study types but limited to cross-sectional studies while socio-economics were the least studied. Only 11% of the theses research transitioned to peer-review publications, taking an average of 2.5 years from theses production to manuscript publication.

Conclusion: Our findings demonstrate increased attention to zoonotic diseases in East Africa but reveal the need to expand the scope, focus and quality of studies to adequately address the public health, social and economic threats posed by zoonoses.

Keywords: Zoonoses, East Africa, Endemic, Epidemic, Research

Background

Nearly two-thirds of human infectious diseases and majority of emerging infectious diseases exerting heavy public health and economic burden to the global community originate from animals [1–3]. Based on their impact and epidemiological characteristics, these zoonotic diseases have been categorized into the more common endemic zoonoses such as salmonellosis, brucellosis and leptospirosis which are responsible for more than 2.2 million human deaths and 2.4 billion cases of illness annually, and the less common epidemic and emerging zoonoses such as anthrax, Rift Valley fever, Ebola, Zika which either occur in sporadic outbreaks in neglected populations or that are new or re-appearing with increased incidence or geographical range [4].

Zoonoses and diseases recently emerged from animals have been estimated to contribute more than a quarter of the disability-adjusted life years (DALYs) lost to infectious diseases in low income settings such as sub-Saharan Africa, and less than 1% in high income countries [5]. The attention given to zoonotic diseases has however focused more on emerging zoonoses that pose global economic and health threats and less on the endemic zoonotic diseases which tend to occur among populations with little political voice [6–8].

The emergence of zoonotic diseases has been accompanied by research to understand when, how, and where

* Correspondence: thumbi.mwangi@wsu.edu
[1]Paul G. Allen School for Global Animal Health, Washington State University, Pullman, USA
[2]Washington State University Global Health Program Kenya, Nairobi, Kenya
Full list of author information is available at the end of the article

they emerge, their pathogenesis and progression, diagnostics and treatment, and strategies for their prevention and control [9, 10]. Taking the example of the recent emergence of HIV, research has played a critical role to understand when and from where HIV emerged, understanding its transmission and pathogenesis, development of anti-retroviral drugs, and prevention modalities that have made its control as a global pandemic possible [10]. Thorough research, environmental, biological, economic and social drivers of disease emergence have been identified [11, 12], hotspots for emergence of wildlife and vector-borne zoonotic diseases identified to be regions in the lower latitudes [3].

Here we focus on East Africa region which has been identified as one of the zoonoses hotspot regions with a high prevalence of endemic zoonotic diseases [4], and where like in the rest of sub-Saharan Africa has a large rural population that lives in close proximity with livestock and wildlife. In order to understand the regional research trends on zoonotic diseases, we conduct a systematic assessment of published literature on zoonotic diseases in the region and theses research in Kenya, characterize the publications, and determine the transition of theses research to peer-reviewed publications.

Methods

Selection of zoonotic diseases and search strategy

We used a list of 36 zoonotic diseases suspected or known to be present in the East Africa region identified by a team of public health and veterinary experts in zoonoses in Kenya (see Table 3 in the referenced article) [13]. Using PubMed, Google scholar and African Journal of Science, we searched for published articles on these zoonotic diseases in Kenya, Uganda, Tanzania, Burundi, Rwanda and Ethiopia for the period between 1920 and 2017. The search terms included a combination of the zoonotic disease and the East Africa region and then in the specific country e.g. 'Anthrax East Africa'; 'Anthrax Kenya'; 'Anthrax Tanzania'; 'Anthrax Uganda'; 'Anthrax Ethiopia'; 'Anthrax Rwanda'; 'Anthrax Burundi'. References in the identified articles were reviewed for additional publications. Only articles in English or in French with an English abstract on research on any of the 36 zoonotic diseases conducted in any of the East Africa countries were considered for further evaluation.

In addition, we conducted a review of MSc and PhD theses submitted to five major universities in Kenya (University of Nairobi, Jomo Kenyatta University of Agriculture and Technology, Moi University, Egerton University and Kenyatta University) that have offered graduate training in either medical, veterinary, or public health for at least 20 years. We included theses research available in two biomedical research institutions in Kenya: the Kenya Medical Research Institute and Institute of Primate Research.

The theses search at the Universities and research institutions was carried out in two stages. The first stage included a systematic search of online repositories of the various study institutions queried using search terms for each of the specific zoonotic diseases of interest e.g. 'Anthrax', 'Trypanosomiasis'. Stage two entailed visiting each institution's library and conducting a physical verification of the theses and dissertations, and updating the list generated in stage-one. Information including thesis title, author names and year of degree award were counter-checked and verified. Researchers at the Kenya Medical Research Institute and the Institute of Primate Research were contacted and requested to provide information on relevant theses and dissertations awarded in any of the five study universities available in their institutions' libraries. The theses and dissertations selected were based on the following inclusion criteria: i) theses and dissertations with data on any of the 36 zoonotic diseases of interest ii) research carried out in Kenya between the period 1970–2016. For diseases such as trypanosomiasis, schistosomiasis and leishmaniasis with both zoonotic and non-zoonotic species, only studies specific to zoonotic species were considered.

Data management and cleaning

Data variables extracted from the identified articles and theses included author, title, country, disease studied, pathogen species, journal, affiliation institution of first author, year of publication/year degree award, University name, subject of the study and study species (human or livestock or wildlife). By comparing details of the theses and journal publications retrieved, we determined theses research that had been published in peer-reviewed journals.

For analysis, the studies were classified into any of three categories: laboratory, epidemiology or socio-economic studies. A study was considered a laboratory study if it was an experimental study conducted within a laboratory setting, or studies developing, testing or comparing diagnostic methods. Studies were considered epidemiological if they determined the distribution, prevalence, incidence, mortality and morbidity rate, associated risk factors, knowledge and practices and control and prevention of the disease. Epidemiological studies were further classified based on the epidemiological study design to determine the most common design methods used. Studies determining the socio-economic impact of zoonotic diseases in either humans, animals or both were classified under socio-economic category. All the data were entered into an Excel spreadsheet, and imported in to R statistical software for analysis [14].

Results

Study selection

A total of 1170 articles were retrieved from PubMed and an additional 10 from Google Scholar and five from African Journals Online databases. Out of the 1185 articles, 390 were removed for being either duplicates, research conducted outside of East Africa or on diseases not selected for this study. A further 24 articles were dropped since full publications or abstracts were unavailable or not in English, remaining with 771 publications for analysis, Fig. 1. The 771 journal articles covered 22 of the 36 zoonotic diseases evaluated, Table 1.

Our search terms identified 326 theses and dissertations from the online digital repositories of the five study universities in Kenya. Physical visits retrieved an additional 12 theses from the university libraries, 36 from the Kenya Medical Research Institute, and 15 from the Institute of Primate Research in Kenya. From the total of 389 theses and dissertations identified, 221 were dropped for either being duplicates or not meeting the inclusion criteria. In total 168 theses covering 21 of the 36 zoonotic diseases evaluated were included in the analysis, Table 1.

Published data research trends

The number of publications on zoonotic diseases from the region has been increasing by year, with 460 (60%) published in the last 10 years. Epidemiological studies were the most common studies accounting for 585 (76%) of all publications reviewed, while laboratory studies were 172 (22%) and socio-economic studies 14 (2%), Fig. 2. By analyzing a random sample of 20% of the studies categorized as epidemiological, we found 75% of the study designs used were cross-sectional or case reports, 15% longitudinal study designs and the remaining case-control studies, reviews and modelling papers.

More than half (52%) of the publications were on four (trypanosomiasis, brucellosis, Rift Valley Fever and rabies) of 22 diseases studied with Kenya, Tanzania, Uganda, Ethiopia, Rwanda and Burundi, contributing 39%, 22%, 21%, 15%, 2% and 1% of the total number of articles published respectively, Fig. 3. Publications on trypanosomiasis were mainly from Kenya and Uganda, Rift Valley fever mainly from Kenya with a few studies in Tanzania, Ebola primarily in Uganda, rabies in Tanzania and Ethiopia, patterns likely related to the incidence of the diseases in specific countries or interests in specific diseases by research groups working in those countries.

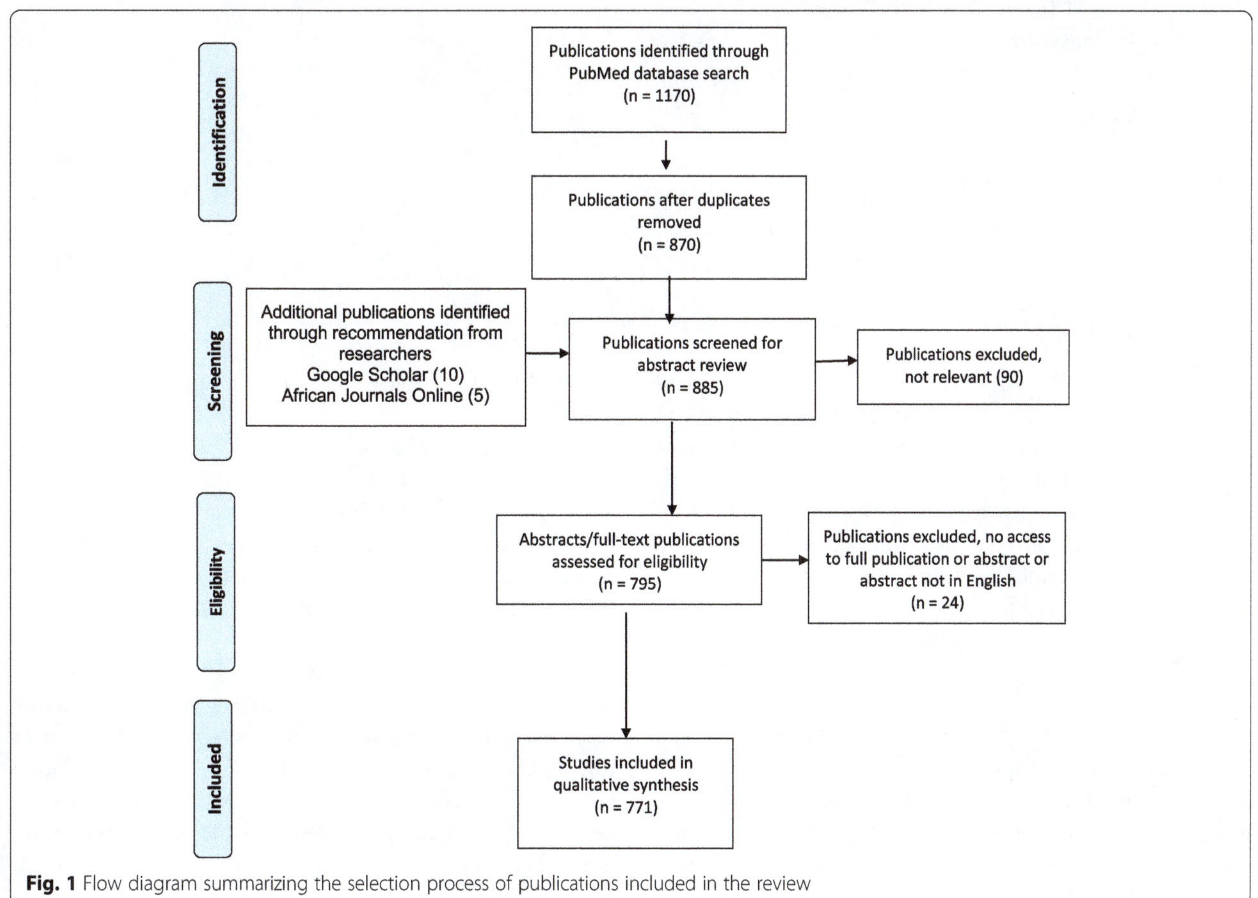

Fig. 1 Flow diagram summarizing the selection process of publications included in the review

Table 1 Summary of the zoonotic diseases from publications in East Africa and theses from Kenyan Universities analysed in this study

	Disease	Publications		Theses	
		Frequency	%	Frequency	%
1	Trypanosomiasis	166	21.5	14	8.3
2	Brucellosis	87	11.3	29	17.3
3	Rift Valley Fever	85	11	17	10.1
4	Rabies	62	8	4	2.4
5	Echinococcosis	56	7.3	21	12.5
6	Cysticercosis	48	6.2	11	6.5
7	Cryptococcosis	44	5.7	1	0.6
8	Campylobacteriosis	40	5.2	5	3
9	Bovine tuberculosis	38	4.9	9	5.4
10	Dengue	31	4	4	2.4
11	Ebola	29	3.8		
12	Leptospirosis	25	3.2	4	2.4
13	Q fever	19	2.5		
14	Anthrax	13	1.7	1	0.6
15	Marburg	9	1.2		
16	Schistosomiasis	5	0.6	1	0.6
17	Mers-Cov	4	0.5		
18	Cyclosporiasis	3	0.4		
19	Crimean-Congo hemorrhagic fever	3	0.4	1	0.6
20	Aspergillosis	2	0.3	6	3.6
21	West Nile	1	0.1		
22	Leishmaniasis	1	0.1	1	0.6
23	Salmonellosis			17	10.1
24	Influenza virus			9	5.4
25	Cryptosporidiosis			9	5.4
26	Toxoplasmosis			3	1.8
27	Rickettsia			1	0.6

Overall, endemic zoonotic diseases accounted for more than 85% of all publications from the region, with publications on epidemic diseases such as Rift Valley fever, Ebola, Marburg and Middle East respiratory syndrome coronavirus associated with years when outbreaks of the diseases occurred in the region or elsewhere in the world (for example the Rift Valley fever epidemics of 2007/2008 in East Africa or MERS-CoV publications after the first reports of the disease in Saudi Arabia in 2012), Fig. 4.

Thesis data research trends

The University of Nairobi, the first university to be established in the country, had 101 (60%) of the theses followed by Kenyatta University 32 (19%), Jomo Kenyatta University of Agriculture and Technology 26 (15%), Moi University 6 (4%) and Egerton University 3 (2%).

The number of theses produced per year increased with 102 (61%) of the theses produced in the last 10 years. Like the published data from the East Africa region, epidemiological studies were the most common accounting for 96 (57%), laboratory studies 70 (42%) and socio-economic 2 (1%) of all theses studies completed, Fig. 5.

Like the published data, majority 150 (89%) of theses on zoonoses in Universities in Kenya were on endemic diseases, with only a few focused on epidemic diseases Rift Valley fever 17 (10%) and Crimean-Congo hemorrhagic fever 1 (1%). By comparing the thesis research data and the published data for Kenya, we found only 11% of the theses research transitioned to peer-review publications.

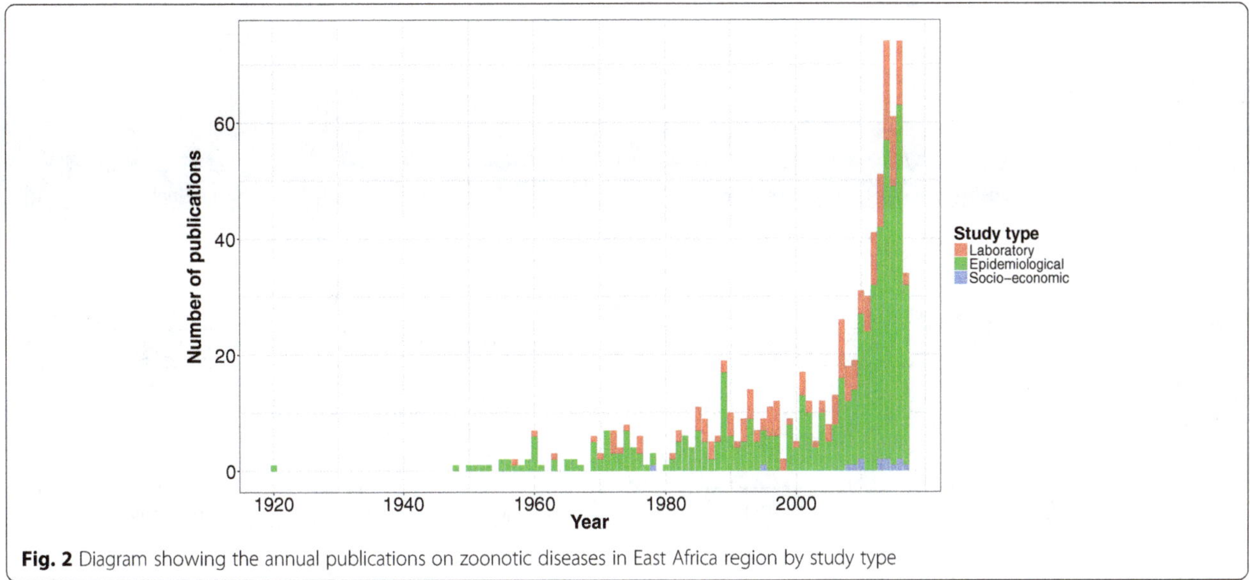

Fig. 2 Diagram showing the annual publications on zoonotic diseases in East Africa region by study type

Among the 11% theses whose data was published in peer-reviewed journals, it took an average of 2.5 years from year the thesis was produced to publication of the manuscript (range 0–8). Figure 6 shows the total number of theses for each of the 21 zoonotic diseases evaluated and the proportion for each that were published in peer-reviewed scientific journals.

Discussion

Our review of research trends on zoonotic diseases in East Africa has revealed a marked increase in publications and theses during the last decade, greater research focus on endemic diseases compared to epidemic diseases whose publications appear associated with specific disease outbreaks, focus on epidemiology type research and little of socio-economic studies, and a low and delayed transition of theses research into peer-reviewed journal publications.

For both journal publications from the East Africa region and theses production from Kenya on zoonotic diseases, two-thirds have come out in the last 10 years. This growth in zoonotic disease research is partly driven by the local and global recognition of the threats from zoonotic diseases and efforts to implement one health approaches in combating the public health and economic threats posed by these diseases. For example, Kenya established a One Health office referred to as the Zoonotic disease unit and one of its mandates is to

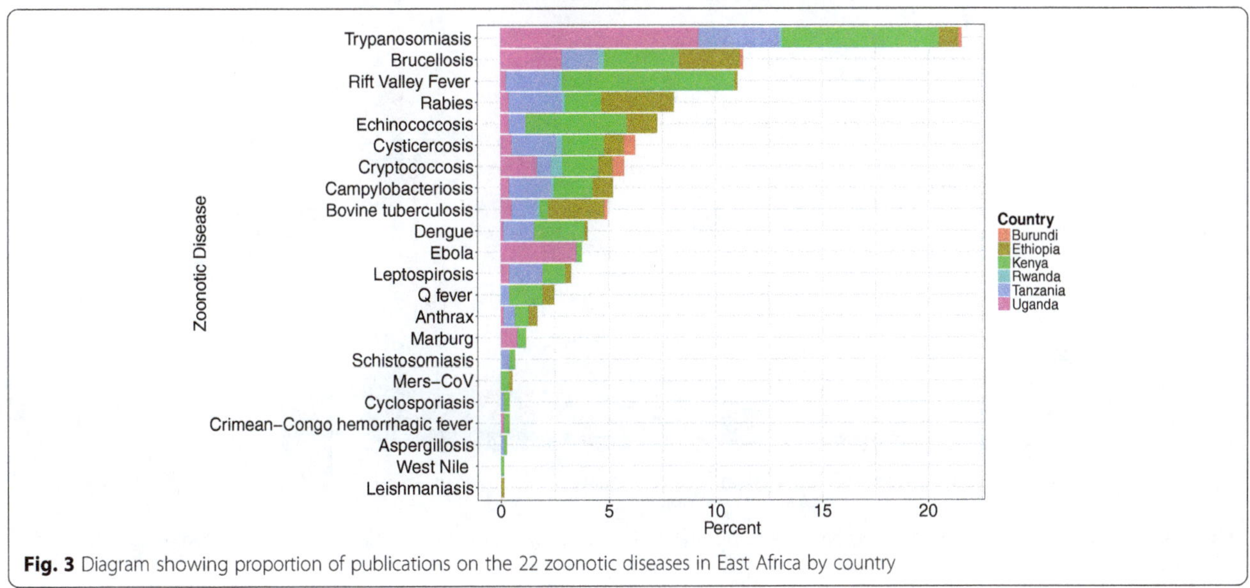

Fig. 3 Diagram showing proportion of publications on the 22 zoonotic diseases in East Africa by country

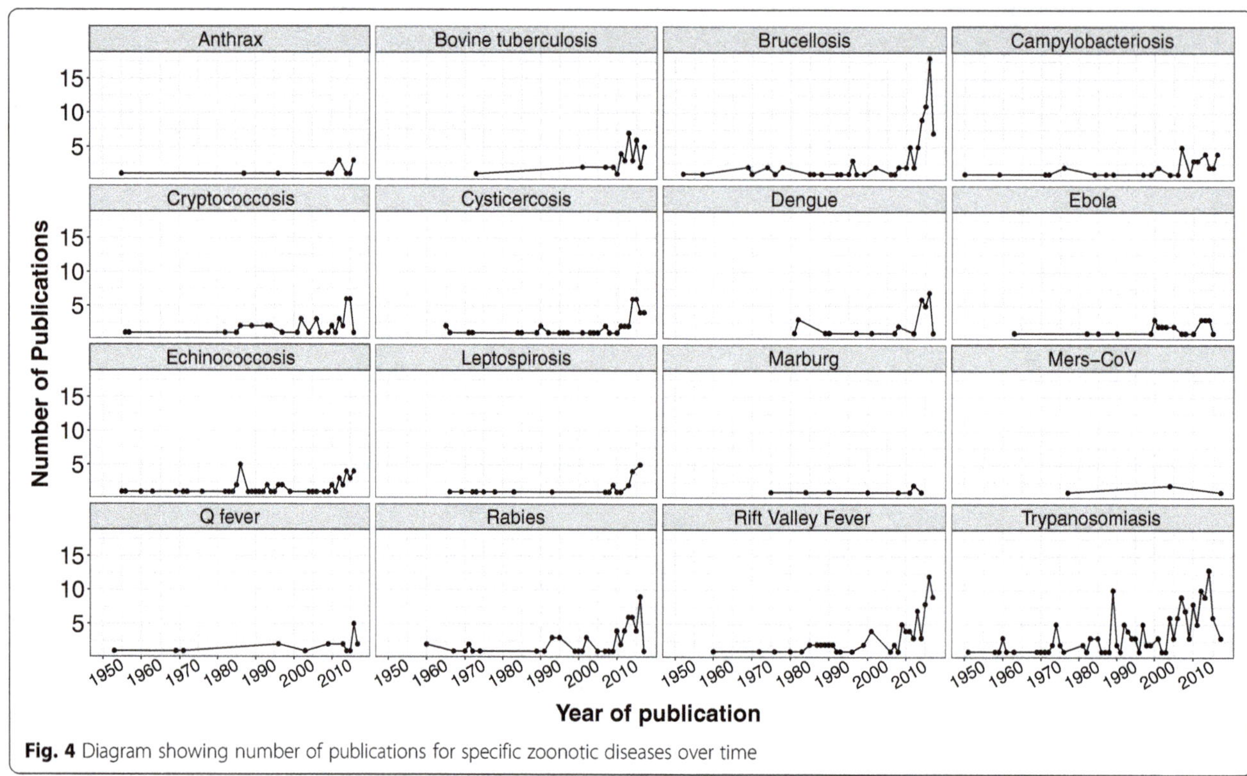

Fig. 4 Diagram showing number of publications for specific zoonotic diseases over time

stimulate and conduct research and training at the human-animal-ecosystem interfaces [15]. Most of the countries involved in this review including Kenya, Tanzania, Uganda, Rwanda and Ethiopia have established similar One Health offices or have organizations and networks created to conduct One Health training, research and outreach [16]. Publication output of countries has been associated with the level of national research spending and English proficiency [17]. These factors could be at play in East Africa region as well, with notable increase in the number of Universities established in the last 20 years [18]. The relatively fewer publications coming from Rwanda and Burundi may be associated with the two countries being French speaking, or political instability during the study period covered in our review.

Although much of the current global focus on zoonoses is mainly directed to emerging and re-emerging

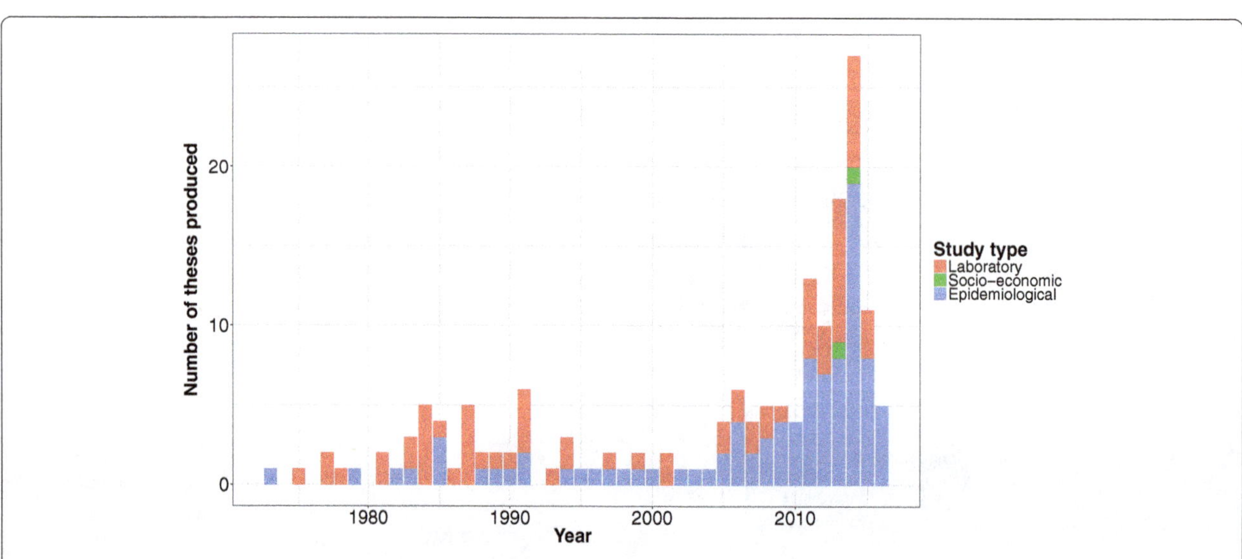

Fig. 5 Diagram showing the number of theses on zoonotic diseases and the study type produced by the five main Kenyan Universities between 1970 and 2017

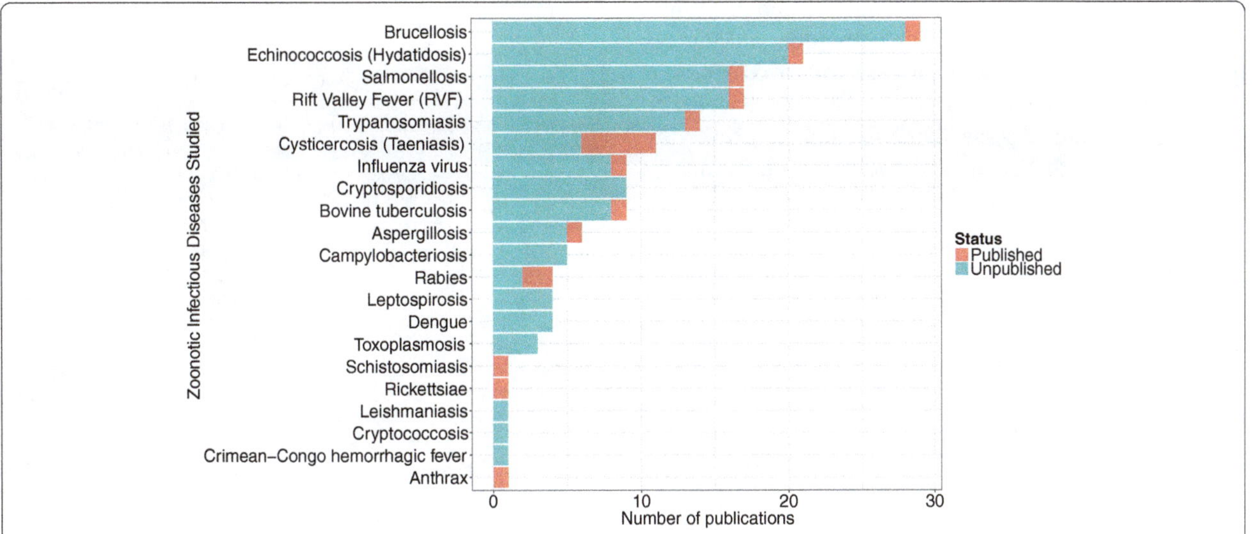

Fig. 6 Figure showing the number of theses produced for each of the 21 zoonotic diseases studied in Kenya, and the number of theses research published in peer-reviewed journals

infectious diseases, our findings from both scientific and theses research highlight the importance of endemic zoonotic diseases compared to the epidemic prone emerging zoonoses such as Ebola, Marburg, highly pathogenic influenza virus and MERS-CoV in the region. This finding is supported by results of zoonotic disease prioritization carried out in Kenya and Ethiopia which have identified endemic zoonotic diseases as top priority [13, 19].

Publications on emerging zoonoses in the region were associated with outbreaks of the disease in the region or elsewhere in the world. Research on Rift Valley Fever heightened following the 2006/2007 outbreaks of the disease that occurred in Tanzania and Kenya [20]. The upward trend in publications on Ebola correspond to the Ebola outbreaks that occurred in various places in Uganda in 2000, 2007, 2011, and 2012 [21–24]. Such peaks in publications associated with disease outbreaks have been reported elsewhere including outbreaks of Severe Acute Respiratory syndrome (SARS) in Asia, Ebola in West Africa and MERS-CoV in the Middle East [25].

Although the bulk of the published research on zoonotic diseases is epidemiological, the finding that three-quarters of the studies were either case reports or cross-sectional studies limits utility of the data to mainly prevalence estimation and determination of associations between exposures and outcomes. Longitudinal studies, although more expensive and taking longer to conduct, allow for estimation of incidence rates, inference of causation and understanding transmission dynamics of infectious diseases [26]. Although both endemic and emerging zoonotic diseases have been associated with large public health and economic losses [3, 4, 27, 28], only a small proportion of the studies from the region have focused on socio-economics. Experiences from recent outbreak in zoonotic diseases in Africa revealed the need for studies that advance disease detection, diagnosis, predicting risk, understanding disease transmission dynamics, pathogen phylogenetics and phylogeography, and inform likely outcomes of available interventions including social and economic factors [20, 29–33].

Our study included review of theses research in Kenyan universities and revealed that up to 89% of the research failed to transition to peer-reviewed publications. Coupled with the 2.5 years average time delay between thesis production and manuscript publication for the 11% that were published, our results demonstrate that a considerable amount of zoonotic research work in the country and probably in the larger East Africa are not widely disseminated or immediately available to public health practitioners or policy makers. It is not clear why such a situation exists but it may be related to researchers' only being keen to obtain an academic qualification or lack of proper academic support towards peer review publication. Recent change in policy on post-graduate education in Kenya making it mandatory for post-graduate students to show evidence of publication before being allowed to graduate may change the trend in dissemination of research findings, including those on zoonotic diseases.

Conclusion

There is a marked increase in the number of research studies on zoonoses in the region mostly focused on endemic diseases, with publications on epidemic diseases triggered by outbreaks. Aspects of diseases such as incidence, economic impact, diagnostics and transmission dynamics are not given much attention and this remains a major knowledge gap. This improved research will lead to better public health interventions that reduce transmission and disease burden, and improve the well-being of both human and livestock populations in the region.

Abbreviations

MERS-CoV: Middle East Respiratory Syndrome Coronavirus; RVF: Rift Valley fever; SARS: Severe Acute Respiratory syndrome

Acknowledgements

NK would like to acknowledge the United States Department of Defense, Defense Threat Reduction Agency (DTRA), Cooperative Biological Engagement Program (CBEP) for their support in presentation of this research in an international forum and grantsmanship training related to this manuscript. The contents of this publication are the responsibility of the authors and do not necessarily reflect the views of DTRA or the United States Government.

Funding

S.M. Thumbi receives funding support from the Wellcome Trust (Grant 110330/Z/15/Z) and the Paul G Allen School for Global Animal Health, Washington State University. The funders had no role in study design, data collection and analysis, decision to publish, or preparation of the manuscript.

Author's contribution

SMT, EM conceived the study. NK collected the data. NK and SMT analysed the data. SMT, NK, EM, MKN, EO, AB contributed to writing and discussion of the manuscript findings. All authors read and approved the final manuscript.

Competing interests

The authors declare that they have no competing interests.

Author details

[1]Paul G. Allen School for Global Animal Health, Washington State University, Pullman, USA. [2]Washington State University Global Health Program Kenya, Nairobi, Kenya. [3]Faculty of Veterinary Medicine, University of Nairobi, Nairobi, Kenya. [4]Food and Agriculture Organization of the United Nations, Nairobi, Kenya. [5]Center for Global Health Research, Kenya Medical Research Institute, Nairobi, Kenya.

References

1. Taylor LH, Latham SM, Woolhouse MEJ. Risk factors for human disease emergence. 2001;
2. Woolhouse MEJ, Gowtage-Sequeria S. Host range and emerging and reemerging pathogens. Emerg Infect Dis. 2005;11:1842–7.
3. Jones KE, Patel NG, Levy MA, Storeygard A, Balk D, Gittleman JL, et al. Global trends in emerging infectious diseases. Nat Lett. 2008;451:990–4.
4. Grace D, Mutua F, Ochungo P, Kruska R, Jones K, Brierley L, et al. Mapping of poverty and likely zoonoses hotspots. Rep. to UK Dep. Int. Dev. 2012.
5. Grace D, Gilbert J, Randolph T, Kang'ethe E. The multiple burdens of zoonotic disease and an ecohealth approach to their assessment. Trop Anim Health Prod. 2012;44:67–73.
6. Molyneux D, Hallaj Z, Keusch GT, McManus DP, Ngowi H, Cleaveland S, et al. Zoonoses and marginalised infectious diseases of poverty: where do we stand? Parasit Vectors. BioMed Central Ltd. 2011;4:106.
7. Seimenis A. Zoonoses and poverty - a long road to the alleviation of suffering. Vet Ital. 2012;48:5–13.
8. Cleaveland S, Sharp J, Abela-Ridder B, Allan KJ, Buza J, Crump JA, et al. One Health contributions towards more effective and equitable approaches to health in low- and middle-income countries. Philos Trans R Soc Lond B Biol Sci. 2017;372(1725):20160168.
9. Woolhouse MEJ, Haydon DT, Antia R. Emerging pathogens: the epidemiology and evolution of species jumps. Trends Ecol Evol. 2005;20:238–44.
10. Morens DM, Fauci AS. Emerging infectious diseases in 2012: 20 years after the Institute of Medicine Report. MBio. 2013;3:1–4.
11. Olson SH, Benedum CM, Mekaru SR, Preston ND, Mazet JAK, Joly DO, et al. Drivers of emerging infectious disease events as a framework for digital detection. Emerg Infect Dis. 2015;21:1285–92.
12. Jones BA, Grace D, Kock R, Alonso S, Rushton J, Said MY, et al. Zoonosis emergence linked to agricultural intensification and environmental change. Proc Natl Acad Sci. 2013;110:8399–404.
13. Munyua P, Bitek A, Osoro E, Pieracci EG, Muema J, Mwatondo A, et al. Prioritization of zoonotic diseases in Kenya., 2015. PLoS One. 2016;11:e0161576.
14. R Core Team. R: A language and environment for statistical computing. Vienna, Austria: R Foundation for Statistical Computing; 2017.
15. Mbabu M, Njeru I, File S, Osoro E, Kiambi S, Bitek A, et al. Establishing a one health office in Kenya. Pan Afr Med J. 2014;19:106.
16. Rwego IB, Babalobi OO, Musotsi P, Nzietchueng S, Tiambo CK, Kabasa JD, et al. One Health capacity building in sub-Saharan Africa. Infect Ecol Epidemiol. 2016;6. https://doi.org/10.3402/iee.v6.34032.
17. Man JP, Weinkauf JG, Tsang M, Sin DD. Why do some countries publish more than others? An international comparison of research funding, English proficiency and publication output in highly ranked general medical journals. Eur J Epidemiol. 2004;19:811–7.
18. Nyangau JZ. Higher education as an instrument of economic growth in Kenya higher education as an instrument of economic growth in Kenya. Forum Int Res Educ. 2014;1:7–25.
19. Pieracci EG, Hall AJ, Gharpure R, Haile A, Walelign E, Deressa A, et al. Prioritizing zoonotic diseases in Ethiopia using a one health approach. One Heal. Elsevier B.V. 2016;2:131–5.
20. Breiman RF, Njenga MK, Cleaveland S, Sharif S, Mbabu M, King L. Lessons from the 2006–2007 Rift Valley fever outbreak in East Africa: implications for prevention of emerging infectious diseases. Future Virol. 2008;3:411–7.
21. Okware SI, Omaswa FG, Zaramba S, Opio A, Lutwama JJ, Kamugisha J, et al. An outbreak of Ebola in Uganda. Tropical Med Int Health. 2002;7:1068–75.
22. Wamala JF, Lukwago L, Malimbo M, Nguku P, Yoti Z, Musenero M, et al. Ebola hemorrhagic fever associated with novel virus strain, Uganda, 2007-2008. Emerg Infect Dis. 2010;16:1087–92.
23. Shoemaker T, MacNeil A, Balinandi S, Campbell S, Wamala JF, McMullan LK, et al. Reemerging Sudan Ebola virus disease in Uganda., 2011. Emerg Infect Dis. 2012;18:1480–3.
24. Albariño CG, Shoemaker T, Khristova ML, Wamala JF, Muyembe JJ, Balinandi S, et al. Genomic analysis of filoviruses associated with four viral hemorrhagic fever outbreaks in Uganda and the Democratic Republic of the Congo in 2012. Virology Elsevier. 2013;442:97–100.
25. Sweileh WM. Global research trends of World Health Organization's top eight emerging pathogens. Global Health. 2017;13:9.
26. Pugh CA, Bronsvoort BMDC, Handel IG, Summers KM, Clements DN. What can cohort studies in the dog tell us? Canine Genet Epidemiol. 2014;1:5.
27. World Bank. People, Pathogens and Our Planet: The Economics of One Health. Washington, DC: © World Bank; 2012. https://openknowledge.worldbank.org/handle/10986/11892.
28. Hampson K, Coudeville L, Lembo T, Sambo M, Kieffer A, Attlan M, et al. Estimating the global burden of endemic canine rabies. PLoS Negl Trop Dis. 2015;9:e0003709.
29. Cascio A, Bosilkovski M, Rodriguez-Morales AJ, Pappas G. The socio-ecology of zoonotic infections. Clin Microbiol Infect. 2011;17:336–42.
30. Woolhouse M. How to make predictions about future infectious disease risks. Philos. Trans. R. Soc. B biol. Sci. 2011;366:2045–54.
31. Woolhouse MEJ, Rambaut A, Kellam P. Lessons from Ebola: Improving infectious disease surveillance to inform outbreak management. Sci. Transl. Med. 2015;7:307rv5.
32. Morse SS, Mazet JAK, Woolhouse M, Parrish CR, Carroll D, Karesh WB, et al. Prediction and prevention of the next pandemic zoonosis. Lancet Elsevier Ltd. 2012;380:1956–65.
33. Halliday JEB, Hampson K, Hanley N, Lembo T, Sharp JP, Haydon DT, et al. Driving improvements in emerging disease surveillance through locally relevant capacity strengthening. Science (80-.). 2017;357:146–8.

9

The interaction between HIV testing social norms and self-efficacy on HIV testing among Chinese men who have sex with men: results from an online cross-sectional study

Peizhen Zhao[1†], Li Liu[2†], Ye Zhang[1], Huanhuan Cheng[3], Bolin Cao[4,5], Chuncheng Liu[4], Cheng Wang[1], Bin Yang[1], Chongyi Wei[6], Joseph D. Tucker[4,5,7] and Weiming Tang[1,4,5,7*]

Abstract

Background: Increasing human immunodeficiency virus (HIV) testing is critical for HIV control. This study aimed to evaluate the interaction between social norms and self-efficacy on HIV testing among Chinese men who have sex with men (MSM).

Methods: We conducted an online survey in eight Chinese cities in Shandong and Guangdong Provinces in July 2016. We included participants who were born as a male, at least 16 years old, currently living in one of the designated cities, and had ever engaged in anal sex with a man. We collected information regarding socio-demographics, high-risk behaviors, and history of HIV and other STI testing. We coded sensitivity to social norms using six items asking participants about their perceived social norm regarding HIV testing. We coded HIV testing self-efficacy using a separate six-item scale. We interpreted higher mean scores as higher sensitivity to social norms and higher self-efficacy, respectively. We conducted logistic regressions to evaluate the interaction between self-efficacy and social norms on HIV testing.

Results: A total of 2105 men completed the survey. The mean age of the participants was 25.97 ± 6.42 years. Over four-fifths (85.9%) of participants were unmarried, 22.7% were students, and 64.6% at least had a college degree. 62.5 and 32.6% of participants ever and tested HIV in the last three months, respectively.
With respect to uptake of HIV testing in the last three months, the adjusted odds ratio was 1.01(95% CI: 0.96–1.06) for higher sensitivity to social norms and 1.09 (95% CI: 1.05–1.14) for higher self-efficacy, with an interaction effect of 1.02 (95% CI: 1.01–1.03), respectively. With respect to uptake of lifetime HIV testing, the adjusted odds ratio was 1.03(95% CI: 0.99–1.07) for higher sensitivity to social norms and 1.15 (95% CI: 1.11–1.19) for higher self-efficacy, with an interaction effect of 1.02 (95% CI: 1.01–1.04), respectively.

Conclusions: Our survey demonstrated that there is a significant association between the uptake of HIV testing with sensitivity to the social norm, higher self-efficacy, as well as the interaction between them. Tailored studies for improving HIV testing among MSM in China can combine these two interventions together.

Keywords: Men who have sex with men (MSM), Social norm, Self-efficacy, HIV testing

* Correspondence: weimingtangscience@gmail.com
†Peizhen Zhao and Li Liu contributed equally to this work.
Peizhen Zhao and Li Liu are co-first authors to this work.
[1]Dermatology Hospital, Southern Medical University, Guangzhou, China
[4]SESH study group of University of North Carolina at Chapel Hill, Guangzhou, China
Full list of author information is available at the end of the article

Introduction

Men who have sex with men have become a key population for HIV infection [1]. Increasing the uptake of HIV testing among MSM is a crucial component of the HIV treatment cascade and the control of the global HIV epidemic [2].

To scale up HIV testing services, the Chinese government has established voluntary counseling and testing (VCT) clinics that offer free HIV testing services and provider-initiated testing and counseling (PITC) [3], but only 60% of Chinese men who have sex with men (MSM) have ever tested for HIV [4]. Among Chinese MSM, potential reasons for low uptake of HIV testing include stigma against HIV, limited access to HIV testing service, and poor sexual orientation disclosure [3, 5, 6]. Identifying potential strategies to reduce these barriers and further improving HIV testing uptake among Chinese MSM is essential.

Studies in China and other countries indicated that HIV testing social norm and self-efficacy are two important psychosocial factors can facilitate HIV testing among MSM [7–9]. Self-efficacy refers to the belief in one's own ability to complete tasks and reach goals [8]. According to the social cognitive theory, self-efficacy plays an important role in the adoption, initiation, and maintenance of health behaviors [8]. HIV testing self-efficacy refers to people's level of confidence to have HIV testing [10]. Social norms are social attitudes of approval or disapproval that specify what ought and ought not to be done and are significant in the context of health [11]. HIV testing social norms refer to people's social attitudes about HIV testing [11]. Improving HIV testing self-efficacy and perceived positive social norms of HIV testing are two intervention strategies for improving uptake of HIV testing among MSM [8, 9, 12].

Even HIV testing social norm and self-efficacy has a positive impact on promoting HIV testing, whether these two can interact with each other and further strengthen the intervention effect is still not clear while knowing this is critical for designing tailored interventions for MSM. Therefore, the aim of this study was to examine whether there exists an interaction effect between perceived HIV testing-related social norm and self-efficacy on HIV testing among Chinese MSM. The hypothesis of this study is that the perceived HIV testing-related social norm and self-efficacy can interact with each other and further improve HIV testing uptake.

Methods

Study population

A nationwide cross-sectional online survey among MSM was conducted in eight Chinese cities: Guangzhou, Shenzhen, Zhuhai, Jiangmen (Guangdong Province, Southern China), Jinan, Qingdao, Jining, and Yantai (Shandong Province, Northern China) in July 2016. These eight cities of Guangdong and Shandong Province were chosen because they were urban cities with the relatively high prevalence of HIV.

We recruited participants online by collaborating with a gay dating application. Banner advertisements with links to the online survey were sent to registered users of the application. Viewers who clicked the survey link were directed to the web survey.

We only included participants who were born biologically as a male, at least 16 years old, and currently living in one of the designated cities who had had anal sex with a man at least once during their lifetime. We also required participants to provide their cell phone numbers for other follow-up purposes and agree to informed consent. All eligible participants received a small phone card reimbursement or WeChat incentive transfer (equivalent to roughly 7.5 USD).

Measures

After screening for eligibility and signing the informed consent, we first collected information on socio-demographic information, including age (which we further categorized into three groups: less than 20, 20–29, or 30 and above), marital status (never married or ever married, including widowed or divorced), occupation (student or not), education (senior high school or below, college/bachelors, or masters or PhD), and monthly income (less than 250 USD, 250–500 USD, 501–800 USD, 801–1250 USD or above 1250 USD). We also asked participants whether they had ever been tested for HIV (including HIV self-testing and facility-based testing) in their lifetime, whether ever self-tested, and whether testing for HIV in the last 3 months. HIV testing in lifetime was measured by asking participants whether they performed any HIV testing in their lifetime, including testing in general hospitals, clinics, the point of care sites or HIV self-testing.The HIV self-testing was defined as people tested HIV in private and interpreted the results on their own [13]. HIV testing in the past 3 months was measured as whether the participants performed any HIV testing in the last 3 months.

HIV testing self-efficacy

HIV testing self-efficacy was measured using six questions that elicited participants' attitudes toward and confidence in receiving HIV testing [14, 15]. The items are shown in Table 2. All items were scored using a 4-point Likert-type response set, with answers ranging from strongly agree (4) to strongly disagree (1). For each participant, a mean score was calculated with 4 as the highest possible score of 4 and 1 as the possible lowest score. Higher mean scores indicated higher HIV testing self-efficacy. The scale assessing respondents' overall levels of HIV testing self-efficacy was found to be reliable (Cronbach's $\alpha = 0\ .792$).

HIV testing social norm

Social norm was measured by six items asking participants about their awareness of social norms about HIV testing [11, 16] (see Table 2). All items were scored using a 4-point Likert-type response set, with answers ranging from strongly agree (4) to strongly disagree (1). For each participant, a mean score was calculated with 4 as the highest possible score of 4 and 1 as the possible lowest score. Higher mean scores indicated higher sensitivity to HIV testing social norms. The Cronbach's α of HIV testing social norm was 0.695.

Statistical analysis

We used descriptive analysis to describe socio-demographics, high-risk behaviors, and self-efficacy among the participants who had been tested for HIV in the past three months and those who had not. We also analyzed the linear assumption through semiparametric regression map (Additional file 1). Spearmen correlation tests were used to identify any association between social norm and self-efficacy. Univariate and multivariable logistic regressions were used to evaluate the association between HIV testing and self-efficacy and HIV testing and sensitivity to social norms. We used a logistic regression multiplication model to analyze the association of the interaction between HIV testing social norm and HIV testing self-efficacy. We used multivariable logistic regression to analyze the influencing factors of HIV testing. Age, education, marital status, and income were a covariate in the model. These variables were chosen based on our prior knowledge, and a directed acyclic graph (DAG) [17] was drawn to assist in this analysis. Throughout all the analyses, results are reported as statistically significant whenever $P < 0.05$. All data were analyzed using SAS 9.4 (SAS Int. Cary, NC, USA).

Results

Socio-demographic characteristics and behaviors

Two thousand one hundred five participants finished the online survey. The mean age of participants was 26.0 ± 6.4 years. 54.4% of the participants were ≤ 25 years old, 14.1% were married, 22.7% were students, 64.6% had a college or above degree, and 71.6% had an annual income less than \$9700 USD (60,000 RMB). Also, 72.4% of the participants self-identified as gay, and 23.6% self-identified as bisexual (Table 1).

HIV testing

Among 2105 participating MSM, 1315 (62.5%) reported being tested for HIV at least once in their lifetime. However, only 687(32.6%) participants had been tested for HIV within the past 3 months. Moreover, 685(32.5%) participants reported having self-tested for HIV at least once in their lifetime.

Table 1 Sociodemographic characteristics of MSM participants ($n = 2105$)

Characteristics	Frequency ($N = 2105$)	Percentage (%)
Age[a]		
≤ 25	1146	54.44
26–35	789	37.48
36–45	149	7.08
≥ 46	21	1.00
Student		
Yes	477	22.66
No	1628	77.34
Marital status		
Not married	1809	85.94
Engaged or Married	187	8.88
Separated or Divorced	106	5.04
Widowed	3	0.14
Education level		
High school or below	746	35.44
College diploma	583	27.70
Undergraduate	697	33.11
Postgraduate (Master/PhD)	79	3.75
Individual monthly income		
<1500 RMB	391	18.57
1500–3000 RMB	425	20.19
3001–5000 RMB	690	32.78
5001–8000 RMB	384	18.24
>8000 RMB	215	10.21
Gender identity		
Male	1999	94.96
Female	33	1.57
Transgender	34	1.62
Unsure/Other	39	1.85
Sexual orientation		
Homosexual	1524	72.40
Bisexual	496	23.56
Heterosexual	11	0.52
Unsure/Other	74	3.52
HIV testing in lifetime		
Yes	1315	62.5
No	790	37.5
HIV Testing in the past 3 months		
Yes	687	32.6
No	1418	67.4
HIV self-testing in lifetime		
Yes	685	32.5
No	1420	67.5

[a]Age: mean = 25.97, SD = ±6.42

Social norm and self-efficacy

In this study, the median(interquartile range, IQR) score of HIV testing social norms was 17.0 (15.0–18.0). While around 75% of participants endorsed all the statements of HIV testing social norms, between 17.2 and 52.2% of participants did not endorse each individual item. For HIV testing self-efficacy, the median (IQR) score was 19.0 (17.0–21.0). A majority of participants endorsed these statements, while a small proportion (2.8–26.8%) did not endorse individual items. (Table 2).

The association between HIV testing with sensitivity to social norms and self-efficacy

Univariate analysis indicated that MSM with higher sensitivity to social norms had a higher proportion of HIV testing in the past 3 months, though the result was not significant (Crude odds ratio (cOR, main effect) = 1.02 [0.96–1.06]). Univariate analysis also indicated that MSM with higher self-efficacy had more HIV testing in the past 3 months, with a cOR (main effect) of 1.09 [1.05–1.13]. We also detected an association of the interaction between sensitivity to HIV testing social norms and self-efficacy with HIV testing in the last 3 months (cOR = 1.02 [1.01,1.04], see Table 3).

Furthermore, univariate analysis indicated that MSM with higher sensitivity to the social norm was more likely to have had HIV testing at least once in their lifetime, though the difference was not significant (cOR = 1.02, [0.98–1.06]). Univariate analysis also revealed that MSM with higher self-efficacy score was more likely to have had HIV testing at least once in their lifetime (cOR = 1.09 [0.96–1.06]). We also detected an association of the interaction between sensitivity to HIV testing social norms and self-efficacy with lifetime HIV testing (cOR = 1.02 [1.01, 1.04], see Table 3).

Univariate analysis demonstrated that MSM with higher sensitivity to social norms had higher lifetime HIV self-testing in a lifetime (cOR =1.12 [1.07, 1.18]). MSM with higher self-efficacy score was more likely to have lifetime HIV self-testing in a lifetime, though the effect was not significant (cOR = 1.03, [0.99–1.07], see Table 3). Similar results were observed after adjusting for potential confounders (age, marital status, education level, and monthly income).

In our multivariate analysis, MSM with higher self-efficacy was more likely to have HIV testing in the past 3 months (adjusted odds ratio, aOR = 1.09 [1.05, 1.14]). For the increasing of every additional self-efficacy score, the HIV testing proportion in the past 3 months increased by 1.09 folds. Further, the interaction between social norm and self-efficacy was also associated with HIV testing in the past 3 months (aOR = 1.02 [1.01, 1.03]). MSM with higher self-efficacy and higher social norm were more likely to have HIV testing in the past 3 months.

In our multivariate analysis, MSM with higher self-efficacy and higher sensitivity to social norms had higher lifetime HIV testing proportion (aOR = 1.15 [1.11, 1.19] and 1.12 [1.06, 1.78], respectively). For every additional increase of self-efficacy score, the HIV testing proportion in the lifetime increased by 1.15 folds. For every additional increase of social norms score, the HIV testing proportion in the lifetime increased by 1.12 folds. Further, the interaction effect between social norm and self-efficacy was also associated with lifetime HIV testing (aOR = 1.02 [1.01, 1.04],

Table 2 Distribution of responses for items related to social norms and self-efficacy

	Strongly agree	Agree	Disagree	Strongly disagree
Social Norm				
Most gay men want to get tested but are afraid to get tested.	513(24.37)	977(46.41)	517(24.56)	98(4.66)
Most gay men who get tested do not want others to find out they were tested.	746(35.44)	969(46.03)	341(16.20)	49(2.33)
Most gay men want to get tested for HIV.	762(36.20)	981(46.60)	345(16.39)	17(0.81)
Most gay men who want to get tested will tell their partners they want to get tested	490(23.28)	995(47.27)	575(27.32)	45(2.14)
Most gay men have been tested for HIV	323(15.34)	684(32.49)	968(45.99)	130(6.18)
Most gay men get tested for HIV only if they are sick or feel uncomfortable	393(18.67)	968(45.99)	634(30.12)	110(5.23)
Self-Efficacy				
You would feel comfortable discussing HIV testing with a potential partner	508(24.13)	1033(49.07)	495(23.52)	69(3.28)
You feel confident that you could refuse to have sex with a partner who did not want to undergo HIV testing	686(32.59)	860(40.86)	447(21.24)	112(5.32)
You feel confident that you could persuade your partner to undergo HIV testing	717(34.06)	1152(54.73)	224(10.64)	12(0.57)
You can get tested for HIV if you wish	1004(47.70)	1043(49.55)	52(2.47)	6(0.29)
You would get tested for HIV even if you are afraid to know the results	925(43.94)	1074(51.02)	91(4.32)	15(0.71)
You have confidence that you will undergo HIV testing regularly	541(25.70)	1028(48.84)	501(23.80)	35(1.66)

Table 3 The association of HIV testing with Social Norms, Self-Efficacy, and their interaction

	Crude Model				Adjusted Model*			
	Coefficient	*SE*	*OR* (95% CI)	*P*-value	Coefficient	*SE*	*OR* (95% CI)	*P*-value
HIV Testing in the past 3 months								
Intercept	−0.16	0.42	–	–	0.82	0.51	–	–
Social norm	0.01	0.02	1.02(0.96,1.06)	0.55	0.01	0.02	1.01(0.96,1.06)	0.75
Intercept	−1.58	0.40	–	–	−0.71	0.48	–	–
Self-efficacy	0.09	0.02	1.09(1.05,1.13)	**< 0.001#**	0.09	0.02	1.09(1.05,1.14)	**< 0.001#**
Intercept	5.10	2.88	–	–	5.47	2.92	–	–
Social norm	−0.40	0.17	0.67(0.48,0.93)	**0.018#**	−0.38	0.17	0.69(0.49,0.96)	**0.029#**
Self-efficacy	−0.23	0.14	0.79(0.60,1.05)	0.11	−0.20	0.15	0.82(0.62,1.09)	0.17
Social norm*Self-efficacy	0.02	0.01	1.02(1.01,1.04)	**0.023#**	0.02	0.01	1.02(1.01,1.03)	**0.042#**
HIV testing in lifetime								
Intercept	0.24	0.35	–	–	−2.20	0.43	–	–
Social norm	0.02	0.02	1.02(0.98,1.06)	0.42	0.03	0.02	1.03(0.99,1.07)	0.20
Intercept	−2.07	0.31	–	–	−4.42	0.41	–	–
Self-efficacy	0.14	0.02	1.15(1,11,1.89)	**< 0.001#**	0.14	0.02	1.15(1.11,1.19)	**< 0.001#**
Intercept					−12.14	2.55	–	–
Social norm	0.39	0.14	1.41(1.10,1.80)	**0.007#**	0.44	0.15	1.48(1.14,1.92)	**0.003#**
Self-efficacy	0.54	0.12	1.64(1.32,2.04)	**< 0.001#**	0.58	0.13	1.70(1.36,2.13)	**< 0.001#**
Social norm*Self-efficacy	0.02	0.01	1.02(1.01,1.04)	**0.001#**	0.03	0.01	1.02(1.01,1.04)	**0.0008#**
Self-HIV testing in lifetime								
Intercept	−1.82	0.43	–	–	−0.53	0.53	–	–
Social norm	0.11	0.03	1.12(1.07,1.18)	**< 0.001#**	0.11	0.03	1.12(1.06,1.18)	**< 0.001#**
Intercept	−0.39	0.39	–	–	0.95	0.49	–	–
Self-efficacy	0.02	0.02	1.03(0.99,1.07)	0.22	0.02	0.02	1.02(0.99,1.07)	0.24
Intercept	2.09	2.81	–	–	3.29	2.87	–	–
Social norm	−0.04	0.17	0.91(0.68,1.22)	0.54	−0.04	0.17	0.92(0.68,1.23)	0.56
Self-efficacy	−0.08	0.14	0.84(0.66,1.07)	0.16	−0.08	0.14	0.84(0.66,1.08)	0.17
Social norm*Self-efficacy	0.04	0.01	1.01(0.99,1.02)	0.16	0.04	0.01	1.01(0.99,1.02)	0.18

*Model adjusted for age (Continuous), marital status (Not married, engaged or Married, separated or widowed), education level (High school or below, college or bachelors, or masters or PhD) and monthly income (<1500 RMB, 1500–3000 RMB, 3001–5000 RMB, 5001–8000 RMB or >8000 RMB). # and bold indicates $P < 0.05$

see Table 3). MSM with higher self-efficacy and higher social norm were more likely to have HIV testing in the life time.

Discussion

Previous studies have shown that HIV testing self-efficacy and social norms had an impact on the uptake of HIV testing. This study extends the existing literature by assessing the relationship between HIV testing and social norms, self-efficacy, and the potential interaction between social norms and self-efficacy.

Our study showed that sensitivity to HIV testing social norms was positively associated with having received an HIV testing within the past 3 months as well as lifetime HIV testing. This is consistent with the findings of previous studies from northern Nigeria and rural Uganda [7]. This finding supports the hypothesis that improving HIV testing social norms can potentially improve the HIV testing uptake among Chinese MSM. Intervention packages aimed at improving HIV testing proportion should consider social norms and perceptions of social norms as an actionable part of the overall intervention strategies.

Our study also indicated that HIV testing self-efficacy was positively associated with lifetime HIV testing. This finding is consistent with previous studies, which have shown that improving HIV testing self-efficacy is useful for promoting HIV testing and medication adherence [18–20]. Our study suggests the importance of developing strategies (i.e. raising the severity perception [14]) to strengthen MSM self-efficacy, thereby improving safe sexual behavior and HIV testing proportion [21]. More importantly, integrating self-efficacy with other ongoing interventions (i.e., HIV self-testing), and further improving the effectiveness of these implementation strategies will be more practical.

Further, our study demonstrated that sensitivity to social norms and self-efficacy interact with each other in promoting HIV testing, and MSM with both higher sensitivity to social norms and self-efficacy were more likely to have HIV testing. This finding is consistent with previous literature that positive social norms and self-efficacy would work together in improving condom use among MSM [22]. There are several potential reasons for this phenomenon. First, MSM with higher sensitivity to social norms may be more likely to discuss HIV testing with friends [23]. This kind of interaction may further increase their self-efficacy and lead to HIV testing. Second, reasoned action theory has shown that when people are aware of their community's support for an act, they will be more likely to carry out such behavior [24]. Third, according to social cognitive theory, people with higher self-efficacy and sensitivity to social norms may make a greater effort to accomplish their goals in the near future [15]. Further implementation studies that can combine the social norms and self-efficacy strategies, and working together to improve HIV testing together would be more effective.

In our study, the prevalence of HIV testing among MSM remained low with 32.6% of participants having been tested for HIV in the last 3 months and 62.5% of participants having been tested for HIV in their lifetime. These testing proportions are higher than those from Thailand in 2014 [25] and Zhejiang, China in 2014 [1], but lower than those from Cambodia in 2015 [26]. The HIV testing proportion is still far behind the UNAIDS target for 90% testing among infected individuals in 2014 [27]. This may be attributable to many factors. First, there is low awareness among MSM of the infection risk associated with sexual behavior [28]. Secondly, even MSM who are willing to be tested often need to travel to other cities for testing in order to avoid social stigma [29]. Thirdly, younger MSM are less likely to have been tested for HIV, potentially due to their fear of HIV testing in healthcare settings [30], in our study about 54.4% of the participants were 25 years old or younger. Lastly, the geographical distribution of HIV testing sites is unbalanced in China [31].

This study has several limitations. Firstly, we recruited participants through a mobile dating application, so participants tended to be younger, more highly educated, with a higher burden of syphilis and HIV [32]. MSM in remote rural areas in China were not included in the study. Secondly, HIV testing in the past 3 months was self-reported, which might lead to social desirability bias. Thirdly, the Cronbach's α of HIV testing social norm and self-efficacy were a bit low. Lastly, like many other online cross-sectional studies, there might be a selection bias in the study, as the online participants are tended to be young and well educated [33].

Conclusions

In summary, our results showed that the prevalence of HIV testing among MSM in China is suboptimal and may result in continuing transmission of HIV. However, most of the MSM who participated in this study were fairly confident in their likelihood of having HIV testing. Our study noted the association of the interaction between sensitivity to HIV testing-related social norms and self-efficacy with HIV testing and self-HIV testing among Chinese MSM. MSM with higher sensitivity to social norms and self-efficacy were more likely to have HIV testing. Future studies should investigate how social norms and self-efficacy are working together in promoting HIV testing. Policies and intervention packages (such as culturally competent sexual health education interventions [34]) should focus on increasing positive social norms and self-efficacy among MSM as an essential component of the overall intervention strategy.

Abbreviations

aOR: Adjusted odds ratio; cOR: Crude odds ratio; DAG: Directed acyclic graph; HIV: Human Immunodeficiency Virus; IQR: Interquartile range; MSM: Men who have sex with men; PITC: Provider-initiated testing and counseling; PLWH: People living with HIV; VCT: Voluntary counseling and testing

Acknowledgments

Thanks to Katherine Li for reviewing a prior version of this manuscript. This work is supported by the National Key Research and Development Program of China (2017YFE0103800), the National Institutes of Health [National Institute of Allergy and Infectious Diseases (NIAID) 1R01AI114310]; University of North Carolina (UNC)-South China STD Research Training Centre [Fogarty International Centre 1D43TW009532]; UNC Center for AIDS Research [NIAID 5P30AI050410]; and the Bill & Melinda Gates Foundation to the Mesh Consortium (BMGF-OPP1120138); National Center for Advancing Translational Sciences [UL1TR001111] at the National Institutes of Health and Medical Scientific Research Foundation of Guangdong Province of China(A2018508). The listed grant funders played no role in any step of this study.

Funding

This work was supported by the National Key Research and Development Program of China (2017YFE0103800), the National Institutes of Health [National Institute of Allergy and Infectious Diseases 1R01AI114310]; UNC-South China STD Research Training Centre [Fogarty International Centre 1D43TW009532]; UNC Center for AIDS Research [National Institute of Allergy and Infectious Diseases 5P30AI050410]; University of California San Francisco Center for AIDS Research [National Institute of Allergy and Infectious Diseases P30 AI027763]; and the Bill & Melinda Gates Foundation to the Mesh Consortium (BMGF-OPP1120138. This publication was also supported by Grant Number UL1TR001111 from the National Center for Advancing Translational Sciences (NCATS) at the National Institutes of Health. Medical Scientific Research Foundation of Guangdong Province of China(A2018508). The listed grant funders played no role in any step of this study.

Authors' contributions

PZ, WT, and LL participated in all stages and wrote the manuscript, BC, CL, CW, and YZ helped collect the data; BY, CW, HC, WT, and JT helped design the study and reviewed the manuscript. All authors read and approved the final manuscript.

Competing interests

The authors declare that they have no competing interests.

Author details

[1]Dermatology Hospital, Southern Medical University, Guangzhou, China. [2]Nanjing Municipal Center for Disease Control and Prevention, Jiangsu, China. [3]The Third Affiliated Hospital, Sun Yat-Sen University, Guangzhou, China. [4]SESH study group of University of North Carolina at Chapel Hill, Guangzhou, China. [5]University of North Carolina at Chapel Hill Project-China, Guangzhou 510095, China. [6]Social and Behavioral Health Sciences, School of Public Health, Rutgers University, Piscataway, NJ, USA. [7]School of Medicine of University of North Carolina at Chapel Hill, Chapel Hill, USA.

References

1. Li R, Pan X, Ma Q, Wang H, He L, Jiang T, Wang D, Zhang Y, Zhang X, Xia S. Prevalence of prior HIV testing and associated factors among MSM in Zhejiang Province, China: a cross-sectional study. BMC Public Health. 2016;16(1):1152.
2. Lui C, Dean J, Mutch A, Mao L, Debattista J, Lemoire J, Howard C, Whittaker A, Hollingdrake O, Fitzgerald L. HIV testing in men who have sex with men: a follow-up review of the qualitative literature since 2010. AIDS Behav. 2018; 22(2):593–605.
3. Tucker JD, Wong FY, Nehl EJ, Zhang F. HIV testing and care systems focused on sexually transmitted HIV in China. Sex Transm Infect. 2012;1;88(2):116-9.
4. Zou H, Hu N, Xin Q, Beck J. HIV testing among men who have sex with men in China: a systematic review and meta-analysis. AIDS Behav. 2012;16(7):1717–28.
5. Evangeli M, Pady K, Wroe AL. Which psychological factors are related to HIV testing? A quantitative systematic review of global studies. AIDS Behav. 2016;20(4):880–918.
6. Chow E, Wilson D, Zhang L. The rate of HIV testing is increasing among men who have sex with men in China. HIV MED. 2012;13(5):255–63.
7. Perkins JM, Nyakato VN, Kakuhikire B, Mbabazi PK, Perkins HW, Tsai AC, Subramanian SV, Christakis NA, Bangsberg DR. Actual versus perceived HIV testing norms, and personal HIV testing uptake: a cross-sectional, population-based study in rural Uganda. AIDS Behav. 2018;22(2):616–28.
8. Prati G, Breveglieri M, Lelleri R, Furegato M, Gios L, Pietrantoni L. Psychosocial correlates of HIV testing among men who have sex with men in Italy: a cross-sectional study. Int J STD AIDS. 2013;25(7):496–503.
9. Babalola S. Readiness for HIV testing among young people in northern Nigeria: the roles of social norm and perceived stigma. AIDS Behav. 2007;11(5):759–69.
10. Safiri S. Knowledge, attitude, self-efficacy and estimation of frequency of condom use among Iranian students based on a crosswise model: more explanation is needed for the crosswise model. Int J Adolesc Med Health. 2017;29(2):20160110.
11. Ahmed A, Weatherburn P, Reid D, Hickson F, Torres-Rueda S, Steinberg P, Bourne A. Social norms related to combining drugs and sex ("chemsex") among gay men in South London. Int J Drug Policy. 2016;38:29–35.
12. Jamil MS, Guy RJ, Bavinton BR, Fairley CK, Grulich AE, Holt M, Smith KS, Chen M, McNulty AM, Conway DP, et al. HIV testing self-efficacy is associated with higher HIV testing frequency and perceived likelihood to self-test among gay and bisexual men. Sex Health. 2017;14(2):170–8.
13. WHO: Consolidated guidelines on HIV testing services. 2015.
14. Jin SS, Bu K, Chen FF, Xu HF, Li Y, Zhao DH, Xu F, Li JY, Han MJ, Wang N, et al. Correlates of condom-use self-efficacy on the EPPM-based integrated model among Chinese college students. Biomed Environ Sci. 2017;30(2):97–105.
15. Ritchwood TD, Penn D, Peasant C, Albritton T, Corbie-Smith G. Condom use self-efficacy among younger rural adolescents:the influence of parent-teen communication, and knowledge of and attitudes toward condoms. J Early Adolesc. 2017;37(2):267–83.
16. Latkin CA, Kuramoto SJ, Davey-Rothwell MA, Tobin KE. Social norms, social networks, and HIV risk behavior among injection drug users. AIDS Behav. 2010;14(5):1159–68.
17. Rothman KJ, Greenland S, Lash TL. Modern. Epidemiology. 2008.
18. Khumsaen N, Stephenson R. Beliefs and perception about HIV/AIDS, self-efficacy, and HIV sexual risk behaviors among young Thai men who have sex with men. AIDS Educ Prev. 2017;29(2):175–90.
19. Zhou G, Li X, Qiao S, Zhou Y, Shen Z. Psychological and behavioral barriers to ART adherence among PLWH in China: role of self-efficacy. AIDS Care. 2017;29(12):1533–7.
20. Sun L, Yang SM, Wu H, Chen B, Wang CJ, Li XF. Reliability and validity of the Chinese version of the HIV treatment adherence self-efficacy scale in mainland China. Int J STD AIDS. 2017;28(8):829–37.
21. Guerra-Ordonez JA, Benavides-Torres RA, Onofre-Rodriguez DJ, Marquez-Vega MA, Guerra-Rodriguez GM, Wall KM. Self-efficacy and coping as correlates of migrant safe sexual behavior to prevent HIV. J Assoc Nurses AIDS Care. 2017;28(5):761–9.
22. Leddy A, Chakravarty D, Dladla S, de Bruyn G, Darbes L. Sexual communication self-efficacy, hegemonic masculine norms and condom use among heterosexual couples in South Africa. AIDS Care. 2015;28(2):228–33.
23. Zhou Q, Wu Y, Hong YA, Yang C, Cai W, Zhu Y, Guo Z, Guo Y. Association between perceived social norm and condom use among people living with HIV/AIDS in Guangzhou, China. AIDS Care. 2017;29(1):91–7.
24. Song F, Yan-ming S, Hong-yan LU, Xiao-yan MA, Hai Y, Li LU, Xiong HE, Wei MA, Xue-feng LI, Yan X, et al. Analysis on the relationship between condom social norms and unprotected anal intercourse among men who have sex with men in Beijing. Chinese J Epidemiol. 2011;32(5):473–6.
25. Sapsirisavat V, Phanuphak N, Keadpudsa S, Egan JE, Pussadee K, Klaytong P, Reuel Friedman M, van Griensven F, Stall R. Psychosocial and behavioral characteristics of high-risk men who have sex with men (MSM) of unknown HIV positive Serostatus in Bangkok, Thailand. AIDS Behav. 2016;20(S3):386–97.
26. Yi S, Tuot S, Chhoun P, Brody C, Pal K, Oum S. Factors associated with recent HIV testing among high-risk men who have sex with men: a cross-sectional study in Cambodia. BMC Public Health. 2015;15(1).
27. UNAIDS. 90–90–90 - an ambitious treatment target to help end the AIDS epidemic. Switzerland: UNAIDS; 2014.
28. Cao B, Liu C, Durvasula M, Tang W, Pan S, Saffer AJ, Wei C, Tucker JD. Social media engagement and HIV testing among men who have sex with men in China: a Nationwide cross-sectional survey. J Med Internet Res. 2017;19(7):e251.
29. Zou H, Zhang L, Chow EPF, Tang W, Wang Z. Testing for HIV/STIs in China: challenges, opportunities, and innovations. Biomed Res Int. 2017;2017:1–3.
30. Wong NS, Tang W, Han L, Best J, Zhang Y. MSM HIV testing following an online testing intervention in China. 2017.
31. Chen W, Zhou F, Hall BJ, Tucker JD, Latkin C, Renzaho AMN, Ling L. Is there a relationship between geographic distance and uptake of HIV testing services? A representative population-based study of Chinese adults in Guangzhou, China. PLOS ONE. 2017;12(7):e180801.
32. Tang W, Best J, Zhang Y, Liu F, Tso LS, Huang S, Yang B, Wei C, Tucker JD. Gay mobile apps and the evolving virtual risk environment: a cross-sectional online survey among men who have sex with men in China. Sex Transm Infect. 2016;92(7):508–14.
33. Zhao P, Tang S, Wang C, Zhang Y, Best J, Tangthanasup TM, Huang S, Yang B, Wei C, Tucker JD, et al. Recreational drug use among Chinese MSM and transgender individuals: results from a National Online Cross-Sectional Study. PLoS One. 2017;12(1):e170024.
34. Cianelli R, Villegas N, McCabe BE, de Tantillo L, Peragallo N. Self-efficacy for HIV prevention among refugee Hispanic women in South Florida. J Immigr Minor Health. 2017;19(4):905–12.

10

The epidemiology of *Taenia* spp. infection and *Taenia solium* cysticerci exposure in humans

Dinh Ng-Nguyen[1,2*], Mark Anthony Stevenson[1], Kathleen Breen[3], Trong Van Phan[4], Van-Anh Thi Nguyen[2], Tinh Van Vo[5] and Rebecca Justine Traub[1]

Abstract

Background: Vietnam is endemic for taeniasis and *T. solium* cysticercosis. Despite this, information on the epidemiological characteristics of the diseases in the Central Highlands of Vietnam are poorly described. The aims of this study were to determine the epidemiological characteristics of taeniasis (*Taenia* spp.) and *T. solium* cysticerci exposure in humans in Dak Lak province in the Central Highlands, Vietnam.

Methods: This cross-sectional study was carried out in six villages in three districts of Dak Lak. A total of 190 households were visited. From each household, between one and five individuals were asked to donate a single faecal and blood sample and respond to a questionnaire. Serum samples were subjected to lentil lectin purified glycoprotein enzyme-linked immunoelectrotransfer blot assay to detect antibodies against *T. solium* cysticerci. Multiplex real-time PCR was used to detect *Taenia* spp. infection in faecal samples. A fixed-effects logistic regression model was developed to identify factors associated with the probability of *Taenia* spp. infection or *T. solium* cysticerci exposure risk. The contribution of each of identified factor was quantified using population attributable fractions.

Results: The prevalence of seroexposure to *T. solium* in Dak Lak was 5% (95% CI 3% to 8%). Consumption of raw vegetables, sourcing drinking water from lakes, streams or ponds and the practice of outdoor defaecation were identified as primary risk factors for the prevalence of *T. solium* cysticerci exposure, while consuming undercooked pork and beef, pork tongue and observing *Taenia* proglottids in stool were associated with *Taenia* spp. infection. Consumption of raw vegetables attributed to 74% of *T. solium* cysticerci exposure-positive cases and consumption of undercooked beef attributed to 77% of taeniasis cases in these communities.

Conclusions: The prevalence of *T. solium* seroexposure in Dak Lak is consistent with those reported in other regions of Vietnam. The identified risk factors associated with the prevalence of *T. solium* seroexposure and taeniasis infection in Dak Lak are modifiable and thus advocate for targeted community intervention programs to mitigating these risks.

Keywords: Epidemiology, Taeniasis, Cysticercosis, Risk factors, Vietnam

Background

Taenia solium cysticercosis and human taeniasis are considered neglected tropical diseases by the World Health Organization [1]. When accidentally ingested either directly, or indirectly via contaminated food and water, eggs of *T. solium* hatch and lodge in the skeletal muscle, under the skin and/or within the central nervous system causing muscular-, subcutaneous- and/or neuro-cysticercosis. Neurocysticercosis is a common cause of epilepsy, syncope, paralysis and chronic headache [2, 3]. Globally, the disease has been estimated to cause approximately 2.8 million DALYs (disability-adjusted life-years) lost and between 2010 and 2015 approximately 300,000 individuals were estimated to be infected globally, resulting in over 28,100 deaths [4]. Consumption of raw or undercooked meat and/or visceral organs containing cysticerci of *T. solium, Taenia*

* Correspondence: ngocn4@student.unimelb.edu.au; theeveret@gmail.com
[1]Faculty of Veterinary and Agricultural Sciences, University of Melbourne, Parkville, VIC 3052, Australia
[2]Faculty of Animal Sciences and Veterinary Medicine, Tay Nguyen University, Dak Lak, Vietnam
Full list of author information is available at the end of the article

saginata or *Taenia asiatica* cause taeniasis. Taeniasis reduces the quality of life, is responsible for diagnostic and treatment costs in infected individuals and indirectly contributes to poverty due to losses in livestock production arising from organ condemnation and loss of market access [5].

Vietnam is considered endemic for taeniasis and *T. solium* cysticercosis [6, 7]. Previous research focusing on these diseases in Vietnam has mostly been carried out in the north of the country. A review of the literature shows that common risk factors for taeniasis and cysticercosis include consumption of raw or undercooked meat and vegetables, lack of functioning latrines, husbandry practices allowing pigs to free-roam and routine use of human waste for fertilizing and irrigating crops [8–12]. Information on the prevalence of and risk factors for taeniasis and *T. solium* cysticercosis in the central and southern areas of Vietnam is scarce and outdated [12]. In Dak Lak province, there is no information available on the infection status of *T. saginata* in livestock, however our research data on the seroprevalence of cysticercosis in pigs was 0.95% [13]. A previous study carried out by our group using a newly developed multiplex real-time PCR found the prevalence of *Taenia solium, T. saginata* and *T. asiatica* taeniasis to be 1.2%, 5.8% and 1.5%, respectively in Dak Lak province [14]. In this study, our aims were to: i) estimate the seroprevalence of *T. solium* cysticerci exposure using the lentil-lectin purified glycoprotein enzyme-linked immunoelectrotransfer blot (LLGP-EITB) assay; ii) identify and quantify risk factors for human *T. solium* cysticerci exposure and taeniasis (*Taenia* spp. infection), that inform optimal risk mitigation measures in studied communities in Dak Lak province, Vietnam.

Methods

Studying site and sampling

The study was deployed in the districts of Buon Don, Krong Nang and M'Drak in the province of Dak Lak in the Central Highlands of Vietnam between May and October 2015. M'Drak is located in the east of Dak Lak province with an average altitude of 400 m to 500 m and has a tropical monsoon climate typical of the Vietnam's Central Coast. Krong Nang is situated in the north of the province at an altitude of 800 m. Buon Don, situated to the west of the province with an average elevation of 330 m and has a hot and dry climate. The standard of living in this area of Vietnam is generally poor. The literacy rate among local residents aged between 15 and 60 in rural areas was low [15]. Open defaecation using outdoor pit latrines is common practice and livestock access to these latrine areas is usually unrestricted. The practice of non-confinement of pigs and cattle is common with slaughter activities often carried out in backyards [12]. The sample size was calculated based on the previous study of Van De at al. [31]. The seroprevalence of *T. solium* cysticerci exposure was assumed to be 7% and there was 95% certainty that this estimate was within 5% of the true population value (i.e. the prevalence ranged from 2% to 12%). Ignoring the tendency for *T. solium* cysticerci exposure to cluster within households we estimated that a total of 100 samples were required. We then assumed the average number of individuals eligible for the study per household was three and the between household (cluster) variance in seroprevalence was around 1.14 times greater than the within household (cluster) variance, returning an intra-class correlation coefficient of 0.07 [16]. Our revised sample size, accounting for the tendency of cluster within households, was 114 for each district and 342 for the whole province

A sampling frame listing the name of all villages in Dak Lak province was obtained from the Sub-Department of Animal Health office within the Ministry of Agriculture. Villages eligible for sampling comprised those with more than 1000 pigs, as recorded by the Sub-Department of Animal Health. All eligible villages within each district were assigned a number and two numbers chosen at random to select villages from each district for inclusion in the study. A list of householder names within each selected village was obtained from each village head person, and household names were assigned a numeric code. The sheet of paper of numeric household codes for each village were cut into pieces and placed face-down on a table. The village head person was asked to select 50 households at random. Each village has a number of households between 200 and 300. All selected households were visited several days before the proposed sampling date to obtain consent from participants to take part in the study. From each household between one and five individuals were requested to take part in the study. Individuals eligible for inclusion in the study were healthy, not pregnant and over seven years of age. Individuals requested to take part in the study signed a consent form. Those that were under 18 years of age were required to provide written consent as well as written consent from either their parents or legal guardians. At the time of consent, each study participant was given a labeled stool container, with instructions that the container would be collected on the date of sampling, several days later. Five mL of venous blood was collected into plain clotting tubes from consenting study participants by local medical staff. The blood was kept at ambient temperature for clotting and then centrifuged at 3200×g for 5 min to collect serum. The serum was stored at – 20 °C until use.

Household questionnaire

Each study participant was requested to answer a prepared questionnaire (Additional File 1). The questionnaire comprised of two sections. The first section collected information at the household level and was completed by the nominated head of the household. Questions included in this section solicited details on housing type, details of the type of latrines in use (if any), the presence and type of backyard pigsties, the source(s) of drinking water and activities associated with cultivation, irrigation and fertilization of home or farm grown vegetables. The second part of the questionnaire solicited details at the individual study participant level including their age, gender, the highest level of education achieved, dietary practices, and hygiene. All questionnaires were conducted in local Vietnamese phraseology and the validity of the questionnaire was pre-tested on thirty individuals in another community in Dak Lak province before application to the field survey. In addition, interviewers were trained before administering the questionnaires.

Laboratory procedures

Detection of antibodies against T. solium cysticerci

Serum samples were subjected to LLGP-EITB assay to detect antibodies against *T. solium* cysticerci. This assay has a diagnostic sensitivity of 98% and a diagnostic specificity of 100%. The assay was performed as previously described by Tsang et al. (1989) [17] and Noh et al. (2014) [18].

Detection of Taenia spp. infection

A total of 342 faecal samples were subject to a multiplex real-time PCR (T3qPCR) to detect all three species of *Taenia*, notably, *T. solium*, *Taenia saginata* and *Taenia asiatica*. The assay has been reported to have a diagnostic sensitivity of 94% and a diagnostic specificity of 98%. The positive results of T3qPCR were confirmed using either a conventional multiplex PCR targeting *T. solium*, *T. saginata* and *T. asiatica* [19] or a singleplex PCR for *Taenia* sp. following DNA sequencing. The methods and results have been described and published elsewhere [14].

Statistical methods

Risk factors for *T. solium* cysticerci exposure and taeniasis (*Taenia* spp. infection) in humans in the communities of Dak Lak province were identified using logistic regression. The outcome of interest for this study was a binary response variable, Y_i, taking the value 1 if an individual was *T. solium* cysticerci exposure-positive using the LLGP-EITB or in the case of taeniasis, was positive for *Taenia* spp. infection by T3qPCR, and 0 otherwise.

This study did not use a simple random sampling design to avoid erroneous point estimates of the strength of the association between hypothesized risk factors and the outcome of interest and their standard errors. The data were analyzed in a manner that respected the three-stage cluster design (villages within districts formed the primary sampling units, households within villages formed the secondary sampling units and individuals within households formed the tertiary sampling units). Sampling weights W_I, provided an estimate of the inverse probability of an individual being selected for study (Lumley 2010) [20] and were quantified for each study participant as follows:

$$w_1 = \frac{V}{v} x \frac{H}{h} x \frac{M}{m} \tag{1}$$

In Eq. 1, V and v represent the total number of villages in each district and the number of sampled villages in each district, respectively; H and h represent the total number of households in each sampled village and the number of sampled households in each village, respectively; and M and m represent the total number of individuals in each sampled household, and the number of sampled individuals in each household, respectively.

Unconditional associations between each of the hypothesized risk factors from the questionnaire and the outcome of interest were computed using the odds ratio. Hypothesized risk factors (explanatory variables) with unconditional associations that were significant at $P < 0.20$ level (2-sided) were selected for multivariable modeling.

A fixed-effects logistic regression model was developed where the probability of an individual being *Taenia*- or *T. solium* cysticerci exposure-positive was parameterized as a function of the explanatory variables with unconditional associations significant at $P < 0.20$, as described above. Explanatory variables that were not statistically significant were removed from the model one at a time, beginning with the least significant, until the estimated regression coefficients for the explanatory variables retained were significant at an alpha level of less than 0.05. Explanatory variables that were excluded at the initial screening stage were tested for inclusion in the final model and were retained if their inclusion changed any of the estimated regression coefficients by more than 20%. Biologically plausible two-way interactions were tested and none were significant at an alpha level of 0.05.

To account for the hierarchical structure of the data, that is, villages within districts and households within villages and study participants within households, we extended the model to include village- and household-level random effect terms using the lme4 package [21] in R version 3.4.3 [22]. This extension to the model was informative because it provided the opportunity to distinguish the influence of unobserved explanatory variables operating at the village, household and individual level on *Taenia*- and *T. solium* cysticerci exposure-positive risk. In our multilevel model the variance of the random effect terms at the village and household level were negligible, and the point estimates of the regression coefficients and standard errors for the explanatory variables were identical to the fixed-effects model. For parsimony, we report the results of the fixed-effects regression model adjusted for the three-stage sampling design using the survey package [23] in R.

The contribution of each of the explanatory variables in the final model on *Taenia*- and *T. solium* cysticerci exposure-positive risk was quantified using the population attributable fraction. The population attributable fraction for a given explanatory variable is the proportional reduction in outcome event incidence expected by either eliminating exposure to the variable or completely preventing the effects of exposure, assuming the explanatory variable is causative and assuming there has been no bias and sampling error in the study population [24]. Using the method of Toschke et al. (2007) [25], adjusted population attributable fractions were calculated for each of the explanatory variables that were significant in the mixed-effects logistic regression model.

Results

General description of study population and data structure

Table 1 presents the structure of the data. In total 342 individuals, from 190 households in six villages in three districts of Dak Lak province consented to take part in the study. A household had, on average, two individuals that consented to take part (minimum 1; maximum 5). In total, only 25% (95% confidence interval (CI) 19% to 32%, 47 of 190) of households possessed a latrine and 25% (95% CI 19% to 32%, 48 of 190) of households sourced their water for daily activities, including drinking, from lakes, streams or ponds. Untreated drinking water was consumed by 60% (95% CI 53% to 67%, 115 of 190) of households (Table 2). The literacy rate among participants was 56% (95% CI 51% to 62%, 193 of 342). Most participants (87%, 95% CI 80% to 88%) listed farming as their main occupational activity (Table 3). The percentage of study participants that did not wash their hands after defaecation or before eating was 35% (95% CI 31% to 41%, 121 of 339) and 44% (95% CI 39% to 50%, 150 of 339), respectively.

Total of 342 serum samples collected from study participants, three were excluded due to hemolysis resulting in 339 samples included for further analysis. Of 339

Table 1 Structure of the data from 342 study participants from six villages in M'Drak, Buon Don and Krong Nang districts

Level	Number	Number at the next highest level	
		Mean	Range
Districts	3	–	–
Villages	6	2	2
Households	190	31	18 to 40
Humans[a]	342	2	1 to 5

[a]A total of 342 individuals participated in this study. The mean of individuals per household was 2 (range 1 to 5)

Table 2 General description of household data

Characteristic	Frequency	Percentage (95% CI)
Number of households	190	
District		
M'Drak	58	30 (24 to 38)
Buon Don	66	35 (28 to 42)
Krong Nang	66	35 (28 to 42)
Owning pigs		
Yes	37	19 (14 to 26)
No	153	81 (74 to 86)
Presence of latrine		
Yes	47	25 (19 to 32)
No	143	75 (68 to 81)
Source of drinking water		
Pipe/well/rain water	142	74 (66 to 79)
Lake/stream/pond	48	26 (19 to 32)
Water treatment		
Yes	75	39 (32 to 47)
No	115	60 (53 to 67)
Are vegetables fertilized?		
Yes	81	43 (35 to 50)
No	109	57 (50 to 64)

Table 3 Demographic data for individual study participants

Characteristic	Frequency	Percentage (95% CI)
Total number of participants	342	
Age (years)		
< 25	63	18 (14 to 23)
25–60	223	65 (60 to 70)
> 60	56	16 (13 to 21)
Sex		
Male	104	30 (26 to 36)
Female	238	70 (64 to 74)
Highest level of education		
None	149	44 (38 to 49)
Primary/secondary	184	54 (48 to 59)
Tertiary	9	2.6 (1.3 to 5.1)
Primary activity		
Farming	298	87 (83 to 90)
Livestock	14	4.1 (2.3 to 6.9)
Civil service	5	1.5 (0.5 to 3.6)
Other	25	7.3 (4.9 to 11)
Ethnicity		
Kinh	40	11 (8.6 to 15)
Ede	302	88 (84 to 91)

serum samples, antibodies against *T. solium* cysticerci were identified in 17 individuals (5%, 95% CI 3% to 8%). Among 342 faecal samples, 23 (6.7%, 95% CI 4.4% to 10%) were positive for *Taenia* spp. Single infection of *T. solium* and *T. saginata* were identified in three and 14 samples, respectively; mixed infections of *T. solium* and *T. saginata* occurred in one samples, and of *T. saginata* and *T. asiatica* in five samples [14].

Risk factors for *T. solium* cysticerci exposure

Of the data recorded using the questionnaire, we identified three factors associated with an individual's likelihood of being exposure-positive to *T. solium* cysticerci based on the results of the LLGP-EITB assay. These were, the frequent consumption of raw vegetables, sourcing drinking water from lakes, streams or ponds and outdoor defaecation.

Estimated regression coefficients for consumption of raw vegetables, the source of drinking water and routine location of defaecation are provided in Table 4. After adjusting for other explanatory variables in the model, the odds of an individual who often consumed raw vegetables being *T. solium* cysticerci exposure-positive was 9.98 (95% CI 2.89 to 34.4) times that of an individual who consumed raw vegetables rarely. The odds ratio for those who routinely defaecated outdoors was similar, at 11.1 (95% CI 2.97 to 42.0). The adjusted population attributable fraction for the consumption of raw vegetables was 74% and thus, reducing the prevalence of raw vegetable consumption in the population is expected to reduce the exposure to *T. solium* cysticerci by a factor of 74%. Similarly, the population attributable fraction estimate for routine location of defaecation was 60%.

The odds of *T. solium* cysticerci exposure for those that routinely sourced their drinking water from streams, ponds or lakes was 3.94 (95% CI 1.29 to 11.9) times higher than the odds of *T. solium* cysticerci exposure for those that sourced their water from wells.

Risk factors for *Taenia* spp. infection

We identified five factors associated with an individual's likelihood of infection with *Taenia* spp. gender, the frequent consumption of pork tongue, the frequent consumption of undercooked pork, frequent consumption of undercooked beef, and observation of *Taenia* proglottids shedding from either themselves, their relatives or neighbors (Table 5).

After adjusting for other explanatory variables in the model, the odds of *Taenia* spp. infection for an individual who frequently consumed pork tongue was 4.62 (95% CI 1.49 to 14.3) times the odds for an individual who consumed pork tongue only rarely. Males had higher odds of being *Taenia* spp. positive compared with females (OR 2.77, 95% CI 1.00 to 7.68).

Among the modifiable risk factors for *Taenia* spp. infection identified in this study, the adjusted population attributable fraction for frequent consumption of undercooked beef was 77%. The population attributable fractions for frequent consumption of undercooked pork and pork tongue were 24% and 26%, respectively. Assuming undercooked beef consumption is a component cause of taeniasis risk, reducing the prevalence of this practice in the population is expected to reduce the overall prevalence of taeniasis by a factor of 77%.

Discussion

The seroprevalence of exposure to *T. solium* in rural communities in Dak Lak in the Central Highlands was 5% (95% CI 3% to 8%). This prevalence is relatively similar to other regions across Vietnam. Phan et al. (2001) [11] reported a 4% seroprevalence of cysticercosis across 22 provinces in the south of Vietnam. For studies in the north and northwest, where *T. solium* is reported to be endemic, the seroprevalence ranged from 2 to 6% [26–29]. In this study, various risk factors were evaluated to

Table 4 Risk factors associated with *T. solium* cysticerci exposure identified by a LLGP-EITB assay

Explanatory variable	Number positive	Number of individuals	Regression coefficient (SE)	*P* value	Adjusted OR (95% CI)
Intercept	17	339	−6.4694 (1.0615)	< 0.01	–
Raw vegetable consumption				< 0.01	
Occasionally	4	226	Reference		1.00
Often	13	113	2.3006 (0.6318)		9.98 (2.89 to 34.4)[a]
Area of defaecation[b]				< 0.01	
Close latrine	5	228	Reference		1.00
Outdoor	12	110	2.4125 (0.6763)		11.1 (2.97 to 42.0)
Source of drinking water				< 0.05	
Other[c]	9	253	Reference		1.00
Stream/Lake/Pond	8	86	1.3702 (0.5684)		3.94 (1.29 to 11.9)

[a]Interpretation: After adjusting for other explanatory variables in the model, the odds of an individual who consumed raw vegetables often being *T. solium* cysticerci exposure was 9.98 (95% CI 2.89 to 34.4) times that of an individual who consumed rare vegetables rarely
[b]A single individual with a missing value for area of defaecation excluded
[c]Drinking water sourced from wells, pipes, rainy and packed water

Table 5 Logistic regression model showing the effect of sex, dietary and observation of proglottids on the odds of a taeniasis case

Explanatory variable	Number positive	Number of individuals	Regression coefficient (SE)	*P* value	Adjusted OR (95% CI)
Intercept	23	342	−6.6069 (1.0365)	< 0.01	–
Sex:				< 0.05	
Female	8	238	Reference		1.00
Male	15	104	1.0183 (0.5209)		2.77 (1.00 to 7.68) [a]
Undercooked pork consumed:				< 0.05	
No	9	241	Reference		1.00
Yes	14	101	1.3023 (0.5695)		3.68 (1.20 to 11.2)
Pork tongue consumed				< 0.01	
Rare	15	305	Reference		1.00
Often	8	37	1.5309 (0.5778)		4.62 (1.49 to 14.3)
Undercooked beef consumed				< 0.01	
No	2	154	Reference		1.00
Yes	21	188	1.935 (0.8070)		6.92 (1.42 to 33.7)
Proglottids observed				< 0.01	
No	12	302	Reference		1.00
Yes	11	40	2.592 (0.5842)		13.36 (4.25 to 41.9)

[a]Interpretation: After adjusting for other explanatory variables in the model, the odds of an individual who is male being taeniasis infection was 2.77 (95% CI 1.00 to 7.68) times that of an individual who is female

determine their association with seroexposure to *T. solium* using the LLGP-EITB assay. Of these, raw vegetable consumption, the source of drinking water and routine location of defaecation were significantly associated with an increase in *T. solium* cysticerci exposure (Table 4). It is known that risk factors for transmission and circulation of *T. solium* cysticercosis are numerous and may vary in different settings. The identified risk factors in Dak Lak were consistent with that of study carried out in the north and south of Vietnam [11, 30]. In contrast to studies in Vietnam's north, the utilisation of night-soil was not associated with the increase in *T. solium* exposure observed in these study communities [12, 31]. Similar to the studies in western Sichuan (China) [32], Mbeya (Tanzania) [26] and northern India [33], routine open defaecation, utilisation of unsafe water sources and consumption of raw vegetables significantly increased the risk of cysticercosis in Dak Lak. However, Cherian et al. (2014) [34] reported that these factors were not contributive in individuals who had epilepsy in Kerala, India. Research on the epidemiological characteristics of human *T. solium* cysticercosis in Nigeria [35], Tanzania [36], and Guatemala [37] found that gender and age [38] were associated with cysticercosis seropositivity, in which the female gender and increased age were significantly linked to the prevalence of *T. solium*. In our study, age and gender did not contribute to seroexposure of *T. solium* cysticerci.

Each of the identified risk factors in this study are eminently modifiable and if effective interventions are deployed, we predict that there will be marked reduction (in the order of 60% to 74%) in the prevalence of exposure to *T. solium* cysticerci in this area of Vietnam. Dak Lak province has a population of approximately 1.8 million [39]; the survey adjusted apparent prevalence of exposure to *T. solium* cysticerci, as estimated in this study, at 5.01% equates to approximately 90,000 exposure-positive individuals. With a population attributable fraction for routine location of defaecation at 60%, and assuming an intervention program to educate inhabitants to practice defaecation indoors, we estimate that the number of exposure-positive individuals will be reduced to approximately 36,000 individuals if the program is 100% successful. Even with 50% efficacy of the intervention program, we estimate the number of exposure-positive individuals would be in the order of 63,000, a substantial reduction from the current prevalence estimate of 90,000. The expected savings to the public health sector (in terms of avoided diagnostics and treatments) is likely to be substantial. If both location of defaecation and raw vegetable consumption practices are modified concurrently, the expected population attributable fraction is 89%. Outdoor defaecation results in the contamination of the environment including water and vegetables; thus, to reduce or mitigate the burden of *T. solium* cysticerci exposure of inhabitants in the communities of Dak Lak province, this factor should be given the highest priority of implementation as an intervention program.

Taenia spp. infection risk in in this study was associated with gender, the consumption of pork tongue, consumption of undercooked pork and beef, and observation of

Taenia proglottids shedding from either themselves, their relatives or neighbors (Table 5). Among these factors, the consumption of pork tongue, and consumption of undercooked pork and beef are modifiable. Consumption of undercooked beef had the highest population attributable fraction of 77% compared to other factors which ranged from 24 to 26%. Thus, an intervention program aimed at discouraging practices of consuming undercooked beef could potentially result in a 77% reduction in the number of cases of taeniasis in the region. The strong association of undercooked beef consumption with *Taenia* positivity could explain the dominant prevalence of *T. saginata* in this study population at 5.8% compared to 1.2% with *T. solium* and 1.5% with *T. asiatica* [14], because beef containing *T. saginata* cysticerci is the cause of *T. saginata* taeniasis in humans.

Males had a higher likelihood of taeniasis compared to females. In rural communities of Dak Lak, males commonly consume undercooked beef, pork, or pork visceral organs while drinking alcohol as part of traditional cultural practices. Thus, educating the community on appropriate consumption of meat, targeting male members of the community is expected to have a substantial impact on the prevalence of taeniasis, although altering cultural dietary practices is recognized as a challenging approach to successful intervention. The most notable limitation of this study was the low prevalence of infection with individual species of *Taenia*, namely, *T. solium*, *T. saginata* and *T. asiatica* in study communities. This deterred our ability to build a model to predict risk factors associated with species-level *Taenia* infection in this study.

A three-stage cluster sampling design was used for this study with villages within districts as the primary sampling unit, households within villages as the secondary sampling unit and individuals within households as the tertiary sampling unit. Given the hierarchical structure of our data it was our a priori belief that observations made on individual study participants were not likely to be independent, justifying the use of regression modelling approaches that accounted for this non-independence. In our mixed-effects logistic regression model the variance of the random effect terms at both the village and individual household levels were negligible. Our inference is that in this population most of the unmeasured *Taenia*/cysticerci-exposure risks resided at the individual (as opposed to either the village or household) level. The practical implications of this finding are that in addition to addressing the modifiable risk factors identified in these analyses, health education programs need to be focused at the individual level.

Since many of the identified risk factors are traditional/behavioural practices in this area of Vietnam, the probability to induce permanent behavioural change from a single education campaign is likely to be small. A One Health approach utilising the expertise of anthropologists might be one way of effecting permanent behavioural change. Long term behavioural change in a population and on-going political support for health interventions occur when aspects of health risk, the economic benefits of disease control and the economic costs associated with disease can be quantified [40]. Financial and human resources are critical factors influencing the success of disease intervention programs. If resources are not available to support an integrated, long-term control and eradication program, a selective approach provides a suitable alternative with the selection of those interventions that provide the most cost-effective return on investment being preferred [41, 42]. The resource for taeniasis, cysticercosis intervention programs in Dak Lak province is limited; therefore, a selective approach is necessary. As discussed above, health education programs involving both the human medical and veterinary health sectors are a feasible intervention option. Choosing a small number of risk factors that make the greatest contribution to the prevalence of taeniasis or cysticercosis are logical targets within an education campaign, for example, indoor latrine construction will ultimately prove the most cost-effective approach.

Conclusions

The prevalence of seroexposure to *T. solium* in the communities of Dak Lak is consistent with that of other regions in Vietnam. Identified risk factors are modifiable, and associated strongly with the prevalence of *T. solium* seroexposure and *Taenia* spp. infection in Dak Lak communities, thus advocating for targeted community intervention programs in mitigating these risks.

Abbreviations

CI: Confidence interval; LLGP-EITB: Lentil lectin purified glycoprotein enzyme-linked immunoelectrotransfer blot assay; OR: Odds ratio; T3qPCR: Multiplex real-time PCR

Acknowledgements

We are grateful to the Institute of Biotechnology and Environment Tay Nguyen University for providing resources and facilities for the fieldwork. We thank Drs. John Noh and Sukwan Handali from the Center for Diseases Control and Prevention, GA, USA for EITB analysis. The Authors are grateful to village medical staff at Buon Don, Krong Nang and M'Drak district for assisting with sample collection. The authors are most thankful to Assoc. Prof. Than Trong Quang, Ms. Nguyen Thi Ngoc Hien, Ms. Long Khanh Linh, and Ms. Nguyen Thi Lan Huong, who assisted with laboratory work and fieldwork.

Funding

This research was self-funded by RJT. This work was done with partial support for travel from the Faculty of Veterinary and Agricultural Sciences, University of Melbourne, Australia. DNN received PhD scholarship from Australia Awards Scholarships, Department of Foreign Affairs and Trade, Australia Government.

Authors' contributions

DNN designed study, analyzed data and wrote manuscript; MAS: assisted with analyses of data and edited paper; KB, TVP, VTN and TW: assisted laboratory work and fieldwork; RJT provided material, supervised study and edited paper. All authors read and approved the final manuscript.

Competing interests
The authors declare that they have no competing interests.

Author details
[1]Faculty of Veterinary and Agricultural Sciences, University of Melbourne, Parkville, VIC 3052, Australia. [2]Faculty of Animal Sciences and Veterinary Medicine, Tay Nguyen University, Dak Lak, Vietnam. [3]Department of Livestock, Montana Veterinary Diagnostic Lab, Bozeman, MT, USA. [4]Faculty of Medicine and Pharmacy, Tay Nguyen University, Dak Lak, Vietnam. [5]Department of Physiology, Pathology and Immunology, Pham Ngoc Thach University of Medicine, Ho Chi Minh, Vietnam.

References
1. FAO/WHO. Multicriterial-based Ranking for Risk Management of Food-borne Parasites. Microbiological risk assessment series no 23. Rome: WHO press; 2014.
2. Ndimubanzi PC, Carabin H, Budke CM, Nguyen H, Qian YJ, Rainwater E, et al. A systematic review of the frequency of neurocyticercosis with a focus on people with epilepsy. PLoS Negl Trop Dis. 2010;4:e870.
3. Garcia HH, Nash TE, Del Brutto OH. Clinical symptoms, diagnosis, and treatment of neurocysticercosis. Lancet Neurol. 2014;13:1202–15.
4. Torgerson PR, Devleesschauwer B, Praet N, Speybroeck N, Willingham AL, Kasuga F, et al. World Health Organization estimates of the global and regional disease burden of 11 foodborne parasitic diseases, 2010: a data synthesis. PLoS Med. 2015;12:e1001920.
5. WHO. Taeniasis/cysticercosis. WHO. 2018. http://www.who.int/news-room/fact-sheets/detail/taeniasis-cysticercosis. Accessed 22 Feb 2018.
6. Aung AK, Spelman DW. *Taenia solium* taeniasis and cysticercosis in Southeast Asia. Am J Trop Med Hyg. 2016;94:947–54.
7. Wu HW, Ito A, Ai L, Zhou XN, Acosta LP, Lee WA. Cysticercosis/taeniasis endemicity in Southeast Asia: current status and control measures. Acta Trop. 2015;165:121–32.
8. NIMPE. Taeniasis and Cysticercosis. In: Review workshop on helminthiasis control activities in the period 2006–2011 and implementing the workplan for the period 2012–2015. Ministry of Health of Vietnam; 2012.
9. Vien HV, Hung NM, Thach DTC, Thuan LK, Dung DT, Hop NT, et al. Investigate *Taenia* infection in two communes of Tan Son district, Phu Tho province. J Malar Parasite Dis Control. 2012;1:69–74.
10. Van Tuan B, Van CN. Situation of *Taenia saginata* infestation and effectiveness of some control measures in Dak Mon commune (Dak Glei) and Yaxier commune (Sa Thay), Kon Tum province. J Malar Parasite Dis Control. 2014;1:41–8.
11. Anh Tuan P, Dung TTK, Nhi VA. Sero-epidemiological investigation of cysticercosis in the southern provinces. J Malar Parasite Dis Control. 2001;4:81–7.
12. Ng-Nguyen D, Stevenson MA, Traub RJ. A systematic review of taeniasis, cysticercosis and trichinellosis in Vietnam. Parasit Vectors. 2017;10:150.
13. Ng-nguyen D, Noh J, Breen K, Stevenson MA, Handali S, Traub RJ. The epidemiology of porcine *Taenia solium* cysticercosis in communities of the Central Highlands in Vietnam. Parasit Vectors. 2018;11:360.
14. Ng-Nguyen D, Stevenson MA, Dorny P, Gabriël S, Van VT, Nguyen VT, et al. Comparison of a new multiplex real-time PCR with the Kato Katz thick smear and copro-antigen ELISA for the detection and differentiation of *Taenia* spp. in human stools. PLoS Negl Trop Dis. 2017;11:e0005743.
15. General statistics office of Viet Nam. Percentage of literate population at 15 years of age and above by province. 2016. https://www.gso.gov.vn/default_en.aspx?tabid=774. Accessed 8 Jan 2018.
16. Lucas LA, Phillip MK, Peter BG, Mark ON, Gerald M, Esther S. A survey of bovine cysticercosis/human taeniosis in Northern Turkana District, Kenya. Preventive Veterinary Medicine. 2009;89(3-4):197–204.
17. Tsang VCW, Brand JA, Boyer AE. An enzyme-linked immunoelectrotransfer blot assay and glycoprotein antigens for diagnosing human cysticercosis (*Taenia solium*). J Infect Dis. 1989;159:50–9.
18. Noh J, Rodriguez S, Lee YM, Handali S, Gonzalez AE, Gilman RH, et al. Recombinant protein- and synthetic peptide-based immunoblot test for diagnosis of neurocysticercosis. J Clin Microbiol. 2014;52:1429–34.
19. Jeon HK, Chai JY, Kong Y, Waikagul J, Insisiengmay B, Rim HJ, et al. Differential diagnosis of *Taenia asiatica* using multiplex PCR. Exp Parasitol. 2009;121:151–6.
20. Lumley T. Complex surveys a guide to analysis using R. New York: Wiley; 2010.
21. Bates D, Machler M, Bolker B, Walker S. Fitting linear mixed-effects models using lme4. J Stat Softw. 2015;67:1–48.
22. Team R Core. R: A Language and Environment for Statistical Computing. 2017. http://www.r-project.org.
23. Lumley T. Analysis of complex survey samples. J Stat Softw. 2004;9:1–19.
24. Whittemore AS. Statistical methods for estimating attributable risk from retrospective data. Stat Med. 1982;1:229–43.
25. Toschke AM, Rückinger S, Böhler E, Von Kries R. Adjusted population attributable fractions and preventable potential of risk factors for childhood obesity. Public Health Nutr. 2007;10:902–6.
26. Trung DD, Praet N, Cam TDT, Lam BVT, Manh HN, Gabriël S, et al. Assessing the burden of human cysticercosis in Vietnam. Trop Med Int Heal. 2013;18:352–6.
27. Somers R, Dorny P, Nguyen VK, Dang TCT, Goddeeris B, Craig PS, et al. *Taenia solium* taeniasis and cysticercosis in three communities in North Vietnam. Trop Med Int Heal. 2006;11:65–72.
28. Doanh NQ, Kim NT, De NV, Lung NL. Result of survey on taeniasis and cysticercosis humans and pigs in Bac Ninh and Bac Kan provinces. Vet Sci Tech. 2002;9:46–9.
29. Erhart A, Dorny P, Van De N, Vien HV, Thach DC, Toan ND, et al. *Taenia solium* cysticercosis in a village in northern Viet Nam: Sero-prevalence study using an ELISA for detecting circulating antigen. Trans R Soc Trop Med Hyg. 2002;96:270–2.
30. Ho ST. Study on genotype of pathogen, clinical, subclinical symptoms, treatment efficacy for taeniasis and cysticercosis patients in National Institute of Malariology, Parasitology and Entomology 2007–2010: Hanoi Medical University; 2013. http://luanan.nlv.gov.vn/luanan?a=d&d=TTcFqWrCyuSa2013.1.4&srpos=1&e=%2D%2D%2D%2D%2D%2D-vi-20%2D%2D1%2D%2Dimg-txIN-H%25e1%25bb%2593+S%25e1%25bb%25b9+Tri%25e1%25bb%2581u
31. Van De N, Le TH, Lien PTH, Eom KS. Current status of taeniasis and cysticercosis in Vietnam. Korean J Parasitol. 2014;52:125–9.
32. Openshaw JJ, Medina A, Felt SA, Li T, Huan Z, Rozelle S, et al. Prevalence and risk factors for *Taenia solium* cysticercosis in school-aged children: a school based study in western Sichuan, People's Republic of China. PLoS Negl Trop Dis. 2018;12:e0006465.
33. Prasad KN, Verma A, Srivastava S, Gupta RK, Pandey CM, Paliwal VK. An epidemiological study of asymptomatic neurocysticercosis in a pig farming community in northern India. Trans R Soc Trop Med Hyg. 2011;105:531–6.
34. Cherian A, Syam UK, Sreevidya D, Jayaraman T, Oommen A, Rajshekhar V, et al. Low seroprevalence of systemic cysticercosis among patients with epilepsy in Kerala-South India. J Infect Public Health. 2014;7:271–6.
35. Rebecca WP, Eugene II, Joshua K. Seroprevalence of antibodies (IgG) to *Taenia solium* among pig rearers and associated risk factors in Jos metropolis, Nigeria. J Infect Dev Ctries. 2013;7:67–72.
36. Mwanjali G, Kihamia C, Kakoko DVC, Lekule F, Ngowi H, Johansen MV, et al. Prevalence and risk factors associated with human *Taenia solium* infections in Mbozi district, Mbeya region, Tanzania. PLoS Negl Trop Dis. 2013;7:e2102.
37. Garcia-Noval J, Moreno E, de Mata F, Soto de Alfaro H, Fletes C, Craig PS, et al. An epidemiological study of epilepsy and epileptic seizures in two rural Guatemalan communities. Ann Trop Med Parasitol. 2001;95:167–75.
38. Edia-Asuke AU, Inabo HI, Mukaratirwa S, Umoh VJ, Whong CM, Asuke S, et al. Seroprevalence of human cysticercosis and its associated risk factors among humans in areas of Kaduna metropolis, Nigeria. J Infect Dev Ctries. 2015;9:799–805.
39. Dak Lak Provincial People's Committee. An overview about Dak Lak province. 2014; 5/8/2014. https://daklak.gov.vn/web/english/about-daklak.
40. Gabriël S, Dorny P, Mwape KE, Trevisan C, Braae UC, Magnussen P, et al. Control of Taenia solium taeniasis/cysticercosis: the best way forward for Sub-Saharan Africa? Acta Trop. 2017;165:252–60.
41. Winskill P, Harrison WE, French MD, Dixon MA, Abela-Ridder B, Basáñez M-G. Assessing the impact of intervention strategies against *Taenia solium* cysticercosis using the EPICYST transmission model. Parasit Vectors. 2017;10:73.
42. O'Neal SE, Moyano LM, Ayvar V, Rodriguez S, Gavidia C, Wilkins PP, et al. Ring-screening to control endemic transmission of *Taenia solium*. PLoS Negl Trop Dis. 2014;8:e3125.

11

Prevalence and anatomical sites of human papillomavirus, Epstein-Barr virus and herpes simplex virus infections in men who have sex with men

Jureeporn Chuerduangphui[1,5], Kanisara Proyrungroj[1,5], Chamsai Pientong[1,5], Saowarop Hinkan[1,5], Jiratha Budkaew[2], Charinya Pimson[3,5], Bandit Chumworathayi[4,5], Ploenpit Hanond[1] and Tipaya Ekalaksananan[1,5*]

Abstract

Background: Human papillomavirus (HPV), Epstein-Barr virus (EBV) and herpes simplex virus (HSV) cause sexually transmitted diseases (STDs) that are frequently found in men who have sex with men (MSM) with human immunodeficiency viral (HIV) infection.

Methods: This study investigated the prevalence of infection and anatomical site distribution of these viruses in asymptomatic MSM. DNA, extracted from cells collected from the anorectum, oropharynx and urethra of 346 participants, was investigated for the presence of EBV, HPV and HSV using real-time PCR. Demographic data from the participants were analyzed.

Results: All three viruses were found in all sampled sites. EBV was the commonest virus, being detected in the anorectum (47.7% of participants), oropharynx (50.6%) and urethra (45.6%). HPV and HSV were found in 43.9% and 2.9% of anorectum samples, 13.8% and 3.8% of oropharynx samples and 25.7% and 2% of urethra samples, respectively. HPV infection of the anorectum was significantly associated with age groups 21–30 (odds = 3.043, 95% CI = 1.643–5.638 and $P = 0.001$) and 46–60 years (odds = 2.679, 95% CI = 1.406–5.101 and $P = 0.03$). EBV infection of the urethra was significantly correlated with age group 21–30 years (odds = 1.790, 95% CI = 1.010–3.173 and $P = 0.046$). EBV/HPV co-infection of the anorectum (odds = 3.211, 95% CI = 1.271–8.110, $P = 0.014$) and urethra (odds = 2.816, 95% CI = 1.024–7.740, $P = 0.045$) was also associated with this age group. Among HIV-positive MSM, there was a significant association between age-group (odds = 21.000, 95% CI = 1.777–248.103, $P = 0.016$) in HPV infection of the anorectum. A failure to use condoms was significantly associated with HPV infection of the anorectum (odds = 4.095, 95% CI = 1.404–11.943, $P = 0.010$) and urethra (odds = 7.187, 95% CI = 1.385–37.306, $P = 0.019$). Similarly, lack of condom use was significantly associated with EBV infection of the urethra (odds = 7.368, 95% CI = 1.580–34.371, $P = 0.011$).

Conclusion: These results indicate that asymptomatic MSM in Northeast Thailand form a potential reservoir for transmission of STDs, and in particular for these viruses.

Keywords: Human papillomavirus, Herpes simplex virus, Epstein-Barr virus, Co-infection, Asymptomatic MSM, Anatomical site

* Correspondence: tipeka@kku.ac.th
[1]Department of Microbiology, Faculty of Medicine, Khon Kaen University, Khon Kaen, Thailand
[5]HPV & EBV and Carcinogenesis Research Group, Khon Kaen University, Khon Kaen, Thailand
Full list of author information is available at the end of the article

Background

Men who have sex with men (MSM) are at higher risk of sexually transmitted diseases (STDs) than other groups. Incidence has been rising due to the practice of various sexual acts including penile–anal, oral–anal, and/or penile–oral contact [1, 2]. HPV is the most common sexually transmitted viral infection and its prevalence is increasing [3]. Human papillomavirus (HPV) is a causative agent of genital warts [4] and the main risk factor for anal cancer in MSM [5]. The incidence of anal cancer is highest in HIV-infected MSM and is increasing annually. HPV is also associated with oropharyngeal and penile cancers, but at lower prevalence than anal cancer [6]. Detection of HPV infection in asymptomatic MSM can be used to monitor and follow-up HPV-persistent infection for HPV-related cancer intervention.

Other viruses are also found in MSM. Epstein-Barr virus (EBV) is one of the most common human viruses found in B-cells and epithelial cells of healthy persons [7]. The presence of EBV in sites such as the anus, oropharynx and urethra can be due not only to intimate contact but also to the movement of EBV-infected B-cells. Most people are infected in childhood and do not develop symptoms, or have very minor symptoms such as a mild infectious mononucleosis syndrome [8]. EBV has been frequently found in the non-genital and genital mucosa, ulcers and urethral discharges and associated with various malignancies including Burkitt's lymphoma, Hodgkin's disease, non-Hodgkin's lymphoma, nasopharyngeal carcinoma, breast cancer, gastric cancer, etc. [9]. It seems likely to be a co-factor in HPV-associated cancers such as anal and penile cancers [10, 11]. Moreover, EBV infection is associated with HPV integration into the host genome, which is a relevant process in cervical cancer progression [12]. In contrast, EBV is more frequently found than HPV in oropharyngeal cancer [13, 14]. Interestingly, the prevalence of EBV in isolated B-cells of MSM is significantly higher than in heterosexual men [15]. MSM appear to be at more risk of EBV infection. Although EBV causes various types of disease, including cancer, its co-prevalence with HPV among asymptomatic MSM at various anatomical sites has been little studied.

Herpes simplex virus (HSV) is one of the commonest sexually transmitted viral infections worldwide. The usual sites of HSV infection are skin and mucosal membranes. Primary infection sites of HSV-1 and HSV-2 are the oropharynx and genital tract, respectively. Infection is often asymptomatic. Even though HSV-2 is predominantly spread via the genital route (in contrast to HSV-1) and its seroprevalence is higher in HIV-positive (> 80%) than HIV-negative MSM [16], HSV-1 is causing an increasing proportion of anogenital herpes worldwide [17, 18]. Anogenital HSV-1 is more common in MSM than heterosexual individuals [19]. Interestingly, HSV infection is associated with increased viral load of HIV in infected MSM [20]. Interestingly, co-infection of HSV and HPV16 in patients with head and neck carcinomas (HNSCC) has the worst disease outcome [21]. In addition, HSV-1 infection may modulate the radiation resistance of HPV16-positive HNSCC cells by improving cell survival after irradiation [22]. Therefore, HSV can be a co-factor of HPV-associated carcinogenesis and may be a main reservoir in MSM. We, therefore, investigated HSV in MSM.

To explore the prevalence and anatomical site distribution of HPV, EBV and HSV infecting asymptomatic MSM in Northeast Thailand, real-time polymerase chain reaction (RT-PCR) was used to detect these viruses from 346 participants at anatomical sites including the oropharynx, urethra and anorectum.

Methods

Specimen and data collection

In total, 358 asymptomatic MSM were enrolled under a cross-sectional study project title of "Factors associated to *Neisseria gonorrhea* infection by anatomic distributions among men who have sex with men, and multidrug resistant patterns of *Neisseria gonorrhea*" at M-Reach STDs clinic in Chatapadung Contracting Medical Unit, and the ARV Clinic, Khon Kaen Hospital, Khon Kaen Province, Thailand from September 2014 to July 2015. Prevalence of *Neisseria gonorrhea* in urethra was published [23, 24], but not in oropharynx and anorectum. Cell samples from anorectum, oropharynx and urethra were collected using sterile Dacron swabs (Puritan, Hardwood Products, Guilford, USA). These swabs were immediately transferred into 2 ml of 10% formalin in normal saline solution and transported to laboratory on ice within 4 h. Three-hundred and forty-six asymptomatic MSM were included whereas 12 MSM were excluded because samples were not collected from all three anatomical sites. Participants provided basic demographic data and information concerning their sexual behavior, including number of sexual partners in the preceding 3 months, condom usage and HIV status. This was done by means of a self-reported questionnaire and data were recorded in an anonymous electronic file. The ethical approval for this study was obtained from Khon Kaen University Ethics Committee in Human Research, No. HE591377.

DNA extraction

Cells from swab samples were pelleted and washed with phosphate buffered saline by centrifugation at 2000 rpm for 5 min. Cells were lysed using lysis buffer (10 mM Tris HCl, 0.1 mM EDTA pH 7.5, 1% SDS and 0.5 M NaCl) supplemented with 50 mg/ml of proteinase K and then incubated at 60 °C for 30 min. Protein was precipitated by addition of protein precipitation buffer (5 M potassium acetate, 11.5 ml of glacial acetic acid and 28.5 ml of distill water, pH 5.5), and then removed by centrifugation at 13,500 rpm for 5 min at 4 °C. DNA was precipitated with an equal volume of isopropanol and collected by centrifugation at 13,500 rpm for 5 min at 25 °C and washed with 70% ethanol. Finally, the DNA pellet was dried at 37 °C for 15–30 min and then resuspended in distilled water. The quality of DNA was checked by amplifying the *GAPDH* gene using specific primers (GAPDH forward: 5′-TCATCAGCAATGCC TCCTGCA-3′ and reverse: TGGGTGGCAGTGAT GGCA-3′ by RT-PCR. Quantity of DNA was assessed using the NanoDrop™ (Thermo Scientific) [25].

Detection of HPV, HSV and EBV infection by RT-PCR

HPV infection was investigated using GP5+/GP6+ primers (forward: 5′-TTTGTTACTGTGGTAGATA CTAC-3′ and reverse: 5′-GAAAAATAAACTGTAAATC ATATTC-3′) by RT-PCR [26] to amplify a 141 bp portion of the L1 viral capsid gene. The reaction mixture had a final volume of 20 μl containing 1× SsoAdvancedTM Universal SYBR® Green Supermix (Bio-Rad, Hercules, CA, USA), 0.2 μM of forward primer, 0.2 μM of reverse primer and DNA template. Thermocycling conditions were a denaturation step of 5 min at 95 °C followed by 45 cycles of 95 °C for 10 s and 42 °C for 30 s in an Applied Biosystems 7500 Fast real-time PCR Instrument (Applied Biosystems, Foster City, CA, USA). DNA from SiHa cells (an HPV16-positive cell line) was used as the positive control for HPV DNA detection.

HSV infection was detected using specific primers: HSV DNA polymerase forward: 5′- GTGTTGTGC CGCGGTCTCAC-3′ and reverse: 5′-GGTGAACGT CTTTTCGAACTC-3′. EBV was detected using EBV DNA polymerase forward: 5′- GGAGAAGGTCTTCT CGGCCTC-3′ and reverse: 5′-TTCAGAGAGCGAGA CCCTGC-3′ [27, 28]. The reaction mixture had a final volume of 20 μl containing 1× SsoAdvancedTM Universal SYBR® Green Supermix (Bio-Rad, Hercules, CA, USA), 0.2 μM of forward primer, 0.2 μM of reverse primer and DNA template. The reaction was performed in an Applied Biosystems 7500 Fast real-time PCR Instrument (ABi). Cycling conditions were; initial 3 min at 95 °C followed by 40 cycles of 95 °C for 10 s, 64 °C for 10 s and 72 °C for 30 s. DNA from HSV-1 kos particles and P3HR1 cells (an EBV-positive cell line) was used as the positive control for HSV DNA and EBV DNA detection, respectively.

HPV genotyping

HPV L1 gene fragments in HPV-positive samples were amplified using GP5/ GP6+ primers labeled with biotin and genotyped by reverse line blot hybridization (RLBH) [29]. Biodyne C blotting membrane (Pall Life Science, Ann Arbor, MI, USA) was activated in 16% (*w*/*v*) 1-ethy-3-(3-dimethylaminopropyl) carbodimide (EDAC) solution (Sigma-Aldrich, St. Louis, MO, USA) at room temperature for 10 min, rinsed with distilled water and placed on a mini blotter. Thirty-seven HPV type-specific 5′-amino linked oligonucleotide probes, including 13 high-risk HPV types (16, 18, 31, 33, 35, 39, 45, 51, 52, 56, 58, 59 and 68); 12 low-risk HPV types (6, 11, 26, 40, 42, 43, 44, 53, 54, 61, 72 and 73); and other HPV types (34, 55, 57, 66, 70, 82MM4, 83MM7, 84MM8, 82IS39, CP6108, 71CP8061 and 81CP8304), were dropped onto the Biodyne C membrane through the wells of the mini blotter in parallel lines. Subsequently, biotin-labeled PCR products were added into the channels of the mini blotter perpendicular to the oligonucleotide probe lines, then hybridized and incubated with streptavidin-peroxidase-conjugate. The HPV types present were detected using chemiluminescence.

Statistical analysis

Bivariate analysis (for comparisons of proportions) was used to investigate the association between EBV, HPV and/or HSV infection and age, number of sex partners, condom usage and HIV status of participants using SPSS software (SPSS Inc., Chicago, IL, USA). Any P–value < 0.05 was considered statistically significant.

Results

Patient characteristics

Table 1 shows demographic data and sexual behavior characteristics of 346 asymptomatic MSM participants. The age range was 18–60 years, with the mode being the 21–30-year-old group. Most participants had only one sexual partner, or no partners, in the previous 3 months and always used condoms. A total of 234 asymptomatic MSM self-revealed HIV status.

Prevalence of EBV, HPV or HSV infecting MSM and anatomical site distribution

Swab samples were obtained from each anatomical site (anorectum, oropharynx and urethra) of 346 asymptomatic MSM participants. HPV, EBV and HSV infection were detected in all three anatomical sites (Fig. 1). EBV infection was common at all three sites, with approximately 50% of samples returning a positive result from each (Fig. 1). The anorectum was the site where HPV infection was most common (43.9%), followed by the urethra (25.7%) and oropharynx (13.9%). HSV was the least prevalent (Fig. 1).

The prevalence of high-risk HPV types were higher than of low-risk HPV in all anatomical sites (Fig. 2). Double/multiple infections of high and low-risk types were particularly frequent in the anorectum (Fig. 2a),

Table 1 Clinical data of MSM ($n = 346$)

Clinical finding	n = 346
Age (years)	
Minimum = 18	60
Maximum = 60	1
Age-range groups	
18–20	76
21–30	139
31–45	106
46–60	25
Number of partners within 3 months	
None	129
1–2	166
> 2	51
Condom usage	
Always	223
Sometimes	64
Never	59
HIV status	
Negative	124
Positive	110
Unknown	112

followed by the urethra (Fig. 2c), but a combination of risk types did not occur in the oropharynx (Fig. 2b). The anorectal site seems to be the main reservoir of infection of HPV high- and low-risk types in MSM.

The highest prevalence of double or multiple infections of any type of HPV was in the anorectum (67/152, 44.1%) followed by the urethra (21/89, 23.6%) and oropharynx (3/48, 6.3%). Infections with double and multiple HPV types were more common than with single HPV types in the anorectum (44.1% vs. 40.1%, with HPV types 18 and 58 being the most common combination), but not in the oropharynx (6.3% vs. 52.1%, with HPV types 39 and 58 being the most common combination) or urethra (23.6% vs. 57.3%, with HPV types 16 and 18 being the most common combination) (Additional file 1: Table S1). HPV 18 was mostly found in the anorectum (42/152, 27.6% followed by HPV 16 and HPV 58 in similar proportions at 25%) and in the urethra (40/89, 44.9% followed by HPV 16 and HPV 58 in 21.3% and 19.1% respectively). HPV 58 was most frequently detected in the oropharynx (18/48, 37.5% followed by HPV types 39, 18 and 53 at 8.3%, 6.3% and 6.3% respectively).

Factors associated with prevalence of HPV, EBV and HSV in the anorectum, oropharynx and urethra among 346 asymptomatic MSM

There were often significant differences between age groups in prevalence and anatomical sites, as shown in Table 2. EBV infection in the urethra (but not the anorectum or oropharynx) was significantly associated with the 21–30 years-old group (odds = 1.790, 95% CI = 1.010–3.173 and $P = 0.046$). HPV infection in the anorectum was significantly associated with the 21–30 years-old group (odds = 3.043, 95% CI = 1.643–5.638 and $P = 0.001$) and also the 46–60 years-old group (odds = 2.679, 95% CI = 1.406–5.101 and $P = 0.03$). HSV infection in the oropharynx was mostly found in the 46–60 years-old group. EBV infection in the oropharynx and urethra was significantly higher among HIV-positive MSM than among HIV-negative MSM (odds = 2.125, 95% CI = 1.257–3.594 and $P = 0.005$ and odds = 2.536, 95% CI = 1.496–4.298 and $P = 0.001$, respectively). Likewise, HPV infection in the anorectum was significantly associated with HIV-infected MSM (odds = 1.935, 95% CI = 1.150–3.257 and $P = 0.013$). In contrast, the incidence of HSV did not differ according to HIV status. This result suggested that HIV-infected MSM might act as reservoirs for transmission of EBV and HPV.

Table 3 shows the correlation between HPV and EBV infection in HIV-infected and uninfected MSM with the associated factors. HPV infection in the anorectum in HIV-positive MSM was significantly associated with increasing age. For the 31–45 years-old group, odds = 10.500, 95% CI = 1.177–93.697, $P = 0.035$; and for the 46–60 years-old group, odds = 21.000, 95% CI = 1.777–248.103, $P = 0.016$. Co-infection of HIV with HPV-infected anorectum (odds = 4.095, 95% CI = 1.404–11.943 and $P = 0.010$), urethra (odds = 7.187, 95% CI = 1.385–37.306, $P = 0.019$) or EBV-infected urethra (odds = 7.368, 95% CI = 1.580–34.371, $P = 0.011$) was significantly associated with an absence of condom usage. HPV infection in the oropharynx wasn't associated with any demographic factors (data not shown). In addition, no association was found between demographic factors and EBV infection in the anorectum and oropharynx among HIV-infected and uninfected MSM (data not shown). This result demonstrated that lack of condom usage was an important factor for HPV infection in the anorectum and urethra as well as EBV infection in the urethra among HIV-positive MSM.

Co-infection with EBV, HPV and/or HSV in three anatomical sites

Co-infection with EBV and HPV was common, especially in the anorectum (17.3%) (Fig. 3). Reflecting its low prevalence generally, co-infection of HSV with either of the other two viruses was uncommon (Fig. 3). All three viruses were found in 0.9% (3/346) of MSM in the anorectum or urethra but not in the oropharynx (Fig. 3). These results demonstrate that co-infection of EBV and HPV common among northeast Thai MSM at all three anatomical sites.

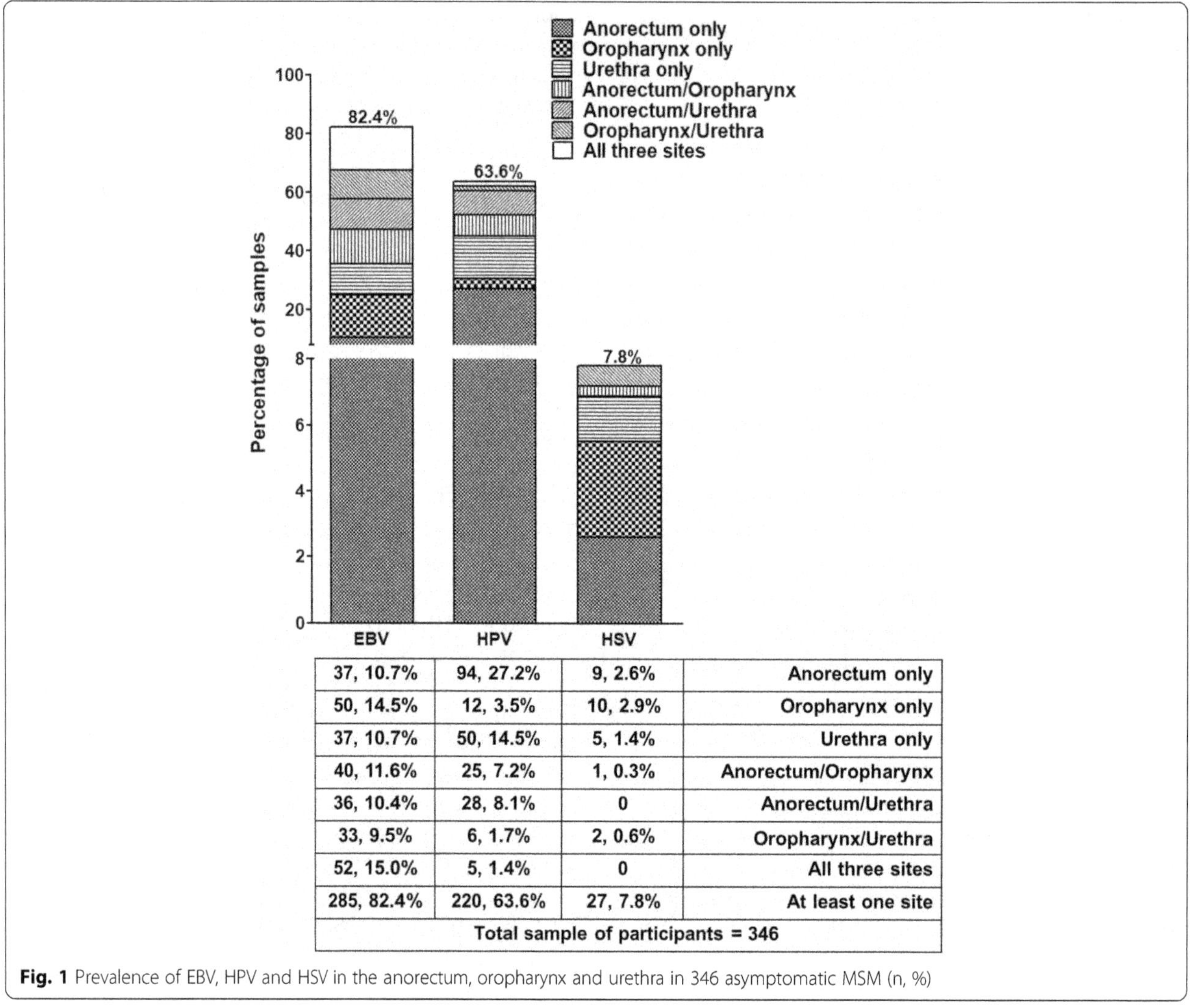

EBV	HPV	HSV	
37, 10.7%	94, 27.2%	9, 2.6%	Anorectum only
50, 14.5%	12, 3.5%	10, 2.9%	Oropharynx only
37, 10.7%	50, 14.5%	5, 1.4%	Urethra only
40, 11.6%	25, 7.2%	1, 0.3%	Anorectum/Oropharynx
36, 10.4%	28, 8.1%	0	Anorectum/Urethra
33, 9.5%	6, 1.7%	2, 0.6%	Oropharynx/Urethra
52, 15.0%	5, 1.4%	0	All three sites
285, 82.4%	220, 63.6%	27, 7.8%	At least one site
Total sample of participants = 346			

Fig. 1 Prevalence of EBV, HPV and HSV in the anorectum, oropharynx and urethra in 346 asymptomatic MSM (n, %)

The association of demographic factors and co-infection of EBV, HPV and HSV in anorectal, oropharyngeal and urethal sites among asymptomatic MSM

Co-infection of HPV with EBV or HSV in all three anatomical sites has not been reported previously. We investigated the association of EBV, HPV and/or HSV co-infection in anorectal, oropharyngeal or urethral sites with demographic factors. Interestingly, co-infection with EBV and HPV at both the anorectum and urethra was significantly associated with the 21–30 years-old group (odds = 3.211, 95% CI = 1.271–8.110, $P = 0.014$ and odds = 2.816, 95% CI = 1.024–7.740, $P = 0.045$ respectively), as shown in Additional file 2: Tables S2 and Additional file 3: Tables S3. In addition, EBV and HPV co-infection in the anorectum and urethra was most found frequently in MSM with current or recent partners and in HIV-positive MSM. Meanwhile, EBV and HPV co-infection at the oropharyngeal site was most frequent in the 45–60 years-old group, as well as in HIV-positive MSM (Additional file 4: Table S4). Co-infections of EBV with HSV, and of HPV with HSV, and of all three viruses together, were not associated with any demographic factors in any anatomical sites (Additional file 2: Tables S2, Additional file 3: Table S3, and Additional file 4: Tables S4). These findings show that co-infection of EBV with HPV was predominately found in the 21–30 years-old group in the anorectum and urethra but not in the oropharynx.

Discussion

In this study, we addressed the prevalence of HPV, EBV and HSV as single and co-infections in different anatomical sites (anorectum, oropharynx and urethra) of 346 MSM in Northeast Thailand. Demographic information was collected from participants, and especially HIV status. Several previous reports exist about the prevalence of EBV in the same anatomical sites of MSM from other countries. EBV infection was found in the anorectum of 29.6% and 32% of HIV-positive German and Swedish MSM, respectively [30, 31]. Oropharyngeal shedding of

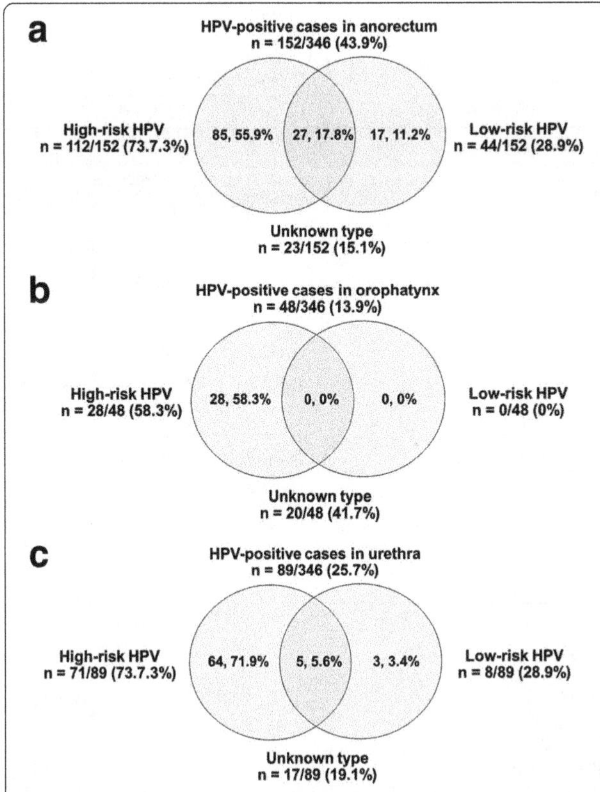

Fig. 2 Site distribution of HPV risk types in HPV-positive cases. **a** HPV-positive cases in anorectum, **b** HPV-positive cases in oropharynx and **c** HPV-positive cases in urethra

EBV was detected in 49–88.8% and 16–56% of HIV-seropositive and seronegative MSM, respectively [32, 33]. In the urethral site, EBV was found in 30.7% of asymptomatic American MSM; notably, EBV prevalence (72.7%) was significantly associated with HIV shedding in semen [34], corresponding to our finding as shown in Table 2. EBV infection of the urethra ranged from 28 to 30.7% among American MSM [34, 35]. Meanwhile, EBV infection of the urethra of American and Spanish men was ranged from 0.4–45% [36]. Most of these published articles demonstrated that EBV had the highest prevalence in the oropharynx, in contrast to the anorectum and urethra, corresponding to our results.

Many studies have demonstrated a high prevalence of HPV infection in the anorectum, ranging from 34.8 to 65.3% [37–39], and was significantly associated with HIV-infected MSM [37, 38], concordant with our results. Prevalence of HPV infection were lower in the oropharynx and urethra (9.6–13.0% and 10.2–16.3%, respectively) [37, 40–42]. As is the case for the anorectum, high prevalence of HPV infection at the oropharynx and urethra were significantly associated with HIV-positive MSM [41, 42].

In Peruvian MSM, the five most common HPV genotypes from the anorectum were 53, 6, 16, 58 and 54 [43]. Similarly, HPV53 was the most frequently found genotype in anorectal samples from HIV-seropositive French MSM [44], but HPV16 was the most frequently found at

Table 2 Prevalence of EBV, HPV or HSV in age range, number of partners within 3 months, condom usage and HIV status in the anorectum, oropharynx and urethra among 346 asymptomatic MSM

Factors	Anorectum, n (%)			Oropharynx, n (%)			Urethra, n (%)		
	EBV	HPV	HSV	EBV	HPV	HSV	EBV	HPV	HSV
Age range (years)									
18–20 (*n* = 76)	35 (46.1)	19 (25.0)	3 (3.9)	41 (53.9)	7 (9.2)	0	28 (36.8)	18 (23.7)	2 (2.6)
21–30 (*n* = 139)	68 (48.9)	70 (50.4)*	3 (2.2)	77 (55.4)	25 (18.0)	3 (2.2)	71 (51.1)*	42 (30.2)	2(1.4)
31–45 (*n* = 106)	51 (48.1)	50 (47.2)	3 (2.8)	44 (41.5)	10 (9.4)	7 (6.6)	48 (45.3)	23 (21.7)	3 (2.8)
46–60 (*n* = 25)	11 (44.0)	13 (52.0) *	1 (4.0)	13 (52.0)	6 (24.0)	3 (12.0)	11 (44.0)	6 (24.0)	0
Number of partners within 3 months									
None (*n* = 129)	56 (43.4)	57 (44.2)	2 (1.6)	74 (57.4)	17 (13.2)	3 (2.3)	66 (51.2)	30 (23.3)	5 (3.9)
1–2 (*n* = 166)	83 (50.0)	78 (47.0)	5 (3.0)	78 (47.0)	28 (16.9)	8 (4.8)	72 (43.4)	45 (27.1)	0
> 2 (*n* = 51)	26 (51.0)	17 (33.3)	3 (5.9)	23 (45.1)	3 (5.9)	2 (3.9)	20 (39.2)	14 (27.5)	2 (3.9)
Condom usage									
Always (*n* = 223)	10 (47.1)	98 (43.9)	7 (3.1)	111 (49.8)	30 (13.5)	7 (3.1)	97 (43.5)	54 (24.2)	5 (2.2)
Sometimes (*n* = 63)	36 (56.3)	23 (35.9)	2 (3.1)	33 (51.6)	6 (9.4)	3 (4.7)	28 (43.8)	21 (32.8)	1 (1.6)
Never (*n* = 60)	24 (40.7)	31 (52.5)	1 (1.7)	31 (52.5)	12 (20.3)	3 (5.1)	33 (55.9)	14 (23.7)	1 (1.7)
HIV status									
Negative (*n* = 124)	60 (48.4)	53 (42.7)	6 (4.8)	56 (45.2)	21 (16.9)	6 (4.8)	45 (36.3)	30 (24.2)	2 (1.6)
Positive (*n* = 110)	53 (48.2)	65 (59.1)*	4 (3.6)	70 (63.6)*	16 (14.5)	5 (4.5)	65 (59.1)*	32 (29.1)	3 (2.7)
Unknown (*n* = 112)	52 (46.4)	34 (30.4)	0	49 (43.8)	11(9.8)	2 (1.8)	48 (42.9)	27 (24.1)	2 (1.8)

* denotes significant difference at $P < 0.05$ by multivariate analysis

Table 3 The association of demographic factors with HPV infection in the anorectum and urethra and with EBV infection in the urethra among HIV-infected MSM

Factors	HPV-infected anorectum		HPV-infected urethra		EBV-infected urethra	
	HIV +	Odds, 95%CI, *P*-value	HIV +	Odds, 95%CI, *P*-value	HIV +	Odds, 95%CI, *P*-value
Age range (years)						
18–20 (n = 76))	1 (12.5)	Reference	0 (0)	-	3 (42.9)	Reference
21–30 (n = 139)	31 (53.5)	8.037, 0.929–69.542, 0.058	18 (53.0)	Reference	35 (61.4)	2.121, 0.433–10.392, 0.354
31–45 (n = 106)	24 (60.0)	10.500, 1.177–93.697, 0.035	9 (50.0)	0.889, 0.283–2.789, 0.840	22 (59.5)	1.956, 0.381–10.026, 0.421
46–60 (n = 25)	9 (75.0)	21.000, 1.777–248.103, 0.016	5 (83.3)	4.444, 0.468–42.175, 0.194	5 (55.6)	1.667, 0.227–12.221, 0.615
No. of partners within 3 mouths						
None (n = 129)	30 (66.7)	Reference	13 (68.4)	Reference	28 (62.2)	Reference
≥ 1 (n = 217)	35 (48.0)	0.461, 0.213–1.000, 0.050	19 (44.2)	0.365, 0.117–1.142, 0.083	37 (56.9)	0.802, 0.369–1.745, 0.579
Condom usage						
Always (n = 223)	40 (50.6)	Reference	16 (41.0)	Reference	38 (52.0)	Reference
Sometimes (n = 63)	4 (30.8)	0.433, 0.123–1.524, 0.193	6 (54.5)	1.725, 0.448–6.637, 0.428	11 (57.9)	1.266, 0.457–3.512, 0.650
Never (n = 60)	21 (80.8)	4.095, 1.404–11.943, 0.010	10 (55.9)	7.187, 1.385–37.306, 0.019	16 (88.0)	7.368, 1.580–34.371, 0.011

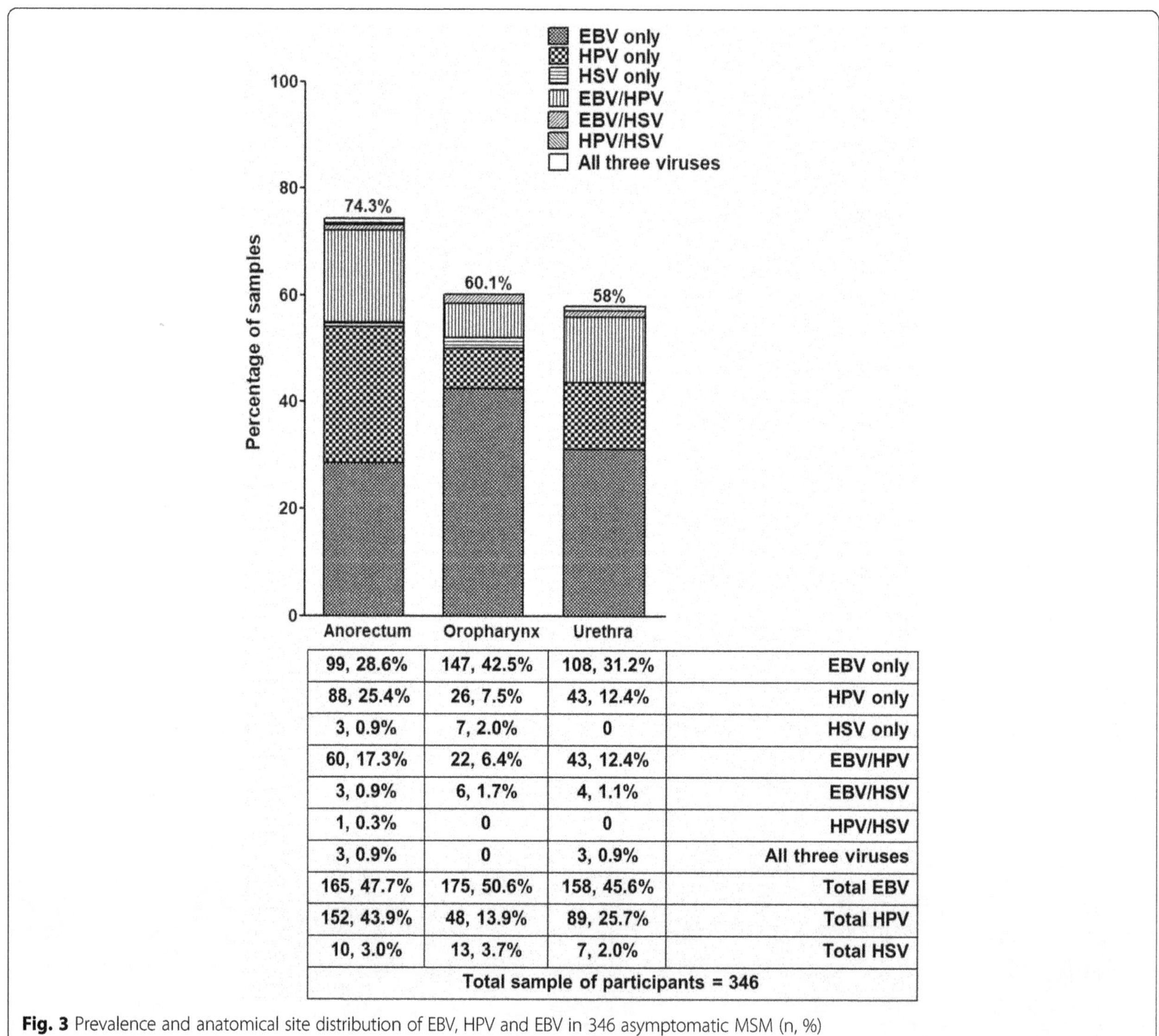

Anorectum	Oropharynx	Urethra	
99, 28.6%	147, 42.5%	108, 31.2%	EBV only
88, 25.4%	26, 7.5%	43, 12.4%	HPV only
3, 0.9%	7, 2.0%	0	HSV only
60, 17.3%	22, 6.4%	43, 12.4%	EBV/HPV
3, 0.9%	6, 1.7%	4, 1.1%	EBV/HSV
1, 0.3%	0	0	HPV/HSV
3, 0.9%	0	3, 0.9%	All three viruses
165, 47.7%	175, 50.6%	158, 45.6%	Total EBV
152, 43.9%	48, 13.9%	89, 25.7%	Total HPV
10, 3.0%	13, 3.7%	7, 2.0%	Total HSV
Total sample of participants = 346			

Fig. 3 Prevalence and anatomical site distribution of EBV, HPV and EBV in 346 asymptomatic MSM (n, %)

this site in Chinese MSM where it was not associated with HIV status. However, HPV6, 18, 31, 39, 45 and 66 were significantly associated with HIV infection in China [39]. HPV16 was the most common genotype found in the anorectum of Italian MSM [45]. However, HPV18 was the most frequently found genotype in the anorectum and urethra of Northeast Thai MSM. In the urethral site, HPV58 was the most common in Italian MSM. HPV16 and HPV58 were the most common infections of the oropharynx of MSM in The Netherlands and Italy respectively [40, 42]. Concordantly, our study has also demonstrated the highest proportion of HPV58 in the oropharynx. Although HPV16 was the most common genotype detected in these three anatomical sites among South African and Dutch MSM [42, 46], there appears to be variation by region and nationality. Co-infections with two or more HPV genotypes are significantly more frequent than single infections [43, 44], consistent with our findings and particularly in the anorectum. Unsurprisingly, high-risk HPV has been more frequently detected than low-risk genotypes among MSM worldwide [39, 44].

Most studies of HSV infection in MSM have reported only seroprevalence (82.5–90%) [47, 48]. However, a few studies have reported prevalence of HSV DNA in the anorectum (ranging from 7.0 to 16.9%), oropharynx (0–7.2%) and urethra (2.3–49.5%) among MSM [11, 34, 49–51]. Consistent with previous studies, we found very low prevalence of HSV in all three sites (Fig. 1).

Our report is the first to find that EBV infection is present in anorectal, oropharyngeal and urethral sites of northeast Thai MSM at higher prevalence than are HPV and HSV. A previous study found high-risk HPV at higher prevalence (90.8%) in the anorectal canal than low-risk-HPV (73.8%), HSV-1 (7.7%), HSV-2 (16.9%) and EBV (7.7%) among HIV-positive Brazilian men [11]. This agreed with a Swedish study of anal cell samples, which found higher HPV infection (76%) among HIV-infected and uninfected MSM than EBV (18.7%) and HSV (9.4%) [30].

HPV was also the most common virus found in anal swabs (44%), followed by semen (7.1%) and pharyngeal swabs (3.8%) in American MSM [35], consistent with our finding that HPV infection was more frequent in the anorectum than in the urethra and oropharynx.

It is well known that HIV-infected MSM have an increased risk of sexually transmitted infections (STIs) and STDs [52]. In addition, HIV infection not only increases susceptibility to persistent HPV but also increases the risk of acquisition of new HPV infections [53]. Similarity, EBV shedding was significantly associated with persistent HPV infection among HIV-infected MSM in the USA [35]. Our finding demonstrated that the presence of HPV in the anorectum was significantly associated with HIV infection in MSM (Table 2). We also found EBV infection of the oropharynx and urethra to be significantly associated with HIV-positive MSM (Table 2). Previous studies suggested that prevalence of EBV, HPV and HSV infection were associated with HIV-infected MSM but not HIV-uninfected MSM [30].

A few studies have reported co-infection of EBV, HPV and/or HSV in asymptomatic MSM. For example, high-risk HPV/HSV-2 co-infections were present in the anorectum of 55% of Brazilian MSM. Corresponding values for other combinations in that study were 27% (high-risk HPV/low-risk HPV/EBV), 9% (high-risk HPV/low-risk HPV/HSV2/EBV) and 9% (high-risk HPV/low-risk HPV/HSV-1/HSV-2/EBV) [11]. HPV and HSV co-infections were found in 4.3% of oral samples from Finnish males [50]. We have demonstrated that co-infection of EBV with HPV was the most common in the anorectum (17.3%), oropharynx (6.4%) and urethra (12.4%) and was significantly associated with the 21–30 years-old group (Fig. 3 and Additional file 2: Tables S2, Additional file 3: Table S3, and Additional file 4: Tables S4).

Different results in prevalence in anatomical sites of three viruses and in the association with any risk factors among various countries may depend on the technique used, site and equipment of sample collection, sample size, sexual behavior, nationality, geography, and particularly questionnaire pattern, etc. (such as a self-report or community based). The strength of our study is that 1) we used swab sample in urethra because this can increase sensitivity of *Neisseria gonorrhea* detection compared with urine sample [24] whereas many previous studies performed EBV, HPV and HSV detection in MSM semen [35, 36]; additionally the cell samples can indicate true infection at each anatomical site instead of movement of EBV infected B cells to each sites; and 2) all participants recruited in our study are collected cell samples from all anatomical sites to compare each participants that can reduce the error of data. However, there was a limitation in our study including self-reporting MSM that may provide invalid answers such as HIV status [54]. This limitation may cause an inaccurate data analysis of demographic information.

Here, we also investigated HIV status among EBV, HPV or HSV-positive MSM. We found that HPV infection of the anorectum increased with age among HIV-infected MSM (Table 3). In addition, failure to use condoms by HIV-positive MSM was significantly associated with HPV infection of the anorectum and urethra as well as with EBV infection of the urethra (Table 3).

Conclusions

EBV and HPV were detected in asymptomatic MSM in Northeast Thailand and were found more frequently than HSV in all three anatomical sites (oropharynx, anorectum and urethra). Oncogenic high-risk HPV genotypes were highly prevalent at these three sites in this population. Therefore, molecular detection and HPV genotyping may be useful for identifying these viruses and facilitating interventions to limit their spread among MSM, especially HIV-infected MSM.

Abbreviations

EBV: Epstein-Barr virus; HIV: human immunodeficiency virus; HNSCC: head and neck carcinomas; HPV: human papillomavirus; HSV: herpes simplex virus; MSM: Men who have sex with men; STD: sexually transmitted disease; STI: sexually transmitted infections

Acknowledgements

We would like to acknowledge Prof. David Blair, for editing the MS via Publication Clinic KKU, Thailand.

Funding

This study was granted by Faculty of Medicine, Khon Kaen University, Thailand (grant number IN59350) and received a scholarship under the Post-Doctoral Training Program from Research Affairs and Graduate School, Khon Kaen University, Thailand (grant number 58443).

Authors' contributions

JC, KP CharP performed the experiment and analyzed the data, JC, ChamP and TE wrote the initial draft of this manuscript. KP, SH, JB, BC and PH managed patients and collected clinical samples required for this study. JC, ChamP and TE critically reviewed and edited the manuscript. All authors read and approved the final manuscript.

Competing interests

The authors declare that they have no conflict of interest.

Author details

[1]Department of Microbiology, Faculty of Medicine, Khon Kaen University, Khon Kaen, Thailand. [2]Department of Social Medicine, Khon Kaen Center Hospital, Khon Kaen, Thailand. [3]Department of Animal Health Science, Faculty of Agro-Industrial Technology, Kalasin University, Kalasin, Thailand. [4]Department of Obstetrics and Gynecology, Faculty of Medicine, Khon Kaen University, Khon Kaen, Thailand. [5]HPV & EBV and Carcinogenesis Research Group, Khon Kaen University, Khon Kaen, Thailand.

References

1. Fenton KA, Imrie J. Increasing rates of sexually transmitted diseases in homosexual men in Western Europe and the United States: why? Clin Infect Dis. 2005;19:311–31.
2. Martin JN, Osmond DH. Invited commentary: determining specific sexual practices associated with human herpesvirus 8 transmission. Am J Epidemiol. 2000;151:225–9.
3. O'mahony C, Law C, Gollnick H, Marini M. New patient-applied therapy for anogenital warts is rated favourably by patients. Int J STD AIDS. 2001;12: 565–70.
4. Trottier H, Franco EL. The epidemiology of genital human papillomavirus infection. Vaccine. 2006;24:S4–S15.
5. van der Loeff MFS, Mooij SH, Richel O, de Vries HJ, Prins JM. HPV and anal cancer in HIV-infected individuals: a review. Curr HIV/AIDS Rep. 2014;11:250–62.
6. Moscicki A-B, Palefsky JM. HPV in men: an update. J Low Genit Tract Dis. 2011;15:231.
7. Tsao SW, Tsang CM, Pang PS, Zhang G, Chen H, Lo KW. The biology of EBV infection in human epithelial cells. Semin Cancer Biol. 2012;22:137–43.
8. Odumade OA, Hogquist KA, Balfour HH. Progress and problems in understanding and managing primary Epstein-Barr virus infections. Clin Microbiol Rev. 2011;24:193–209.
9. Thompson MP, Kurzrock R. Epstein-Barr virus and cancer. Clin Cancer Res. 2004;10:803–21.
10. Afonso LA, Moyses N, Alves G, Ornellas AA, Passos MRL, Oliveira LHS, et al. Prevalence of human papillomavirus and Epstein-Barr virus DNA in penile cancer cases from Brazil. Mem Inst Oswaldo Cruz. 2012;107:18–23.
11. Guimarães AGDP, JRd A, RVd A, CMd C, Galvão RS, Hada AL, et al. Coinfection of Epstein-Barr virus, cytomegalovirus, herpes simplex virus, human papillomavirus and anal intraepithelial neoplasia in HIV patients in Amazon, Brazil. J Coloproctol (Rio J). 2012;32:18–25.
12. Kahla S, Oueslati S, Achour M, Kochbati L, Chanoufi MB, Maalej M, et al. Correlation between ebv co-infection and HPV16 genome integrity in Tunisian cervical cancer patients. Braz J Microbiol. 2012;43:744–53.
13. Deng Z, Uehara T, Maeda H, Hasegawa M, Matayoshi S, Kiyuna A, et al. Epstein-Barr virus and human papillomavirus infections and genotype distribution in head and neck cancers. PLoS One. 2014;9:e113702.
14. Polz-Gruszka D, Morshed K, Stec A, Polz-Dacewicz M. Prevalence of human papillomavirus (HPV) and Epstein-Barr virus (EBV) in oral and oropharyngeal squamous cell carcinoma in South-Eastern Poland. Infect Agent Cancer. 2015;10:37.
15. van Baarle D, Hovenkamp E, Dukers NH, Renwick N, Kersten MJ, Goudsmit J, et al. High prevalence of Epstein-Barr virus type 2 among homosexual men is caused by sexual transmission. J Infect Dis. 2000;181:2045–9.
16. Lama JR, Lucchetti A, Suárez L, Laguna-Torres VA, Guanira JV, Pun M, et al. Association of herpes simplex virus type 2 infection and syphilis with human immunodeficiency virus infection among men who have sex with men in Peru. J Infect Dis. 2006;194:1459–66.
17. Kortekangas-Savolainen O, Vuorinen T. Trends in herpes simplex virus type 1 and 2 infections among patients diagnosed with genital herpes in a Finnish sexually transmitted disease clinic, 1994–2002. Sex Transm Dis. 2007;34:37–40.
18. Ryder N, Jin F, Mcnulty AM, Grulich AE, Donovan B. Increasing role of herpes simplex virus type 1 in first-episode anogenital herpes in heterosexual women and younger men who have sex with men, 1992–2006. Sex Transm Infect. 2009;85:416–9.
19. Lafferty WE, Downey L, Celum C, Wald A. Herpes simplex virus type 1 as a cause of genital herpes: impact on surveillance and prevention. J Infect Dis. 2000;181:1454–7.
20. Stamm WE, Handsfield HH, Rompalo AM, Ashley RL, Roberts PL, Corey L. The association between genital ulcer disease and acquisition of HIV infection in homosexual men. JAMA. 1988;260:1429–33.
21. Rautava J, Kuuskoski J, Syrjänen K, Grenman R, Syrjänen S. HPV genotypes and their prognostic significance in head and neck squamous cell carcinomas. J Clin Virol. 2012;53:116–20.
22. Turunen A, Hukkanen V, Nygårdas M, Kulmala J, Syrjänen S. The combined effects of irradiation and herpes simplex virus type 1 infection on an immortal gingival cell line. Virol J. 2014;11:125.
23. Budkaew J, Chumworathayi B, Pientong C, Ekalaksananan T. Conventional culture versus nucleic acid amplification tests for screening of urethral Neisseria gonorrhea infection among asymptomatic men who have sex with men. Pragmat Obs Res. 2017;8:167.
24. Budkaew J, Chumworathayi B, Peintong C, Ekalaksananan T. Endourethral swab versus urine collection for real-time PCR with TaqMan probe based detection of gonorrheal infection among men who have sex with men. J Med Assoc Thail. 2018;101:323–9.
25. Namwat N, Amimanan P, Loilome W, Jearanaikoon P, Sripa B, Bhudhisawasdi V, et al. Characterization of 5-fluorouracil-resistant cholangiocarcinoma cell lines. Chemotherapy. 2008;54:343–51.
26. Zehbe I, Wilander E, Delius H, Tommasino M. Human papillomavirus 16 E6 variants are more prevalent in invasive cervical carcinoma than the prototype. Cancer Res. 1998;58:829–33.
27. Tenorio A, Echevarría JE, Casasa I, Echevarría J, Tabarés E. Detection and typing of human herpesviruses by multiplex polymerase chain reaction. J Virol Methods. 1993;44:261–9.
28. Panagiotakis SH, Soufla G, Baritaki S, Sourvinos G, Passam A, Zagoreos I, et al. Concurrent CMV and EBV DNAemia is significantly correlated with a delay in the response to HAART in treatment-naive HIV type 1-positive patients. AIDS Res Hum Retrovir. 2007;23:10–8.
29. van den Brule AJ, Pol R, Fransen-Daalmeijer N, Schouls LM, Meijer CJ, Snijders PJ. GP5+/6+ PCR followed by reverse line blot analysis enables rapid and high-throughput identification of human papillomavirus genotypes. J Clin Microbiol. 2002;40:779–87.

30. Lowhagen G, Bergbrant I, Bergstrom T, Voog E. PCR detection of Epstein-Barr virus, herpes simplex virus and human papillomavirus from the anal mucosa in HIV-seropositive and HIV-seronegative homosexual men. Int J STD AIDS. 1999;10:615–8.
31. Naeher H, Lenhard B, Wilms J, Nickel P. Detection of Epstein-Barr virus DNA in anal scrapings from HIV-positive homosexual men. Arch Dermatol Res. 1995;287:608–11.
32. Ferbas J, Rahman MA, Kingsley LA, Armstrong JA, Ho M, Zhou SY, et al. Frequent oropharyngeal shedding of Epstein-Barr virus in homosexual men during early HIV infection. AIDS. 1992;6:1273–8.
33. Diaz-Mitoma F, Ruiz A, Flowerdew G, Houston S, Romanowski B, Kovithavongs T, et al. High levels of Epstein-Barr virus in the oropharynx: a predictor of disease progression in human immunodeficiency virus infection. J Med Virol. 1990;31:69–75.
34. Gianella S, Smith DM, Vargas MV, Little SJ, Richman DD, Daar ES, et al. Shedding of HIV and human herpesviruses in the semen of effectively treated HIV-1–infected men who have sex with men. Clin Infect Dis. 2013;57:441–7.
35. Gianella S, Ginocchio CC, Daar ES, Dube MP, Morris SR. Genital Epstein Barr virus is associated with higher prevalence and persistence of anal human papillomavirus in HIV-infected men on antiretroviral therapy. BMC Infect Dis. 2016;16:24.
36. Kaspersen MD, Höllsberg P. Seminal shedding of human herpesviruses. Virol J. 2013;10:226.
37. Van Der Snoek EM, Niesters HG, Mulder PG, Van Doornum GJ, Osterhaus AD, van der Meijden WI. Human papillomavirus infection in men who have sex with men participating in a Dutch gay-cohort study. Sex Transm Dis. 2003;30:639–44.
38. Breese PL, Judson FN, Penley KA, Douglas JM Jr. Anal human papillomavirus infection among homosexual and bisexual men: prevalence of type-specific infection and association with human immunodeficiency virus. Sex Transm Dis. 1995;22:7–14.
39. Hu Y, Qian H-Z, Sun J, Gao L, Yin L, Li X, et al. Anal human papillomavirus infection among HIV-infected and uninfected men who have sex with men in Beijing, China. J Acquir Immune Defic Syndr. 2013;64:103.
40. Ucciferri C, Tamburro M, Falasca K, Sammarco ML, Ripabelli G, Vecchiet J. Prevalence of anal, oral, penile and urethral human papillomavirus in HIV infected and HIV uninfected men who have sex with men. J Med Virol. 2018;90:358–66.
41. Read TR, Hocking JS, Vodstrcil LA, Tabrizi SN, McCullough MJ, Grulich AE, et al. Oral human papillomavirus in men having sex with men: risk-factors and sampling. PLoS One. 2012;7:e49324.
42. Van Rijn VM, Mooij SH, Mollers M, Snijders PJ, Speksnijder AG, King AJ, et al. Anal, penile, and oral high-risk HPV infections and HPV seropositivity in HIV-positive and HIV-negative men who have sex with men. PLoS One. 2014;9: e92208.
43. Quinn R, Salvatierra J, Solari V, Calderon M, Ton TG, Zunt JR. Human papillomavirus infection in men who have sex with men in Lima, Peru. AIDS Res Hum Retrovir. 2012;28:1734–8.
44. Damay A, Fabre J, Costes V, Didelot J-M, Didelot M-N, Boulle N, et al. Human papillomavirus (HPV) prevalence and type distribution, and HPV-associated cytological abnormalities in anal specimens from men infected with HIV who have sex with men. J Med Virol. 2010;82:592–6.
45. Sammarco ML, Ucciferri C, Tamburro M, Falasca K, Ripabelli G, Vecchiet J. High prevalence of human papillomavirus type 58 in HIV infected men who have sex with men: a preliminary report in Central Italy. J Med Virol. 2016;88:911–4.
46. Müller EE, Rebe K, Chirwa TF, Struthers H, McIntyre J, Lewis DA. The prevalence of human papillomavirus infections and associated risk factors in men-who-have-sex-with-men in Cape Town, South Africa. BMC Infect Dis. 2016;16:440.
47. Hill C, McKinney E, Lowndes C, Munro H, Murphy G, Parry J, et al. Epidemiology of herpes simplex virus types 2 and 1 amongst men who have sex with men attending sexual health clinics in England and Wales: implications for HIV prevention and management. Eur Secur. 2009;14:19418.
48. Russell DB, Tabrizi SN, Russell JM, Garland SM. Seroprevalence of herpes simplex virus types 1 and 2 in HIV-infected and uninfected homosexual men in a primary care setting. J Clin Virol. 2001;22:305–13.
49. Kapranos N, Petrakou E, Anastasiadou C, Kotronias D. Detection of herpes simplex virus, cytomegalovirus, and Epstein-Barr virus in the semen of men attending an infertility clinic. Fertil Steril. 2003;79:1566–70.
50. Mäki J, Paavilainen H, Kero K, Hukkanen V, Syrjänen S. Herpes simplex and human papilloma virus coinfections in oral mucosa of men—a 6-year follow-up study. J Med Virol. 2018;90:564–70.
51. Kiviat NB, Critchlow CW, Hawes SE, Kuypers J, Surawicz C, Goldbaum G, et al. Determinants of human immunodeficiency virus DNA and RNA shedding in the anal-rectal canal of homosexual men. J Infect Dis. 1998;177:571–8.
52. Aggarwal P, Bhattar S, Sahani SK, Bhalla P, Garg VK. Sexually transmitted infections and HIV in self reporting men who have sex with men: a two-year study from India. J Infect Public Health. 2016;9:564–70.
53. Parisi SG, Cruciani M, Scaggiante R, Boldrin C, Andreis S, Dal Bello F, et al. Anal and oral human papillomavirus (HPV) infection in HIV-infected subjects in northern Italy: a longitudinal cohort study among men who have sex with men. BMC Infect Dis. 2011;11:150.
54. McDonald JD. Measuring personality constructs: the advantages and disadvantages of self-reports, informant reports and behavioural assessments. Enquire. 2008;1:1–19.

12

Characteristics and management of bone and joint tuberculosis in native and migrant population in Shanghai during 2011 to 2015

Yun Qian[1†], Qixin Han[2,3†], Wenjun Liu[4,5†], Wei-En Yuan[6*] and Cunyi Fan[1,4*]

Abstract

Background: China had the third highest burden of tuberculosis population in the world. Bone and joint tuberculosis was a major part and its characteristics were rarely discussed before. This study was designed to review the characteristics and management of bone and joint tuberculosis among native and migrant population in Shanghai, China during 2011–2015.

Methods: A retrospective analysis of the patient clinical records on their demographic information, clinical features and treatment was conducted from three tertiary referral hospitals. Analysis of continuous variables included calculation of the median value with interquartile range. Categorical variables were displayed as percentages and compared using the Fisher's exact test and chi-square test. All continuous variables were compared using Student's unpaired t-test and Mann Whitney U test.

Results: One hundred fifteen patients with bone and joint tuberculosis were involved in this study. Native people were generally older ($p = 0.003$) and had more comorbidities like hypertension (40.74% vs. 16.39%, $p = 0.004$), diabetes mellitus (38.89% vs. 13.11%, $p = 0.001$), and cancer (31.48% vs. 14.75%, $p = 0.032$) than migrants. Migrant patients generally experienced a longer period of uncomfortable feelings before going to doctor than native people ($p = 0.007$). Spine was a major infection site in comparison with other peripheral joints. Radiological evaluation displayed increased osteolytic reaction in migrant patients compared with native people ($p = 0.031$). The mean time for anti-tuberculosis treatment was significantly longer in native Shanghai patients (8.96 months vs. 7.94 months, $p = 0.003$). The curative ratio displayed a significant difference between native and migrant patients (88.24%vs.75.93%, $p = 0.009$).

Conclusion: Bone and joint tuberculosis exhibited a poorer outcome in migrant people, who also had longer period of manifestation, more severe osteolytic reaction from CT scan and higher recurrent rate than native people. The surgical treatment in addition to anti-tuberculosis drug therapy had great implications for bone and joint tuberculosis recovery.

Keywords: Bone and joint tuberculosis, Native, Migrant, Surgery, Anti-tuberculosis, Shanghai

* Correspondence: yuanweien@sjtu.edu.cn; cyfan@sjtu.edu.cn
[†]Yun Qian, Qixin Han and Wenjun Liu contributed equally to this work.
[6]Engineering Research Center of Cell & Therapeutic Antibody, Ministry of Education, and School of Pharmacy, Shanghai Jiao Tong University, Shanghai 200240, China
[1]Department of Orthopedics, Shanghai Jiao Tong University Affiliated Sixth People's Hospital, 600 Yishan Road, Shanghai 200233, People's Republic of China
Full list of author information is available at the end of the article

Background

In 2015, new tuberculosis cases were estimated to reach 10.4 million in the whole world, and six nations had around 60% of all incidences, among which were India, Indonesia, China, Nigeria, Pakistan and South Africa [1]. China had the third highest burden of tuberculosis population in the world, with approximately 0.93 million new cases in 2015, according to the statistics released by National Health and Family Planning Commission of China [2].

The bone and joint tuberculosis (BJTB) represents approximately 2–5% in all TB cases, and 10% in extra-pulmonary tuberculosis (EPTB), ranking the third common location of all TB infection [3]. Osteoarticular involvement primarily contains spine, shoulder, elbow, wrist, hip, knee, ankle and foot [4, 5]. Although great efforts have been made to control this serious public health issue, very limited achievements were made even in major metropolises in China due to many migrant workers from less developed regions and failure to successful diagnosis with atypical presentation. Besides, classic drug therapy is not really efficacious for those patients who are at advanced stages with specific joint activity restriction. The efficient treatment calls for a combination of surgical removal and drug therapy [6].

There is very limited published literature on the epidemiology, clinical features and diagnosis, as well as treatment of BJTB in Shanghai, the most prosperous city in China with the most complicated population proportion. In this study, BJTB was comprehensively evaluated based on data from three tertiary referral centers in Shanghai from 2011 to 2015, including their demographic information, clinical features and treatment.

Methods

All data for BJTB cases were collected from the medical history system and database from three tertiary referral hospitals in Shanghai from the year 2011 to 2015. In this study, patients were classified into native Shanghai people group and migrant group. Migrants are defined as floating population who leave their birthplaces and live in another city without local identity. Native people are considered as resident population who live and have local residency [7]. We defined TB patients using laboratory examinations, radiographs and biopsies. The patient records included their demographic features, duration of disease onset, clinical manifestation and symptoms, concomitant diseases, laboratory and radiological examination, treatment and follow-up. Part of the patients' medical documents which were incomplete or incorrect were removed from this study. The suggestive laboratory tests involve neutrophils, erythrocyte sedimentation rate (ESR), C-reactive protein (CRP), hemoglobin, T-SPOT, and sputum culture. Relevant radiological examination includes chest X-ray, diseased bone or joint X-ray, computed tomography (CT) scan or magnetic resonance imaging (MRI). For different stages of bone and joint tuberculosis, we treated patients with different procedures, either conservative medication therapy and minimally invasive practices or open surgeries. The relative standards for open surgical treatment include advanced stage of TB, major limitations in bone and joint activity, and patients' willingness to accept surgeries. Tubercular masses and regional lesions were removed for pathological evaluation. Besides, the open surgery provided us with clear vision and possibly full recovery of joint motion. However, extended clearance of surrounding tissues and bones were not recommended in order not to spread the pathogen. In those severe cases with vast devastation of structures, osteotomy and orthopedic operations were also required. For spine TB patients, spinal fusion was adopted for reconstruction of stable joints via a direct lateral interbody fusion manner using minimal invasive operations. For those who experienced stiff joint and limitations in activity, joint arthrolysis was carried out basically including capsule release, muscle and tendon repair as well as bone reconstruction [8].Biopsy of bone or soft tissue was conducted in partial patients.

For peripheral BJTB patients who accepted surgeries, they needed to follow passive and active joint motion practice. For instance, elbow TB patients were required to regain elbow range of motion by extension of 0° and flexion of 120°. At the same time, celecoxib or indomethacin were given to patients for oral intake thrice a day for heterotopic ossification prevention. Proper antibiotic therapy was used in all patients.

Statistical analysis

Analysis of continuous variables included calculation of the median value with interquartile range. Categorical variables were displayed as percentages and compared using the Fisher's exact test and chi-square test. All continuous variables were compared using Student's unpaired t-test and Mann Whitney U test. A p value less than 0.05 was considered statistical significance.

Results

Epidemiological analysis

After a general examination of all patients' medical documents, a total of 136 patients were diagnosed with bone and joint tuberculosis, among which 115 patients were included in this study (Fig. 1). Of all the patients, 54 patients were native Shanghai people, while 61 were migrant from other provinces in China. Among these migrants, 18 were from Heilongjiang, and the second largest immigration came from Guizhou with 12 patients, followed by Hunan (9), Hubei (6), Guangxi (4), and Jiangxi (3) (Fig. 2). The male/female ratio was 37/17 and 42/19 in native people and migrants respectively. The median age of these patients was 55.89, ranging from 25 to 83 in native people. However, the mean age was 46.84 in migrants, varying from 16 to 85 (p =

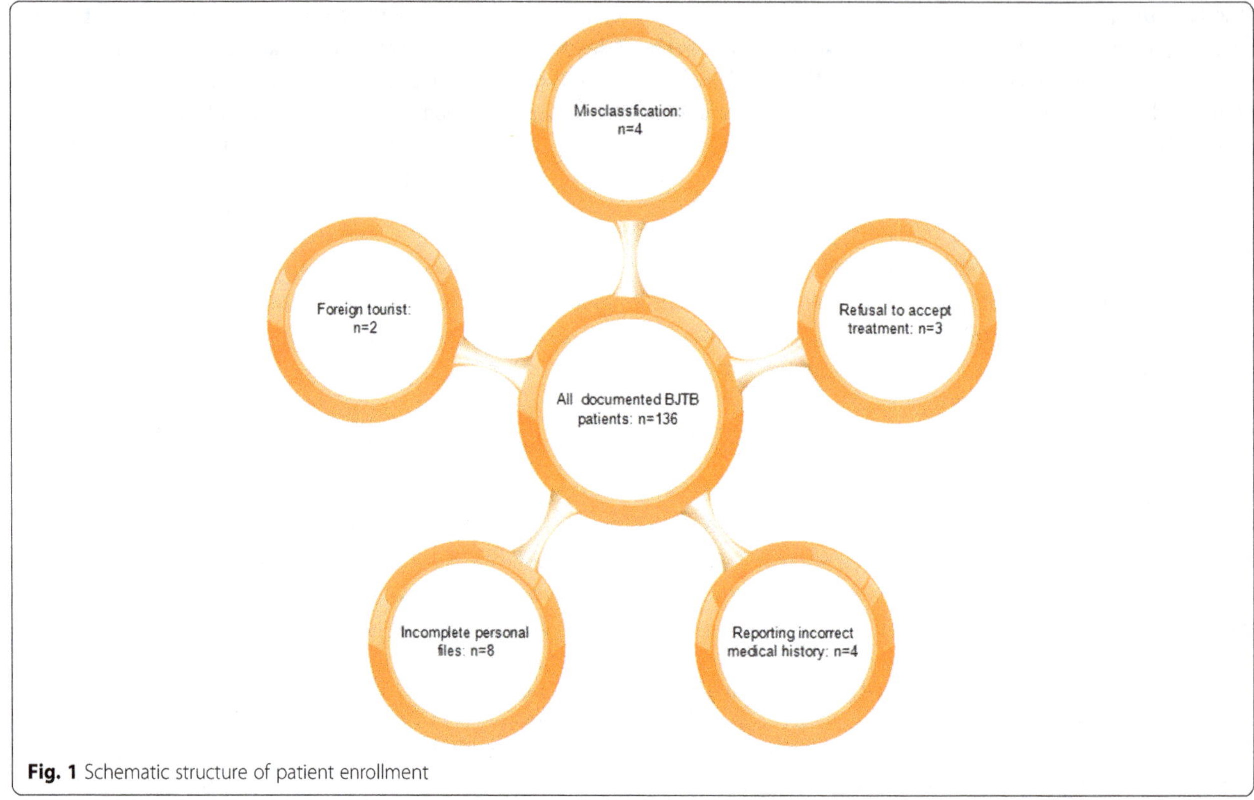

Fig. 1 Schematic structure of patient enrollment

0.003). The curative ratio displayed a significant difference between native people and migrants, with 45 out of 51 (88.24%) and 41 out of 54 (75.93%) ($p = 0.009$). In those recurrent cases, there was 1 death case (1.96%) in native people within 1 year from initial diagnosis. In contrast, 4 migrant patients (7.41%) died during the same period of time. The general demographic data were displayed in Table 1 according to population classification.

Clinical evaluation

Clinical manifestation and presentation of BJTB patients normally involved pain (92.59% vs. 95.08%), night sweat

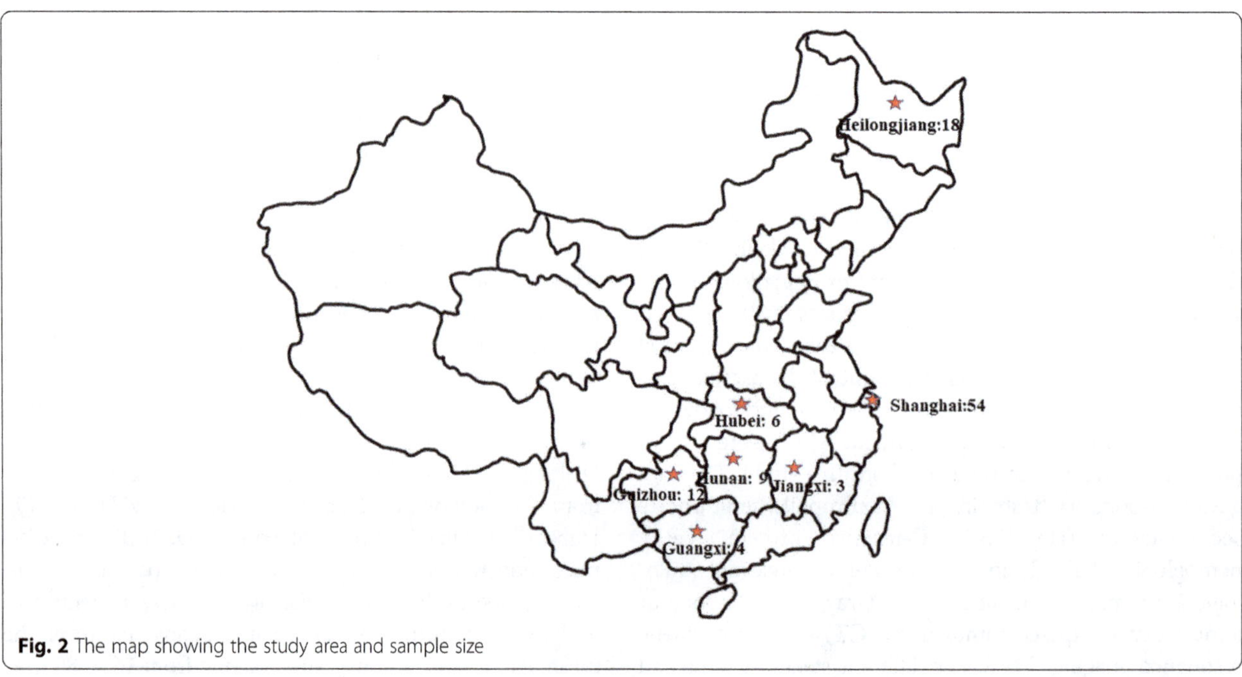

Fig. 2 The map showing the study area and sample size

Table 1 Demographic information of bone and joint tuberculosis patients from 2011 to 2015 in Shanghai

Demographic information	Native people	Migrant people	*P* value
Patients	54	61	/
Male/female	37/17	42/19	0.969
Age	55.89(25–83)	46.84(16–85)	0.003[a]
Recurrent(Alive)	5(9.80%)	9(16.67%)	0.009[b]
Dead	1(1.96%)	4(7.41%)	
Cured	45(88.24%)	41(75.93%)	

[a]Man whitney U test
[b]Fischer Exact test

(27.78% vs. 19.67%), fever (44.44% vs. 40.98%), cough (12.96% vs. 18.03%), weight loss (22.22% vs. 16.39%), paraplegia (5.56% vs. 14.75%), and limitations in activity (42.59% vs. 31.15%) in native and migrant patients respectively, with a major complaint in pain at infection site. It did not show any significant difference between people from Shanghai and other provinces (Table 2). The average duration of symptom onset to hospital was 5.63 months, varying from 1 to 72 months in native Shanghai patients. Nevertheless, migrants experienced uncomfortable feelings and symptoms for a much longer period, with an average duration of 8.57 months, varying from 1 to 36 months ($p = 0.007$). Partial peripheral joint infection patients experienced limitations in joint range of motion (ROM), especially in elbow, hip, shoulder and knee TB infection. Some patients had comorbidities, including hypertension (HT, 40.74% vs. 16.39%), diabetes mellitus (DM, 38.89% vs. 13.11%), Human Immunodeficiency Virus (HIV, 5.56% vs. 4.92%), Rheumatoid Arthritis (RA, 11.11% vs. 8.20%), syphilis (5.56% vs. 3.28%), previous tuberculosis (9.26% vs. 11.48%) and cancer (31.48% vs. 14.75%) in two groups (Table 2). Migrants were younger and had less concomitant diseases than native patients. BJTB accompanied by pulmonary tuberculosis was noticed (40.74% vs. 44.26%), while other types of EPTB were also found, including lymph nodes (3.70% vs. 4.92%) and urinary tract and kidney (3.70% vs. 8.20%). There was no notable difference between native people and migrants either ($p = 0.888$). For BJTB types, there were 75 spinal tuberculosis cases, and the other types contained knee (11), hip (10), shoulder (7), elbow (6), ankle/foot (4) and wrist (2). In spine tuberculosis, lumbar infection was the most common (32). Thoracic and cervical vertebra infection was next to it, with 24 and 16 cases respectively, followed by paravertebral abscess (3). No cases were reported to have over one infection location. Migrant-dependent details were displayed in Table 2. No significant differences were found in laboratory examination or drug resistance patterns between groups (Table 2). Twenty-one patients were reported severe infection findings, like osteolytic reaction in native Shanghai people, compared with 36 in migrants in CT scan ($p = 0.031$), in spite of insignificant differences in other radiological examinations (Figs. 3, 4, 5).

The median time for anti-tuberculosis treatment showed a significant difference between two groups. It was 8.96 months in native Shanghai patients compared with 7.94 months in migrant patients ($p = 0.003$). The treatment outcome at 1 year (including dead cases within 1 year) was achieved in 51 of 54 native patients and 54 of 61 migrants. The average follow-up time was 15.16 months and 13.63 months in native and migrant groups respectively ($p = 0.011$). Ten patients were lost in follow-up or unwilling to report their conditions. Curative ratio was 88.24% (45 out of 51) in native patients and 75.93% (41 out of 54) in immigration patients.

Discussion

Tuberculosis is generally considered as an economic and sanitary condition-related infectious disease, with high prevalence in developing countries [9]. Bone and joint tuberculosis has a relatively lower incidence. Shanghai is a major metropolis in the world, which has a comparable economic and health care level with Chicago, Seoul, Hong Kong, Singapore, and so forth [10]. Besides, established health care system has enabled people to enjoy a higher quality of life in Shanghai [11]. Even under this environment, the overall BJTB incidence is still much higher than it in other big cities, like Paris [12]. It is estimated that the complex population proportion and migration from underdeveloped provinces are major causes for tuberculosis incidences [13]. The statistics showed that older people were more prone to being infected with BJTB than young people from native group. And the majority of infected migrants were younger than native people, which probably resulted from their status of migrant workers. The age-related characteristics were also observed in other researches [14, 15]. This study was based on the BJTB cases occurring between the year 2011 and 2015, during which time sick immigration patients were mainly from several provinces of high TB incidences, like Heilongjiang, Guizhou, Hunan, Hubei, Guangxi, and Jiangxi. These areas have occupied the top places in the list of TB incidence in China for many years due to low economic and health care development [16]. Although the overall infected patients were declining from 2011 to 2015 by year, the proportion of migrants was increased every year [17]. Besides, as for the types of BJTB cases, spinal TB was a leading type [18]. Migrants had a higher incidence of spinal TB, accounting for 70.49%. It is consistent to the data of other places reporting BJTB cases, like United Kingdom 92% [19], Holland 66% [20], and France 68% [21]. To evaluate the difference between two population groups, we decided to follow a population classification based analysis in the

Table 2 Clinical evaluation of bone and joint tuberculosis patients from 2011 to 2015 in Shanghai

Clinical features			Native people	Migrant people	*P* value
Duration of symptom onset to hospital			5.63(1–72)	8.57(1–36)	0.007[a]
Symptom	Pain		50(92.59%)	58(95.08%)	0.705[b]
	Night sweat		15(27.78%)	12(19.67%)	0.306
	Fever		24(44.44%)	25(40.98%)	0.708
	Cough		7(12.96%)	11(18.03%)	0.455
	Weight loss		12(22.22%)	10(16.39%)	0.428
	Paraplegia		3(5.56%)	9(14.75%)	0.107
	Limitations in activity		23(42.59%)	19(31.15%)	0.203
Laboratory exam	Neutrophils (%)		61.57(39.10–79.40)	62.40(42.40–79.60)	0.659
	ESR(mm/h)		17.51(7.60–25.90)	16.75(7.50–25.20)	0.346
	CRP(mg/l)		13.57(9.22–20.22)	13.13(8.45–21.23)	0.358[a]
	Hemoglobin(g/l)		111.98(86–143)	112.89(80–139)	0.733
	T-SPOT		24(64.86%)	25(44.64%)	0.056
	Sputum culture		31(73.81%)	35(71.43%)	0.800
	Biopsies		0	2	/
Radiological exam	Chest	negative	24(44.44%)	32(52.46%)	0.442
		moderate	23(42.59%)	19(31.15%)	
		severe	7(12.96%)	10(16.39%)	
	Joint	negative	0	0	0.031
		moderate	33(61.11%)	25(40.98%)	
		severe	21(38.89%)	36(59.02%)	
Infection site	Peripheral	Shoulder	3(5.56%)	4(6.56%)	0.639
		Elbow	3(5.56%)	3(4.92%)	
		Wrist	1(1.85%)	1(1.64%)	
		Hip	4(7.41%)	6(9.84%)	
		Knee	8(14.81%)	3(4.92%)	
		Ankle/foot	3(5.56%)	1(1.64%)	
	Spine	Cervical	7(12.96%)	9(14.75%)	0.649
		Thoracic	8(14.81%)	16(26.23%)	
		Lumbar	16(29.63%)	16(26.23%)	
		Paravertebral abscess	1(1.85%)	2(3.28%)	
Concomitant TB	Pulmonary		22(40.74%)	27(44.26%)	0.888
	Lymph nodes		2(3.70%)	3(4.92%)	
	Urinary tract and kidney		2(3.70%)	5(8.20%)	
Comorbidity	HT		22(40.74%)	10(16.39%)	0.004
	DM		21(38.89%)	8(13.11%)	0.001
	RA		6(11.11%)	5(8.20%)	0.596
	HIV		3(5.56%)	3(4.92%)	1.000
	Syphilis		3(5.56%)	2(3.28%)	0.664
	Previous TB		5(9.26%)	7(11.48%)	0.698
	Cancer		17(31.48%)	9(14.75%)	0.032
Drug resistant pattern	Isoniazid		14(25.93%)	18(29.51%)	0.669[c]
	Rifampin		8(14.81%)	11(18.03%)	0.643[c]

Table 2 Clinical evaluation of bone and joint tuberculosis patients from 2011 to 2015 in Shanghai *(Continued)*

Clinical features		Native people	Migrant people	*P* value
	Ethambutol	6(11.11%)	8(13.11%)	0.743[c]
	Streptomycin	10(18.52%)	11(18.03%)	0.946[c]
	Multidrug resistance	0	2(3.28%)	0.497[b]
Surgical intervention		34(62.96%)	32(52.46%)	0.256
Infection		5(9.26%)	8(13.11%)	0.515
Drug		40(74.08%)	46(75.41%)	0.869
Mean time for anti-tuberculosis treatment		8.96(6–12) [d1]	7.94(4–12) [d2]	0.003
Follow-up duration		15.16(12–24)[d1]	13.63(12–23)[d2]	0.011[a]

ESR erythrocyte sedimentation rate, *CRP* C-reactive protein, *HT* hypertension, *DM* diabetes mellitus, *RA* rheumatoid arthritis, *HIV* Human Immunodeficiency Virus, *TB* tuberculosis
[a]Mann Whitney U test
[b]Fischer Exact test
[c]Pearson chi square test
[d1]3 patients were lost in the follow-up
[d2]7 patients were lost in the follow-up

following data. The mean duration between disease onset and clinical treatment was 5.63 and 8.57 months in two groups respectively. This was much shorter than a report conducted in Iran, with 12.94 months in average (1 to 108 months) [22], and relatively longer than that from Denmark research [23].

The comorbidities like DM, HT, and cancer could compromise the immune system of these patients, leading to their vulnerable exposure to TB pathogen and BJTB onset. The clinical manifestation generally was characteristic of TB pathogen infection, and pain was the most common symptom among all, which originated from bone erosion and nerve irritation. This result was much higher than that from Western countries with neurological complaints varying from 20 to 50% [23]. Other symptoms like cough, fever, and sweat were related to respiratory system infection. BJTB accompanied pulmonary TB was 40.74% and 44.26% in native and migrant groups respectively in this study, which was higher than the average data from developed regions in the world, ranging from 23 to 35% [11].

As is known to all, only a small portion of the laboratory examination has direct relationship with TB diagnosis, like T-SPOT and sputum culture as well as pathological examination. All the patients had at least one positive result from the above three tests to confirm TB infection, in addition to radiological findings as well as clinical presentation. As tuberculosis is getting increasingly resistant to drug, the anti-tuberculosis drug resistant pattern was evaluated as well for proper drug selection. Many patients displayed monoresistance to a single drug. Two patients from migrant group experienced multidrug resistant. One patient had previous TB history. The other patient had concomitant kidney tuberculosis. It was believed that their multidrug resistant condition was also because they received irregular anti-tuberculosis treatment before tuberculosis diagnosis. This is in

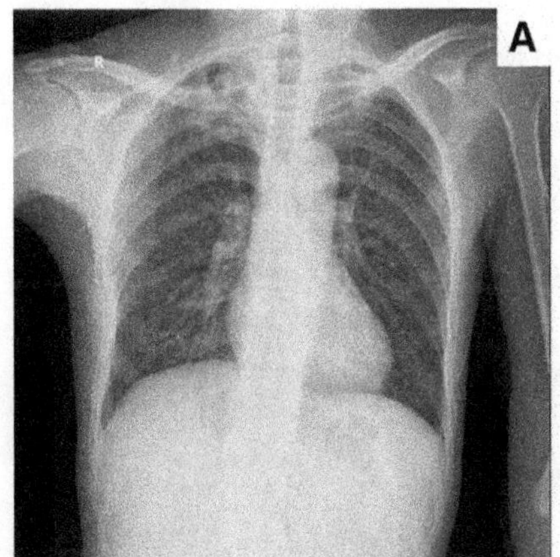

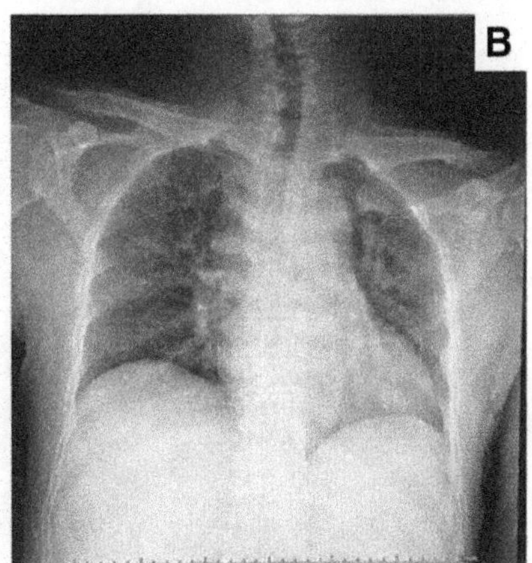

Fig. 3 X-ray of pulmonary tuberculosis. **a** Moderate infection; **b** Severe infection

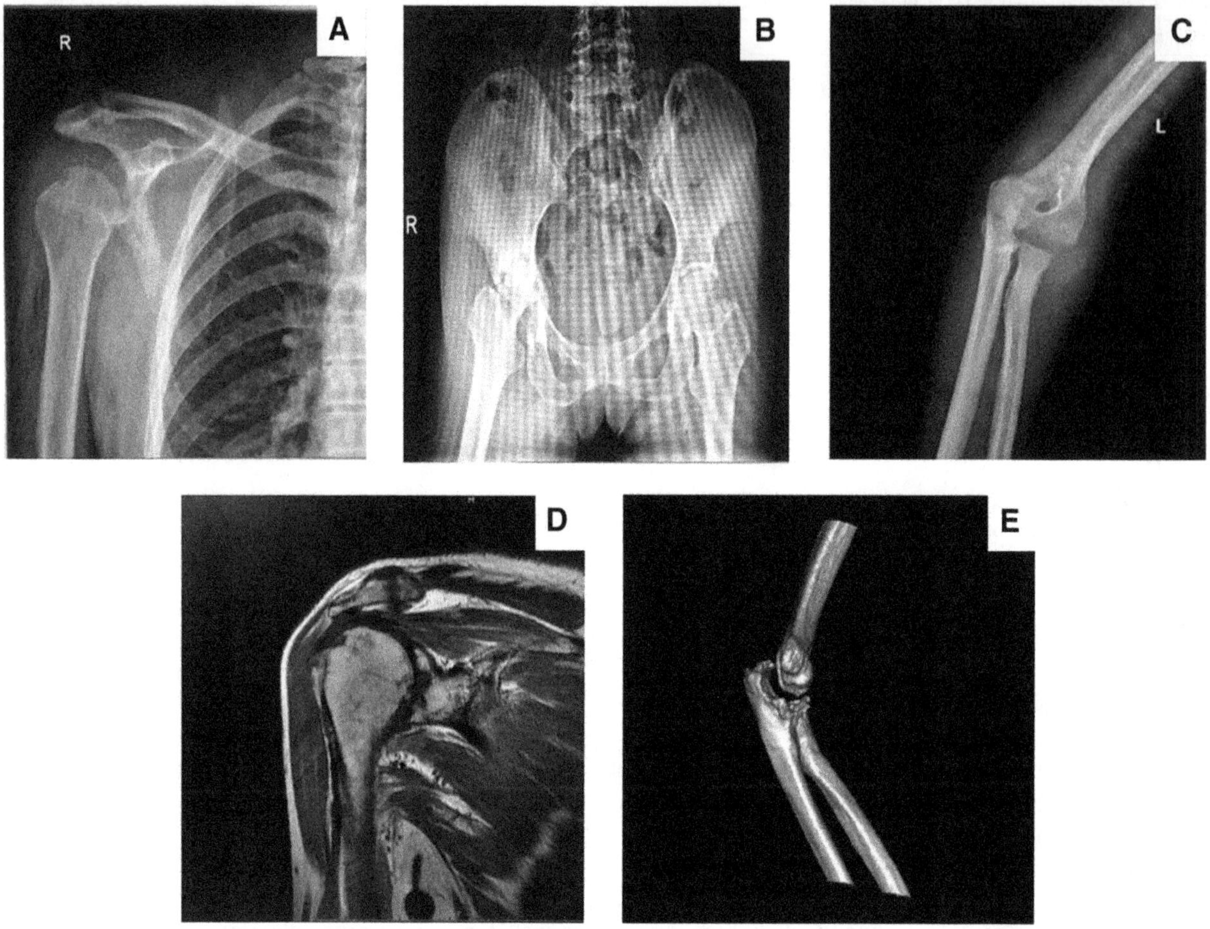

Fig. 4 X-ray, CT and MR of different peripheral bone and joint tuberculosis. **a** X-ray of shoulder TB; **b** X-ray of hip TB; **c** X-ray of elbow TB; **d** MR of shoulder TB; **e** CT of elbow TB

consistent with the conclusion of a previous research. Chen and colleagues conducted a nationwide BJTB research and collected 113 cases for bacterial evaluation. They discovered 17 multidrug resistance cases and among them, 2 cases were extremely severe resistant. Like our patients, those people had either concomitant tuberculosis, past tuberculosis infection or irregular anti-tuberculosis treatment before final diagnosis [24, 25]. The radiological examination is of vital importance for supplementary diagnosis. In X-rays, bone defects were noticed. CT provided us with a three dimensional structure of bone erosion. Moreover, MRI offered a more comprehensive presentation of osteoarthritis changes,

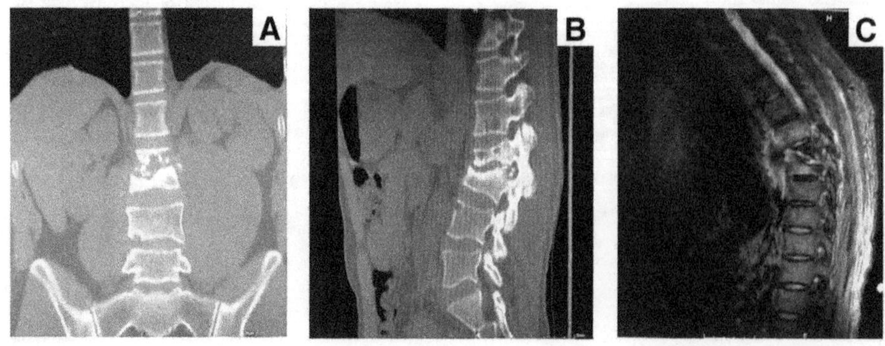

Fig. 5 CT and MR of spine tuberculosis. **a** CT of spine TB: anterioposterior position; **b** CT of spine TB: lateral position; **c** MR of spine TB

with bone devastation, mass edema and abscess formation. It was mainly applied in spinal TB patients. Correct and timely diagnosis is of great significance to final treatment and recovery for BJTB patients.

Surgical treatment remained a primary procedure for BJTB in this study. Although BJTB patients sometimes had pulmonary TB at the same time, early symptoms were generally atypical and they went for medical treatment at an advanced level. Because the structure of bone and joints was severely damaged by TB pathogen, simple anti-tuberculosis drugs were unable to restore functional activity. Moreover, the erosive remnants were at high risk of further collapsing and deformation. Therefore, proper surgical intervention was extremely necessary, including arthroplasty and arthrolysis. Joint arthrolysis typically fit those cases with limited joint range of motion [26, 27]. Arthroplasty was more appropriate for complete devastation of joint structure, with limited choices of reconstruction except artificial joint replacement [28]. For spine TB patients, they also received intervertebral disc fusion via minimal invasive operations [29]. In this study, 66 patients received joint arthrolysis and no arthroplasty was performed. These patients received anti-tuberculosis drugs just like those who received conservative therapy. In addition, postoperative active and passive exercise was of vital significance to functional recovery for patients, for instance, in elbow stiffness [30]. Celecoxib or indomethocin was taken for prevention of heterotopic ossification occurrence.

Standard anti-tuberculosis therapy was initiated in partial patients immediately after surgery. In contrast, other patients were recommended to start their anti-tuberculosis treatment at specialized infectious disease department or hospital. They needed systematic evaluation of anti-tuberculosis treatment from professionals of infectious diseases. In China, we suggest the entire treatment should last for 6 to 12 months, which is similar to common practices in Western world [31]. However, the mean time for anti-tuberculosis treatment showed a significant difference between two groups. Migrant patients generally received anti-tuberculosis drugs irregularly for a shorter period of time.

The general treatment success rate was 81.90% in all patients, with 88.24% in native patients and 75.93% in migrants. The relatively higher recurrent rate and poorer outcome in migrants were estimated due to their migrant characteristics, disobedience to self-supervision on anti-tuberculosis drugs intake as well as failure in receiving medical treatment because of heavy economic burden [17]. These people migrated frequently due to job insecurity. Therefore, they tended to overlook taking medication regularly. Meanwhile, in our long-term follow-ups, some of migrant patients considered medication was insignificant since they regained functional joint activity after surgery. These people refused to supervise themselves on anti-tuberculosis drugs intake. More importantly, the poor outcomes also resulted from huge economic burden on migrant patients because many of them were not covered by local medical insurance. Insufficient government budget outlay in public health, especially for severe infectious diseases, is a common problem in developing countries. In China, TB patients need to cover 30–44% of total medical expense by themselves. It means more for migrants. However, the general successful result was already close to that from developed countries in Europe, like Denmark [23]. Johansen and colleagues retrospectively reviewed 282 cases of bone and joint tuberculosis in 17 years. Their general success rate was 83%. However, 15 patients died within 1 year of follow-up in their study. Besides, only 44% of all BJTB patients received open surgeries because they did not consider surgery as a major contributing factor for final successful treatment. It was especially valuable in such a big city with over 24 million people and highly complicated population proportion. The population mobility was used to evaluate the attraction of a major city, which also may bring about potential risks in transmitting infectious diseases [32]. This was one important reason proposed previously for the high incidence of BJTB in Shanghai. However, experienced medical team and sophisticated treatment protocol as well as timely diagnosis and treatment has contributed to successful rehabilitation in BJTB patients. More emphasis on medical care reforms will improve the overall tuberculosis treatment in Shanghai and nationwide.

Conclusion

BJTB was not uncommon in large developed cities, like Shanghai. The migrants had a higher risk of recurrence and exhibited a relatively poorer outcome than native patients. The typical BJTB patients displayed bone defects and erosion at lesion site from X-ray, CT or MRI examination. The diagnosis could be assisted by T-SPOT, sputum culture and biopsy. The surgical intervention and postoperative management was vital to restore functional joint activity and ensured final recovery.

Abbreviations

BJTB: bone and joint tuberculosis; CRP: C-reactive protein; CT: computed tomography; DM: diabetes mellitus; EPTB: extra-pulmonary tuberculosis; ESR: erythrocyte sedimentation rate; HIV: Human Immunodeficiency Virus; HT: hypertension; MRI: magnetic resonance imaging; RA: Rheumatoid Arthritis; ROM: range of motion; UCLA: University of California, Los Angeles

Acknowledgments

We would also like to thank the reviewers whose comments and suggestions greatly improved this manuscript.

Funding
The study was supported by Projects of the Shanghai Committee of Science and Technology, China (No. 12XD1403800), SUMHS seed foundation project (No. HMSF-16-21-010), and Funds for Interdisciplinary Projects of Medicine and Engineering of Shanghai Jiao Tong University (No. YG2014QN06 and YG2015MS06), and Science and Technology Development Foundation of Pudong New District, Shanghai, China (PKJ2016-Y55 and PWZxq2017-03).

Authors' contributions
YQ, QXH, WJL, WEY and CYF participated in its design, searched databases, extracted and assessed studies and helped to draft the manuscript. WEY and CYF conceived the initial idea and the conceptualization and participated in the data extraction and analysis. YQ wrote and revised the manuscript. All authors read and approved the final manuscript.

Competing interests
The authors declare that they have no competing interests.

Author details
[1]Department of Orthopedics, Shanghai Jiao Tong University Affiliated Sixth People's Hospital, 600 Yishan Road, Shanghai 200233, People's Republic of China. [2]Center for Reproductive Medicine, Renji Hospital, School of Medicine, Shanghai Jiao Tong University, Shanghai 200135, China. [3]Shanghai Key Laboratory for Assisted Reproduction and Reproductive Genetics, Shanghai 200135, China. [4]Department of Orthopedics, Shanghai Sixth People's Hospital East Affiliated to Shanghai University of Medicine & Health Sciences, Shanghai 201306, China. [5]Taishan Medical University, Taian 271016, China. [6]Engineering Research Center of Cell & Therapeutic Antibody, Ministry of Education, and School of Pharmacy, Shanghai Jiao Tong University, Shanghai 200240, China.

References
1. World Health Organization. Tuberculosis fact sheet. Geneva, Switzerland: World Health Organization. 2017. https://www.cdc.gov/tb/publications/factsheets/ Accessed 1 October 2017.
2. An J, Gao M, Chu N, Huang H, Pang Y, Li L. Transregional movement of multidrug-resistant tuberculosis in North China: an underlying threat to tuberculosis control. Sci Rep. 2016;6:29727.
3. Cormican L, Hammal R, Messenger J, Milburn HJ. Current difficulties in the diagnosis and management of spinal tuberculosis. Postgrad Med J. 2006;82(963):46–51.
4. Talbot JC, Bismil Q, Saralaya D, Newton DA, Frizzel RM, Shaw DL. Musculoskeletal tuberculosis in Bradford – a 6-year review. Ann R Coll Surg Engl. 2007;89(4):405–9.
5. Pigrau-Serrallach C, Rodríguez-Pardo D. Bone and joint tuberculosis. Eur Spine J. 2013;22(Suppl 4):556–66.
6. Bao YC, Li YL, Ning GZ, Wu Q, Feng SQ. Forked osteotomy arthroplasty for elbow tuberculosis: six years of follow-up. Eur J Orthop Surg Traumatol. 2014;24(6):857–62.
7. Department of Disease Control, Ministry of Health. Guidelines for Implementing the National TB Control Program in China. Beijing, China: Ministry of Health. 2009; ISBN 978-7-81136-190-2/R.190.
8. Qian Y, Han Q, Wang W, Ouyang Y, Yuan W, Fan C. Surgical release for tubercular elbow stiffness. Infect Drug Resist. 2017;11:9–16.
9. Fair E, Miller CR, Ottmani SE, Fox GJ, Hopewell PC. Tuberculosis contact investigation in low- and middle-income countries: standardized definitions and indicators. Int J Tuberc Lung Dis. 2015;19(3):269–72.
10. China Institute of city competitiveness. Global city economic competitiveness list. 2016. http://news.sina.com.cn/w/sy/2017-10-30/doc-ifynhhay9107171.shtml. Accessed October 30 2017.
11. Wei X, Li H, Yang N, Wong SY, Chong MC, Shi L, Wong MC, Xu J, Zhang D, Tang J, Li DK, Meng Q, Griffiths SM. Changes in the perceived quality of primary care in Shanghai and Shenzhen, China: a difference-in-difference analysis. Bull World Health Organ. 2015; 93(6):407–16.
12. Wibaux C, Moafo-Tiatsop M, Andrei I, Biver E, Cotten A, Cortet B, Duquesnoy B, Flipo RM. Changes in the incidence and management of spinal tuberculosis in a French University hospital rheumatology department from 1966 to 2010. Joint Bone Spine. 2013;80(5):516–9.
13. Gilbert RL, Antoine D, French CE, Abubakar I, Watson JM, Jones JA. The impact of immigration on tuberculosis rates in the United Kingdom compared with other European countries. Int J Tuberc Lung Dis. 2009;13(5):645–51.
14. Autzen B, Elberg JJ. Bone and joint tuberculosis in Denmark. Acta Orthop Scand. 1988;59(1):50–2.
15. Jabalameli M, Ameri E. Bone and joint tuberculosis, review of the patients treated in the Shafa Yahiaian hospital, 1350-74. Tehran University Medical Journal. 1998;56(4):62–6.
16. Tang SJ. Tang shenjie Chinese yearbook of. Tuberculosis. 2015.
17. Chen J, Qi L, Xia Z, Shen M, Shen X, Mei J, DeRiemer K, Zheng'an Y. Which urban migrants default from tuberculosis treatment in Shanghai, China? PLoS One. 2013;8(11):e81351.
18. Wang Y, Wang Q, Zhu R, Yang C, Chen Z, Bai Y, Li M, Zhai X. Trends of spinal tuberculosis research (1994–2015): a bibliometric study. Medicine (Baltimore). 2016;95(38):e4923.
19. Kenyon PC, Chapman AL. Tuberculous vertebral osteomyelitis: findings of a 10-year review of experience in a UK centre. J Inf Secur. 2009;59(5):372–3.
20. Pertuiset E, Beaudreuil J, Lioté F, Horusitzky A, Kemiche F, Richette P, Clerc-Wyel D, Cerf-Payrastre I, Dorfmann H, Glowinski J, Crouzet J, Bardin T, Meyer O, Dryll A, Ziza JM, Kahn MF, Kuntz D. Spinal tuberculosis in adults. A study of 103 cases in a developed country, 1980-1994. Medicine (Baltimore). 1999;78(5):309–20.
21. Jutte PC, van Loenhout-Rooyackers JH, Borgdorff MW, van Horn JR. Increase of bone and joint tuberculosis in the Netherlands. J Bone Joint Surg Br. 2004;86(6):901–4.
22. Hadadi A, Rasoulinejad M, Khashayar P, Mosavi M, Maghighi Morad M. Osteoarticular tuberculosis in Tehran, Iran: a 2-year study. Clin Microbiol Infect. 2010;16(8):1270–3.
23. Johansen IS, Nielsen SL, Hove M, Kehrer M, Shakar S, Wøyen AV, Andersen PH, Bjerrum S, Wejse C, Andersen ÅB. Characteristics and clinical outcome of bone and joint tuberculosis from 1994 to 2011: a retrospective register-based study in Denmark. Clin Infect Dis. 2015;61(4):554–62.
24. Colmenero JD, Jiménez-Mejías ME, Reguera JM, Palomino-Nicás J, Ruiz-Mesa JD, Márquez-Rivas J, Lozano A, Pachón J. Tuberculous vertebral osteomyelitis in the new millennium: still a diagnostic and therapeutic challenge. Eur J Clin Microbiol Infect Dis. 2004;23(6):477–83.
25. Chen ST, Zhao LP, Dong WJ, Gu YT, Li YX, Dong LL, Ma YF, Qin SB, Huang HR. The clinical features and bacteriological characterizations of bone and joint tuberculosis in China. Sci Rep. 2015;5:11084.
26. Kodde IF, van Rijn J, van den Bekerom MP, Eygendaal D. Surgical treatment of post-traumatic elbow stiffness: a systematic review. J Shoulder Elb Surg. 2013;22(4):574–80.
27. Pujol N, Boisrenoult P, Beaufils P. Post-traumatic knee stiffness: surgical techniques. Orthop Traumatol Surg Res. 2015;101(1 Suppl):S179–86.
28. Ollivier M, Parratte S, Argenson JN. Results and outcomes of unicompartmental knee arthroplasty. Orthop Clin North Am. 2013; 44(3):287–300 vii-viii.
29. Gan F, Jiang J, Xie Z, Huang S, Li Y, Chen G, Tan H. Minimally invasive direct lateral interbody fusion in the treatment of the thoracic and lumbar spinal tuberculosisMini-DLIF for the thoracic and lumbar spinal tuberculosis. BMC Musculoskelet Disord. 2018;19(1):283.
30. Yu S, Chen M, Fan C. Team approach: elbow contracture due to heterotopic ossification. JBJS Rev 2017;5(1). pii: 01874474-201701000-00004.
31. World Health Organization. Stop TB Dept. treatment of tuberculosis: guidelines. 4th edition. Geneva: World Health Organization, 2010. http://www.who.int/tb/publications/9789241547833/en/
32. Neiderud CJ. How urbanization affects the epidemiology of emerging infectious diseases. Infect Ecol Epidemiol. 2015;5:27060.

13

Prevalence and antibiotic susceptibility pattern of CTX-M type extended-spectrum β-lactamases among clinical isolates of gram-negative bacilli

Ahmed Zeynudin[1,2,3†], Michael Pritsch[1,4,5†], Sören Schubert[1], Maxim Messerer[6], Gabriele Liegl[1], Michael Hoelscher[3,4,5], Tefara Belachew[2] and Andreas Wieser[1,2,4,5*]

Abstract

Background: The prevalence of extended-spectrum β-lactamases (ESBLs) have been reported in clinical isolates obtained from various hospitals in Ethiopia. However, there is no data on the prevalence and antibiotic susceptibility patterns of CTX-M type ESBL produced by Gram-negative bacilli. The aim of this study was to determine the frequency and distribution of the bla_{CTX-M} genes and the susceptibility patterns in ESBL producing clinical isolates of Gram-negative bacilli in Jimma University Specialized Hospital (JUSH), southwest Ethiopia.

Methods: A total of 224 non-duplicate and pure isolates obtained from clinically apparent infections, were included in the study. Identification of the isolates was performed by MALDI-TOF mass spectrometry. Susceptibility testing and ESBL detection was performed using VITEK® 2, according to EUCAST v4.0 guidelines. Genotypic analysis was performed using Check-MDR CT103 Microarrays.

Results: Of the total 112 (50.0%) isolates screen positive for ESBLs, 63.4% (71/112) tested positive for ESBL encoding genes by Check-MDR array, which corresponds to 91.8% (67/73) of the total *Enterobacteriaceae* and 10.3% (4/39) of nonfermenting Gram-negative bacilli. Among the total ESBL gene positive isolates, 95.8% (68/71) carried bla_{CTX-M} genes with CTX-M group 1 type15 being predominant (66/68; 97.1% of CTX-M genes). The bla_{CTX-M} carrying *Enterobacteriaceae* ($n = 64$) isolates showed no resistance against imipenem and meropenem and a moderate resistance rate against tigecycline (14.1%), fosfomycin (10.9%) and amikacin (1.6%) suggesting the effectiveness of these antibiotics against most isolates. On the other hand, all the bla_{CTX-M} positive *Enterobacteriaceae* showed a multidrug resistant (MDR) phenotype with remarkable co-resistances (non-susceptibility rates) to aminoglycosides (92.2%), fluoroquinolones (78.1%) and trimethoprim/sulfamethoxazol (92.2%).

Conclusions: This study demonstrates a remarkably high prevalence of bla_{CTX-M} genes among ESBL-producing isolates. The high level of resistance to β-lactam and non-β-lactam antibiotics as well as the trend to a MDR profile associated with the bla_{CTX-M} genes are alarming and emphasize the need for routine diagnostic antimicrobial susceptibility testing for appropriate choice of antimicrobial therapy.

Keywords: Gram-negative bacilli, Extended-spectrum beta-lactamase, CTX-M, Antimicrobial susceptibility, Ethiopia

* Correspondence: wieser@mvp.uni-muenchen.de
†Ahmed Zeynudin and Michael Pritsch contributed equally to this work.
[1]Chair of Medical Microbiology and Hospital Epidemiology, Max von Pettenkofer Institute, Faculty of Medicine, LMU Munich, Marchioninistr. 17, 81377 Munich, Germany
[2]Institute of Health Sciences, Jimma University, Jimma, Ethiopia
Full list of author information is available at the end of the article

Background

Extended-spectrum β-lactamases (ESBLs) are a predominant cause of β-lactam resistance in Gram-negative bacilli (GNB) [1, 2]. Incidences of infections caused by ESBLs producing GNB are increasing in prevalence worldwide, both in the healthcare as well as community settings, posing significant therapeutic challenges [3–5]. ESBLs are most often a plasmid mediated heterogeneous group of β-lactamase enzymes, that confer resistance to a wide range of commonly used β-lactam antibiotics including third generation cephalosporins (e.g., ceftriaxone, cefotaxime and ceftazidime) as well as monobactams (aztreonam) [6]. TEM and SHV type ESBLs used to be the dominant ESBL genotypes [7]. However, in the past decade, the CTX-M type ESBLs have become the most widely distributed and globally dominant genotypes [8].

The CTX-M type enzymes are a group of class A ESBLs that in general exhibit much higher levels of activity against cefotaxime and ceftriaxone than ceftazidime [6, 9]. The presence of CTX-M type ESBLs is often associated with co-resistance phenotypes in particular to fluoroquinolones and aminoglycosides, in addition to tetracycline, and trimethoprim/sulfamethoxazole co-resistance, which is commonly observed among TEM and SHV type ESBLs [10, 11]. The group of CTX-M type ESBLs currently constitutes more than 170 allelic variants, which cluster into five major groups based on sequence homologies. The five CTX-M groups are: CTX-M-1, CTX-M-2, CTX-M-8, CTX-M-9 and CTX-M-25 [12]. Each group consists of a number of particular variants with dominant variants being restricted in distribution to specific geographic areas, while few others are globally distributed. CTX-M-14 and CTX-M-15 were the most commonly isolated variants worldwide [10, 13].

In Africa, CTX-M-15 (of the CTX-M-1 group) is the most frequently reported variant, although some other variants were also detected in the region [14, 15]. CTX-M type ESBLs have now spread and could be detected among many different bacterial strains of clinical importance. This is particularly true for *Enterobacteriaceae* revealing an ESBL phenotype such as *Escherichia coli* and *Klebsiella pneumoniae*, which often cause potentially serious infections in the hospital as well as community setting [13].

In Ethiopia, multiple studies have reported prevalence of ESBLs ranging from 25 to 38.5% among *Enterobacteriaceae* in clinical samples obtained from various hospitals, including Jimma University Specialized Hospital (JUSH) [16–19]. However, there is no data on the prevalence and antibiotic susceptibility patterns of CTX-M type ESBLs produced by GNB. Therefore, the aim of the present study was to determine the relative frequency and distribution of the $bla_{\text{CTX-M}}$ genes, as well as the overall susceptibility patterns in ESBL producing clinical isolates of GNB in JUSH, southwest Ethiopia.

Methods

Study setting and clinical specimens

A total of 224 randomly selected, non-duplicate, pure and clinically relevant Gram-negative bacilli isolates recovered from various clinical specimens submitted to the bacteriology laboratory for routine culture and antimicrobial susceptibility testing at JUSH during March to October 2014 were included in the study. The isolates were stored in − 20 °C freezers until transport and subsequently shipped to the Department of Bacteriology, Max von Pettenkofer-Institute (LMU), Munich, Germany for further screening and molecular analysis. The specimens were sent from different inpatient and outpatient units of JUSH, the only teaching and referral hospital in the southwestern part of Ethiopia, providing health services for approximately 15 million people in the catchment area. The specimens included wound swabs, urine, biopsies, sputum and others (see Additional file 1). All inpatient clinical specimens were obtained after more than 48 h of hospitalization of the patient. Along with the specimens, basic demographic and medical data were recorded using standard clinical and laboratory record forms.

Bacterial isolation, identification and susceptibility testing

Isolation and identification of the bacterial isolates was performed using standard microbiological techniques in use at the bacteriology laboratory in JUSH [20]. At the Max von Pettenkofer-Institute (LMU), all isolates were identified to the species level by MALDI-TOF mass spectrometry (MALDI Biotyper, Bruker Daltonik, Bremen, Germany, Biotyper software package, version 3.0) [21], and then retested for antibiotic susceptibilities using VITEK® 2 compact automated system (N215 and N248, bioMérieux, France), according to the instructions of the manufacturers. Software supplied by the manufacturer in compliance with the EUCAST v4.0 guidelines was used. The system included an Advanced Expert System (AES) that analysed growth patterns and detected the phenotype of organisms. Calculated MICs of piperacillin, piperacillin-tazobactam, cefotaxime, ceftazidime, cefepime, aztreonam, imipenem, meropenem, amikacin, gentamicin, ciprofloxacin, tobramycin, moxifloxacin, fosfomycin, tigecycline, colistin and trimethoprim/sulfamethoxazole were determined and interpreted according to EUCAST v4.0 guidelines [22].

ESBL screening and phenotypic tests

All *Enterobacteriaceae* isolates with reduced susceptibility or resistance to ceftazidime and/or cefotaxime and/or aztreonam [23] and all non-fermenting GNB with multi-resistant phenotype [24] were considered as ESBL-screen positive and subjected to phenotypic and genotypic analysis. Phenotypic detection of ESBL production was performed with the VITEK® 2 compact automated systems (bioMérieux, France).

Detection and molecular characterization of β-lactamase genes

Detection and molecular characterization of the β-lactamase genes was performed on all ESBL-screen positive isolates using Check-MDR CT103 Microarray Kits (Check-Points B.V., Wageningen, The Netherlands) following the manufacturer's instructions. With this assay, mutation analysis of TEM and SHV genes was performed to separate wild type (WT) alleles from ESBL variants, further AmpC β-lactamases (CMY-I/MOX, ACC, DHA, ACT/MIR, CMY-II, FOX) and carbapenemases (KPC, NDM, VIM, IMP, OXA-48-like) were investigated. Finally, CTX-M group ESBLs 1, 2, 8 plus 25, and 9 are also detected with the chip. To further define the type of CTX-M group – 1 and – 9 genes specifically, all positive isolates were amplified with primers suggested by Kim et al. [25]. For CTX-M-1 group, the primers with the sequence 5-cgt cacgctgttgttaggaa-3 and 5-acggctttctgccttaggtt-3 were used at 55 °C annealing temperature to yield a 780 bp fragment. CTX-M-9 group genes were amplified with the primers 5-tattgggagtttgagatggt-3 and 5-tccttcaactcagcaaaagt-3 at 50 °C annealing temperature to yield a 932 bp fragment. The fragments were sequenced for allele type identification. In combination with the Check-MDR hybridization the CTX-M subtypes can thereby be identified with high confidence, although a theoretical uncertainty remains, as the gene is not completely covered by the sequencing.

Quality control

For ESBL testing, *K. pneumoniae* ATCC 700603 (ESBL positive), *E. coli* CCUG62975 (ESBL positive), *E. coli* ATCC 25922 (ESBL negative) and *P. aeruginosa* (ATCC 27853) were used as quality control (QC) in all tests.

Statistical analyses

Statistical significance for comparison of proportions was calculated by the chi-squared test using Statistical Package for Social Sciences (SPSS, version 23, SPSS, Chicago, IL, U.S.A.). A value of $P < 0.05$ was considered as statistically significant.

Ethical considerations

The study was approved by Jimma University Ethical Review Board.

Results

Clinical bacterial isolates and specimens

Of the total 224 Gram-negative bacterial strains, 112 (50%) isolates were considered as screen positive for ESBLs. These isolates consisted of 73 *Enterobacteriaceae* (31 *Klebsiella pneumoniae,* 2 *Klebsiella oxytoca,* 14 *Enterobacter cloacae,* 13 *Escherichia coli,* 5 *Providencia stuartii,* 4 *Proteus mirabilis,* 3 *Morganella morganii,* and 1 *Escherichia hermanii)* and 39 non-fermenting Gram-negative bacilli (14 *Acinetobacter baumanii,* 2 *Acinetobacter pittii,* 1 *Acinetobacter haemolyticus,* 14 *Pseudomonas aeruginosa,* 3 *Alcaligenes faecalis,* 4 *Stenotrophomonas maltophilia* and 1 *Bordetella bronchiseptica*). The majority of these isolates was recovered from inpatients (83.9%, $n = 94$) mainly from surgical wards (60.6%, $n = 57$) followed by medical wards (21.3%, $n = 20$) and from two types of specimens; wound (54.5%, $n = 61$) and urine samples (26.8%, $n = 30$), which together account for 81.3% ($n = 91$) of the total isolates (see also Additional file 1). The total 112 screen positive isolates were collected from 100 patients; 90 (90%) of patients yielded one isolate for inclusion whereas ten (10%) patients yielded multiple species (eight patients with two species and two patients with three species).

Phenotypic detection of ESBLs

Phenotypic ESBL production was observed in 62.5% ($n = 70$) of the total screen positive isolates ($n = 112$) using VITEK® 2 compact automated system (bioMérieux, France).

Genotypic detection of ESBL encoding genes

Of the total 112 screen positive isolates, 63.4% ($n = 71$) were positive for ESBL encoding genes by Check-MDR array. This corresponds to 91.8% (67/73) of the total *Enterobacteriaceae* and 10.3% (4/39) of non-fermenting Gram-negative bacilli, namely 3 *P. aeruginosa* and 1 *A. faecalis* isolate. No ESBL alleles were detected among *Acinetobacter* spp., *S. maltophilia* and *B. bronchiseptica* (Table 1). Specimen wise, 60.7% ($n = 37$) of isolates from wound samples, 63.3% ($n = 19$) from urine, 66.7% ($n = 8$) from biopsy samples and all the isolates obtained from sputum samples ($n = 6$) as well as eye discharge ($n = 1$) were positive for ESBL encoding genes. Among total inpatient ($n = 94$) and outpatient ($n = 18$) isolates, ESBL genes were detected in 68.1% and 38.9% of the isolates respectively. The comparison of the difference in proportion should be taken with caution as convenient sampling was used and most specimens were obtained from inpatients. Four patients had two different ESBL-positive isolates (*E. cloacae* and *K. pneumoniae* in two cases cases, *E. coli* and *M. morganii*, and *P. aeruginosa* and *A. faecalis* in one case each). One of the four patients had an SHV 238S + 240 K mutation bearing *E. cloacae* and a

Table 1 Frequency, distribution and combinations of *bla* genes among screen and ESBL gene positive Gram-negative isolates

Screen positive species	Total ESBL		Among ESBL gene positive isolates							
			SHV E240K + G238S alone		CTX-M alone		CTX-M + SHV E240K + G238S		Total CTXM	
	n:	%	n:	%	n:	%	n:	%	n:	%
E. coli (*n* = 13)	13	100	0	0	12	92.3	1	7.7	13	100
K. pneumoniae (*n* = 31)	30	96.8	0	0	29	96.7	1	3.3	30	100
E. cloacae (*n* = 14)	12	85.7	3	25.0	9	75.0	0	0	9	75.0
other *Enterobacteriaceae*[a] (*n* = 15)	12	80.0	0	0	12	100	0	0	12	100
P. aeruginosa (*n* = 14)	3	21.4	0	0	3	100	0	0	3	100
other Non-fermenters[b] (*n* = 25)	1	4	0	0	1	100	0	0	1	100
Total (*n* = 112)	71	63.4	3	4.2	66	92.9	2	2.8	68	95.8

[a]includes 3 *M. morganii*, 4 *P. mirablis*, 5 *P. stuartii*, 2 *K. oxytoca* and 1 *E. hermanii*
[b]includes 17 *Acinetobacter* species (14 *A. baumanii*, 2 *A. pittii* and 1 *A. haemolyticus*), 3 *A. faecalis*, 4 *S. maltophilia* and 1 *B. bronchiseptica*

CTX-M-15 positive *K. pneumoniae* in the specimen, whereas the three other patients each had two different species each positive for CTX-M-15.

Frequency and distribution of *bla*$_{CTX-M}$ genes

From a total of 71 isolates carrying ESBL encoding genes, 68 (95.8%) carried CTX-M genes either alone or in combination with SHV and/or TEM genes. Sixty-four out of 67 (95.5%) *Enterobacteriaceae* and all non-fermenting GNB (*n* = 4) which carried ESBL encoding genes, were positive for CTX-M genes. The remaining three isolates negative for CTX-M (4.2%) carried SHV-type ESBLs (G238S + E240K) genes and were found to be *E. cloacae* obtained from wound samples. All TEM and SHV β-lactam genes detected were wild type except five G238S + E240K SHV type ESBLs. Three of the five were detected in *E. cloacae* in combination with wild type TEM. The other two were found in one *E. coli* and *K. pneumoniae* isolate along with CTX-M genes (Table 1).

Combinations of *bla*$_{CTX-M}$ with other β-lactamase genes

Multiple β-lactamase genes in a single strain were observed in 83.1% (*n* = 59) of the total isolates carrying ESBL encoding genes. From a total of 68 CTX-M positive isolates, 12 (17.6%) harbored CTX-M alone. The remaining 56 (82.4%) isolates carried CTX-M in combination with wild type TEM and/or SHV (except two SHV E240K + G238S) in different frequencies, which is partly explained due to the general presence of β-lactamases in some strains e.g. in *Klebsiella* spp. (Table 1).

Frequency and distribution of CTX-M groups and types

CTX-M group 1 was the most dominant CTX-M group detected in 66 of 68 CTX-M positive isolates (97.1%), either alone (*n* = 63, 92.6%) or in combination with other groups (*n* = 3, 4.5%). All CTX-M-1 genes were sequenced and all were found to be allele CTX-M-15. The remaining two (2.9%) CTX-M positive isolates carried CTX-M group 9 (Table 2) genes which upon sequencing were identified as allele CTX-M-24.

Antibiotic susceptibility pattern of CTX-M positive gram-negative bacilli isolates

The antibiotic susceptibility testing for CTX-M-positive *Enterobacteriaceae* isolates demonstrated a MIC in the respective susceptible range in < 2% of cases against cephalosporins according to EUCAST guidelines. Susceptibilities to carbapenems and a few other substances were found to be much higher. In terms of non-susceptibility, the highest level of antibiotic resistances was observed as expected against β-lactams such as piperacillin and cephalosporins, but also against trimethoprim-sulfamethoxazole (92.2%), gentamicin (89.1%), and quinolones (75%). No isolates showed full resistance to imipenem or meropenem, and only 3.1% and 1.6% tested intermediate for these substances, respectively (Table 3). One *E. coli* isolate tested positive for CTX-M-15 but was measured susceptible to third generation cephalosporins using VITEK 2 as well as disc diffusion tests.

Co-resistance (co-non-susceptibility) to non-β-lactam antibiotics

All the CTX-M-positive *Enterobacteriaceae* (*n* = 64, 100%) and *P. aeruginosa* (*n* = 3, 100%) were non-susceptible to ≥1 agent in ≥3 antimicrobial categories and hence defined as multidrug resistant (MDR) according to the international expert proposal for interim standard definitions for acquired resistance promoted by the European Centre for Disease Prevention and Control (ECDC) [26]. About 92.2%, 78.1% and 92.2% of the total CTX-M-positive *Enterobacteriaceae* were found to be non-susceptible (co-resistant) to aminoglycosides, fluoroquinolones and trimethoprim-sulfamethoxazole, respectively (Fig. 1).

Table 2 Frequency and distribution of CTX-M groups among CTX-M positive Gram-negative bacilli isolates

CTX-M positive species	CTX-M groups (total)								CTX-M group combinations									
	CTX-M-1		CTX-M-2		CTX-M-8 + 25		CTX-M-9		CTX-M-1 alone		CTX-M-1 + 2		CTX-M-1 + 9		CTX-M-1 + 2 + 8 + 25		CTX-M-9 alone	
	n:	%	n:	%	n:	%	n:	%	n:	%	n:	%	n:	%	n:	%	n:	%
E. coli (*n* = 13)	12	92.3	0	0	0	0	2	15.4	11	84.6	0	0	1	7.7	0	0	1	7.7
K. pneumoniae (*n* = 30)	30	100	1	3.3	0	0	0	0	29	96.7	1	3.3	0	0	0	0	0	0
E. cloacae (*n* = 9)	9	100	0	0	0	0	0	0	9	100	0	0	0	0	0	0	0	0
Other *Enterobacteriaceae*[a] (*n* = 12)	11	91.7	0	0	0	0	1	8.3	11	91.7	0	0	0	0	0	0	1	8.3
P. aeruginosa (*n* = 3)	3	100	1	33.3	1	33.3	0	0	2	66.7	0	0	0	0	1	33.3	0	0
Other Non-Fermenters[b] (*n* = 1)	1	100	0	0	0	0	0	0	1	100	0	0	0	0	0	0	0	0
Total (*n* = 68)	66	97.1	2	2.9	1	1.5	3	4.4	63	92.6	1	1.5	1	1.5	1	1.5	2	2.9

[a]includes 3 *M. morganii*, 4 *P. mirablis*, 2 *P. stuartii*, 2 *K. oxytoca* and 1 *E. hermanii*
[b]includes 1 *A. faecalis*

Non-susceptibility pattern in CTX-M and non-CTX-M carrying isolates

Both CTX-M (n = 64) and non-CTX-M-producing (n = 119) *Enterobacteriaceae* isolates have comparable non-susceptibility patterns to piperacillin/tazobactam, imipenem, meropenem, fosfomycin, and colistin/polymyxin B ($P > 0.05$). However, the non-susceptibility rate to all other antibiotics tested were all significantly higher among CTX-M-positive isolates compared to non-CTX-M ESBL-carrying isolates ($P < 0.001$) (Fig. 2). All the CTX-M negative isolates were also non-ESBLs except for three isolates expressing SHV type ESBLs. Unlike seen with CTX-M ESBLs, this did not affect the other non-susceptibilities.

Discussion

The present study is the first report describing the molecular epidemiology of ESBL-encoding genes in Ethiopia. We demonstrate a high level of prevalence of CTX-M-type ESBLs among all ESBL positive isolates at JUSH. In total, 95.8% of all ESBL genes detected were of CTX-M type, and almost unanimously CTX-M-1 group variant type 15 (97.1% of all CTX-M positive isolates). These findings are in accordance with the fact that the CTX-M type ESBLs are the most widely distributed and globally dominant ESBL genotypes to date [13, 27, 28]. Of the groups, CTX-M-1 was also described to be highly prevalent in Italy [29], India [30], Switzerland [31], Saudi-Arabia [32], Syria [33], Pakistan [34] and China [35].

Table 3 In vitro antimicrobial resistance pattern of CTX-M-positive Gram-negative isolates

Species	CTX-M positive isolate % resistance																
	PI	PIT	CTX	CAZ	CPM	AT	IMP	MRP	AK	HLG	TOB	CIP	MOX	FO	TGC	CL	COT
E. coli (*n* = 13)	100	30.8	92.3	92.3	92.3	92.3	0	0	7.7	76.9	76.9	92.3	84.6	7.7	0	7.7	84.6
K. pneumoniae (*n* = 30)	100	60	100	96.7	96.7	96.7	0	0	0	90	96.7	66.7	80	0	0	0	93.3
E. cloacae (*n* = 9)	100	0	100	100	100	100	0	0	0	88.9	88.9	22.2	77.8	0	0	0	100
M. morganii (*n* = 3)	100	0	100	100	100	100	0	0	0	100	100	66.7	100	100	IR	IR	100
P. mirablis (*n* = 4)	100	0	100	100	100	100	0	0	0	100	100	25	25	50	IR	IR	75
P. stuartii (*n* = 2)	100	0	100	100	100	100	0	0	0	IR	IR	50	50	50	IR	IR	100
K. oxytoca (*n* = 2)	100	50	100	100	100	100	0	0	0	100	100	0	50	0	0	0	100
E. hermanii (*n* = 1)	R	R	R	R	R	R	S	S	S	R	R	R	R	S	S	S	R
Total *Enterobacteriaceae* (*n* = 64)	100	35.9	98.4	96.9	96.9	96.9	0	0	1.6	89.1	92.2	59.4	75	10.9	14.1	15.6	92.2
P. aeruginosa (*n* = 3)	66.7	66.7	IR	33.3	66.7	66.7	0	0	33.3	66.7	66.7	100	100	100	IR	0	IR
A. faecalis (*n* = 1)	R	S	IE	IE	IE	R	S	S	S	S	S	IE	S	IE	IE	IE	IE
Total GNB (*n* = 68)	98.5	36.8	97.1	92.6	94.1	95.6	0	0	2.9	88.2	91.2	60.3	76.5	14.7	17.6	14.7	91.2

Key: PI piperacillin, *PIT* piperacillin/tazobactam, *CTX* cefotaxime, *CAZ* ceftazidime, *CPM* cefepime, *AT* aztreonam, *IMP* imipenem, *MRP* meropenem, *AK* amikacin, *HLG* gentamicin, *TOB* tobramycin, *CIP* ciprofloxacin, *MOX* moxifloxacin, *FO* fosfomycine, *TGC* tigecycline, *CL* colistin, *COT* trimethoprim/sulfamethoxazole
n number of isolates, *S* sensitive, *R* resistant, *IR* intrinsic resistance, *IE* insufficient evidence

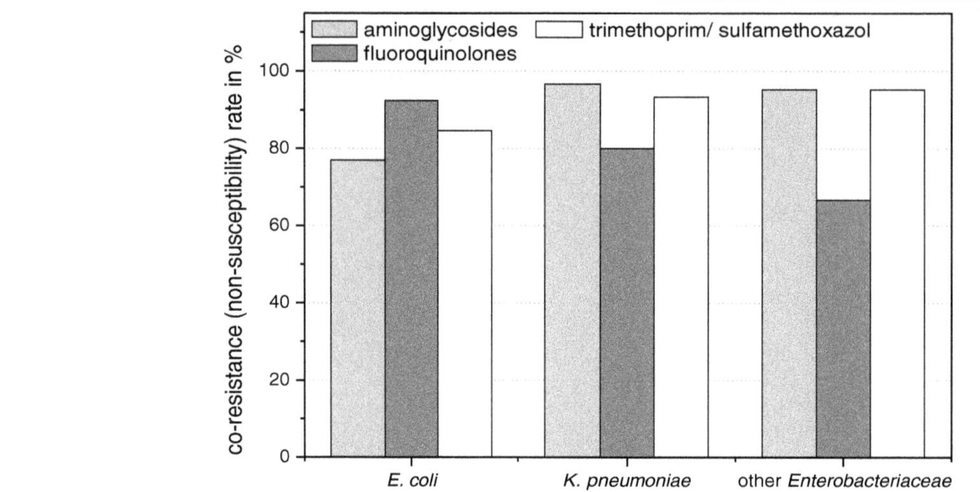

Fig. 1 Bar graph showing the non-susceptibility pattern of the CTX-M positive *E. coli* (n = 13), *K. pneumoniae* (n = 30) and other *Enterobacteriaceae* (n = 21) against aminoglycosides, fluoroquinolones and trimethoprim-sulfamethoxazole

Factors and mechanisms which contribute to the emergence and increasing prevalence of CTX-M ESBLs of all groups are complex and may involve both, plasmid dissemination as well as clonal spread of bacterial strains [36, 37]. In addition, the selective pressure exerted by the frequent use of wide spectrum cephalosporins may promote their epidemiological success [10, 28, 38]. Especially in Ethiopia, the widespread misuse and overuse of cephalosporins may contribute to the selection and spread of CTX-M gene carrying clones [39–41]. The frequency of the CTX-M genotype among the ESBL gene-positive *Enterobacteriaceae* isolates was also remarkably high (95.5%) compared to similar findings among clinical *Enterobacteriaceae* isolates with prevalence rates of 91% in Brazil [42], 80.3% in Germany [43] and 79% in Switzerland [31].

Other than *E. coli* (92.3% CTX-M-15) and *K. pneumoniae* (100% CTX-M-15), CTX-M were also detected among other members of ESBL producing *Enterobacteriaceae (K. oxytoca, M. morganii, P. mirablis, P. stuartii, E. hermannii* and *E. cloacae)* as well as non-fermenting GNB *(P. aeruginosa* and *A. fecalis)* in 87.5% (n = 21) and 100% (n = 4), respectively. Out of all screen positive isolates (112) 41 were found to be non-ESBL producers. Thereby, most (35/41) were lactose non-fermenting GNB with

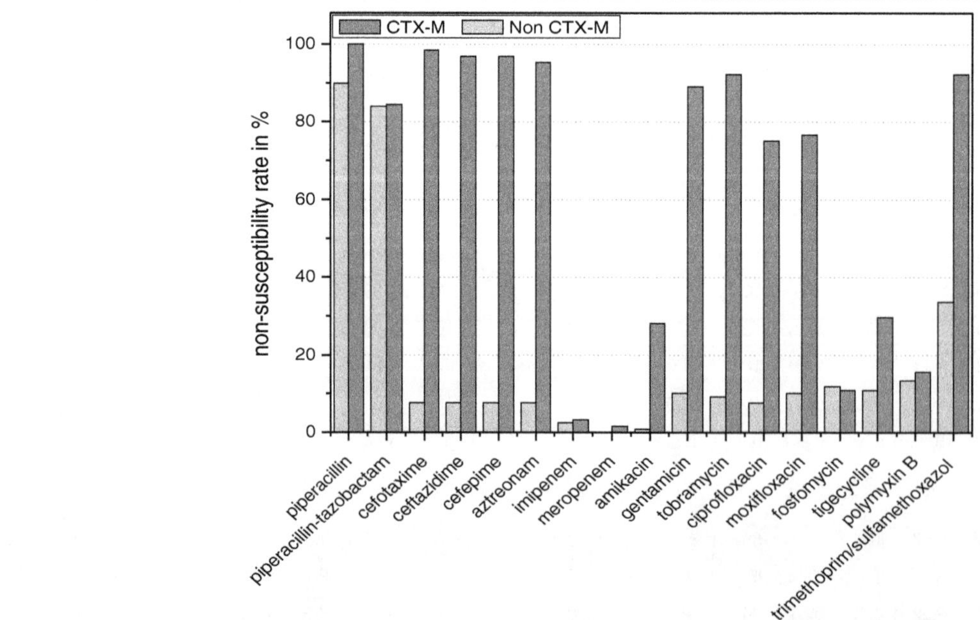

Fig. 2 Comparison of non-susceptibility patterns of $bla_{CTX\text{-}M}$ (n = 64) and non-$bla_{CTX\text{-}M}$ (n = 119) *Enterobacteriaceae* isolates against the 17 different antibiotics tested

known extensive intrinsic resistance mechanisms. Other isolates may be resistant due to genes not tested within this study, or due to derepression of wild type β-lactamases or even permeability defects. Among screen positive *Enterobacteriaceae* isolates, 92% (67/73) were also positive for an ESBL gene tested within this study.

Although, this study was small, it indicates the dissemination of the CTX-M genes to other GNB besides *Enterobacteriaceae* in Jimma. Similar findings have been reported in Switzerland [31], Argentina [44], Netherlands [45] and Japan [13]. The frequency of ESBL gene positive *Pseudomonas aeruginosa* was low (21.4%, $n = 3$) when compared to other GNB. This is probably due to the fact that most resistance mechanisms in *Pseudomonas aeruginosa* are mediated by the overproduction of AmpC β-lactamases as well as acquired metallo-β-lactamases, decreased permeability and efflux pumps [46]. In addition, plasmid incompatibility and host range of ESBL encoding plasmids might also play a role in our setting [13]. The emergence and spread of CTX-M-producing isolates in the community, particularly among *E. coli* in urinary tract infections (UTI), were reported from China [47], Brazil [48] and the UK [49]. A trend in this direction can also be seen in our study, as all the outpatient urine isolates of *E. coli* ($n = 2$), *K. pneumoniae* ($n = 2$), *M. morganii* ($n = 1$), *P. mirablis* ($n = 1$) and *E. cloacae* ($n = 1$) with an ESBL gene were shown to carry CTX-M genes. However, the total sample size of outpatient isolates in the present study is small compared to the inpatient sample number.

The overall resistance pattern of the total CTX-M positive *Enterobacteriaceae* is very high for most antibiotics tested in the present study. The carbapenems (0% resistance) followed by amikacin (3% resistance) were found to have the highest susceptibility rates. However, all CTX-M-positive isolates identified in this study showed a MDR phenotype as well as remarkably high rates of co-resistance to fluoroquinolones, aminoglycosides, and trimethoprim/sulfamethoxazole. Only one *E. coli* isolate positive for an ESBL gene (CTX-M-15) was not resistant against third generation cephalosporins, while still maintaining an MDR phenotype. In this particular case, the CTX-M operon seems to be non-functional perhaps due to mutations. These findings are consistent with studies from Ghana [50], Lebanon [51] and India [52] which propose imipenem and amikacin as possible drugs for the management of infection caused by CTX-M-producing isolates. The results are also in accordance with findings of high prevalence of MDR phenotype (88.4%) among ESBL-producing *E. coli* and *K. pneumoniae* isolates in a previous phenotypic characterization of strains in JUSH [17]. Comparably high rates of co-resistance to non-β-lactam antibiotics were also reported from Brazil [42], South Korea [53] and Indian hospitals [54].

Surprisingly, colistin/polymyxin, which is not available in Ethiopia, showed resistance rates of above 10%. However, this rate has to be interpreted with caution, as the data based on VITEK® 2 testing system is unreliable for detecting colistin resistance [55], and results obtained by these methods may be overrated and require confirmation by ISO-standard broth microdilution method as nowadays recommended by EUCAST [56, 57]. As the respective recommendation was issued after completion of the study, it was not taken into consideration.

In the present study, only clinically relevant isolates of in- and outpatients were used, a screening upon admission, or screening of healthy controls was not performed. However, the high rates of ESBL positive organisms in outpatients without contact to the health care system within the last 3 months, argues for considerable ESBL carrier rates among the general population. Within the study population, mainly samples from internal medicine, pediatrics and ICU were ESBL positive and MDR, whereas in the surgical patient group many patients were found to harbor non-fermenters with MDR phenotype which are negative for the ESBL and carbapenemase genes tested within this study (see Additional file 2).

This conclusion is supported by a study conducted at black lion hospital in Addis Ababa (Ethiopia) reporting a high gastrointestinal colonization rate with ESBL producing *Enterobacteriaceae* among hospitalized patients [58]. It is well known, that many of the patients who develop health care-associated ESBL infections have preceding colonization of the gastrointestinal tract [59, 60]. A combination based on lack of hygiene and high colonization rates with ESBL positive organisms are likely to drive the ESBL rates in JUSH.

Within the sample group, other prominent resistance determinants were also investigated as part of the CT103 panel. Thereby, no KPC, NDM-1, VIM, IMP or Oxa48-like coding organism was detected. Previously, we could demonstrate the presence of NDM-1 in *Acinetobacter baumannii* in the area [61]. NDM-1 gene transfer to other isolates seems not to have occurred in relevant numbers. However, the presence of CTX-M-15 genes in different species in such high prevalence argues for horizontal gene transfer currently or in the past. The transfer might have occurred by plasmid exchange, which is especially common among *Enterobacteriaceae*, or by less frequent recombination events, e.g. involving IS elements. How recent or frequent such events have been cannot be elucidated given the methodology used, as the genes are found in numerous different species and isolates, it certainly cannot be explained simply by local clonal expansion of one strain.

Conclusions

This study demonstrates a remarkably high level of CTX-M genes in GNB isolated in JUSH. The most predominant group was CTX-M-1 allele 15 and a few percent CTX-M-9 allele 24 among all the ESBLs gene positive clinical isolates. In South Africa, CTX-M-2 and -3 group are most prevalent, and CTX-M-14 and -15 in Egypt [62]. Meropenem, imipenem, colistin and amikacin were found to have the highest in vitro efficacy against the CTX-M-producing isolates. The high level of resistance to β-lactam and non-β-lactam antibiotics as well as the trend of a MDR profile associated with the CTX-M genes are alarming and emphasize the need for diagnostic antimicrobial susceptibility testing for appropriate choice of antimicrobial therapy and limiting the spread of antimicrobial resistance in Ethiopia and in the region.

Acknowledgements

We thank Gabriele Liegl for excellent technical assistance as well as Dr. A.-C. Neumann for excellent support with figure generation.

Funding

The study was supported by Jimma University (to AZ and AW) and the German Center for Infection Research (DZIF) (AW, MH) as well as the Else Kröner-Fresenius-Stiftung (EKFS) to AW.

Authors' contributions

AZ, SS, TB and AW designed the study and protocol. AZ, MP, GL, MH and AW performed laboratory work. AZ, MP, SS, MH, TB, MM and AW analyzed the data and wrote the manuscript. All authors read and approved the final manuscript.

Competing interests

The authors declare that they have no competing interests.

Author details

[1]Chair of Medical Microbiology and Hospital Epidemiology, Max von Pettenkofer Institute, Faculty of Medicine, LMU Munich, Marchioninistr. 17, 81377 Munich, Germany. [2]Institute of Health Sciences, Jimma University, Jimma, Ethiopia. [3]Center for International Health (CIH), University of Munich (LMU), 80802 Munich, Germany. [4]Division of Infectious Diseases and Tropical Medicine, Medical Center of the University of Munich (LMU), 80802 Munich, Germany. [5]German Center for Infection Research (DZIF), Partner Site Munich, 80802 Munich, Germany. [6]Plant Genome and Systems Biology, Helmholtz Center Munich, German Research Center for Environmental Health, 85764 Neuherberg, Germany.

References

1. Ruppé É, Woerther PL, Barbier F. Mechanisms of antimicrobial resistance in gram-negative bacilli. Ann Intensive Care. 2015;5(1):1.
2. Sutton SS. What are extended-spectrum beta-lactamases? JAAPA. 2014;27(3): 14–7.
3. Chong Y, Shimoda S, Yakushiji H, Ito Y, Miyamoto T, Kamimura T, et al. Community spread of extended-spectrum β-lactamase-producing Escherichia coli, Klebsiella pneumoniae and Proteus mirabilis: a long-term study in Japan. J Med Microbiol. 2013;62(7):1038–43.
4. Kassakian SZ, Mermel LA. Changing epidemiology of infections due to extended spectrum beta-lactamase producing bacteria. Antimicrob Resist Infect Control. 2014;3(1):9.
5. WHO. Antimicrobial resistance: global report on surveillance. 2014. http://www.who.int/drugresistance/documents/surveillancereport/en/. Accessed 17 Feb 2018.
6. Ghafourian S, Sadeghifard N, Soheili S, Sekawi Z. Extended spectrum beta-lactamases: definition, classification and epidemiology. Curr Issues Mol Biol. 2015;17:11–21.
7. Thenmozhi S, Moorthy K, Sureshkumar B, Suresh M. Antibiotic resistance mechanism of ESBL producing Enterobacteriaceae in clinical field: a review. Int J Pure Appl Biosci. 2014;2(3):207–26.
8. Adamski CJ, Cardenas AM, Brown NG, Horton LB, Sankaran B, Prasad BV, et al. Molecular basis for the catalytic specificity of the CTX-M extended-spectrum β-lactamases. Biochemistry. 2014;54(2):447–57.
9. Shaikh S, Fatima J, Shakil S, Rizvi SMD, Kamal MA. Antibiotic resistance and extended spectrum beta-lactamases: types, epidemiology and treatment. Saudi J Biol Sci. 2015;22(1):90–101.
10. Lahlaoui H, Khalifa ABH, Moussa MB. Epidemiology of Enterobacteriaceae producing CTX-M type extended spectrum β-lactamase (ESBL). Med Mal Infect. 2014;44(9):400–4.
11. Östholm Balkhed Å, Tärnberg M, Monstein HJ, Hällgren A, Hanberger H, Nilsson LE. High frequency of co-resistance in CTX-M-producing Escherichia coli to non-beta-lactam antibiotics, with the exceptions of amikacin, nitrofurantoin, colistin, tigecycline, and fosfomycin, in a county of Sweden. Scand J Infect Dis. 2013;45(4):271–8.
12. Bush K, Palzkill T, Jacoby G. ß-lactamase classification and amino acid sequences for TEM, SHV and OXA extended-Spectrum and inhibitor resistant enzymes: Lahey Clinic; 2015. https://www.lahey.org/Studies/. Accessed 20 Feb 2018
13. Zhao WH, Hu ZQ. Epidemiology and genetics of CTX-M extended-spectrum β-lactamases in gram-negative bacteria. Crit Rev Microbiol. 2013;39(1):79–101.
14. Storberg V. ESBL-producing Enterobacteriaceae in Africa–a non-systematic literature review of research published 2008–2012. Infect Ecol Epidemiol. 2014;4. https://doi.org/10.3402/iee.v4.20342.
15. Ehlers MM, Veldsman C, Makgotlho EP, Dove MG, Hoosen AA, Kock MM. Detection of blaSHV, blaTEM and blaCTX-M antibiotic resistance genes in randomly selected bacterial pathogens from the Steve Biko academic hospital. FEMS Immunol Med Microbiol. 2009;56(3):191–6.
16. Mulisa G, Selassie L, Jarso G, Shiferew T, Zewdu A. Prevalence of extended Spectrum Beta-lactamase producing Enterobacteriaceae: a cross sectional study at Adama hospital, Adama, Ethiopia. J Emerg Infect Dis. 2016;1(102):2.
17. Siraj SM, Ali S, Wondafrash B. Extended-spectrum-lactamase production and antimicrobial resistance in Klebsiella pneumoniae and Escherichia coli among inpatients and outpatients of Jimma University specialized hospital, south-west, Ethiopia. Afr J Microbiol Res. 2014;8(43):3687–94.
18. Seid J, Asrat D. Occurrence of extended spectrum β-lactamase enzymes in clinical isolates of Klebsiella species from Harar region, eastern Ethiopia. Acta Trop. 2005;95(2):143–8.
19. Mulualem Y, Kasa T, Mekonnen Z, Suleman S. Occurrence of extended spectrum beta lactamases in multi-drug resistant Escherichia coli isolated from a clinical setting in Jimma University specialized hospital, Jimma, southwest Ethiopia. East Afr J Public Health. 2012;9(2):58–61.
20. Vandepitte J, Verhaegen J, Engbaek K, Rohner P, Piot P, Heuck C. Basic laboratory procedures in clinical bacteriology: World Health Organization; 2003. http://apps.who.int/iris/bitstream/10665/42696/1/9241545453.pdf. Accessed 20 Feb 2018
21. Wieser A, Schneider L, Jung J, Schubert S. MALDI-TOF MS in microbiological diagnostics—identification of microorganisms and beyond (mini review). Appl Microbiol Biotechnol. 2012;93(3):965–74.
22. European Committee on Antimicrobial Susceptibility Testing. Breakpoint tables for interpretation of MICs and zone diameters. Version 4.0, valid from 2014-01-01. EUCAST. https://asmsig.files.wordpress.com/2014/11/breakpoint_table_v_4-01-2014.pdf. Accessed 20 Feb 2018.
23. European Committee on Antimicrobial Susceptibility Testing. EUCAST guidelines for detection of resistance mechanisms and specific resistances of clinical and/or epidemiological importance. Version 1.0: EUCAST; 2013. http://www.eucast.org/fileadmin/src/media/PDFs/EUCAST_files/Resistance_mechanisms/EUCAST_detection_of_resistance_mechanisms_v1.0_20131211.pdf. Accessed 20 Feb 2018
24. Dally S, Lemuth K, Kaase M, Rupp S, Knabbe C, Weile J. DNA microarray for genotyping antibiotic resistance determinants in Acinetobacter baumannii clinical isolates. Antimicrob Agents Chemother. 2013;57(10):4761–8.
25. Kim J, Lim YM, Jeong YS, Seol SY. Occurrence of CTX-M-3, CTX-M-15, CTX-M-14, and CTX-M-9 extended-spectrum beta-lactamases in Enterobacteriaceae clinical isolates in Korea. Antimicrob Agents Chemother. 2005;49(4):1572–5.

26. Magiorakos AP, Srinivasan A, Carey R, Carmeli Y, Falagas M, Giske C, et al. Multidrug-resistant, extensively drug-resistant and pandrug-resistant bacteria: an international expert proposal for interim standard definitions for acquired resistance. Clin Microbiol Infect. 2012;18(3):268–81.
27. Canton R, Coque TM. The CTX-M beta-lactamase pandemic. Curr Opin Microbiol. 2006;9(5):466–75.
28. Rossolini GM, D'Andrea MM, Mugnaioli C. The spread of CTX-M-type extended-spectrum beta-lactamases. Clin Microbiol Infect. 2008;14(Suppl 1):33–41.
29. Mugnaioli C, Luzzaro F, De Luca F, Brigante G, Perilli M, Amicosante G, et al. CTX-M-type extended-spectrum β-lactamases in Italy: molecular epidemiology of an emerging countrywide problem. Antimicrob Agents Chemother. 2006;50(8):2700–6.
30. Singh A, Shahid M, Sobia F, Khan HM. Occurrence and molecular epidemiology of Bla CTX-M, including co-occurrence of bla TEM and Bla SHV genes, and sul1 association in Indian Enterobacteriaceae. Int J Antimicrob Agents. 2012;39(2):184–5.
31. Lartigue MF, Zinsius C, Wenger A, Bille J, Poirel L, Nordmann P. Extended-spectrum β-lactamases of the CTX-M type now in Switzerland. Antimicrob Agents Chemother. 2007;51(8):2855–60.
32. Al-Agamy MH, Shibl AM, Hafez MM, Al-Ahdal MN, Memish ZA, Khubnani H. Molecular characteristics of extended-spectrum β-lactamase-producing Escherichia coli in Riyadh: emergence of CTX-M-15-producing E. coli ST131. Ann Clin Microbiol Antimicrob. 2014;13(1):1.
33. Ibrahim AS, Youssef N. Prevalence of CTX-M, TEM and SHV Beta-lactamases in clinical isolates of Escherichia Coli and Klebsiella Pneumoniae isolated from Aleppo University Hospitals, Aleppo, Syria. Arch Clin Infect Dis. 2015;10(2):e22540.
34. Khan E, Schneiders T, Zafar A, Aziz E, Parekh A, Hasan R. Emergence of CTX-M Group 1-ESBL producing Klebsiella pneumonia from a tertiary care Centre in Karachi, Pakistan. J Infect Dev Ctries. 2010;4(08):472–6.
35. Shi H, Sun F, Chen J, Ou Q, Feng W, Yong X, Xia P. Epidemiology of CTX-M-type extended-spectrum beta-lactamase (ESBL)-producing nosocomial-Escherichia coli infection in China. Ann Clin Microbiol Antimicrob. 2015; 14(1):1.
36. Cantón R, González-Alba JM, Galán JC. CTX-M enzymes: origin and diffusion. Front Microbiol. 2012;3:110.
37. D'Andrea MM, Arena F, Pallecchi L, Rossolini GM. CTX-M-type β-lactamases: a successful story of antibiotic resistance. Int J Med Microbiol. 2013;303(6): 305–17.
38. Gelband H, Miller-Petrie M, Pant S, Gandra S, Levinson J, Barter D, et al. State of the World's Antibiotics 2015: Center for Disease Dynamics, Economics & Policy; 2015. https://www.cddep.org/wp-content/uploads/2017/06/swa_edits_9.16.pdf. Accessed 20 Feb 2018
39. Shimels T, Bilal AI, Mulugeta A. Evaluation of ceftriaxone utilization in internal medicine wards of general hospitals in Addis Ababa, Ethiopia: a comparative retrospective study. J Pharm Policy Pract. 2015;8(1):1.
40. Worku S, G/Mariam A. Practice of self medication in Jimma town. Ethiop J Health Dev 2003;17:111–116.
41. Ayinalem GA, Gelaw BK, Belay AZ, Linjesa JL. Drug use evaluation of ceftriaxone in medical ward of Dessie referral hospital, north East Ethiopia. Int J Basic Clin Pharmacol. 2013;2(6):711–7.
42. Seki LM, Pereira PS, de Souza Conceição M, Souza MJ, Marques EA, Carballido JM, et al. Molecular epidemiology of CTX-M producing Enterobacteriaceae isolated from bloodstream infections in Rio de Janeiro, Brazil: emergence of CTX-M-15. Braz J Infect Dis. 2013;17(6):640–6.
43. Schmiedel J, Falgenhauer L, Domann E, Bauerfeind R, Prenger-Berninghoff E, Imirzalioglu C, Chakraborty T. Multiresistant extended-spectrum β-lactamase-producing Enterobacteriaceae from humans, companion animals and horses in Central Hesse, Germany. BMC Microbiol. 2014;14(1):1.
44. Quinteros M, Radice M, Gardella N, Rodriguez M, Costa N, Korbenfeld D, et al. Extended-spectrum β-lactamases in Enterobacteriaceae in Buenos Aires, Argentina, public hospitals. Antimicrob Agents Chemother. 2003; 47(9):2864–7.
45. Al Naiemi N, Bart A, De Jong M, Vandenbroucke-Grauls C, Rietra P, Debets-Ossenkopp Y. Widely distributed and predominant CTX-M extended-spectrum β-lactamases in Amsterdam, the Netherlands. J Clin Microbiol. 2006;44(8):3012–4.
46. Noyal M, Menezes G, Harish B, Sujatha S, Parija S. Simple screening tests for detection of carbapenemases in clinical isolates of nonfermentative gram-negative bacteria. Indian J Med Res. 2009;129(6):707–12.
47. Xia S, Fan X, Huang Z, Xia L, Xiao M, Chen R, et al. Dominance of CTX-M-type extended-spectrum β-lactamase (ESBL)-producing Escherichia coli isolated from patients with community-onset and hospital-onset infection in China. PLoS One. 2014;9(7):e100707.
48. Minarini LA, Poirel L, Trevisani NA, Darini ALC, Nordmann P. Predominance of CTX-M–type extended-spectrum β-lactamase genes among enterobacterial isolates from outpatients in Brazil. Diagn Microbiol Infect Dis. 2009;65(2):202–6.
49. Woodford N, Ward M, Kaufmann M, Turton J, Fagan E, James D, et al. Community and hospital spread of Escherichia coli producing CTX-M extended-spectrum β-lactamases in the UK. J Antimicrob Chemother. 2004;54(4):735–43.
50. Hackman HK, Brown CA, Twum-Danso K, Bu K. Antibiotic Resistance Profile of CTX-M-type Extended-Spectrum Beta-Lactamases in *Escherichia coli* and *Klebsiella pneumoniae* in Accra, Ghana. J Nat Sci Res. 2014;4(12):24–29.
51. Sana T, Rami K, Racha B, Fouad D, Marcel A, Hassan M, et al. Detection of genes TEM, OXA, SHV and CTX-M in 73 clinical isolates of *Escherichia coli* producers of extended spectrum Betalactamases and determination of their susceptibility to antibiotics. Int Arab J Antimicrob Agents. 2011;1(1). https://doi.org/10.3823/704.
52. Upadhyay S, Hussain A, Mishra S, Maurya AP, Bhattacharjee A, Joshi SR. Genetic environment of plasmid mediated CTX-M-15 extended Spectrum Beta-lactamases from clinical and food borne Bacteria in north-eastern India. PLoS One. 2015;10(9):e0138056.
53. Shin J, Ko KS. Comparative study of genotype and virulence in CTX-M-producing and non-extended-spectrum-β-lactamase-producing Klebsiella pneumoniae isolates. Antimicrob Agents Chemother. 2014;58(4):2463–7.
54. Ensor V, Shahid M, Evans J, Hawkey P. Occurrence, prevalence and genetic environment of CTX-M β-lactamases in Enterobacteriaceae from Indian hospitals. J Antimicrob Chemother. 2006;58(6):1260–3.
55. Tan TY, Ng SY. Comparison of Etest, Vitek and agar dilution for susceptibility testing of colistin. Clin Microbiol Infect. 2007 May;13(5):541–4.
56. European Committee on Antimicrobial Susceptibility Testing. Breakpoint tables for interpretation of MICs and zone diameters. Version 6.0: EUCAST; 2016. http://www.eucast.org/fileadmin/src/media/PDFs/EUCAST_files/Breakpoint_tables/v_6.0_Breakpoint_table.pdf. Accessed 20 Feb 2018
57. European Committee on Antimicrobial Susceptibility Testing. Recommendations for MIC determination of colistin (polymyxin E) as recommended by the joint CLSI-EUCAST Polymyxin Breakpoints Working Group EUCAST. http://www.eucast.org/fileadmin/src/media/PDFs/EUCAST_files/General_documents/Recommendations_for_MIC_determination_of_colistin_March_2016.pdf. Accessed 20 Feb 2018.
58. Desta K, Woldeamanuel Y, Azazh A, Mohammod H, Desalegn D, Shimelis D, et al. High gastrointestinal colonization rate with extended-Spectrum β-lactamase-producing Enterobacteriaceae in hospitalized patients: emergence of Carbapenemase-Producing K. pneumoniae in Ethiopia. PLoS One. 2016;11(8):e0161685.
59. Christiaens G, Ciccarella Y, Damas P, Hayette MP, Melin P, Nys M, De Mol P. Prospective survey of digestive tract colonization with enterobacteriaceae that produce ESBLs in intensive care units. J Hosp Infect. 2006;62(3):386–8.
60. Falagas M, Karageorgopoulos DE. Extended-spectrum β-lactamase-producing organisms. J Hosp Infect. 2009;73(4):345–54.
61. Pritsch M, Zeynudin A, Messerer M, Baumer S, Liegl G, Schubert S, Löscher T, Hoelscher M, Belachew T, Rachow A, Wieser A. First repot on blaNDM-1-producing Acinetobacter baumannii in three clinical isolates from Ethiopia. BMC Infect Dis. 2017;17(1):180.
62. Hawkey PM, Jones AM. The changing epidemiology of resistance. J Antimicrob Chemother. 2009 Sep;64(Suppl 1):i3–10.

14

Multidrug resistant *Pseudomonas aeruginosa* in Estonian hospitals

Kaidi Telling[1*], Mailis Laht[2], Age Brauer[3], Maido Remm[3], Veljo Kisand[2], Matti Maimets[4], Tanel Tenson[2] and Irja Lutsar[1]

Abstract

Background: We aimed to identify the main spreading clones, describe the resistance mechanisms associated with carbapenem- and/or multidrug-resistant *P. aeruginosa* and characterize patients at risk of acquiring these strains in Estonian hospitals.

Methods: Ninety-two non-duplicated carbapenem- and/or multidrug-resistant *P. aeruginosa* strains were collected between 27th March 2012 and 30th April 2013. Clinical data of the patients was obtained retrospectively from the medical charts. Clonal relationships of the strains were determined by whole genome sequencing and analyzed by multi-locus sequence typing. The presence of resistance genes and beta-lactamases and their origin was determined. Combined-disk method and PCR was used to evaluate carbapenemase and metallo-beta-lactamase production.

Results: Forty-three strains were carbapenem-resistant, 11 were multidrug-resistant and 38 were both carbapenem- and multidrug-resistant. Most strains (54%) were isolated from respiratory secretions and caused an infection (74%).

Over half of the patients (57%) were ≥ 65 years old and 85% had ≥1 co-morbidity; 96% had contacts with healthcare and/or had received antimicrobial treatment in the previous 90 days.

Clinically relevant beta-lactamases (OXA-101, OXA-2 and GES-5) were found in 12% of strains, 27% of which were located in plasmids. No Ambler class B beta-lactamases were detected. Aminoglycoside modifying enzymes were found in 15% of the strains. *OprD* was defective in 13% of the strains (all with CR phenotype); carbapenem resistance triggering mutations (F170 L, W277X, S403P) were present in 29% of the strains. Ciprofloxacin resistance correlated well with mutations in topoisomerase genes gyrA (T83I, D87N) and parC (S87 L). Almost all strains (97%) with these mutations showed ciprofloxacin-resistant phenotype.

Multi-locus sequence type analysis indicated high diversity at the strain level – 36 different sequence types being detected. Two sequence types (ST108 (n = 23) and ST260 (n = 18)) predominated. Whereas ST108 was associated with localized spread in one hospital and mostly carbapenem-resistant phenotype, ST260 strains occurred in all hospitals, mostly with multi-resistant phenotype and carried different resistance genotype/machinery.

Conclusions: Diverse spread of local rather than international *P. aeruginosa* strains harboring multiple chromosomal mutations, but not plasmid-mediated Ambler class B beta-lactamases, were found in Estonian hospitals.

Keywords: Carbapenem resistance, Outbreak, WGS (whole-genome sequencing), Beta-lactamases

* Correspondence: kaidi.telling@ut.ee
[1]Department of Microbiology, Institute of Biomedicine and Translational Medicine, University of Tartu, Ravila 19, 50411 Tartu, Estonia
Full list of author information is available at the end of the article

Background

Pseudomonas aeruginosa (PA) is an opportunistic pathogen present in many ecological settings. It can survive in living (humans, animals, plants) and non-living (water, soil, artificial surfaces) sources [1], but is rarely found in the microbiota of healthy humans [2]. The colonization rate by PA significantly increases (reaching up to 80%) in patients with chronic illnesses (e.g. cystic fibrosis, severe burns) or extensive exposure to healthcare facilities involving interruption of protective barriers [3–5].

PA is exceptionally flexible, using different regulatory and metabolic mechanisms to adapt to antibiotic pressure. It has an intrinsic resistance to wide range of antimicrobial agents, and a high capacity to attain resistance mutations and mobile genetic elements [6].

According to the European Centre for Disease Prevention and Control (ECDC) in 2016, resistance of PA in most European countries exceeded 10% of all antimicrobials investigated. Furthermore, the prevalence of MDR-PA is rising globally, a phenomenon mainly associated with the spread of high-risk clones (e.g. multi-locus sequence types ST235, ST111, ST175) associated with nosocomial outbreaks and transferable resistance mechanisms, especially horizontally-acquired beta-lactamases [7]. Despite the low antibiotic consumption comparable to other North European countries [8], the resistance rates of PA in Estonia, especially to carbapenems, are much higher than in other low-end usage countries, with the trends becoming alarming. In 2012, 12.5% of the strains reported to the ECDC were carbapenem-resistant (CR), but this had risen above 20% by 2016 [9, 10].

Although main trigger associated with CR in PA is production of plasmid-mediated beta-lactamases/carbapenemases, mutational resistance mechanisms in chromosomal genes – e.g. altered expression of outer membrane porins or efflux systems and increased chromosomal cephalosporinase (AmpC) activity, may all have affected the development of resistance [7].

Unfortunately data provided by the ECDC reflects just a fraction of the actual situation, as only invasive strains and the phenotypic resistance are reported. This leaves a gap in terms of non-invasive infections, and in genetic information of the spreading bacterial lineages and resistance machinery they carry. Previous studies conducted in Estonia are no exception; they have included only certain patient groups (intensive care units) [11] or blood-stream infections [12] without any information at the molecular level. Both knowledge of main risk groups and genetic data of strains is essential in understanding resistance transfer, and to take actions needed to stop it.

Methods

We aimed to characterize hospitalized patients carrying carbapenem- or/and multidrug- resistant *P. aeruginosa* (CR/MDR-PA), identifying the main spreading clones and describing the most important resistance mechanisms, including the occurrence of clinically relevant beta-lactamases.

Study design and settings

The study was conducted in 5 major Estonian hospitals treating both pediatric and adult patients - 2 3rd level multidisciplinary referral hospitals (Tartu University Hospital and North Estonia Medical Centre), 2 central hospitals (West Tallinn Central Hospital and East-Tallinn Central Hospital) and 1 private hospital specializing in plastic and vascular surgery (The Hospital of Reconstructive Surgery).

During the study period all consecutive PA strains isolated from hospitalized patients taken by discretion of treating physicians on suspicion or confirmed infection and identified as CR and/or MDR by the microbiology laboratories of the hospitals were collected, with a target of 100 strains. Only one strain was included from each patient (invasive strain or firstly isolated strain). Strains from ambulatory patients and clinics were excluded. The collection lasted from 27th of March 2012 to 30th of April 2013.

Clinical data collection

Hospital records of patients with eligible PA strains were reviewed retrospectively to obtain demographic data (age, gender), the presence of major co-morbidities and predisposing clinical conditions, date and reason of admission, site of infection, in-hospital movement, presence of infection or colonization caused by CR/MDR-PA, and the outcome.

Specifically, we recorded the presence of invasive devices, surgery within the previous 30 days, hospitalization, or time spent in a long-term care facility, and antimicrobial therapy in the previous 90 days.

Sampling and microbiological methods

Standard clinical laboratory methods were used to isolate and identify PA from clinical specimens. Briefly, urine was plated on cysteine lactose electrolyte-deficient agar, respiratory samples on blood and chocolate agar, which were incubated at 37 °C for 24 to 48 h. Tissue biopsies were homogenized and incubated in thioglycolate broth at 37 °C for 14 days. Blood, cerebrospinal, pleural and abdominal fluids were processed and monitored with a BACTEC 9240 blood culture system (Becton Dickinson, Sparks, MD, USA). One colony with *Pseudomonas*-like morphology was identified using classical biochemical tests (catalase and oxidase reactions) and VITEK2 Compact or API tests (bioMérieux, Marcy l'Etoile, France).

Finally, all PA isolates were confirmed by using matrix-assisted laser desorption ionization time-of-flight mass spectrometry (Bruker Daltonics, Bremen, Germany).

Only one isolate per patient was included in the final analysis, giving preference to more invasive strains (blood or cerebrospinal fluid).

Phenotypic susceptibility testing

The MIC for 9 antipseudomonal antibiotics (ceftazidime, cefepime, meropenem, imipenem, piperacillin/tazobactam, amikacin, gentamicin, tobramycin and ciprofloxacin) for each strain was measured with an epsilometer (E-test, bioMérieux, Marcy l'Etoile, France), with the quality control strain ATCC® 27,853™ being routinely used. Antibiotic susceptibility was determined using EUCAST breakpoints and definitions [13, 14]. Strains non-susceptible to at least one tested carbapenem were designated CR, whereas those not susceptible to 3 or more antibiotic classes were defined as MDR [13].

Forty-seven CR strains were screened for *Klebsiella pneumoniae* carbapenemase (KPC) and metallo-beta-lactamase (MBL) production by combined-disk method using disks containing 10 μg imipenem, 10 μg imipenem with phenylboronic acid, 10 μg imipenem with cloxacillin high, 10 μg imipenem with dipicolinic acid and imipenem with EDTA (Rosco Diagnostica, Taastrup, Denmark). Quality control strains were *P. aeruginosa* CCUG59626, *K. pneumoniae* BAA1705 and *E. coli* ATCC® 25,922™.

PCR-based test for detection of genes encoding carbapenemases was used according to Poirel et al. [15] on the same 47 strains for double-control. Three different multiplex reaction mixtures were defined and evaluated for the detection of MBL-encoding genes ($\boldsymbol{bla}_{\mathrm{IMP}}$, $\boldsymbol{bla}_{\mathrm{VIM}}$, $\boldsymbol{bla}_{\mathrm{GIM}}$ and $\boldsymbol{bla}_{\mathrm{NDM}}$), class A carbapenemase gene $\boldsymbol{bla}_{\mathrm{KPC}}$ and class D carbapenemase gene $\boldsymbol{bla}_{\mathrm{oxa\text{-}48}}$. The following control strains were used - Swedish Institute for Communicable Disease Control (Sweden) carbapenemases detection control set: OXA-48-positive *K. pneumoniae* Oxa241, KPC-positive *K. pneumoniae* K271, NDM-1-positive *K. pneumoniae* K275, IMP-positive *P. aeruginosa* CCUG59626, VIM-positive *K. pneumoniae* CCUG58547, GIM-positive *P. aeruginosa;* and KPC-positive *K. pneumoniae* BAA1705.

DNA extraction

A modified GuSCN-silica protocol was used for the DNA extraction from a single colony [16]. Briefly, cells were transferred into a solution containing 570 μl TE (pH 7.6) buffer (TRIS-EDTA) and 30 μL 10% SDS, with ~ 0.5 g zirconium beads (0.1 mm diameter), which was processed by 5 min on bead beater (Minibead beater, Bio-Spec Products, Bartlesville, USA), followed by centrifugation at 10000 rpm for 1 min. Cells were lysed by combining the supernatant with lysis buffer L6 (5.25 M GuSCN, 100 mM Tris – HCl, pH 6.4, 20 mM EDTA, 1.3% Triton X-100). Custom-prepared silica suspension (40 μl) was added before incubation for 5 min at room temperature and centrifugation at 5000 rpm for 10 s. The supernatant was discarded and the pellet washed with buffer L2 (5 M GuSCN) and 50% ethanol. The silica pellet was briefly dried and the DNA eluted in ultra-pure water (milli-Q). The extracted DNA was stored at – 20 °C until analyzed.

Whole genome sequencing

Total bacterial DNA was quantified using a Qubit® 2.0 Fluorometer (Invitrogen, Grand Island, USA) and 2200 TapeStation (Agilent Technologies, Santa Clara, USA). Ten nanograms of sample DNA was processed using an Illumina Nextera XT sample preparation kit (Illumina, San Diego, USA). The resulting DNA libraries were validated by qPCR using a Kapa Library Quantification Kit (Kapa Biosystems, Woburn, USA) to optimize cluster generation.

Ninety-two ssDNA Nextera XT libraries originating from 92 different clones were pooled and sequenced in one rapid-output run of HiSeq2500 (Illumina, San Diego, USA), with paired-end, 150-bp reads. Demultiplexing was done with CASAVA 1.8.2. (Illumina, San Diego, USA), allowing one mismatch in the index reads.

Draft assembly of whole genome sequences (WGS), multilocus sequence typing (MLST) and phylogeny analysis

All Illumina reads were assembled de novo using the SPAdes genome assembler (ver 3.5.0), together with the MismatchCorrector [17].

A BLAST-based tool from https://cge.cbs.dtu.dk/services/MLST/ was run to annotate the MLST fragments within the WGS data [18]. To identify the sequence types (ST), the batch profile query from the pubMLST website for PA (http://pubmlst.org/paeruginosa) together with their locus/sequence definitions was used.

Sequences were aligned using global genome alignment to determine the core genomes. Thereafter, recombinations in the core genomes were detected using BratNextGen software [19]. For phylogenetic analysis, recombination-free alignments were created by masking all significant recombinant segments as missing data in the input alignment. These alignments were used to reconstruct a maximum likelihood phylogenetic tree with RaxML, using the GTR-GAMMA model.

As core genome alignment and MLST analysis resulted in similar clustering, the data are presented according to STs of MLST.

Identifying resistance genes

Antibiotic resistance genes were identified using a homology search against the collection of antibiotic resistance protein sequences from The Comprehensive Antibiotic Resistance Database (CARD, http://arpcard.mcmaster.ca/, version 1.1.0) and beta-lactamases from http://www.lahey.org/

studies/. *GyrA, ParC, OprD, Rmt and Arm* sequences were retrieved from the NCBI protein database. Identity and coverage thresholds were set to 90%.

Clinical relevance of found beta-lactamases was assessed as suggested by Potron et al. [20]

The chromosomal or plasmid origin of beta-lactamase genes was determined using a blastn search of corresponding contigs against the NCBI nt/nr database. Top matches were also examined manually to determine whether they were plasmid or chromosomal sequences. We could not decide whether the beta-lactamase gene was located in plasmid or chromosome for very short contigs and/or contigs with low coverage matches, or matches against both chromosomal and plasmid sequences. Contigs matching only against chromosomal genome sequences were not considered to be plasmid-related, whereas contigs matching with high coverage (> 95%) and identity (> 98%) to only plasmid sequences were considered as possibly originating from the plasmids.

Definitions and statistical analysis

For the analysis of demographic and clinical characteristics, patients were categorized as infected and colonized according to following criteria. Colonization was defined as absence of clinical signs of infection on day of isolation PA in the anatomical site were microorganism was detected. Infections were classified by their most probable origin of acquisition to community and hospital-acquired. ECDC definitions for hospital-acquired infections were used [21]. The Charlson weighted index of comorbidity was calculated using an updated (ICD-10 diagnosis-based) version [22].

Descriptive analysis used R 2.8.1 [23]. Chi-square or Fisher's exact tests were run where appropriate for categorical and the Kolmogorov-Smirnov test for continuous variables. Adjustment for multiple testing was made using the Bonferroni method.

Results

The local microbiology laboratories identified a total of 118 CR/MDR-PA strains, of which 26 were excluded from the final analysis (16 from ambulatory patients, 6 were duplicates from the same patient, and 4 were not PA according to MALDI-TOF). Of the 92 strains, 43 were CR, 11 were MDR, and 38 were both MDR and CR.

The most frequently represented sources were respiratory secretions (n = 50; 54%), followed by wound aspirates (n = 22; 24%), urine (n = 12; 13%) and materials retrieved during intra-abdominal or vaginal procedures or surgeries (n = 7; 8%). One strain originated from the bloodstream.

The median time elapsed between hospital admission and CR/MDR-PA isolation was 13 days (IQR: 6–27 days).

Study population and characteristics

Sixty-eight (74%) patients had infections, whereas 24 (26%) were classified as asymptomatic carriers. The most common infections were pneumonia (n = 34; 50%), skin and soft tissue (n = 14; 21%), surgical site (n = 6; 9%), and intra-abdominal infections (n = 5; 7%). About half the patients (n = 44; 47%) had hospital-acquired infections (Additional file 1: Table S1).

The demographic and clinical characteristics of patients that had CR/MDR-PA are presented in Table 1.

Over half of the patients were elderly (≥65 years) with multiple co-morbidities (average (±SD), Charlson comorbidity index (2.6 ± 2.1). About 85% patients had at least one co-morbidity. There were no patients < 18 years old.

Congestive cardiac insufficiency was commonly present (32%), followed by renal failure (23%) and diabetes mellitus (22%). Although 17 patients had chronic pulmonary disease, none had cystic fibrosis.

Most of the patients (n = 88; 96%) had preceding contact with the healthcare and/or received antibacterial treatment within the previous 90 days; beta-lactams were by far the most commonly used antibiotics (Additional file 2: Table S2).

There were no statistically significant differences detected in risk factors of colonized and infected patients probably due to small sample size and great variety in population analyzed. It might be assumed that factors affecting exposure to PA and leading from colonization to infection are quite diverse and need further research in more precisely selected groups to draw adequate conclusions.

Eighteen patients (20%) died during their hospital stay. The mortality rates in the 7 day, 30 day and 1 year after PA isolation were 2, 14 and 44%, respectively.

Antibiotic susceptibility of PA

The MIC values together with the interpretations are shown in Table 2. The highest resistance rates were observed to imipenem and the lowest to amikacin (59.8 and 7.6%, respectively).

CR was detected in 81 (88%) strains but no production of KPC or MBL was found by using combined-disk method and PCR in 47 randomly selected CR strains (Fig. 1).

Genetic relationship and spread

Ninety-two CR/MDR-PA strains were assigned to 36 different sequence types (Fig. 1), of which 9 strains were novel to the MLST database.

The most prevalent sequence types were ST108 (n = 23; 25%) and ST260 (n = 18; 20%). ST108 strains were found throughout the study, indicating an endemic spread in 6 different wards (mostly in 2 ICUs) of one hospital. Eleven patients carrying ST108 had nosocomial infection, mostly

Table 1 The most important clinical characteristics of patients with CR/MDR-PA infection or colonization

	All (*n* = 92)	Infection (*n* = 68)	Colonization (*n* = 24)	OR (95% CI)
Demographic characteristics				
Male sex (%)	56 (61)	44 (65)	12 (52)	1.8 (0.7–4.7)
Age: median; years (IQR)	68 (52–74)	69 (51–74)	66 (52–75)	
Patients ≥65 years (%)	52 (57)	37 (54)	15 (63)	0.7 (0.3–1.9)
Previous contact with health care system				
Hospitalization within 90 days (%)	35 (38)	25 (37)	10 (42)	0.8 (0.3–2.1)
Long-term healthcare facilities stay within 90 days (%)	5 (5)	4 (6)	1 (4)	1.4 (0.2–13.5)
Antibiotic therapy in previous 90 days (%)	82 (89)	60 (88)	22 (92)	0.7 (0.1–3.5)
Surgery in previous 30 days (%)	53 (58)	38 (56)	15 (63)	0.8 (0.3–2.0)
Intensive care unit stay; duration in days: median (IQR)	57 (62); 15 (8–24.5)	40 (59)	17 (71)	0.6 (0.2–1.6)
Invasive procedures in previous 30 days				
Bronchoscopy	30 (33)	25 (37)	5 (21)	2.2 (0.7–6.7)
Hemodialysis	17 (19)	13 (19)	4 (17)	1.2 (0.3–4.1)
Endoscopy	17 (18)	14 (21)	3 (13)	1.8 (0.5–7.0)
Other	16 (17)	10 (15)	6 (25)	0.5 (0.2–1.6)
Invasive device use on the microorganism isolation day				
Mechanical ventilation of the lungs	47 (51)	34 (50)	13 (54)	0.8 (0.3–2.2)
Central venous catheter	48 (52)	33 (49)	15 (63)	0.6 (0.2–1.5)
Urinary catheter	51 (55)	38 (56)	13 (54)	1.1 (0.4–2.7)
Epicystostomy	9 (10)	7 (10)	2 (8)	1.3 (0.2–6.5)
Co-morbidities				
Congestive cardiac insufficiency	29 (32)	21 (31)	8 (33)	0.9 (0.3–2.4)
Chronic renal failure	21 (23)	16 (24)	5 (21)	1.2 (0.4–3.6)
Diabetes mellitus	20 (22)	15 (22)	5 (21)	1.1 (0.3–3.4)
Chronic pulmonary disease	17 (18)	12 (18)	5 (21)	0.8 (0.3–2.6)
Malignant tumor	16 (16)	9 (13)	7 (25)	0.4 (0.1–1.1)
Hemiplegia	14 (16)	11 (16)	3 (13)	1.4 (0.3–5.3)
Myocardial infarct	13 (14)	9 (13)	4 (17)	0.8 (0.2–2.8)
Cerebrovascular disease	12 (13)	11 (16)	1 (4)	4.4 (0.5–36.4)
Other[a]	34 (37)	27 (40)	7 (29)	1.6 (0.6–4.4)

[a]HIV, AIDS, hematologic malignancy, dementia, connective tissue disease, liver disease, peripheral vascular disease, ulcer disease, neutropenia, trauma, burn

ventilator-associated pneumonia (10 cases). All ST108 strains were CR (22 resistant to imipenem and 18 to meropenem) and 9 strains were MDR.

ST260 was found in all participating hospitals, but almost half of the strains (*n* = 7; 39%) belonging to this ST were isolated from a single hospital that was linked to one ICU. In most of cases (*n* = 14; 78%) ST260 caused infection and was phenotypically tested as MDR.

Only one strain belonged to the so-called high-risk international clone (ST235).

Resistance genes

Beta-lactamases

Clinically relevant beta-lactamases (OXA-101, OXA-2 and GES-5) were found in 12% of the strains. Oxacillinases belonging to class D were found in 10 isolates, with OXA-101 (*n* = 9; 10%) being the most frequent and isolated only in ST260. No class B beta-lactamases (IMP, VIM; SPM; GIM, NDM, FIM) were present. None of the strains produced carbapenemases.

Plasmid encoded β-lactamases were present in 3 (3%) of the strains. Only one plasmid encoded class A beta-lactamase, GES-5; an isolate that belongs to the previously well-known high-risk, clone ST235.

Aminoglycoside modifying enzymes (AME) and 16S rRNA methyltransferases

Clinically relevant AME genes were found in 14 (15%) strains, the most frequent being ANT(2")-Ia, present in 11 (12%) strains, 9 of which belonged to ST260.

Table 2 Minimal inhibitory concentrations and antibiotic susceptibility interpretations of PA (n = 92)

Antibiotic	MIC range (mg/L)	MIC_{50} (mg/L)	MIC_{90} (mg/L)	S (%)	I (%)	R (%)
Beta-lactams						
Imipenem	0.5–32	24	32	19.6	20.7	59.8
Piperacillin/tazobactam	0.5–256	16	256	50.0	0	50.0
Meropenem	0.125–32	8	32	28.3	25.0	46.7
Cefepime	0.5–256	6	32	70.7	0	29.3
Ceftazidime	0.75–256	2	64	73.9	0	26.1
Ciprofloxacin	0.064–32	0.5	32	53.3	0	46.7
Aminoglycosides						
Gentamicin	0.125–256	2	48	80.4	0	19.6
Amikacin	1–256	6	16	75.0	17.4	7.6
Tobramycin	0.125–256	1	4	90.2	0	9.8

Abbreviations: MIC_{50} minimal inhibitory concentration inhibiting 50% of isolates, MIC_{90} minimal inhibitory concentration inhibiting 90% of isolates, *S* susceptible, *I* intermediately susceptible, *R* resistant

The AAC(6′)-Ib-cr cassette mediating resistance to both aminoglycosides and fluoroquinolones was found in one isolate belonging to ST235 phenotypically resistant to ciprofloxacin and amikacin, but sensitive to gentamicin and tobramycin.

No 16S rRNA methyltransferase coding genes were found.

Mutational resistance mechanisms

The *oprD* gene was defective in 12 strains (13%; 8 resistant to both imipenem and meropenem; 1 imipenem and 1 meropenem resistant, and 2 with carbapenem-susceptible) and mutated in 77 strains (84%). We found 3 previously described mutations triggering CR – F170 L (n = 18; 20%), S403P (n = 8; 9%) and W277X (n = 2; 2%). Statistical analysis showed an association between defective *oprD* and non-susceptibility to meropenem (9 meropenem resistant vs 3 meropenem sensitive strains; $p < 0.05$).

Having researched fluoroquinolone resistance-associated mutations in topoisomerase genes *gyrA* (T83I, D87N) and *parC* (S87 L), we found T83I mutation was present in 27 (29%) strains, of which 23 were ciprofloxacin resistant. D87N was found in one and *parC* S87 L substitution in 6 ciprofloxacin resistant strains. Both gyrA T83I and parC S87 L mutations correlated well with ciprofloxacin resistance (23 resistant vs 4 sensitive strains; $p < 0.0001$, and 4 resistant vs 2 sensitive strains; $p < 0.01$, respectively).

Discussion

This is the first study that addresses clinical risk factors alongside with the presence of resistance mechanisms in a mixed population of hospitalized patients infected or colonized with CR/MDR-PA and covers all major Estonian hospitals. The observations show that: (1) the vast majority of affected patients were elderly and had a history of previous contact with healthcare institutions and/or multiple co-morbidities confirming results of previous studies [24]; (2) the 2 predominant STs (ST108 and ST260) we described had good spreading potential and have rarely been recorded in previous studies, suggesting high ST variability within PA and minimal entry of internationally spreading strains into Estonian hospitals; (3) most of the CR strains lacked clinically relevant beta-lactamases including carbapenemases and metallo-beta-lactamases, suggesting that CR is encoded by a selection of mutations in chromosomal genes; (4) correlation between *gyrA* T83I and *parC* S83 L mutations and quinolone resistance were in support of previous studies [25–27].

Considering the high rate of patients with advanced age, the high rate of contact with healthcare facilities, and association with multiple courses of prior antibiotic therapy, it is not unsurprising that they have been previously described as risk factors for PA infection [28]. However, none of these patients belonged to typical risk groups, such as burns, cystic fibrosis or febrile neutropenia, but more commonly had congestive cardiac insufficiency. Similarly, other studies have shown decreasing trends of PA in burn and oncologic patients in Europe and North-America [29]. The reason for these trends is not entirely clear, but the fact that most of the empirical treatment regimens include anti-pseudomonal antibiotics may be a contributing factor.

The high rate of patients with congestive heart disease is more difficult to explain. It may be a concomitant finding and not directly related to the colonization of CR/MDR-PA. This also highlights the fact that PA infection is not a disease strictly associated with people that have severe disturbances of immune or barrier systems, because it can also affect patients without obvious immune defects, such as the elderly.

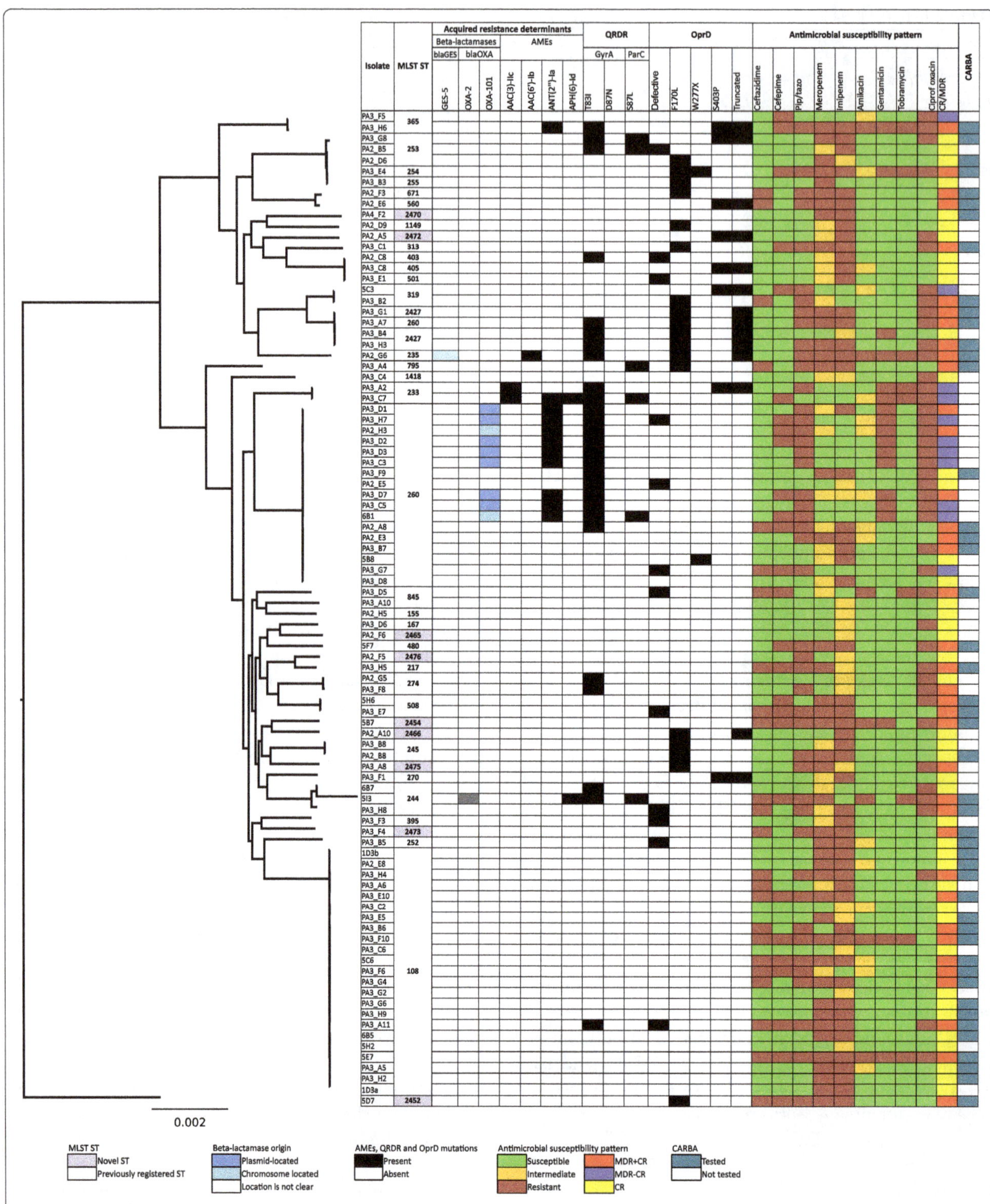

Fig. 1 Analysis of 92 sequenced carbapenem or/and multiresistant *P.aeruginosa* genomes. A maximum-likelihood tree and MLST analysis, presence of beta-lactamases and their location (either in plasmid or chromosome) and aminoglycoside modifying enzymes, selected mutations in quinolone resistance-determining region (QRDR) and OprD. Tested antimicrobial susceptibilities are presented as follows: green color – susceptible; orange color – intermediate and red – resistant strain. CARBA represents coordinated results of phenotypic testing of class B beta-lactamases by combined-disk method and PCR where tested strains are marked with a dark blue color

We found that the pattern of antibiotic resistance is largely driven but 2 STs (ST108 and ST265) causing hospital-acquired infections (mainly ventilator-associated pneumonia) and at least 2 outbreaks. Neither of these strains belonged to well-known internationally spreading clones [7]. ST108 was mostly associated with a singularly CR phenotype and spread only in one hospital. On the other hand, ST260 strains were much more diffused in hospitals. These strains usually had multiresistant phenotypes and carried some resistance machinery (ANT(2″)-Ia, OXA-101 and GyrA T83I mutation). Hence ST may have the potential for becoming a new high-risk clone. ST260 has been previously described in different human settings and in different geographical regions; it is mostly associated with MDR or XDR phenotype, but never with outbreaks [30–33].

CR of PA, reaching up to 20.4% has been a problem within Estonian hospitals for years [34]; however, potential resistance mechanisms have remained unidentified [11], and unfortunately we do not have definite answers from this study. In contrast to other European studies in which the most important trigger of resistance is the production of horizontally-acquired beta-lactamases (mainly belonging to Ambler class B), we found none of these strains, only a few clinically relevant beta-lactamases, of which only one (GES-5) has been described as having carbapenemase activity [20]. We detected a correlation between defective *oprD* and meropenem-resistance in 10 strains and a single mutation previously associated with carbapenem resistance in 25 strains [27]. These mechanisms, however, did not explain resistant phenotype of the remaining 46 strains. Probably a cascade of mutations that were not addressed in this study, including structural modifications in AmpC, peptidoglycan recycling genes and mutations leading to efflux pump overexpression, are required to facilitate phenotypic resistance.

Our data indicates the importance of 2 locally spread resistant clones in spite of low antibiotic consumption; tackling the main spreading routes of these clones could significantly reduce the burden of CR/MDR-PA. Because both the spreading clones had been isolated from respiratory secretions and associated with mechanical ventilation or bronchoscopy, the procedures related to the maintenance of the airway should be the focal point in the prevention of colonization and infections with CR/MDR-PA. Updating both the knowledge and skills of basic hand hygiene and isolation methods, improving oral hygiene practices, and revising bronchoscope cleaning techniques, including disinfection processes, can be effective in aborting PA outbreaks [35]. Infection control measures could be significantly improved by implementing high resolution molecular identification techniques (egg. WGS, MLVA) into everyday practice for rapid detection of outbreaks and stopping the spread of multiresistant microorganism and thus should be encouraged [36].

Some limitations of our study should be noted. Because samples were identified by microbiology laboratories and taken on discretion of treating physicians, there is a possibility that some patients, especially asymptomatic carriers, were not sampled. This leaves a gap in our understanding of how MDR-PA circulates in Estonian hospitals. Secondly, E-test was used for susceptibility measurement instead of microdilution that is EUCAST suggested reference method. Still, E-test results have correlated well with MICs generated by the dilution methods [37] and thus we believe that our results are reliable. Despite these limitations we believe that our results allow us to draw adequate conclusions.

Conclusions

PA is a pathogen that affects not only immunocompromised, but also elderly multi-morbid patients. It is characterized by wide genetic diversity and spread via local rather than global clones in Estonian hospitals. The resistance machinery of PA is complex with only few certain correlations between genotypic and phenotypic resistance. Many different genetic changes may be required to develop the resistance pattern observed in phenotypic tests. High resolution genotyping methods are very valuable for tracking the spread of outbreaks, and therefore it is crucial to encourage the use of sequence-based methods in everyday practice.

Abbreviations

AME: Aminoglycoside modifying enzymes; CR: Carbapenem resistant; CR/MDR-PA: Carbapenem and/or multidrug resistant *P. aeruginosa*; ECDC: European Centre for Disease Prevention and Control; EUCAST: European Committee on Antimicrobial Susceptibility Testing; I: Intermediately susceptible; KPC: *K.pneumoniae* carbapenemase; MBL: Metallo-beta-lactamase; MDR: Multidrug-resistant; MDR-PA: Multidrug-resistant *Pseudomonas aeruginosa*; MIC: Minimal inhibitory concentration; MIC_{50}: Minimal inhibitory concentration at 50%; MIC_{90}: Minimal inhibitory concentration at 90%; MLST: Multi-locus sequence typing; PA: *Pseudomonas aeruginosa*; QRDR: Quinolone resistance-determining region; R: Resistant; S: Susceptible; ST: Sequence type; WGS: Whole genome sequencing; XDR: Extremely drug resistant

Acknowledgements

We are grateful to all infection control specialists and microbiologists involved in this project from the Tartu University Hospital, North Estonia Medical Centre, West Tallinn Central Hospital, and East-Tallinn Central Hospital. We are especially thankful to Anastasia Pavelkovich. Marina Ivanova, Paul Naaber and Tiiu Rööp for their help with quality control strains and methodology for carbapenemase testing. We thank BioMedES UK (www.biomedes.biz) for improvement of the final manuscript.

Funding

This work was supported by Estonian Research Council (IUT2-22) and the European Union from the European Regional Development Fund through the Centre of Excellence in Molecular Cell Engineering and Estonian Program for Health Sciences (ABRESIST). Age Brauer and Maido Remm were funded by institutional grant IUT34-11 from the Estonian Ministry of Education and Research and the European Regional Development Fund through Centre of

Excellence in Genomics and Translational Medicine (grant No. 2014–2020.4.01.15–0012). Veljo Kisand was funded by a personal research grant (PUT-134) from the Estonian Ministry of Education and Research. The funder had no role in the study design, data collection, analysis, decision to publish, or preparation of the manuscript.

Authors' contributions

KT was a principal investigator and has contributed to all sections (implementation of study protocol, data collection, laboratory analyses, statistical analyses, first draft manuscript, final manuscript revision). ML participated in laboratory analyses and manuscript revision. AB did bioinformatical analysis, contributed to the results and discussion sections, as also to manuscript revision. MR gave bioinformatical advice and participated in manuscript revision. VK participated in laboratory analyses (WGS, MLST) and manuscript revision. MM contributed to developing the study protocol and revision of manuscript. TT and IL helped developing the study protocol, drafting first version of the manuscript, and revising all sections in the manuscript. All authors have read and approved the final manuscript

Competing interests

The authors declare that they have no competing interests.

Author details

[1]Department of Microbiology, Institute of Biomedicine and Translational Medicine, University of Tartu, Ravila 19, 50411 Tartu, Estonia. [2]Institute of Technology, University of Tartu, Tartu, Estonia. [3]Institute of Molecular and Cell Biology, University of Tartu, Tartu, Estonia. [4]Department of Infection Control, Tartu University Hospital, Tartu, Estonia.

References

1. Silby MW, Winstanley C, Godfrey SA, Levy SB, Jackson RW. Pseudomonas genomes: diverse and adaptable. FEMS Microbiol Rev. 2011;35(4):652–80.
2. Estepa V, Rojo-Bezares B, Torres C, Saenz Y. Faecal carriage of Pseudomonas aeruginosa in healthy humans: antimicrobial susceptibility and global genetic lineages. FEMS Microbiol Ecol. 2014;89(1):15–9.
3. Ciofu O, Tolker-Nielsen T, Jensen PO, Wang H, Hoiby N. Antimicrobial resistance, respiratory tract infections and role of biofilms in lung infections in cystic fibrosis patients. Adv Drug Deliv Rev. 2015;85:7–23.
4. Wolf SE, Phelan HA, Arnoldo BD. The year in burns 2013. Burns. 2014;40(8): 1421–32.
5. Gomez-Zorrilla S, Camoez M, Tubau F, Periche E, Canizares R, Dominguez MA, Ariza J, Pena C. Antibiotic pressure is a major risk factor for rectal colonization by multidrug-resistant Pseudomonas aeruginosa in critically ill patients. Antimicrob Agents Chemother. 2014;58(10):5863–70.
6. Acharya M, Joshi PR, Thapa K, Aryal R, Kakshapati T, Sharma S. Detection of metallo-beta-lactamases-encoding genes among clinical isolates of Pseudomonas aeruginosa in a tertiary care hospital, Kathmandu, Nepal. BMC Res Notes. 2017;10(1):718.
7. Oliver A, Mulet X, Lopez-Causape C, Juan C. The increasing threat of Pseudomonas aeruginosa high-risk clones. Drug Resist Updat. 2015;21-22: 41–59.
8. Antimicrobial consumption database (ESAC-Net) [http://ecdc.europa.eu/en/antimicrobial-consumption/surveillance-and-disease-data/database].
9. Antimicrobial resistance surveillance in Europe 2016 [http://ecdc.europa.eu/en/publications-data/antimicrobial-resistance-surveillance-europe-2016].
10. Antimicrobial resistance surveillance in Europe 2012 [http://ecdc.europa.eu/en/publications-data/antimicrobial-resistance-surveillance-europe-2012].
11. Loivukene K, Sepp E, Adamson V, Mitt P, Kallandi U, Otter K, Naaber P. Prevalence and antibiotic susceptibility of Acinetobacter baumannii, Pseudomonas aeruginosa and Klebsiella pneumoniae in Estonian intensive care units in comparison with European data. Scand J Infect Dis. 2006; 38(11–12):1001–8.
12. Mitt P, Adamson V, Loivukene K, Lang K, Telling K, Paro K, Room A, Naaber P, Maimets M. Epidemiology of nosocomial bloodstream infections in Estonia. J Hosp Infect. 2009;71(4):365–70.
13. Magiorakos AP, Srinivasan A, Carey RB, Carmeli Y, Falagas ME, Giske CG, Harbarth S, Hindler JF, Kahlmeter G, Olsson-Liljequist B, et al. Multidrug-resistant, extensively drug-resistant and pandrug-resistant bacteria: an international expert proposal for interim standard definitions for acquired resistance. Clin Microbiol Infect. 2012;18(3):268 81.
14. EUCAST: Clinical breakpoints [http://www.eucast.org/clinical_breakpoints/].
15. Poirel L, Walsh TR, Cuvillier V, Nordmann P. Multiplex PCR for detection of acquired carbapenemase genes. Diagn Microbiol Infect Dis. 2011;70(1):119–23.
16. Boom R, Sol C, Wertheim-van Dillen P. Rapid purification of ribosomal RNAs from neutral agarose gels. Nucleic Acids Res. 1990;18(8):2195.
17. Bankevich A, Nurk S, Antipov D, Gurevich AA, Dvorkin M, Kulikov AS, Lesin VM, Nikolenko SI, Pham S, Prjibelski AD, et al. SPAdes: a new genome assembly algorithm and its applications to single-cell sequencing. J Comput Biol. 2012;19(5):455–77.
18. Larsen MV, Cosentino S, Rasmussen S, Friis C, Hasman H, Marvig RL, Jelsbak L, Sicheritz-Ponten T, Ussery DW, Aarestrup FM, et al. Multilocus sequence typing of total-genome-sequenced bacteria. J Clin Microbiol. 2012;50(4):1355–61.
19. Marttinen P, Hanage WP, Croucher NJ, Connor TR, Harris SR, Bentley SD, Corander J. Detection of recombination events in bacterial genomes from large population samples. Nucleic Acids Res. 2012;40(1):e6.
20. Potron A, Poirel L, Nordmann P. Emerging broad-spectrum resistance in Pseudomonas aeruginosa and Acinetobacter baumannii: mechanisms and epidemiology. Int J Antimicrob Agents. 2015;45(6):568–85.
21. Point prevalence survey of healthcare-associated infections and antimicrobial use in European acute care hospitals 2011-2012 [http://ecdc.europa.eu/en/publications/_layouts/forms/Publication_DispForm.aspx?List=4f55ad51-4aed-4d32-b960-af70113dbb90&ID=865].
22. Sundararajan V, Henderson T, Perry C, Muggivan A, Quan H, Ghali WA. New ICD-10 version of the Charlson comorbidity index predicted in-hospital mortality. J Clin Epidemiol. 2004;57(12):1288–94.
23. R Core Team (2013). R: A language and environment for statistical computing. R Foundation for Statistical Computing, Vienna, Austria. URL http://www.R-project.org/. In.
24. Lin KY, Lauderdale TL, Wang JT, Chang SC. Carbapenem-resistant Pseudomonas aeruginosa in Taiwan: prevalence, risk factors, and impact on outcome of infections. J Microbiol Immunol Infect. 2016;49(1):52–9.
25. Kos VN, Deraspe M, McLaughlin RE, Whiteaker JD, Roy PH, Alm RA, Corbeil J, Gardner H. The resistome of Pseudomonas aeruginosa in relationship to phenotypic susceptibility. Antimicrob Agents Chemother. 2015;59(1):427–36.
26. Cabot G, Ocampo-Sosa AA, Dominguez MA, Gago JF, Juan C, Tubau F, Rodriguez C, Moya B, Pena C, Martinez-Martinez L, et al. Genetic markers of widespread extensively drug-resistant Pseudomonas aeruginosa high-risk clones. Antimicrob Agents Chemother. 2012;56(12):6349–57.
27. Del Barrio-Tofino E, Lopez-Causape C, Cabot G, Rivera A, Benito N, Segura C, Montero MM, Sorli L, Tubau F, Gomez-Zorrilla S, et al. Genomics and Susceptibility Profiles of Extensively Drug-Resistant Pseudomonas aeruginosa Isolates from Spain. Antimicrob Agents Chemother. 2017;61(11): e01589–17.
28. Cohen R, Babushkin F, Cohen S, Afraimov M, Shapiro M, Uda M, Khabra E, Adler A, Ben Ami R, Paikin S. A prospective survey of Pseudomonas aeruginosa colonization and infection in the intensive care unit. Antimicrob Resist Infect Control. 2017;6:7.
29. Mikulska M, Viscoli C, Orasch C, Livermore DM, Averbuch D, Cordonnier C, Akova M. Aetiology and resistance in bacteraemias among adult and paediatric haematology and cancer patients. J Inf Secur. 2014;68(4):321–31.
30. Chen SH, Chen RY, Xu XL, Chen HT. Multilocus sequencing typing of Pseudomonas aeruginosa isolates and analysis of potential pathogenicity of typical genotype strains from occupational oxyhelium saturation divers. Undersea Hyperb Med. 2014;41(2):135–41.
31. Mudau M, Jacobson R, Minenza N, Kuonza L, Morris V, Engelbrecht H, Nicol MP, Bamford C. Outbreak of multi-drug resistant Pseudomonas aeruginosa bloodstream infection in the haematology unit of a south African academic hospital. PLoS One. 2013;8(3):e55985.
32. Pobiega M, Maciag J, Chmielarczyk A, Romaniszyn D, Pomorska-Wesolowska M, Ziolkowski G, Heczko PB, Bulanda M, Wojkowska-Mach J. Molecular characterization of carbapenem-resistant Pseudomonas aeruginosa strains isolated from patients with urinary tract infections in southern Poland. Diagn Microbiol Infect Dis. 2015;83(3):295–7.
33. Samuelsen O, Toleman MA, Sundsfjord A, Rydberg J, Leegaard TM, Walder M, Lia A, Ranheim TE, Rajendra Y, Hermansen NO, et al. Molecular epidemiology of metallo-beta-lactamase-producing Pseudomonas aeruginosa isolates from Norway and Sweden shows import of international clones and local clonal expansion. Antimicrob Agents Chemother. 2010;54(1):346–52.

15

Clinical characteristics, organ failure, inflammatory markers and prediction of mortality in patients with community acquired bloodstream infection

Vu Quoc Dat[1,2,3*], Nguyen Thanh Long[1], Vu Ngoc Hieu[4], Nguyen Dinh Hong Phuc[1], Nguyen Van Kinh[3], Nguyen Vu Trung[3,4], H. Rogier van Doorn[2,5], Ana Bonell[2] and Behzad Nadjm[2,5]

Abstract

Background: Community acquired bloodstream infection (CABSI) in low- and middle income countries is associated with a high mortality. This study describes the clinical manifestations, laboratory findings and correlation of SOFA and qSOFA with mortality in patients with CABSI in northern Vietnam.

Methods: This was a retrospective study of 393 patients with at least one positive blood culture with not more than one bacterium taken within 48 h of hospitalisation. Clinical characteristic and laboratory results from the first 24 h in hospital were collected. SOFA and qSOFA scores were calculated and their validity in this setting was evaluated.

Results: Among 393 patients with bacterial CABSI, approximately 80% (307/393) of patients had dysfunction of one or more organ on admission to the study hospital with the most common being that of coagulation (57.1% or 226/393). SOFA performed well in prediction of mortality in those patients initially admitted to the critical care unit (AUC 0.858, 95%CI 0.793–0.922) but poor in those admitted to medical wards (AUC 0.667, 95%CI 0.577–0.758). In contrast qSOFA had poor predictive validity in both settings (AUC 0.692, 95%CI 0.605–0.780 and AUC 0.527, 95%CI 0.424–0.630, respectively). The overall case fatality rate was 28%. HIV infection (HR = 3.145, $p = 0.001$), neutropenia (HR = 2.442, $p = 0.002$), SOFA score 1-point increment (HR = 1.19, $p < 0.001$) and infection with Enterobacteriaceae (HR = 1.722, $p = 0.037$) were independent risk factors for in-hospital mortality.

Conclusions: Organ dysfunction was common among Vietnamese patients with CABSI and associated with high case fatality. SOFA and qSOFA both need to be further validated in this setting.

Keywords: Bloodstream infection, Organ failure, Sequential organ failure assessment score, SOFA, qSOFA, Inflammatory markers, Procalcitonin, C-reactive protein

Background

Bloodstream infection (BSI) is a common cause of sepsis and is associated with significant morbidity and in-hospital mortality worldwide [1]. It is ranked the 11th leading cause of death among adults in USA in 2014, with an age-adjusted death rate of 10.7 per 100,000 standard population [2]. In South and Southeast Asia, the incidence rate of community-acquired BSI in the period of 2004–2010 increased from 16.7 to 38.1 per 100,000 people per year and the 30 days mortality rate can reach up to 37.5% [3].

In patients with BSI, an increasing number of organs with dysfunction is correlated with increased morbidity and mortality [4]. Multiple organ dysfunction is a leading cause of morbidity and mortality in patients admitted to intensive care units (ICUs) in Europe, with an in-hospital mortality of 34.2% [5]. Sequential organ failure assessment (SOFA) score, and the related qSOFA (quickSOFA) score have been recently recommended for

* Correspondence: datvq@hmu.edu.vn; quocdat181@yahoo.com
[1]Department of Infectious Diseases, Hanoi Medical University, no 1 Ton That Tung street, Dong Da district, Hanoi, Vietnam
[2]Wellcome Trust Major Overseas Programme, Oxford University Clinical Research Unit, Hanoi, 78 Giai Phong street, Dong Da district, Hanoi, Vietnam
Full list of author information is available at the end of the article

identifying sepsis and predicting outcome by the Third International Consensus Definitions for Sepsis and Septic Shock (Sepsis-3) [6]. qSOFA was originally designed for use outside the ICU, but it's simplicity, brevity and lack of laboratory results, make it compelling for use in emergency departments and resource-constrained setting. However the validation of qSOFA is not consistent among studies quantifying the risk of death in those presenting with suspected infection in critical care [6–9]. Development and validation of these scores were mostly carried out in high income countries, with limited data on their validity in low- and middle income countries (LMICs) [7, 8, 10]. Additionally there have been few studies looking specifically at patients with BSI, a population with an associated increase in mortality.

This study aims to describe the clinical manifestations and associated organ dysfunctions as described by Sequential [Sepsis-related] Organ Failure Assessment (SOFA) scores and its correlation with mortality in patients with community acquired bloodstream infection at the time of presenting to a large teaching hospital in Vietnam, and their associated mortality.

Methods

Study design

This was a retrospective, cohort study of patients hospitalised at the National Hospital for Tropical Diseases (NHTD) (a tertiary referral infectious disease hospital) in northern Vietnam between January 2011 and December 2013. As a referral centre, this hospital often receives patients with specific infections (eg. central nervous system infections), complicated infections and those with severe infections who have failed on treatment elsewhere. Additionally, at the time of the study, the hospital had not establish a separate emergency department and intensive care unit (ICU), therefore we refer to the critical care unit (CCU) for the unit with both ventilated and unventilated beds, available haemodynamic support and renal replacement therapy. A convenience sampling method was used to select medical notes from the list of all hospitalised patients with positive bacterial blood cultures during the study period. The inclusion criteria were having a blood culture, taken within 48 h of hospitalisation (to any institution) for the current admission, positive for a recognised pathogen according to the US CDC's National Healthcare Safety Network (NHSN) list [11]. Patients with infection with more than one bacterium were excluded, as were cases considered to be pseudobacteraemia [12].

Data collection

Data was extracted from patients' medical notes using a case-report form that captured patient demographics, reported history of prior medical illness, clinical manifestations, laboratory results, inflammatory markers within the first 24 h of admission to the study hospital and outcome at hospital discharge.

BSI with concurrent meningitis was defined in bacteremic patients who had cerebrospinal fluid examination within 24 h of blood drawn for microorganism isolation showing at least one of the following criteria: (1) turbid appearance; (2) leukocytosis (> 100 cells/mm3) or (3) leukocytosis from 10 to 100 cells/ mm3) and either an elevated protein (> 100 mg/dl) or decreased glucose (< 40 mg/dl) [13]. BSI with concurrent pneumonia was confirmed by radiology within 24 h of blood drawn for microorganism isolation. Gastrointestinal tract infection and urine tract infection were defined by the CDC/NHSN Surveillance Definitions for Specific Types of Infections [14]. Sequential [Sepsis-related] Organ Failure Assessment (SOFA) score, and quick SOFA (qSOFA) score were calculated using the worst parameters recorded within the first 24 h of admission to the study hospital and missing values were considered to be normal [6]. Organ dysfunction was defined by organ-specific SOFA scores ≥1. Failure of kidney function was further evaluated using the RIFLE criteria with RIFLE-F (Failure) defined as patients with a serum creatinine greater than three times the age adjusted upper limit of serum creatinine [15]. Neutropenia was defined as an absolute neutrophil count < 1500 cells/mm^3, severe anemia as hemoglobin concentration was < 80 g/L and thrombocytopenia as a platelet count below 100×10^3 cells/mm^3.

The outcome at hospital discharge was defined as death for those who died in hospital or were palliatively discharged (discharged home for palliative care with the expectation of an early death, as per common practice in Vietnam) and 'survived' in all other cases.

Data analysis

Data was analysed using IBM SPSS Statistics for Windows (IBM Corp., Armonk, NY). Depending on the distribution, continuous data were presented as mean (95% confidence interval) or median (interquartile range) and categorical data as number (percentage). To evaluate the predictive value of SOFA, qSOFA score, white blood cell counts, C-Reactive Protein (CRP) and procalcitonin levels, a receiver operating characteristic (ROC) curve and the area under the curve (AUC) were calculated along with the sensitivity, specificity, positive and negative predictive values, positive and negative likelihood ratios associated with the cut-off value that gave the highest difference between sensitivity and (1-specificity) (Youden index). Since procalcitonin level was obtained by a semi-quantitative test that was only quantitatively measured for levels under 100 ng/mL, the result of "above 100 ng/mL" was considered as 100 ng/mL. The Mann Whitney U test and Kruskal Wallis test were used to analyze continuous variables and the Chi-square and Fisher's exact were used for bivariate analyses as appropriated. Logistic regression models were used to calculate unadjusted odds ratios (ORs) and 95% confidence intervals (CIs) for associations between clinical, laboratory characteristics and case fatality rate. Comparison of AUC between different ROC curves was performed using a nonparametric approach [16]. Cox proportional hazards regression was used to identify variables that predicted clinical outcomes. Variables for inclusion were selected by review of the literature (age, HIV infection status, neutropenia, SOFA score and aetiology of CABSI). All tests were two-tailed and differences were considered statistically significant at p values ≤0.05.

Results

Among 400 patients with community acquired bloodstream infections (CABSI) there were 393 patients with infection with one bacterium included in this analysis, 7 dual infection cases were excluded (including 3 HIV infected cases with co-infection of *T. marneffei* and *S. aureus, Escherichia hermannii* or *Salmonella group D*; 1 case with *S. aureus* and *K. pneumoniae*, 1 case with *Enterococcus faecalis* and viridans streptococci, 1 case with *E. coli* and *K. pneumoniae* and 1 case with *S. aureus* and *E. coli* co-infection). Gram-negative bacteria dominated (70.7%, 278/393), comprising *Enterobacteriaceae* (50.9%, 200/393) and non-*Enterobacteriaceae* Gram-negative bacteria (19.8%, 78/393) followed by Gram-positive bacteria 29.3% (115/393).

Clinical characteristics, aetiology of CABSI and organ failure

The median age of patients included was 48 years (IQR 36–60), with 271 males and a male to female ratio of 2.2:1. There was a history of chronic disease in 27% of patients, with the highest prevalence in patients with *Enterobacteriaceae* BSI, 34% (38/200). Thirty-eight percent (150/393) of patients were transferred from another hospital (< 48 h) for the current illness episode. The median time from onset of illness to hospitalisation at the study site was 5 days and 36.9% (145/393) were admitted directly to critical care.

Concurrent meningitis was confirmed in 18.3% (72/393) and pneumonia in 24.9% (98/393) of patients, with both conditions occurring in 2.8% (11/393) of patients with CABSI. Gram-positive organisms were isolated from 72.2% (52/72) of those with meningitis, *Enterobacteriaceae* in 18.1% (13/72) and non-*Enterobacteriaceae* Gram-negative bacteria in 9.7% (7/72), see Table 1 for details. Concurrent meningitis was found in 6.5% (13/200) patients with *Enterobacteriaceae* BSI, 9.0% (7/71) patients with non-*Enterobacteriaceae* Gram-negative bacteria BSI and 45.2% (52/115) patients with gram positive BSI. In the 98 cases of pneumonia the causative pathogens isolated from blood were *Enterobacteriaceae* (46.9%, 46/98), non-*Enterobacteriaceae* Gram-negative bacteria (25.5%, 25/98) and Gram-positive bacteria (27.6%, 27/98) (see Additional file 1: Table S1).

A further 8.4% (33/393) of patients presented with or developed at least one abscess, of which 2 patients (6.1%) had 2 abscess foci and 1 patient (3.0%) had 3 abscess foci in different locations. The locations were 16/37 (43.2%) liver, 8 (21%) skin, 4 (10.8%) muscle, 3 (8.1%) brain, 3 (8.1%) spleen, 2 (5.4%) lung, 1 (2.7%) eyelid. Endocarditis was confirmed by echocardiography in 4.1% (16/393) patients. These were due to *Staphylococcus aureus* (7/16, 43.8%), viridans group *streptococci* (4/16, 28.6%), *Enterococcus* species (3/16, 18.8%), *Klebsiella pneumoniae* (1/16, 6.25%) and *Pseudomonas aeruginosa* (1/16, 6.25%). The distribution of aetiology by the foci of infection is presented in Additional file 1: Table S1.

On the day of admission to the study hospital, BSI patients had a median SOFA score of 3 (IQR 1–7) and 78.1% (307/393) of patients had dysfunction of at least one organ. The SOFA score differed significantly between patients admitted direct to CCU (median of 7, IQR 4–12) and medical wards (median of 2, IQR 0–4) ($p < 0.001$). *Enterobacteriaceae* BSIs accounted for most cases with SOFA score above 12 (74% or 28/38, vs. 48% (172/355) in patients with SOFA score ≤ 12, $p = 0.003$) or more than 3 organ dysfunctions (60% or 47/78, vs. 49% or 153/315 in patients with ≤3 organ dysfunctions, $p = 0.065$). qSOFA score was ≥2 in 28.6% (71/248) of patients that were initially admitted to medical wards. The unadjusted associations between clinical factors and case fatality are presented in Table 1.

Laboratory results and inflammatory markers

The proportions of patients with white blood cells count $< 4 \times 10^9$/l, 4–12 × 10^9/l and > 12 × 10^9/l were 11.8% (46/389), 47% (183/389) and 41.1% (160/389) respectively. Neutropenia, severe anaemia and thrombocytopenia was presented in 7.2% (28/388), 8% (31/389) and 43.4% (169/389) patients with BSI on admission to the study hospital, respectively. The proportion of patients with RIFLE-F, increased lactate, procalcitonin or CRP were not significantly different when classified by bacterial aetiology (*Enterobacteriaceae,* non-*Enterobacteriaceae* and Gram-positive). Lactate levels were only available for 73 patients and 52/73 (69.9%) patients had lactate level ≥ 2 mmol/L on admission. The median lactate level increased significantly with increasing SOFA score; from 1.23 mmol/L (IQR: 0.99–2.04 mmol/L) in those with a SOFA score < 6, to 7.89 mmol/L (IQR: 3.7–10.38) in those with a SOFA score > 12 ($p < 0.001$, Kruskal Wallis test). There was no significant difference between median lactate levels in those with qSOFA < 2 and qSOFA≥2 ($p = 0.055$, Mann-Whitney U test). Laboratory factors associated with case mortality was showed in

Table 1 Clinical characteristic on admission of patients with bloodstream infection

Factor	Proportion	Case fatality rate	Unadjusted odds ratios (95%CI) for case fatality	P values
Age (yrs)				
≤ 40 years old	122/393 (31%)	27 (22.1%)	1	
41–55 years old	152/393 (38.7%)	46 (30.3%)	1.527 (0.881–2.646)	0.131
≥ 56 years old	119/393 (30.3%)	37 (31.1%)_	1.588 (0.891–2.828)	0.117
Male sex (%)	271/393 (69.0%)	84 (31.0%)	1.659 (1.002–2.746)	0.049
Any previous hospitalisation (%)	150/393 (38.2%)	62 (41.3%)	2.862 (1.819–4.503)	< 0.001
Any antibiotic prior to NHTD hospitalisation (%)	50/150 (33.3%)	23 (46.0%)	1.332 (0.671–2.646)	0.412
Time from onset to current hospitalisation < 5 days	217/393 (55.2%)	57 (26.3%)	0.827 (0.532–1.286)	0.399
Direct ICU admission	145/393 (36.9%)	68 (46.9%)	4.331 (2.720–6.898)	< 0.001
Any history of medical disease	106/393 (27.0%)	44 (41.5%)	2.376 (1.479–3.818)	< 0.001
HIV	19/393 (4.8%)	10 (52.6%)	3.044 (1.202–7.710)	0.019
Moderate or severe liver disease	53/393 (13.5%)	25 (47.2%)	2.679 (1.481–4.844)	0.001
Diabetes	25/393 (6.4%)	7 (28.0%)	1.001 (0.406–2.466)	0.999
Concurrent foci of infection				
Radiology-confirmed pneumonia on admission	98/393 (24.9%)[a]	29 (29.6%)	1.11 (0.671–1.837)	0.684
Lumbar puncture confirmed meningitis on admission	72/393 (18.3%)[b]	19 (26.4%)	0.906 (0.509–1.614)	0.738
Heart valve vegetations during hospitalisation	16/393 (4.1%)	4 (25.0%)	0.852 (0.269–2.701)	0.786
Any abscess during hospitalisation	33/393 (8.4%)[c]	6 (18.2%)	0.547 (0.219–1.364)	0.196
Organ dysfunction on admission				
Cardiovascular	65/393 (16.5%)	52 (80.0%)	18.621 (9.522–36.415)	< 0.001
Respiratory	87/393 (22.1%)	53 (60.9%)	6.81 (4.057–11.431)	< 0.001
CNS	105/393 (26.7%)	55 (52.4%)	4.66 (2.876–7.551)	< 0.001
Hepatic	146/393 (37.2%)	57 (39.0%)	2.344 (1.494–3.678)	< 0.001
Renal	153/393 (38.9%)	66 (43.1%)	3.379 (2.139–5.339)	< 0.001
Coagulation	226/393 (57.5%)	85 (37.6%)	3.424 (2.070–5.663)	< 0.001

[a]Isolates from blood in patients with pneumonia were *K. pneumoniae* (22.4%, 22/98), *E. coli* (16.3%, 16/98), *S. maltophilia* (11.2%, 11/98), *Burkholderia pseudomallei* (8.2%, 8/98), *S. aureus* (7.1%, 7/98) and *S. suis* (7.1%, 7/98) and other pathogens (23.5%, 27/98)

[b]Isolates from blood in patients with meningitis were *S. suis* (40/72, 55.6%), *K. pneumoniae* (8/72, 11.1%), *Stenotrophomonas maltophilia* (7/72, 9.7%), *S. aureus* (5/72, 6.9%). *Enterococcus* species (2/72, 2.8%), *Listeria* species (2/72, 2.8%), *E. coli* (2/72, 2,8%), *Salmonella enterica (2/72,2.8%)* and each of *S. pneumoniae*, beta hemolytic *Streptococcus*, *viridans* group *Streptococcus* and *Enterobacter* species (1/72, 1.4%)

[c]There were 16 cases with liver abscess with isolates from blood were *K. pneumoniae* (8/16 or 50%), *E. coli* and *Salmonella enterica* (2/16 of each, or 12.5%), *Aeromonas* species, *Enterobacter* species, *S. suis* and *viridans* group *streptococci* (1/16 of each, 6.3%)

Table 2. There was no unadjusted associated between procalcitonin and CRP levels with case fatality rates.

Mortality and associated factors

The overall case-fatality of CABSI was 28% (110/393), of which 71.8% (79/110) occurred within 7 days of admission to the study hospital. Case fatality rates in patients with CABSI due to *Enterobacteriaceae*, non-*Enterobacteriaceae* Gram-negative bacteria and Gram-positive bacteria were 33.5%, 25.6% and 20%, respectively. Among the most common isolates, the case fatality was 35.2% (31/88) in *K. pneumoniae*, 32.8% (21/64) in *Escherichia coli*, 9.3% (4/43) in *Streptococcus suis*, 15.4% (6/39) in *Stenotrophomonas maltophilia* and 32.4% (11/34) in *S. aureus*. The case-fatality in patients directly admitted to CCU was 46.9% (68/145).

Organ dysfunction was associated with higher risk of in-hospital mortality (33.2% patients with at least one organ dysfunction on admission to the study hospital vs 9.3% patients without, $p < 0.001$). Case fatality rate increased with increasing SOFA score (Fig. 1). The mortality in patients with 1, 2, 3 and more than 4 organs dysfunction was 17% (17/100), 19.5% (16/82), 31.9% (15/47) and 69.2% (54/78), respectively. The highest case fatality rates were observed in patients with cardiovascular, respiratory and central nervous system (CNS) dysfunction, 80% (52/65), 60.9% (53/87), 52.4% (55/105), respectively. qSOFA < 2 was associated with lower mortality compared with qSOFA ≥2, 18.8% (26/138) vs 40.6% (63/155), $p < 0.001$. Among patients admitted directly to CCU, SOFA performed well at predicting in-hospital mortality (AUC 0.858, 95%CI 0.793–0.922)

Table 2 Laboratory characteristics on admission

	Proportion	Case fatality	Unadjusted odds ratios (95%CI) for case fatality	*P* values
Neutropenia (< 1500 cell/mm^3) (%)	28/388 (7.2%)	22 (78.6%)	11.682 (4.588–29.746)	< 0.001
Hemoglobin< 80 g/L	31/389 (8.0%)	11 (35.5%)	1.459 (0.675–3.156)	0.337
RIFLE criteria				
No renal dysfunction	283/386 (73.3%)	56 (19.8%)	1	
RIFLE-risk	50/386 (13.0%)	16 (32.0%)	1.908 (0.984–3.699)	0.056
RIFLE-failure	52/386 (13.5%)	35 (67.3%)	8.346 (4.361–15.971)	< 0.001
Hypoalbuminemia (albumin ≤30 g/L)	72/245 (29.4%)	39 (54.2%)	3.263 (1.839–5.789)	< 0.001
Aspartate Aminotransferase (AST) ≥ 2 ULN	153/379 (40.4%)	65 (42.5%)	3.435 (2.150–5.487)	< 0.001
Alanine aminotransferase (ALT) ≥ 2 ULN	109/378 (28.8%)	45 (41.3%)	2.449 (1.520–3.947)	< 0.001
Platelet < 100 × 10^3/mm^3	169/389 (43.4%)	70 (41.4%)	3.282 (2.068–5.208)	< 0.001
Procalcitonin				
PCT ≤ 0.005 ng/mL (%)	6/239 (2.5%)	2 (33.3%)	1	
PCT > 0.005–2 ng/mL (%)	83/239 (34.7%)	11 (13.3%)	0.306 (0.050–1.871)	0.2
PCT > 2–10 ng/mL (%)	59/239 (24.7%)	20 (33.9%)	1.026 (0.173–6.087)	0.978
PCT > 10–100 ng/mL (%)	69/239 (28.9%)	29 (42.0%)	1.45 (0.249–8.457)	0.68
PCT > 100 ng/mL (%)	22/239 (9.2%)	14 (63.6%)	3.5 (0.520–23.559)	0.198
C-reactive protein (CRP) (median, IQR) (mg/L)				
CRP less than 5 mg/L (%)	14/341 (4.1%)	4 (28.6%)	1	
CRP from 5.01 to 20 mg/L (%)	26/341 (7.6%)	4 (15.4%)	0.455 (0.094–2.195)	0.326
CRP from 20.001 to 100 mg/L (%)	112/341 (32.8%)	29 (25.9%)	0.873 (0.254–3.001)	0.83
CRP more than 100 mg/L (%)	189/341 (55.4%)	56 (29.6%)	1.053 (0.317–3.498)	0.933

ULN upper limit of normal; *RIFLE* Risk, Injury, Failure, Loss of kidney function, and End-stage kidney disease

while qSOFA was a poor predictor (AUC 0.692, 95%CI 0.605–0.780) in this population. However, outside of CCU, regardless of eventual CCU admission, both SOFA and qSOFA had poor predictive validity (AUC 0.667, 95%CI 0.577–0.758 and AUC 0.527, 95%CI 0.424–0.630, respectively).

Table 3 shows the prognostic validity of the Youden index of SOFA, qSOFA, WBC, CRP and PCT on admission to NHTD in all patients. The SOFA score was more accurate than qSOFA in predicting mortality (AUC = 0.795 vs 0.658, $p < 0.001$); PCT (AUC = 0.703), and WBC (AUC = 0.642) was more accurate than CRP (AUC =

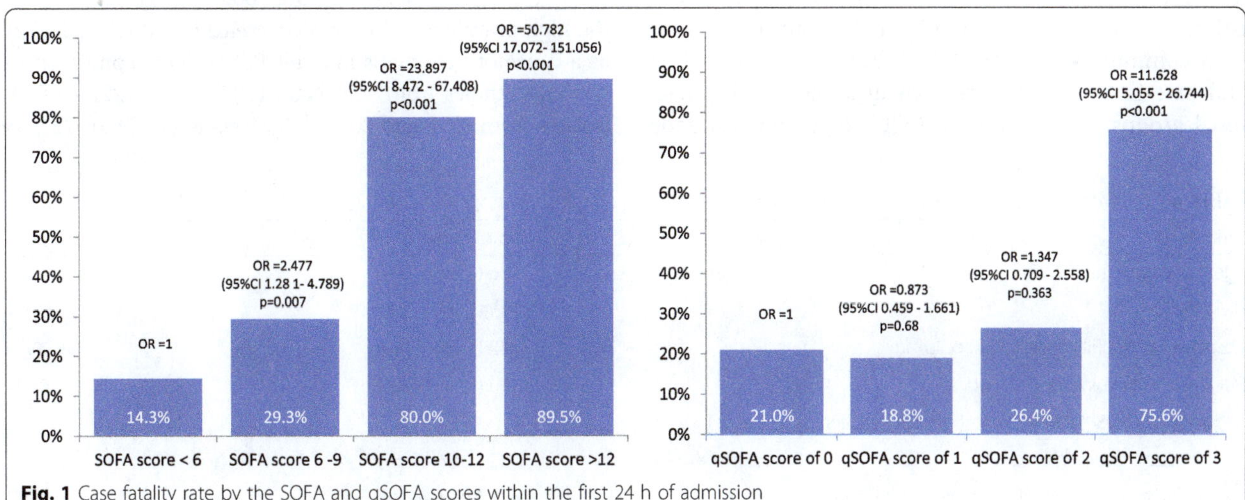

Fig. 1 Case fatality rate by the SOFA and qSOFA scores within the first 24 h of admission

Table 3 Performance of initial SOFA score, qSOFA score, white blood cells, C-reactive protein and procalcitonin, in prediction of in-hospital mortality

	SOFA (n = 393)	qSOFA (n = 393)	WBC (n = 389)	CRP (n = 341)	Procalcitonin (n = 239)
AUC (95% CI)	0.795 (0.741–0.850)	0.658 (0.595–0.721)	0.642 (0.576–0.708)	0.561 (0.492–0.630)	0.703 (0.629–0.776)
Cut-off value	≥ 9	≥ 3	≤ 7.39	≥ 210	≥ 5.49
Sensitivity	53.6%	30.9%	77.9%	35.5%	69.7%
Specificity	94.7%	96.1%	49.5%	75.8%	63.2%
Positive predictive value	79.7%	75.6%	79.9%	35.5%	46.9%
Negative predictive value	84.0%	78.2%	46.6%	75.8%	81.8%
Positive likelihood ratio	10.1194	7.9521	1.5430	1.4667	1.8945
Negative likelihood ratio	0.4896	0.7189	0.4470	0.8511	0.4789

SOFA Sequential Organ Failure Assessment, *qSOFA* quick Sequential Organ Failure Assessment, *WBC* white blood cell, *CRP* C-reactive protein

0.561) in predicting mortality ($P < 0.001$ and $P = 0.0498$ respectively).

In unadjusted association analysis, higher mortality was associated with male sex, any previous hospitalisation, direct CCU admission, history of HIV infection, moderate severe liver diseases and. Analysis, male sex, previous hospitalisation prior to NHTD admission, any history of chronic disease, history of moderate or severe liver diseases, HIV infection, organ dysfunctions on admission, neutropenia, haemoglobin < 80 g/L, RIFLE failure (RIFLE-F), hypoalbuminemia (< 30 g/L), elevated liver enzymes (> 2 times the upper limit of normal), thrombocytopenia ($< 100 \times 10^3$/mm^3) and were associated with increased in-hospital mortality (p values < 0.05). In Cox regression proportional hazards model, HIV infection (HR = 3.145, p = 0.001), neutropenia (HR = 2.442, p = 0.002), SOFA score 1-point increment (HR = 1.19, p < 0.001) and infection with *Enterobacteriaceae* (HR = 1.722, p = 0.037) were significant risk factors for in-hospital mortality (Table 4).

Discussion

This retrospective study describes the clinical characteristics and outcomes in this high-risk group of patients with community acquired BSI. Multi-organ dysfunction and case-fatality rates were high in all aetiological bacterial groups. SOFA score on CCU admission had good prognostic accuracy for in-hospital mortality whilst qSOFA, WBC, CRP and PCT did not.

BSI patients admitted directly to CCU in our study had a median SOFA score of 7 (IQR 4–12), comparable with large-scale validation studies of Sepsis-3 criteria in the US (median of 6, IQR 3–9) [10] and Australia and New Zealand (median of 5, IQR 3–8) [7]. The proportion of bacteraemic patients with qSOFA of 2 or above in our study (39.4%) was also higher than in studies of sepsis conducted in high income countries (10–27%) [8, 10]. The percentage of patients with pneumonia in our CABSI cohort (24.9%) was lower than or similar to other studies on CABSI (24–38%) [17–19]. *K. pneumoniae* was the most common pathogen isolated from bacteremic patients with pneumonia in our study, reflecting its role here as an important cause of community acquired pneumonia [20]. We also confirmed the role of *S. suis* as the leading pathogen causing BSI associated with meningitis in Viet Nam [21]. Our findings further confirmed the reduction of *Neisseria meningitidis* in Viet Nam which was reported in 0.5% of blood isolates [22] and around 4.4% of cerebral spinal fluid (CSF) isolates before 2005 [23]. We also report the high prevalence of *Enterobacteriacaea* (18.1% or 13/72) as a cause of meningitis in adult BSI patients compared to previous studies from Viet Nam (13.5% or 30/222 of CSF isolates from 1996 and 2005) [23], Iceland (11.3% or 12/106

Table 4 Cox proportional hazards model of factors associated with all-cause in-hospital case fatality

Variable	Hazard ratio (95% CI)	P-value
Age (each increase of 1 year)	1.006 (0.994–1.019)	0.321
HIV infection	3.145 (1.569–6.305)	0.001
Absolute neutrophil count < 1500 cells/mm^3	2.442 (1.381–4.319)	0.002
SOFA score (each increase of 1 point)	1.190 (1.146–1.235)	< 0.001
Aetiology of CABSI (gram-positive bacterial infection as reference)		
Enterobacteriaceae infections	1.722 (1.034–2.869)	0.037
Non *Enterobacteriaceae* Gram-negative infections	1.528 (0.824–2.834)	0.178

of positive CSF cultures during 1995–2010) [24] and Denmark (6.1% or 88/1437 during 1991–2000) [25]. The high prevalence of meningitis associated with *Enterobacteriaceae* in this setting may be related to *Strongyloides* hyperinfection, given the evidence for high seroprevalence of *Strongyloides* infection in this population [26].

A review of CABSI in south and Southeast Asia from 1990 to 2010 showed the most frequent isolates in adult patients were *Salmonella enterica* (37.8%), *S. aureus* (12.6%) and *E. coli* (12%) with an overall case fatality rate of 9% [27]. In North America and Europe, there was a significant increase in bloodstream infection caused by Gram-negative bacteria, and case fatality rates in the period 1992–2008 were 13–20.6% in patients with CABSI [1]. The overall case fatality of 28% in our CABSI patients was lower than in a study in Thailand [3] from 2004 and 2010 (37.5%) where the most common pathogens were *E. coli* (23.1%), *Burkholderia pseudomallei* (19.3%), and *S. aureus* (8.2%) but higher than in Cambodia (22.1%) where there was a predominance of *E. coli* (29.7%), *Salmonella* spp. (14.4%) and *B. pseudomallei* (12.6%) in the period of 2007–2010) [28]. The higher case fatality in Thailand and our study may relate to the shift in the aetiology of CABSI from *Salmonella* to other Gram-negative bacteria observed since the last decade.

Organ dysfunction is strongly associated with in-hospital mortality. In a multicentre study of severe sepsis in Spain, case fatality in patients with more than 4 organs with dysfunction was 78.4% [29]. From a large prospective European study, case fatality in patients with more than 3 organs with dysfunction was 58% and the, highest in-hospital mortality rates were observed in patients with coagulation failure (45%) [5]. In high income settings, among ICU patients with suspected infection, the predictive accuracy for in-hospital mortality is higher using SOFA than qSOFA (AUC = 0.74; 95% CI, 0.73–0.76; vs AUC = 0.66; 95% CI, 0.64–0.68) whilst outside of ICU, the predictive validity of qSOFA (AUC = 0.81; 95% CI, 0.80–0.82) was better than SOFA (AUC = 0.79; 95% CI, 0.78–0.80; $P < 0.001$) [10]. In a prospective study of patients with suspected infection admitted to an emergency department in Norway, the qSOFA had poor performance to predict 7-day and 30-day mortality with AUCs < 0.6 in both multiple imputation and complete case analysis [30]. The usefulness of qSOFA in low- and middle income countries has not been well established. Procalcitonin levels can serve as a useful marker to rule out sepsis and discriminate contamination from true bloodstream infection [31, 32]. Our study shows a poor prediction of initial PCT and CRP in prediction of mortality.

Our study has some major limitations. Firstly, as the study site is a referral hospital specialising in infectious diseases, the aetiologies, clinical manifestations, severity and response to the treatment may be different from those presenting to a general hospital. Secondly, SOFA and qSOFA was calculated based on the worst parameters within 24 h of admission to the study hospital which may not accurately present the severity of infection at arrival. Thirdly, due to the retrospective design, the data collection was incomplete and unbalanced distribution of missing data can be a bias in the prediction models The utilisation of SOFA and qSOFA needs to be validated prospectively in other setting at different time points of assessment.

Conclusions

In conclusion, community acquired BSI has a high rate of organ dysfunction and mortality in this setting. SOFA performed well at predicting those at risk of death admitted directly to CCU, whilst qSOFA performed poorly. Further prospective validation in low- and middle income settings is needed.

Abbreviations

AUC: Area under the curve; BSI: Bloodstream infection; CABSI: Community acquired bloodstream infection; CCU: Critical care unit; CI: Confidence interval; CNS: Central nervous system; CRP: C-reactive protein; CSF: Cerebral spinal fluid; HR: Hazard ratio; ICU: Intensive care unit; IQR: Interquartile range; LMICs: Low- and middle income countries; NHSN: National Healthcare Safety Network; NHTD: National Hospital for Tropical Diseases; OR: Odds ratio; PCT: Procalcitonin; qSOFA: Quick sequential organ failure assessment; ROC: Receiver operating characteristic; SOFA: Sequential organ failure assessment

Acknowledgments

We gratefully acknowledge the General Planning Department in National Hospital for Tropical Diseases for providing the list of medical records. We also thank Nguyen The Hung, Nguyen Thi Hoa, Bui Linh Chi and Hoang Bao Long for their assistance with data collection.

Funding

This study was funded by the Wellcome Trust of Great Britain.

Availability of data and materials

The datasets used and/or analysed during the current study are available from the corresponding author on reasonable request.

Authors' contributions

VQD designed the study, collected & analysed the data and wrote the first & final draft; NTL, VNH, NDHP collected, entered data, drafted sections of the manuscript; NTL was responsible for cleaning data, analysis and drafted sections of the manuscript; NVT, NVK contributed to study design and were responsible for laboratory and clinical care, provided revisions of the manuscript edited the final draft; HRvD and AB helped with interpretation of the data, revision of the manuscript and edited the final draft; BN involved to design the study, interpreted the data, revised the manuscript and edited the final draft. All authors approved of the final draft.

Competing interests

HRvD is a member of the editorial board (Associate Editor) of the BMC Infectious Diseases. The authors otherwise declare that they have no competing interests.

Author details

[1]Department of Infectious Diseases, Hanoi Medical University, no 1 Ton That Tung street, Dong Da district, Hanoi, Vietnam. [2]Wellcome Trust Major Overseas Programme, Oxford University Clinical Research Unit, Hanoi, 78 Giai Phong street, Dong Da district, Hanoi, Vietnam. [3]National Hospital for Tropical Diseases, 78 Giai Phong street, Dong Da district, Hanoi, Vietnam. [4]Department of Microbiology, Hanoi Medical University, no 1 Ton That Tung

street, Dong Da district, Hanoi, Vietnam. [5]Nuffield Department of Clinical Medicine, Centre for Tropical Medicine, University of Oxford, Oxford, UK.

References

1. Goto M, Al-Hasan MN. Overall burden of bloodstream infection and nosocomial bloodstream infection in North America and Europe. Clin Microbiol infect off Publ Eur Soc Clin Microbiol. Infect Dis. 2013;19:501–9.
2. Kochanek KD, Murphy SL, Xu J, Deaths T-VB. Final data for 2014. Natl vital stat rep cent dis control Prev Natl cent health stat Natl vital stat. Syst. 2016; 65:1–122.
3. Kanoksil M, Jatapai A, Peacock SJ, Limmathurotsakul D. Epidemiology, Microbiology and mortality associated with community-acquired bacteremia in Northeast Thailand: a multicenter surveillance study. PLoS One. 2013;8:e54714.
4. El-Menyar A, Thani HA, Zakaria ER, Zarour A, Tuma M, AbdulRahman H, et al. Multiple organ dysfunction syndrome (MODS): is it preventable or inevitable? Int J Clin Med. 2013;03:722.
5. Sakr Y, Lobo SM, Moreno RP, Gerlach H, Ranieri VM, Michalopoulos A, et al. Patterns and early evolution of organ failure in the intensive care unit and their relation to outcome. Crit Care Lond Engl. 2012;16:R222.
6. Singer M, Deutschman CS, Seymour CW, Shankar-Hari M, Annane D, Bauer M, et al. The third international consensus definitions for Sepsis and septic shock (Sepsis-3). JAMA. 2016;315:801.
7. Raith EP, Udy AA, Bailey M, McGloughlin S, MacIsaac C, Bellomo R, et al. Prognostic accuracy of the SOFA score, SIRS criteria, and qSOFA score for in-hospital mortality among adults with suspected infection admitted to the intensive care unit. JAMA. 2017;317:290–300.
8. Freund Y, Lemachatti N, Krastinova E, Van Laer M, Claessens Y-E, Avondo A, et al. Prognostic accuracy of Sepsis-3 criteria for in-hospital mortality among patients with suspected infection presenting to the emergency department. JAMA. 2017;317:301–8.
9. Churpek MM, Snyder A, Han X, Sokol S, Pettit N, Howell MD, et al. Quick Sepsis-related organ failure assessment, systemic inflammatory response syndrome, and early warning scores for detecting clinical deterioration in infected patients outside the intensive care unit. Am J Respir Crit Care Med. 2017;195:906–11.
10. Seymour CW, Liu VX, Iwashyna TJ, Brunkhorst FM, Rea TD, Scherag A, et al. Assessment of clinical criteria for Sepsis: for the third international consensus definitions for Sepsis and septic shock (Sepsis-3). JAMA. 2016;315: 762–74.
11. Centers for Disease Control and Prevention. NHSN Organism List. 2017. https://www.cdc.gov/nhsn/xls/master-organism-com-commensals-lists.xlsx. Accessed 7 Oct 2017.
12. Dat VQ, Vu HN. Nguyen the H, Nguyen HT, Hoang LB, vu Tien Viet D, et al. bacterial bloodstream infections in a tertiary infectious diseases hospital in northern Vietnam: aetiology, drug resistance, and treatment outcome. BMC Infect Dis. 2017;17:493.
13. World Health Organization. Invasive Bacterial Vaccine Preventable Diseases (IB-VPD) Surveillance Network Case definitions. 2012. http://www.who.int/immunization/monitoring_surveillance/resources/IB-VPD_Case_Defs.pdf. Accessed 7 Oct 2017.
14. Centers for Disease Control and Prevention. CDC/NHSN Surveillance Definitions for Specific Types of Infections. 2018. https://www.cdc.gov/nhsn/pdfs/pscmanual/17pscnosinfdef_current.pdf. Accessed 29 Aug 2018.
15. Uchino S, Bellomo R, Goldsmith D, Bates S, Ronco C. An assessment of the RIFLE criteria for acute renal failure in hospitalized patients. Crit Care Med. 2006;34:1913–7.
16. DeLong ER, DeLong DM, Clarke-Pearson DL. Comparing the areas under two or more correlated receiver operating characteristic curves: a nonparametric approach. Biometrics. 1988;44:837–45.
17. Zahar J-R, Timsit J-F, Garrouste-Orgeas M, Français A, Vesin A, Vesim A, et al. Outcomes in severe sepsis and patients with septic shock: pathogen species and infection sites are not associated with mortality. Crit Care Med. 2011;39:1886–95.
18. Park HK, Kim WY, Kim MC, Jung W, Ko BS. Quick sequential organ failure assessment compared to systemic inflammatory response syndrome for predicting sepsis in emergency department. J Crit Care. 2017;42:12–7.
19. Artero A, Zaragoza R, Camarena JJ, Sancho S, González R, Nogueira JM. Prognostic factors of mortality in patients with community-acquired bloodstream infection with severe sepsis and septic shock. J Crit Care. 2010; 25:276–81.
20. Peto L, Nadjm B, Horby P, Ngan TTD, van Doorn R, Kinh NV, et al. The bacterial aetiology of adult community-acquired pneumonia in Asia: a systematic review. Trans R Soc Trop Med Hyg. 2014;108:326–37.
21. Huong V, Ha N, Huy N, Peter H, Nghia H, Thiem V, et al. Epidemiology, clinical manifestations, and outcomes of Streptococcus suis infection in humans. Emerg Infect Dis. 2014;20:1105–14.
22. Hoa NT, Diep TS, Wain J, Parry CM, Hien TT, Smith MD, et al. Community-acquired septicaemia in southern Viet Nam: the importance of multidrug-resistant Salmonella typhi. Trans R Soc Trop Med Hyg. 1998;92:503–8.
23. Mai NTH, Chau TTH, Thwaites G, Chuong LV, Sinh DX, Nghia HDT, et al. Dexamethasone in Vietnamese adolescents and adults with bacterial meningitis. N Engl J Med. 2007;357:2431–40.
24. Thornórðardóttir A, Erlendsdóttir H, Sigurðardóttir B, Harðardóttir H, Reynisson IK, Gottfreðsson M, et al. Bacterial meningitis in adults in Iceland, 1995-2010. Scand J Infect Dis. 2014;46:354–60.
25. Meyer CN, Samuelsson IS, Galle M, Bangsborg JM. Adult bacterial meningitis: aetiology, penicillin susceptibility, risk factors, prognostic factors and guidelines for empirical antibiotic treatment. Clin Microbiol Infect. 2004;10: 709–17.
26. Diep NTN, Thai PQ, Trang NNM, Jager J, Fox A, Horby P, et al. Strongyloides stercoralis seroprevalence in Vietnam. Epidemiol Infect. 2017;145(15):3214–8.
27. Deen J, von Seidlein L, Andersen F, Elle N, White NJ, Lubell Y. Community-acquired bacterial bloodstream infections in developing countries in south and Southeast Asia: a systematic review. Lancet Infect Dis. 2012;12:480–7.
28. Vlieghe ER, Phe T, Smet BD, Veng HC, Kham C, Lim K, et al. Bloodstream infection among adults in Phnom Penh, Cambodia: key pathogens and resistance patterns. PLoS One. 2013;8:e59775.
29. Blanco J, Muriel-Bombín A, Sagredo V, Taboada F, Gandía F, Tamayo L, et al. Incidence, organ dysfunction and mortality in severe sepsis: a Spanish multicentre study. Crit Care. 2008;12:R158.
30. Askim Å, Moser F, Gustad LT, Stene H, Gundersen M, Åsvold BO, et al. Poor performance of quick-SOFA (qSOFA) score in predicting severe sepsis and mortality – a prospective study of patients admitted with infection to the emergency department. Scand J Trauma Resusc Emerg Med. 2017;25:56.
31. Riedel S, Melendez JH, An AT, Rosenbaum JE, Zenilman JM. Procalcitonin as a marker for the detection of bacteremia and Sepsis in the emergency department. Am J Clin Pathol. 2011;135:182–9.
32. Schuetz P, Mueller B, Trampuz A. Serum Procalcitonin for discrimination of blood contamination from bloodstream infection due to coagulase-negative staphylococci. Infection. 2007;35:352.

16

Using simultaneous amplification and testing method for evaluating the treatment outcome of pulmonary tuberculosis

Liping Yan[†], Heping Xiao[†] and Qing Zhang[*]

Abstract

Background: To evaluate the utility of Simultaneous Amplification and Testing (SAT-TB) Method for monitoring anti-TB treatment response.

Methods: Serial morning sputum specimens were obtained from 377 active pulmonary tuberculosis (PTB) cases at baseline, weeks 2, months 2, 5 and 6 (newly diagnosed patients) or 8 (previously treated patients) for AmpSure assay, smear fluorescence microscopy (FM) and BACTEC MGIT 960 culture assay.

Results: After treatment of 2 weeks, sputum culture was positive in 280 patients (74.27%). Among whom, 219 patients tested positive for SAT-TB assay and 143 patients smear FM positive. The detection rate of SAT-TB (78.21%) was significantly higher than sputum FM (51.07%, $\chi2 = 45.128$, $P < 0.001$). At the end of the second month of treatment, 157 patients (41.64%) were still culture-positive, 115 patients of them SAT-TB positive and 79 smear FM positive. The difference of detection rate between SAT-TB (73.25%) and sputum FM (50.32%) was significant ($\chi2 = 17.480$, $P < 0.001$). When patients underwent five months of treatment, 65 patients (17.24%) with sputum culture positive was defined as treatment failure. Among whom, 60 patients (92.31%) were SAT-TB positive and 38 patients (58.46%) were smear FM positive. The detection rate of SAT-TB assay was significantly higher than sputum FM ($\chi2 = 17.333$, $P < 0.001$).

Conclusion: Results of AmpSure assays for monitoring treatment responses can be obtained without waiting for the results of BACTEC MGIT 960 assays and most patients with treatment failures could be detected after 5 months.

Keywords: SAT-TB assay, Pulmonary tuberculosis, Culture test, Smear test, Tuberculosis treatment

Background

Tuberculosis (TB) is the leading cause of death from a single infectious disease [1]. Drug resistance further aggravates the problem. Effective drug treatment of active pulmonary tuberculosis (PTB) patients is critical for TB control. New TB patients are treated with 2HRZE/4HR regimen according to recommendation of World Health Organization (WHO) and 2HRZES/6HRE regimen are used in previously treated patients with drug-susceptible pulmonary TB [2]. All patients in the treatment of TB should be monitored to evaluate their response to treatment by sputum examination. Monitor the patient by chest radiography is not reliable and wasteful of resources. Sputum culture conversion (SCC) is commonly used as a microbiological endpoint in the treatment of tuberculosis [3]. 2-month, 5-month and 6-month or 8-month SCC status is proxy marker for treatment outcome. However, Sputum culture is not convenient in routine clinical practice [4]. It will take weeks to obtain the results. Smear microscopy is widely used in most undeveloped

* Correspondence: zhangingbm123@163.com
[†]Liping Yan and Heping Xiao contributed equally to this work.
Department of Tuberculosis, Shanghai Pulmonary Hospital, Tongji University School of Medicine, 507 Zhengmin Road, Shanghai 200433, People's Republic of China

countries. Sputum smear is performed at the end of the 2nd month (the intensive phase of treatment), the 5th month and treatment completion [5]. If smear is positive at month 2, sputum smear is repeated at month 3. If smear is positive at month 2 or at month 5, sputum culture and drug susceptibility testing (DST) should be obtained [5]. Smear positive at the end of the 2nd month indicates the patient may have drug-resistant M. tuberculosis. Smear-positivity at the end of the fifth month is defined as treatment failure and it is necessary to change the present treatment regimen. However, its sensitivity being unacceptably flawed [6] and non-viable bacteria remain visible by microscopy. In addition, microscopy could not distinguish tuberculos mycobacteria (NTM) from Mycobacterium tuberculosis complex (MTBC) [5].

An increasing number of molecular methods, that is more rapid and sensitive than existing conventional tests, have become available [7–9]. Simultaneous amplification and testing methods for detection of MTBC (SAT-TB assay), that is based on nucleic acid isolation, real-time fluorescence simultaneous isothermal RNA amplification and fluorescence-labeled hybridization probes testing has the advantage of rapid, simple and good reproducibility. The results could be obtained within 120 min.

Moreover, the SAT-TB assay is intended for point-of-care testing for TB [10]. Recent researches showed that sensitivity of the SAT-TB assay for the diagnosis of PTB with sputum samples was from 39.2 to 93% [11, 12]. In patients with sputum-scarce, the sensitivity of the SAT-TB test using bronchial alveolar lavage fluid (BALF) specimens was 50.75% [13]. However, studies using the SAT-TB assay to evaluate anti-TB treatment outcome have not been reported.

For the above reasons, we designed a prospective study to investigate the efficacy of SAT-TB assays for monitoring response to anti-TB therapy with sputum specimens from new PTB patients and previously treated patients in China.

Methods

Patients

This prospective study was approved by The Ethics Committee of the Shanghai Pulmonary Hospital. Each participant gave written informed consent before enrollment.

We prospectively screened all confirmed active PTB patients based on culture positive in Shanghai Pulmonary Hospital from January 2016 to January 2017. Informations about sex; age; TB contacts; symptoms of TB; history of anti-TB treatment; comorbidities and concurrent therapies were routinely collected from each patient by attending physicians using a questionnaire. The standard 2HRZE/4HR regimen are used in newly PTB patients according to recommendation of WHO and 2HRZES/6HRE regimen in previously treated patients under direct observed treatment (DOT) strategy [2]. The exclusion criteria included: (1) HIV test positive; (2) aged more than 17 years; (3) inability to provide sputum for examinations; (4) with concomitant extra-pulmonary TB; (5) resistant to any drug of the two regimens; (6) participate in other clinical researches at the same time; (7) had a history of poor adherence in other clinical trials before.

Examinations

Morning sputum specimens were obtained from enrolled patients at baseline (at the time of diagnosis before initiation of the treatment) (T0) and at the end of 2-week (T1), 2-month (T2), 5-month (T3) and 6-month (initially diagnosed patients) or 8-month (previously treated patients) (T4) after treatment initiation. M. tuberculosis detection was performed using smear fluorescence microscopy (FM), bacteriological analysis and the AmpSure assay. Smear positive grade 1 was the detection threshold of a positive sputum smear. Bacteriological analysis was done using the BACTEC MGIT 960 System (Becton Dickinson Diagnostic Systems, Sparks, MD, USA), according to WHO guidelines [14]. The SAT-TB assay was performed by means of the AmpSure assay (Shanghai Rendu Biotechnology, Shanghai China) according to the protocol of manufacturer, which was described previously [15]. Initial MTB isolates obtained from patients at the time of 2-month were subjected to DST for ofloxacin (Ofx),

Isoniazid (H), rifampicin (Rfp), ethambutol (E), streptomycin (Sm), amikacin (Am), and capreomycin (Cm) using BACTEC MGIT 960 System according to WHO guidlines [14]. All of the above tests were performed in a tuberculosis reference laboratory of Shanghai Pulmonary Hospital. Quality control was performed routinely following the Manual of procedures of the National Tuberculosis Control program. Sputum specimens were given identification laboratory numbers, and technicians who carried out bacteriological investigations were blinded to the patients.

Computed tomography (CT) scans was taken on all study participants at baseline, months 2 and the end of the course or anytime if necessary. Two radiologists and a physician independently evaluated all images. A standard format was followed to make sure the radiological readings were optimized for interpretation.

Definitions

End-of-treatment outcomes were assigned according to WHO definitions [3], namely, cure: a negative sputum smear or culture result in the last month of the therapy and on previous occasion at least once; treatment completed: completed the therapy but without a sputum smear- or culture- result in the last month of the therapy and on previous occasion at least once; failure: have a positive sputum smear or culture result at the 5th month or later or a multidrug-resistant (MDR) strain was found at anytime during the treatment; died: died due to any cause during the treatment; default: treatment was suspended for ≥2 consecutive months; transfer out: transferred to other registration department. Cure or treatment completion was defined as treatment success [3].

MDR is defined as resistance to at least isoniazid and rifampin. Extensively drug-resistant tuberculosis (XDR-TB), by definition, is a form of MDR-TB plus resistance to at least one drug in both of the two most significant groups of drugs in an MDR-TB schedule: fluoroquinolones (FQs) and second-line injectable agents (amikacin, capreomycin or kanamycin). Pre-XDR-TB is defined as MDR-TB plus resistance to either a FQs or a second-line injectable agent.

Statistical analyses

SPSS 18.0 software for Windows (Version 18.0, SPSS Inc., Chicago) was used to analyze the data. Numerical variables were shown as the mean ± standard deviation. Fisher exact test or Pearson chi-squared analysis was used to analyze categorical variables. $P \leq 0.05$ was set as the level of statistical significance.

Results

We enrolled 400 suspected active PTB patients, prospectively. Twenty-three of them were excluded from our analysis because of NTM. The remaining 377 confirmed patients including 200 initially diagnosed TB cases and 177 previously treated cases with a mean age of 46.4 ± 17.5 years were eligible for this analysis and were followed during the standard anti-TB treatment (Fig. 1). These patients were predominantly males (69.5%) with a mean body mass index (BMI) of 19.0 kg/m^2. The participants had typical CT findings that suggested active TB, including cavitary lesions, tree-in-bud appearance and lung nodules. There are 1820 sputum specimens collected for examinations. The demographic and clinical characteristics of 377 patients were summarized in Table 1.

After treatment of 2 weeks, sputum culture was positive in 280 patients (74.27%). Among whom, 219 patients tested positive for SAT-TB assay and 143 patients smear FM positive. The detection rate of SAT-TB (78.21%) was significantly higher than sputum FM (51.07%, $X^2 = 45.128$, $P = 0.000$). At the end of the second month of treatment, 157 patients (41.64%) were still culture-positive, 115 patients of them SAT-TB positive and 79 smear FM positive. The difference of detection rate between SAT-TB (73.25%) and sputum FM (50.32%) was significant ($X2 = 17.480$, $P = 0.000$). When patients underwent five months of treatment, 65 patients (17.24%) with sputum culture positive was defined as treatment failure. Among whom, 60 patients (92.31%) were SAT-TB positive and 40 patients (61.54%) were smear FM positive. The detection rate of SAT-TB assay was significantly higher than sputum FM ($X2 = 17.333$, $P < 0$ .001). Ultimately, 312 patients (82.76%) cured with culture clearing and imaging improvement. The results of SAT-TB assay, smear FM, and BACTEC MGIT 960 culture at different time points were summarized in Table 2.

The overall sensitivity of SAT-TB assay was 86.92%, which was significantly higher than that of smear FM (56.43%) ($P < 0.001$). The overall specificity of SAT-TB assay was 100%, which was also higher than that of smear FM (99.69%) ($P = 0.156$). The PPV and NPV of SAT-TB assay was 100% and 84.55%, respectively. The PPV and NPV of smear FM was 99.6% and 62.28%, respectively. The difference between PPV had no statistical significance ($P = 0.080$), but the difference between NPV had statistical significance ($P < 0.001$) (Fig. 2).

Initial MTB isolates obtained from positive culture of 157 patients at the end of the second month of treatment were subjected to DST. The DST results were summarized in Table 3. There were 6 XDR-TB, 9 pre-XDR-TB, 32 MDR-TB and 6 mono-drug resistant (resistant to

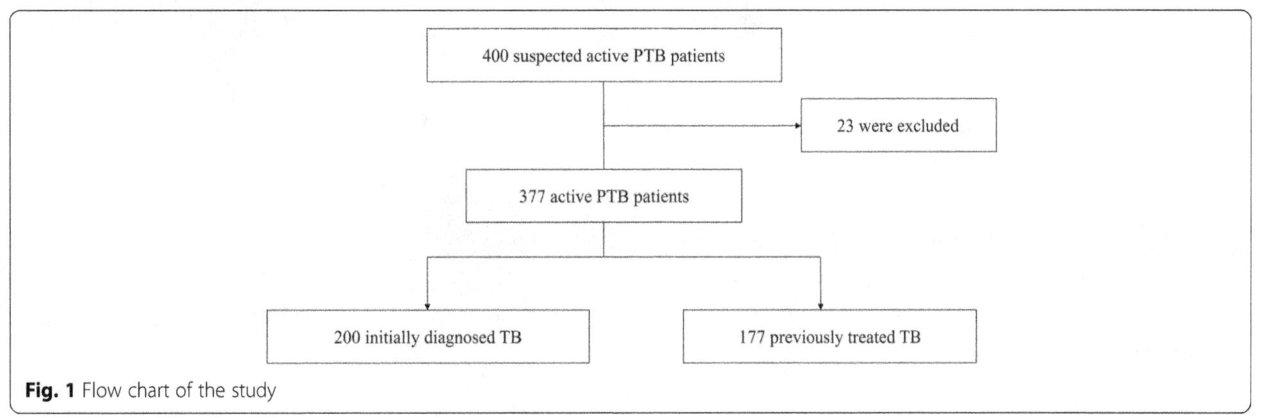

Fig. 1 Flow chart of the study

Table 1 Patient characteristics

Variable	New PTB (*n* = 200)	Previously treated (*n* = 177)	Total (*n* = 377)
Men (n [%])	135 (67.5)	127 (71.75)	262
Women (n [%])	65 (32.5)	50 (28.25)	115
Age (y) (median) (range)	44.6 ± 17.7	47.4 ± 19.7	46.4 ± 17.5
Body mass index (median) (range)	19.1 (13–27)	18.9 (13–27)	
Cured cases	173	139	312
Failed cases	27	38	65

streptomycin) TB patients. All of the 47 MDR/XDR-TB and 3 mono-drug resistant as well as 15 susceptible TB patients failed.

Discussion

In the current study, we used SAT-TB assay to evaluate treatment outcome in Chinese PTB patients compared with smear FM and BACTEC MGIT 960 at different time points, and observed that the SAT-TB assay is preferred. All the patients that was in the treatment of TB should be monitored the response to treatment. If sputum smear is positive at month 2, sputum smear is repeated at month 3. If smear is positive at month 3, sputum culture and DST should be obtained. Smear-positivity or culture-positivity at the end of the fifth month is defined as treatment failure [3]. Unfortunately, sputum smear and culture have significant limitations. The technological development of nucleic acid amplification has led to advances in the early detection of tubercle bacilli. The GeneXpert assay (Cepheid, Sunnyvale, CA) was introduced currently in China. The high price of the GeneXpert assay and the requirement of costly especial instrument for the MTD test (Gen-Probe; San Diego, CA, USA) prevent these assays from being a routine test in resource-limited countries [16, 17]. The SAT-TB assay has another advantage over PCR, as the detection objective is rRNA. RNA is much more unstable than DNA, so a positive result indicates the presence of viable MTBC. Therefore the false positive rate decreased. In addition, the SAT-TB assay can be performed on real-time PCR instruments, which can be found in most clinical laboratories.

The SAT-TB assay was demonstrated to have better sensitivity and high specificity for the detection of tubercle bacilli in our study. Over the intensive phase of therapy, 73.25% of culture-positive patients could be detected with the SAT-TB assay within 2 h. Month-2 culture conversion is generally used as substitute index of anti-TB treatment efficiency [18]. Detection of tubercle bacilli at the end of the intensive phase remains important as it may indicate that the patient may have multidrug-resistant M. tuberculosis and DST should be performed. If we use sputum smear for monitoring the treatment response, only about half of culture-positive patients (50.32%) could be detected. If we use the SAT-TB assay, DST could be performed in three-quarters of these patients. The number of patients in need of DST was increased by about a quarter. Drug-resistant tuberculosis (DR-TB) should be identified as early as possible not only for achieving the best treatment outcome but also for controlling the spread of DR-TB. Smear-positivity at the end of the fifth month is defined as treatment failure and it is necessary to change the present treatment regimen. In this study, 65 patients with sputum culture positive were defined as treatment failure. Among whom, 60 patients were SAT-TB assay positive. This means that if we use the SAT-TB assay for monitoring the treatment response, 92.31% of patients with treatment failure can be found timely and changed to appropriate therapy. However, only 58.46% of these culture-positive patients were sputum smear positive. After a month or three, physicians may mistakenly declare the treatment successful for 41.54% of these failure patients. It's worth mentioning that two sputum smear

Table 2 Summary of SAT-TB, smear FM, and culture results

		SAT-TB (+)		SAT-TB (−)	
		Smear (+)	Smear (−)	Smear (+)	Smear (−)
before treatment	Mt-culture (+)	236 (62.6%)	134 (35.55%)	0	7 (1.86%)
	Mt-culture (−)	0	0	0	0
2nd week	Mt-culture (+)	143 (51.07%)	76 (27.15%)	0	61 (21.78%)
	Mt-culture (−)	0	0	0	97 (25.73%)
2nd month	Mt-culture (+)	79 (50.32%)	36 (22.93%)	0	42 (26.75%)
	Mt-culture (−)	0	0	0	220 (59.46%)
5th month	Mt-culture (+)	38 (58.46%)	22 (33.84%)	0	5 (7.7%)
	Mt-culture (−)	0	0	2 (0.65%)	310 (99.35%)
6th/8th month	Mt-culture (+)	0	0	0	0
	Mt-culture (−)	0	0	0	312 (82.76%)

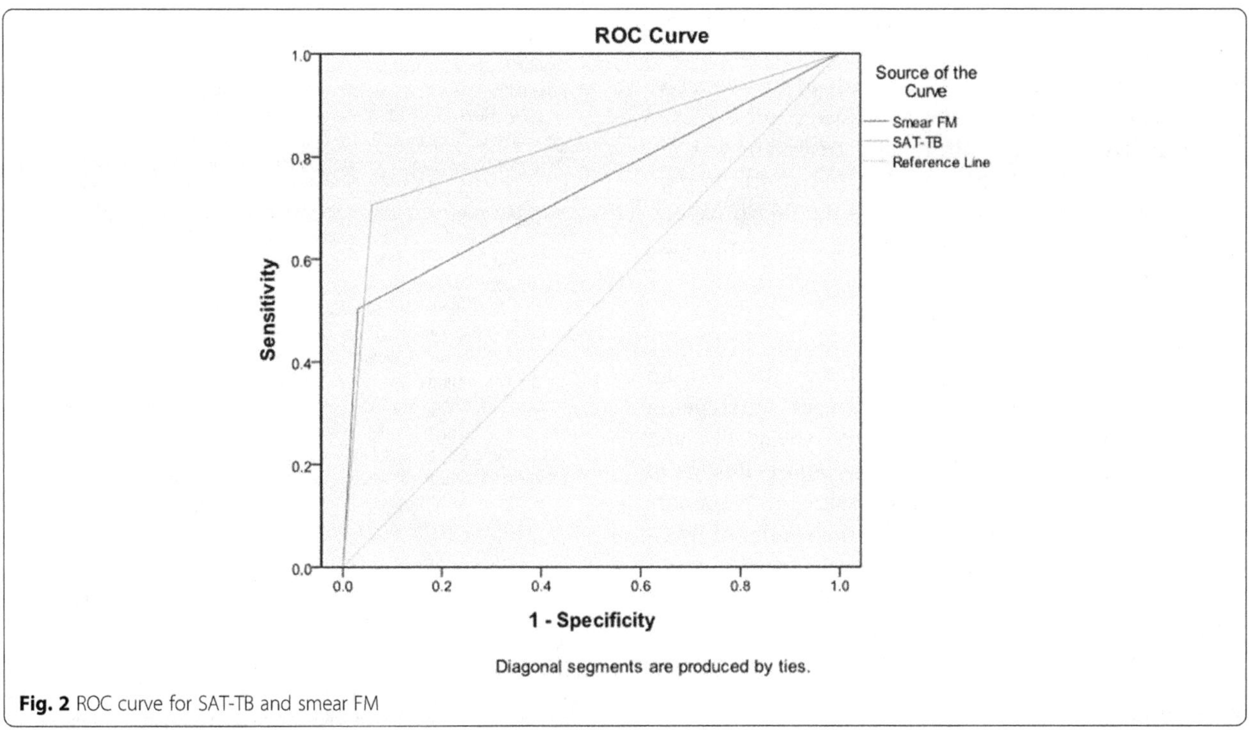

Fig. 2 ROC curve for SAT-TB and smear FM

positive were identified as false-positives or laboratory contamination according to culture and SAT-TB assay negative and imaging improvement at the end of the fifth month. Ultimately, the treatment success rate in this study was 82.76%, which was comparable to the average success rate in the world. Globally, the treatment success rate for the 5.9 million new and relapse cases was 83% in 2015 [1]. False-negative findings, however, are inevitable with the current technology [19–21]. In addition, the major barrier in applying molecular detection method in evaluating treatment response is the problem of false positive rather than false negative. In our research, there was no false positive (sputum culture-negative but SAT-TB assay positive) for SAT-TB assay.

Treatment outcome of anti-TB treatment in bacteriologically confirmed PTB patients is evaluated principally by serial bacteriologic examinations [2], whereas Treatment outcome in clinically diagnosed PTB patients are usually monitored clinically or radiographically. To overcome these shortcomings, numerous biomarkers have been evaluated [4, 22], although most of the markers do not have high levels of validity. More and more studies confirmed that the possible function of plasma-based IFN-γ-release assays (IGRAs) for evaluation of reaction to anti-TB therapy is objectionable [23]. The IGRA is less useful in terms of treatment monitoring, given that the IGRA is based on the TB antigen-stimulated immunologic reaction, which tends to persist and shows blunted fluctuations during the longitudinal monitoring of TB [24]. Lago et al. observed a consistent decrease in IL-10 levels in active PTB patients at all times of therapy, suggesting that this cytokine could be used as a helpful biomarker for evaluating disease progression [25]. Therefore, novel accessing means of anti-TB therapy outcome are required to make anti-TB therapy better in some clinical circumstances.

Table 3 Summary of drug susceptibility testing results of 157 patients

		XDR	Pre-XDR	MDR	Sm-resistant	Susceptible	Total
New PTB	cure	0	0	0	1	34	35
	failure	0	2	9	1	15	27
Previously treated	cure	0	0	0	2	55	57
	failure	6	7	23	2	0	38
Total		6	9	32	6	104	157

In this study, 65% of patients were male. Men seem to be more affected with TB than women with a male/female ratio of 1.86 for the worldwide case notification rate in 2017 [26]. This excess of male pulmonary TB cases is seen in almost all countries of the world, and this gender effect is thought to be related to many factors, such as access to healthcare, nutritional status, socioeconomic and cultural factors. TB disease is not gender specific. Male and female are equally susceptible.

There are several limitations in this study. First, the number of patients with microbiological diagnosed active TB is relatively small. Second, this study was limited to only HIV-negative PTB patient group, which limits its generalization to the HIV-infected group.

HIV-positive cases, a clinically significant population, were removed from this study as they must be shifted to special hospitals in China. Third, a few variables such as chest imaging manifestations were not explored in this analysis. Finally, culture after treatment was not followed up in this study. Despite these shortcomings, as far as we know, this is likely to be the first prospective study to evaluate the utility of SAT-TB assays to access TB therapy outcome.

Conclusions

In summary, our research suggests that the SAT-TB assay is preferred to evaluate treatment outcome in Chinese PTB patients compared with smear FM and BACTEC MGIT 960 at different time points. Results of AmpSure assays for monitoring treatment responses can be obtained without waiting for the results of BACTEC MGIT 960 assays and most patients with treatment failures could be detected after 5 months. Whether SAT-TB assays can be used to access TB therapy outcome needs to be explored further.

Abbreviations

Am: Amikacin; BALF: Bronchial alveolar lavage fluid; Cm: Capreomycin; CT: Computed tomography; DOT: Direct observed treatment; DR-TB: Drug-resistant tuberculosis; DST: Drug susceptibility testing; E: Ethambutol; FM: Fluorescence microscopy; FQs: Fluoroquinolones; H: Isoniazid; IGRAs: IFN-γ-release assays; MDR: Multidrug-resistant; MTBC: Mycobacterium tuberculosis complex; NTM: Non- tuberculos mycobacteria; Ofx: Ofloxacin; PTB: Pulmonary tuberculosis; Rfp: Rifampicin; SAT-TB assay: Simultaneous amplification and testing methods for detection of MTBC; SCC: Sputum culture conversion; Sm: Streptomycin; TB: Tuberculosis; WHO: World Health Organization; XDR-TB: Extensively drug-resistant tuberculosis

Funding

This work was supported by a grant from the National Key Scientific and Technical Program (Grant No. 2013ZX10003009).

Authors' contributions

QZ and HX were responsible for the conception and design of the study. All author were responsible for acquisition and analysis of data; furthermore, LY and QZ were in charge of statistical analysis. All authors drafted the manuscript; QZ revised and approved the final version of the manuscript. All authors read and approved the final manuscript.

Competing interests

The authors declare that they have no competing interests.

References

1. WHO: Global Tuberculosis Report 2017. In Geneva: World Health Organization; 2017.
2. WHO. Guidelines for treatment of drug-susceptible tuberculosis and patient care, 2017 update. Geneva: World Health Organization; 2017.
3. Wallis RS, Kim P, Cole S, Hanna D, Andrade BB, Maeurer M, et al. Tuberculosis biomarkers discovery: developments, needs, and challenges. Lancet Infect Dis. 2013;13(4):362–72.
4. Ritchie SR, Harrison AC, Vaughan RH, Calder L, Morris AJ. New recommendations for duration of respiratory isolation based on time to detect Mycobacterium tuberculosis in liquid culture. Eur Respir J. 2007;30(3):501–7.
5. Eurosurveillance editorial team. WHO revised definitions and reporting framework for tuberculosis. Euro Surveill. 2013;18(16):20455.
6. Desikan P. Sputum smear microscopy in tuberculosis: is it still relevant? Indian J Med Res. 2013;137(3):442–4.
7. Dinnes J, Deeks J, Kunst H, Gibson A, Cummins E, Waugh N, et al. A systematic review of rapid diagnostic tests for the detection of tuberculosis infection. Health Technol Assess. 2007;11(3):1–196.
8. Piersimoni C, Scarparo C, Piccoli P, Rigon A, Ruggiero G, Nista D, et al. Performance assessment of two commercial amplification assays for direct detection of Mycobacterium tuberculosis complex from respiratory and extrapulmonary specimens. J Clin Microbiol. 2002;40(11):4138–42.
9. Yan L, Xiao H, Zhang Q. Systematic review: comparison of Xpert MTB/RIF, LAMP and SAT methods for the diagnosis of pulmonary tuberculosis. Tuberculosis. 2016;96:75–86.
10. Mdivani N, Li H, Akhalaia M, Gegia M, Goginashvili L, Kernodle DS, et al. Monitoring therapeutic efficacy by real-time detection of Mycobacterium tuberculosis mRNA in sputum. Clin Chem. 2009;55(9):1694–700.
11. Cui Z, Wang Y, Fang L, Zheng R, Huang X, Liu X, et al. Novel real-time simultaneous amplification and testing method to accurately and rapidly detect Mycobacterium tuberculosis complex. J Clin Microbiol. 2012;50(3):646–50.
12. Fan L, Zhang Q, Cheng L, Liu Z, Ji X, Cui Z, et al. Clinical diagnostic performance of the simultaneous amplification and testing methods for detection of the Mycobacterium tuberculosis complex for smear-negative or sputum-scarce pulmonary tuberculosis in China. Chin Med J. 2014; 127(10):1863–7.
13. Yan L, Zhang Q, Xiao H. Clinical diagnostic value of simultaneous amplification and testing for the diagnosis of sputum-scarce pulmonary tuberculosis. BMC Infect Dis. 2017;17(1):545.
14. WHO. Guidelines for surveillance of drug resistance in tuberculosis In. 4th ed. Geneva: World Health Organization; 2009.
15. Yan L, Tang S, Yang Y, Shi X, Ge Y, Sun W, et al. A large cohort study on the clinical value of simultaneous amplification and testing for the diagnosis of pulmonary tuberculosis. Medicine. 2016;95(4):e2597.
16. Du J, Huang Z, Luo Q, Xiong G, Xu X, Li W, et al. Rapid diagnosis of pleural tuberculosis by Xpert MTB/RIF assay using pleural biopsy and pleural fluid specimens. J Res Med Sci. 2015;20(1):26–31.
17. Jonas V, Alden MJ, Curry JI, Kamisango K, Knott CA, Lankford R, et al. Detection and identification of Mycobacterium tuberculosis directly from sputum sediments by amplification of rRNA. J Clin Microbiol. 1993;31(9): 2410–6.
18. Mitchison D, Davies G. The chemotherapy of tuberculosis: past, present and future. Int J Tuberc Lung Dis. 2012;16(6):724–32.
19. Boehme CC, Nabeta P, Hillemann D, Nicol MP, Shenai S, Krapp F, et al. Rapid molecular detection of tuberculosis and rifampin resistance. N Engl J Med. 2010;363(11):1005–15.
20. Boehme CC, Nicol MP, Nabeta P, Michael JS, Gotuzzo E, Tahirli R, et al. Feasibility, diagnostic accuracy, and effectiveness of decentralised use of the Xpert MTB/RIF test for diagnosis of tuberculosis and multidrug resistance: a multicentre implementation study. Lancet. 2011;377(9776):1495–505.
21. Sethi S, Singh S, Dhatwalia SK, Yadav R, Mewara A, Singh M, et al. Evaluation of in-house loopmediated isothermal amplification (LAMP) assay for rapid diagnosis of M. tuberculosis in pulmonary specimens. J Clin Lab Anal. 2013; 27(4):272–6.
22. Mihret A, Bekele Y, Bobosha K, Kidd M, Aseffa A, Howe R, et al. Plasma cytokines and chemokines differentiate between active disease and non-active tuberculosis infection. J Infect. 2013;66(4):357–65.
23. Chiappini E, Fossi F, Bonsignori F, Sollai S, Galli L, de Martino M. Utility of interferongamma release assay results to monitor anti-tubercular treatment in adults and children. Clin Ther. 2012;34(5):1041–8.
24. Denkinger CM, Pai M, Patel M, Menzies D. Gamma interferon release assay for monitoring of treatment response for active tuberculosis: an explosion in the spaghetti factory. J Clin Microbiol. 2013;51(2):607–10.
25. Lago PM, Boéchat N, Migueis DP, Almeida AS, Lazzarini LC, Saldanha MM, et al. Interleukin-10 and interferon-gamma patterns during tuberculosis treatment: possible association with recurrence. Int J Tuberc Lung Dis. 2012; 16(5):656–9.
26. Khan KB. Understanding the gender aspects of tuberculosis: a narrative analysis of the lived experiences of women with TB in slums of Delhi, India. Health Care Women Int. 2012;33(1):3–18.

17

Comparative study of virulence factors among methicillin resistant *Staphylococcus aureus* clinical isolates

Ons Haddad[1,2*], Abderrahmen Merghni[2], Aida Elargoubi[1,2], Hajer Rhim[1,2], Yosr Kadri[1,2] and Maha Mastouri[1,2]

Abstract

Background: Methicillin resistant *Staphylococcus aureus* (MRSA) is recognized worldwide as a leading cause of hospital and community infections. Biofilm formation by MRSA is an extremely important virulence factor to be understood. Our aim was to establish phenotypic and genotypic characterization of virulence factors among 43 MRSA clinical isolates in a Tunisian hospital.

Methods: We investigated enzymatic profiles, biofilm production and prevalences of genes encoding intracellular adhesion molecules (*icaA* and *icaD*), Microbial Surface Components Recognizing Adhesive Matrix Molecules genes (*fnbA*, *fnbB* and *cna*) and exoenzymes genes (*geh*, *sspA* and *sspB*).

Results: Our findings revealed that caseinase, gelatinase, lipase and lecithinase activities were detected in 100%, 100%, 76.6% and 93.3% of cases respectively. This study showed that 23 strains (76.7%) were slime producers on Congo red medium. Furthermore, 46.5% and 53.5% of isolates were respectively highly and moderately biofilm-forming on polystyrene. Significant association was found between both biofilm tests. PCR detection showed that 74.4%, 18.6%, 69.8%, 65.1% and 74.4% of isolates harbored *fnbA*, *fnbB*, *icaA*, *icaD* and *cna* genes respectively. In addition, 34.9%, 18.6% and 30.2% of MRSA strains were found positive for *sspA*, *sspB* and *geh* genes respectively. Further, statistical data showed that the presence of the *fnbA* and *fnbB* genes was significantly associated with a high biofilm production on polystyrene. However, no statistical association was observed for the *icaA*, *icaD* and *cna* genes.

Conclusions: This study indicates that the detection of *fnbA* and *fnbB* contributing to the first step of biofilm formation has been predictable of high biofilm production. As studied factors contribute to MRSA virulence, this research could be of value in orienting towards the development of new preventive and therapeutic measures.

Keywords: *Staphylococcus aureus*, methicillin, biofilm, virulence, adhesion molecules

Introduction

Methicillin resistant *Staphylococcus aureus* (MRSA) is recognized worldwide as an important bacterial pathogen causing a wide range of infections ranging from skin and soft tissue lesions to lethal infections (osteomyelitis, endocarditis, pneumonia and septicaemia). It is regarded as a major world health threat with a substantial increase in morbidity and mortality [1]. In addition to resistance, the pathogenicity of MRSA is an extremely important feature to be understood. The pathogenesis of this bacterium depends on a combination of extracellular factors and biofilm forming ability [2]. The adherence of *S. aureus* to biotic and abiotic surfaces stage is mediated by a protein family of staphylococcal Microbial Surface Components Recognizing Adhesive Matrix Molecules (MSCRAMMs). Whereas the cell aggregation is led by the synthesis of polysaccharide intercellular adhesin (PIA) molecule encoded by the intracellular adhesion (*ica*) [3–6].

Our aim was to establish a phenotypic characterization of virulence factors among MRSA clinical isolates in a Tunisian Hospital, to determine prevalences of genes encoding intracellular adhesion molecules (*icaA* and *icaD*),

* Correspondence: onshadad@gmail.com
[1]Laboratoire de Microbiologie, CHU Fatouma Bourguiba de Monastir, Monastir, Tunisie
[2]Laboratoire des Maladies Transmissible et Substances Biologiquement Actives, LR99ES27, Faculté de Pharmacie de Monastir, Université de Monastir, Monastir, Tunisie

MSCRAMMs genes (*fnbA*, *fnbB*, *cna*) and exoenzymes genes (*geh*, *sspA* and *sspB*), and to investigate the involvement of these genes in biofilm forming ability.

Materials and methods

Bacterial strains

A total of 43 non-redundant MRSA clinical isolates were obtained from the Laboratory of Microbiology of the University hospital of Monastir-Tunisia. These strains were obtained from bacteriological samples in hospitalized patients and/or consultants at the University Hospital of Monastir-Tunisia during the period (January 2016 - June 2016). Two reference strains (*S. aureus* ATCC 6538 and ATCC 43300) were used as controls. Bacterial identification was performed using Gram staining, catalase test, tube coagulase, DNase agar, mannitol salt agar and API ID 20 STAPH galleries (bio-Merieux, France). To confirm the identity of the isolate as *S. aureus*, the *Sa442* gene was amplified by a PCR-based method. Extraction of genomic DNA was performed using a standard phenolechloroform technique. The PCR mixture (25 µl) for all genes contained 1 mM forward and reverse primers, dNTP mix (100 mM each of dATP, dCTP, dGTP and dTTP), 1 U of Go Taq DNA polymerase (Promega), 5 ml green Go Taq buffer (5X), and DNA template (50 ng). PCR conditions were the following: an initial temperature of 96°C (3min), followed by denaturation at 95°C (1min), annealing at 55°C (30s), elongation at 72°C (3min), and a final elongation step at 72°C (4min). Amplicons of the expected size (108 bp) were obtained. Methicillin resistance was confirmed using a cefoxitin disk (30 µg) on Mueller-Hinton agar plates (Bio-Rad, France) as recommended by the French Society of Microbiology and by the European Committee on Antimicrobial Susceptibility Testing. The *mecA* gene was detected by PCR. PCR conditions were the following : an initial temperature of 95°C (1min), denaturation at 95°C (15s), annealing at 45°C (15 s), and elongation at 72°C (30s), with a final extension at 72°C (4min). Amplicons of the expected size (162 bp) were obtained [7]. PCR primers were chosen as listed in Table 1.

Amplified PCR products were analyzed on 2% (wt/v) agarose gel stained with ethidium bromide (0.5 µg ml^{-1}), visualized under ultraviolet transillumination and photographed using Gel Doc XR apparatus (Biorad, USA).

Characterization of the enzymatic activity

The ability to produce hydrolytic enzymes was determined after inoculation of cultures on TSA-1 media (Biorad) supplemented with: 1% (wt/vol) skim milk for caseinase; 1% (wt/vol) gelatin for gelatinase; Tween 80 for lipase and 5% (vol/vol) egg yolk for lecithinase. The presence of a clear halo around the colonies indicates the presence of the hydrolytic enzyme. The haemolytic activity was evaluated on bacteriological agar supplemented with 5% sheep's blood [8].

Phenotypic determination of slime production

Phenotypic qualitative characterization of slime producing strains was carried out by the cultivation of the

Table 1 List of primers used for bacterial identification and detection of MSCRAMMs genes (*fnbA*, *fnbB* and *cna*), biofim control genes (*icaA* and *icaD*) and exoenzymes genes (*sspA*, *sspB* and *geh*)

Target gene	Sequence (5'-3')	aT (°C)	Amplified fragment	Amplicon size (bp)	Reference
Sa442	5'-AATCTTTGTCGGTACACGATATTCTTCACG-3' 5'-CGTAATGAGATTTCAGTAAATACAACA-3'	55	Sa442 protein	108	[7]
mecA	5'-ACCAGATTACAACTTCACCAGG-3' 5'-CCACTTCATATCTTGTAACG-3'	45	Penicillin binding protein 2a	162	[7]
icaA	5'-ACACTTGCTGGCGCAGTCAA-3' 5'-TCTGGAACCAACATCCAACA-3'	55	Intercellular adhesion A	188	[24]
icaD	5'-ATGGTCAAGCCCAGACAGAG-3' 5'-AGTATTTTCAATGTTTAAAGCAA-3'	55	Intercellular adhesion D	198	[24]
Can	5'-GTCAAGCAGTTATTAACACCAGAC-3' 5'-AATCAGTAATTGCACTTTGTCCACTG-3'	62	Collagen adhesion	192	[36]
fnbA	5'-CATAAATTGGGAGCAGCATCA-3' 5'-ATCAGCAGCTGAATTCCCATT-3'	62	Fibronectin binding protein A	191	[36]
fnbB	5'-GTAACAGCTAATGGTCGAATTGATACT-3' 5'-CAAGTTCGATAGGAGTACTATGTTC-3'	62	Fibronectin binding protein B	201	[36]
sspA	5'-GACAACAGCGACACTTGT 3' 3'-AGTATCTTTACCTACAACTACA-5'	45	Serine protease	292	[40]
sspB	5'-TGAAGAAGATGGCAAAGTTAG-3' 3'-TTGAGATACACTTTGTGCAAG-5'	47	Cysteine protease	493	[40]
Geh	5'-GCACAAGCCTCGG -3' 3'-GACGGGGGTGTAG-5'	40	Lipase	473	[45]

aT annealing temperature

isolates on Congo red agar (CRA) plate made by mixing 36 g of sucrose (Sigma Chemical Company, St. Louis, MO) with 0.8 Congo red in 1L of brain heart infusion agar (Biorad, USA) as previously described [9]. The strains were incubated at 37°C for 24 hours under aerobic conditions followed by subsequent storage at room temperature. The Congo red dye interacts directly with certain bacterial polysaccharides forming a slime and giving black colonies in contrast to the non-producing colonies which remain red. After 48-72 hours, the results were interpreted as follows: strains producing intensive black, black, and reddish black colonies with a rough, dry, and crystalline consistency were classified as slime producers, whereas red and Bordeaux red with smooth colonies were considered to be non slime producers [9].

Semi-quantitative adherence assay

Biofilm production by MRSA strains, grown in Brain Heart Infusion with 1% glucose, was quantified using a semi-quantitative adherence assay on 96-well tissue culture plates as described previously [10]. Adherent bacteria were fixed with 95% ethanol and stained with 100 mL of 1% crystal violet (Merck, France) for 5 min. The microplates were air-dried and the optical density of each well was measured at 570 nm (OD570) using an automated Multiskan reader (GIO. DE VITA E C, ome, Italy). This assay was performed for each strain in triplicate. The background was determined by using noninoculated media as a control. The cut-off value (ODC) of noninoculated media at an optical density of 570 nm (OD570) was considered the deadline point to define biofilm quantities [cut-off (ODC) = mean OD + 3 standard deviation (SD) of negative control]. Biofilm formation was interpreted as highly positive (OD570> = 4 * ODC), moderately positive (2 * ODC <= OD570 <4 * ODC), weakly positive (ODC <= OD570 <2 * ODC) or negative (OD570 < ODC). These criteria were established by Stepanovic et al. [11].

Detection of *icaA, icaD, fnbA, fnbB, cna, sspA, sspB* and *geh* genes

PCR primers were chosen as listed in Table 1. Amplifications of *icaA, icaD, fnbA, fnbB, cna, sspA, sspB* and *geh* genes were performed according to the following cycle conditions: an initial denaturation at 94°C for 5 min was followed by 30 cycles of denaturation at 94°C for 30s, annealing for 30s at temperature determined for each gene as described in Table 1 and elongation at 72°C for 45s, followed by 10 min of final extension at 72°C.

Statistical analysis

The data from this study were captured, recorded and analyzed by SPSS 17.0 software. The non-parametric Mann Whitney U test was used to compare biofilm production assays (Congo red test and polystyrene adherence assay). The same statistical test was used to evaluate correlations of MSCRAMMs genes (*fnbA, fnbB* and *cna*), biofilm production control genes (*icaA* and *icaD*) and exoenzymes genes (*sspA, sspB* and *geh*) to the level of biofilm production on polystyrene. All factors with p values of less than 0.20 were included in multivariate ordinal logistic regression analysis. *P* values of less than 0.05 were considered to indicate significant difference.

Results

Distribution of isolates

A total of 43 MRSA strains were collected (i.e. a rate of 21.4% of all S. aureus isolates in the laboratory of Microbiology at the University Hospital of Monastir-Tunisia during the same period). Samples were gathered from different organs and systems: pus (58.1%), blood (25.6%), respiratory samples (11.6%) and catheters (4.7%). They were collected from patients admitted in surgery units (44.2%), intensive care units (25.6%), medical units (13.9%), Pediatrics/Neonatology (9.3%) and Gynecology (7.0%).

Characterization of the enzymatic activity

Our results showed that 51.1% and 48.9% of isolates were respectively beta and alpha-hemolytic. All isolates were protease producers (caseinase and gelatinase). Lipase and lecithinase secretion were found in 93.0% and 79.1% of cases respectively (Table 2).

Phenotypic determination of slime production

Out of 43 MRSA isolates, 30 strains (69.8%) were slime producers on the CRA plate. They were black or reddish black color colony producers. Slime production was noted in 16 out of 25 strains isolated from suppurations and in 9 out of 11 blood culture isolates (Table 3).

Semi-quantitative adherence assay

The results of OD570 presented in Table 3, showed that 46.5% and 53.5% strains were respectively highly and moderately biofilm-formers on polystyrene. No isolate was weakly or non-biofilm producer on polystyrene. We detected 5/11 blood culture isolates and 10/25 pus isolates considered as highly biofilm formers. Both reference strains *S. aureus* ATCC 6538 and ATCC 43300 were highly biofilm-forming on polystyrene.

Detection by PCR of icaA, icaD, fnbA, fnbB, cna, sspA, sspB and geh genes

The *icaA* and the *icaD* genes were present in 69.8% and 65.1% of MRSA isolates respectively. A concomitant presence of both genes was detected in 55.8% of the strains. Our results revealed that 74.4% and 18.6% of

Table 2 Exoenzymes production and hemolysis of studied strains

Strains	Exoenzymes expression				Hemolysis type
	Lecithinase	Lipase	Caseinase	Gelatinase	
ATCC6538	+	+	+	+	Beta
1	+	+	+	+	Alpha
2	+	+	+	+	Alpha
3	+	+	+	+	Alpha
4	+	+	+	+	Alpha
5	+	+	+	+	Beta
6	+	+	+	+	Beta
7	+	+	+	+	Beta
8	-	-	+	+	Beta
9	+	+	+	+	Alpha
10	+	+	+	+	Beta
11	+	+	+	+	Alpha
12	+	+	+	+	Beta
13	+	+	+	+	Beta
14	+	-	+	+	Alpha
15	+	+	+	+	Alpha
16	+	-	+	+	Beta
17	+	-	+	+	Beta
18	+	+	+	+	Alpha
19	+	+	+	+	Beta
20	+	+	+	+	Alpha
21	+	+	+	+	Beta
22	+	+	+	+	Alpha
23	-	-	+	+	Beta
24	+	+	+	+	Alpha
25	+	+	+	+	Alpha
26	+	+	+	+	Beta
27	+	+	+	+	Beta
28	+	+	+	+	Alpha
29	+	+	+	+	Alpha
30	-	-	+	+	Beta
31	+	+	+	+	Beta
32	+	+	+	+	Alpha
33	+	+	+	+	Alpha
34	+	+	+	+	Alpha
35	+	+	+	+	Beta
36	+	-	+	+	Alpha
37	+	+	+	+	Beta
38	+	+	+	+	Beta
39	+	+	+	+	Alpha
40	+	-	+	+	Beta
41	+	+	+	+	Alpha
42	+	+	+	+	Beta
43	+	-	+	+	Beta
% expression	93,0%	79,1%	100%	100%	48.9%(alpha);51.1%(beta)

Table 3 Slime production and adherence assay of methicillin resistant *Staphylococcus aureus* isolates

Strains	Biofilm phenotype (CRA)	OD570 ± SD	Adherence state
ATCC 6538	S+	2.90±0.05	highly positive
ATCC 43300	S+	0.71±0.15	highly positive
1	S-	0.19±0.05	moderately positive
2	S-	0.12±0.03	moderately positive
3	S+	0.13±0.02	moderately positive
4	S+	0.59±0.11	highly positive
5	S+	0.46±0.02	highly positive
6	S+	0.26±0.01	highly positive
7	S+	0.22±0.08	moderately positive
8	S+	0.42±0.01	highly positive
9	S-	0.15±0.02	moderately positive
10	S+	0.80±0.03	highly positive
11	S+	2.96±0.08	highly positive
12	S-	0.15±0.04	moderately positive
13	S-	0.15±0.07	moderately positive
14	S+	1.77±0.02	highly positive
15	S+	0.22±0.01	moderately positive
16	S+	0.17±0.03	moderately positive
17	S+	2.62±0.01	highly positive
18	S+	0.24±0.02	highly positive
19	S+	0.13±0.05	moderately positive
20	S+	0.62±0.03	highly positive
21	S+	0.12±0.03	moderately positive
22	S+	0.21±0.39	moderately positive
23	S+	0.14±0.06	moderately positive
24	S+	0.14±0.01	moderately positive
25	S+	0.14±0.01	moderately positive
26	S+	1.00±0.12	highly positive
27	S-	0.18±0.13	moderately positive
28	S+	0.16±0.30	moderately positive
29	S-	0.26±0.60	highly positive
30	S+	0.14±0.02	moderately positive
31	S-	0.20±0.03	moderately positive
32	S+	1.51±0.08	highly positive
33	S+	0.41±0.09	highly positive
34	S+	0.40±0.07	highly positive
35	S+	0.27±0.06	highly positive
36	S+	0.31±0.04	highly positive
37	S+	0.23±0.02	highly positive
38	S+	0.37±0.05	highly positive
39	S-	0.18±0.02	moderately positive
40	S-	0.16±0.03	moderately positive
41	S-	0.22±0.04	moderately positive
42	S-	0.25±0.05	highly positive
43	S-	0.12±0.03	moderately positive

isolates respectively harbored the *fnbA* and *fnbB* genes. The *cna* gene coding for adhesin to collagen was detected in 32 strains (74.4%). Among the tested strains, 15 (34.9%), 8 (18.6%) and 13 (30.2%) were positive for *sspA*, *sspB* and *geh* genes.

Statistical analysis

Association between Congo red phenotypic test and adherence assay

Out of 20 highly-biofilm producing isolates, 18 showed a positive slime phenotype on Congo red agar. The nonparametric test of Mann Whitney U demonstrated that high biofilm production on polystyrene was significantly correlated with a positive Congo red phenotypic test (p = 0.017).

Association between biofilm production on polystyrene and biofilm related genes

Table 4 shows prevalence rates of MSCRAMMs genes (*fnbA*, *fnbB* and *cna*) and biofilm production control genes (*icaA* and *icaD*) depending on biofilm production. Univariate analysis followed by multivariate analysis showed that *fnbA* and *fnbB* genes were significantly associated with high biofilm production on polystyrene. However, no difference was observed in prevalence rates of *icaA*, *icaD* and *cna* genes between highly and moderately biofilm producing groups.

Association between biofilm production on polystyrene and exoenzymes genes

Table 5 details the prevalence rates of genes encoding serine protease (*sspA*), cysteine protease (*sspB*) and lipase (*geh*) in moderate and high biofilm-producing groups. Analysis showed that the presence of *sspB* gene was significantly associated with high biofilm production on polystyrene (p=0.003). However, no differences were found in prevalence rates of *sspA* and *geh* genes between both groups (Table 5).

Discussion

S. aureus has emerged in recent decades as one of the leading causes of hospital and community infections [12]. Its virulence is a multifactorial process requiring the use of a variety of components regulated in a coordinated manner [2]. In this study, we noted that all isolates were alpha or beta-hemolytic. This finding agrees with the results of Barretti et al [13]. Hemolysin-α has pore-forming and pro-inflammatory properties. It binds to a membrane receptor and disrupts the integrity of host cells [14]. As for β-toxin, it is known to be the "hot-cold" hemolysin with a sphingomyelinase and a biofilm ligase activities [15–17].

Protease, lipase and lecithinase secretion were detected in most tested strains. Similar results were found by

Table 4 Association between biofilm production on polystyrene and biofilm related genes

Genes		Moderately bioflm producers (*n*=23)	Highly biofilm producers (*n*=20)	P (univariate analysis)	P (multivariate analysis)
MSCRAMMs genes	*fnbA*+	14/23	18/20	0,001[a]	0,040
	fnbB+	2/23	6/20	0,002[a]	0,003
	cna+	15/23	17/20	0,154[a]	0,981
Biofilm production control genes	*icaA*+	13/23	17/20	0,143[a]	0,661
	icaD+	14/23	13/20	0,546	-

[a] Factor studied in mutivariate analysis

many reports [13, 18, 19]. *S. aureus* uses proteolytic and lipolytic exoenzymes to invade, damage the host tissue components and even spread to other sites [20]. They also protect against the innate immune system and are key mediators of secreted and cell wall-associated virulence determinant stability [21].

Biofilm formation is a major virulence factor. It provides inter-bacterial contact, accumulation of bacteria in superimposed layers, protection against the host immunity and acquisition of significant multiresistance [22, 23]. Our study showed that the majority of strains were slime producers on CRA. Several reports noted lower frequencies [13, 24–30]. In addition, all isolates were highly or moderately biofilm-forming on polystyrene. According to other studies, adhesion capacity was weaker [1, 4, 9, 10, 27, 28, 31–34]. This variability in adhesion capacity between MRSA strains can be explained by inter-strain variability of surface associated proteins and of biofilm production regulatory genes [23]. Significant association between biofilm production on polystyrene and Congo red test in our study highlights the performance of this non-costly phenotypic test to detect potential virulent *S. aureus* clinical isolates. Similarly, previous reports showed a high consistency between both tests [28, 30, 31].

Biofilm formation in *S. aureus* isolates occurs through the polysaccharide intercellular adhesin (PIA) as well as the MSCRAMMs. These structures provide initial binding of *S. aureus* to host tissues and biomaterials [29]. After the step of adhesion and colonization of host cells and mucous membranes, a phase of tissue invasion occurs. It was demonstrated that fibronectin binding proteins FnbA and FnbB are involved in bacterial invasion of the endothelial cells in vivo and in vitro [35]. Prevalences of *fnbA* and *fnbB* genes were higher in other studies [36, 37]. Moreover, the intracellular adhesion (*ica*) operon is essential for the control of biofilm production. The synthesis of polymer matrix exopolysaccharides is monitored by the *icaADBC* operon, which encodes three membrane proteins (IcaA, IcaD, and IcaC) with enzymatic activity and one extracellular protein (IcaB). The PIA, encoded by this operon, plays also an important role in adhesion to epithelial cells and allows escaping the immune system of the host. Frequencies of *icaA* and *icaD* genes were also higher in several previous studies [4, 24, 26–28, 35, 37]. Our results showed that *icaA* and *icaD* genes were not present in all highly biofilm formers. This discrepancy between biofilm phenotype and genotype could be due to the fact that *ica* expression is dependent on environmental conditions [38].

Adhesion to collagen plays an important role in the pathogenesis induced by *S. aureus* [36]. The collagen binding protein Cna is the second most important adhesion molecule. Furthermore, the recombinant Cna can even be designed as an effective vaccine component and antibodies raised against Cna are protective in a mouse model of *S. aureus* induced septic death [39]. Most of studied isolates were positive for *cna* gene. Other reports revealed lower rates [4, 35, 37, 40].

The complexity of bacterial tools used for cell adherence and invasion ranges from single monomeric proteins to intricate multimeric macromolecules that perform highly sophisticated functions [41]. In contrast with this study, *sspA*, *sspB* and *geh* genes were harbored by all strains of another report [40].

- With regard to the complexity and the variability of the biofilm phenotype, genetic studies identified numerous genes involved in biofilm formation.

Table 5 Association between biofilm production on polystyrene and exoenzymes genes

Exoenzymes genes	Moderately bioflm producers (*n*=23)	Highly biofilm producers (*n*=20)	P (univariate analysis)	P (bivariate analysis)
geh+	8/23	5/20	0,791	-
sspA+	6/23	9/20	0,117[a]	0,223
sspB+	1/23	5/20	0,013[a]	0,003

[a] Factor studied in bivariate analysis

However, their relative importance is still unclear [42]. In the light of this, our multivariate analysis showed that the presence of *fnbA* and *fnbB* genes was significantly associated with a high biofilm production on polystyrene. This consolidates the alleged role of these genes in biofilm formation. Comparably, some studies suggested that detection of some adhesion factors is more practical for the prediction of biofilm formation [4, 31, 43]. Other reports have shown the decisive role of the *ica* gene [32, 33]. However, no statistical difference was found in the distribution of genes by some researchs [28, 31]. Such investigations aim to find new attractive targets for antivirulence therapy by overcoming biofilm formation [31].

We also found a significant association between the presence of *sspB* gene and biofilm production. In fact, a number of soluble extracellular proteins can affect biofilm formation. The relationship between staphylococcal enzymes activities and biofilm formation was reported by some studies. However, it remains to be elucidated and merits further investigation [44].

Conclusion

In summary, most of our MRSA isolates were highly biofilm producers with elevated prevalences of some MSCRAMMs genes and biofilm production control genes. The present study indicates that the detection of the adhesion factors (*fnbA* and *fnbB* genes) contributing to the first step of biofilm formation can be used as a biofilm formation marker in *S. aureus*. Further in-depth research could be of value in the development of new preventive and therapeutic measures of staphylococcal infections.

Abbreviations

ATCC: American Type Culture Collection; Cna: Collagen binding protein; CRA: Congo red agar; DNA: Deoxyribonucleic acid; Fnb: Fibronectin binding protein; Ica: Intracellular adhesion; MRSA: Methicillin resistant *Staphylococcus aureus*; MSCRAMMs: Microbial Surface Components Recognizing Adhesive Matrix Molecules; OD: Optical density; PCR: Polymerase chain reaction; PIA: Polysaccharide intercellular adhesion; TSA: Trypticase soja agar

Acknowledgements

Not applicable.

Funding

This work was financed by the Higher education and scientific research in Tunisia through the laboratory of Transmissible Diseases and Biologically Active Substances, LR99ES27, Faculty of Pharmacy, Monastir University, street Avicenne 5000 Monastir (Tunisia).

Authors' contributions

OH, YK and MM collected and cultured the strains. OH, AM, AE and MM designed the experiments. OH, AM and HR carried out the experiments. OH and AE analyzed the data. OH, AM and MM prepared the manuscript. All authors read and approved the final manuscript.

Competing interests

The authors declare that they have no competing interests.

References

1. Naicker PR, Karayem K, Hoek KG, Harvey J, Wasserman E. Biofilm formation in invasive *Staphylococcus aureus* isolates is associated with the clonal lineage. Microb Pathog. 2016;90:41–9 https://doi.org/10.1016/j.micpath.2015.10.023.
2. Dinges MM, Orwin PM, Schlievert PM. Exotoxins of *Staphylococcus aureus*. Clin Microbiol Rev. 2000;13:16–34.
3. Donlan RM. Biofilms: microbial life on surfaces. Emerg Infect Dis. 2002;8:881–90 https://doi.org/10.3201/eid0809.020063.
4. Khoramian B, Jabalameli F, Niasari-Naslaji A, Taherikalani M, Emaneini M. Comparison of virulence factors and biofilm formation among *Staphylococcus aureus* strains isolated from human and bovine infections. Microb Pathog. 2015;88:73–7 https://doi.org/10.1016/j.micpath.2015.08.007.
5. Abraham NM, Jefferson KK. A low molecular weight component of serum inhibits biofilm formation in *Staphylococcus aureus*. Microb Pathog. 2010;49: 388–91 https://doi.org/10.1016/j.micpath.2010.07.005.
6. Dobinsky S, Kiel K, Rohde H, Bartscht K, Knobloch JK, Horstkotte MA, et al. Glucose-related dissociation between icaADBC transcription and biofilm expression by *Staphylococcus epidermidis*: evidence for an additional factor required for polysaccharide intercellular adhesin synthesis. J Bacteriol. 2003; 185:2879–86.
7. Milheiriço C, Oliveira DC, de Lencastre H. Multiplex PCR strategy for subtyping the staphylococcal cassette chromosome mec type IV in methicillin-resistant *Staphylococcus aureus*: 'SCCmec IV multiplex'. J Antimicrob Chemother. 2007;60:42–8 https://doi.org/10.1093/jac/dkm112.
8. Stulik L, Malafa S, Hudcova J, Rouha H, Henics BZ, Craven DE, et al. α-Hemolysin activity of methicillin-susceptible *Staphylococcus aureus* predicts ventilator-associated pneumonia. Am J Respir Crit Care Med. 2014;15:1139–48 https://doi.org/10.1164/rccm.201406-1012OC.
9. Kouidhi B, Zmantar T, Hentati H, Bakhrouf A. Cell surface hydrophobicity, formation, adhesives properties and molecular detection of adhesins genes in *Staphylococcus aureus* associated to dental caries. Microb Pathog. 2010; 49:14–22 https://doi.org/10.1016/j.micpath.2010.03.007.
10. Manago K, Nishi J, Wakimoto N, Miyanohara H, Sarantuya J, et al. Biofilm formation by and accessory gene regulator typing of methicilin-resistant *Staphylococcus aureus* strains recovered from patient with nosocomial infections. Infect Control Hosp Epidemiol. 2006;27:188–90 https://doi.org/10.1086/500620.
11. Stepanovic S, Vukovic D, Dakic I, Savic B, Svabic-Vlahovic M. A modified microtiter-plate test for quantification of staphylococcal biofilm formation. J Microbiol Methods. 2000;40:175–9.
12. Gould I. Costs of hospital-acquired methicillin-resistant *Staphylococcus aureus* (MRSA) and its control. Int J Antimicrob Agents. 2006;28:379–84 https://doi.org/10.1016/j.ijantimicag.2006.09.001.
13. Barretti P, Montelli AC, Batalha JE, Caramori JC, Cunha Mde L. The role of virulence factors in the outcome of staphylococcal peritonitis in CAPD patients. BMC Infect Dis. 2009;9(212) https://doi.org/10.1186/1471-2334-9-212.
14. Inoshima N, Wang Y, Wardenburg JB. Genetic requirement for ADAM10 in severe *Staphylococcus aureus* skin infection. J Invest Dermatol. 2012;132: 1513–6 https://doi.org/10.1038/jid.2011.
15. Salgado-Pabón W, Herrera A, Vu BG, Stach CS, Merriman JA, et al. *Staphylococcus aureus* β-toxin production is common in strains with the β-toxin gene inactivatedby bacteriophage. J Infect Dis. 2014;210:784–92 https://doi.org/10.1093/infdis/jiu146.
16. Diep BA, Carleton HA, Chang RF, Sensabaugh GF, Perdreau-Remington F. Roles of 34 virulence genes in the evolution of hospital- and community-associated strains of methicillin-resistant *Staphylococcus aureus*. J Infect Dis. 2006;193:1495–503 https://doi.org/10.1086/503777.
17. Huseby MJ, Kruse AC, Digre J, et al. Beta toxin catalyzes formation of nucleoprotein matrix in staphylococcal biofilms. Proc Natl Acad Sci USA. 2010;107:14407–12 https://doi.org/10.1073/pnas.0911032107.

18. Wu PZ, Zhu H, Thakur A, Willcox MD. Comparison of potential pathogenic traits of staphylococci that may contribute to corneal ulceration and inflammation. Aust N Z J Ophthalmol. 1999;27:234–6.
19. Lakshmi HP, Prasad UV, Yeswanth S, Swarupa V, Prasad OH, Narasu ML, et al. Molecular characterization of α-amylase from *Staphylococcus aureus*. Bioinformation. 2013;9:281–5. https://doi.org/10.6026/97320630009281.
20. Kolar SL, Ibarra JA, Rivera FE, Mootz JM, Davenport JE, et al. Extracellular proteases are key mediators of *Staphylococcus aureus* virulence via the global modulation of virulence-determinant stability. Microbiologyopen. 2013;2:18–34 https://doi.org/10.1002/mbo3.55.
21. Donlan RM, Costerton JW. Biofilms: survival mechanisms of clinically relevant microorganisms. Clin Microbiol Rev. 2002;15:167–93.
22. Pozzi C, Waters E, Rudkin J, Schaeffer C, Lohan A, Tong P, et al. Methicillin Resistance Alters the Biofilm Phenotype and Attenuates Virulence in *Staphylococcus aureus* Device-Associated Infections. PLoS Pathog. 2012;8: 1002626 https://doi.org/10.1371/journal.ppat.1002626.
23. Mulcahy ME, Geoghegan JA, Monk IR, O'Keeffe KM, Walsh EJ, Foster TJ, et al. Nasal colonisation by *Staphylococcus aureus* depends upon clumping factor B binding to the squamous epithelial cell envelope protein loricrin. PLoS Pathog. 2012;8:1003092 https://doi.org/10.1371/journal.ppat.1003092.
24. El-Mahallawy HA, Loutfy SA, El-Wakil M, El-Al AK, Morcos H. Clinical implications of icaA and icaD genes in coagulase negative staphylococci and *Staphylococcus aureus* bacteremia in febrile neutropenic pediatric cancer patients. Pediatr Blood Cancer. 2009;52:824–8 https://doi.org/10.1002/pbc.21964.
25. Elkhatib WF, Khairalla AS, Ashour HM. Evaluation of Different Microtiter Plate-Based Methods for the Quantitative Assessment of *Staphylococcus aureus* Biofilms. Future Microbiol. 2014;9:725–35 https://doi.org/10.2217/fmb.14.33.
26. Arciola CR, Baldassarri L, Montanaro L. Presence of icaA and icaD genes and slime production in a collection of staphylococcal strains from catheter-associated infections. J Clin Microbiol. 2001;39:2151–6 https://doi.org/10.1128/JCM.39.6.2151-2156.2001.
27. Lindsay JA, Moore CE, Day NP, Peacock SJ, Witney AA, Stabler RA. Microarrays reveal that each of the ten dominant lineages of *Staphylococcus aureus* has a unique combination of surface-associated and regulatory genes. J Bacteriol. 2006;188:669–76 https://doi.org/10.1128/JB.188.2.669-676.2006.
28. Grinholc M, Wegrzyn G, Kurlenda J. Evaluation of biofilm production and prevalence of the icaD gene in methicillin-resistant and methicillin-susceptible *Staphylococcus aureus* strains isolated from patients with nosocomial infections and carriers. FEMS Immunol Med Microbiol. 2007;50: 375–9 https://doi.org/10.1111/j.1574-695X.2007.00262.x.
29. Jain A, Agarwal A. Biofilm production, a marker of pathogenic potential of colonizing and commensal staphylococci. J Microbiol Methods. 2009;76:88–92. https://doi.org/10.1016/j.mimet.2008.09.017.
30. Arciola CR, Campoccia D, Baldassarri L, Donati ME, Pirini V, Gamberini S, et al. Detection of biofilm formation in *Staphylococcus epidermidis* from implant infections. Comparison of a PCR-method that recognizes the presence of ica genes with two classic phenotypic methods. J Biomed Mater Res A. 2006;76:425–30.
31. Cha JO, Yoo JI, Yoo JS, Chung HS, Park SH, Kim HS, et al. Investigation of Biofilm Formation and its Association with the Molecular and Clinical Characteristics of Methicillin-resistant *Staphylococcus aureus*. Osong Public Health Res Perspect. 2013;4:225–32 https://doi.org/10.1016/j.phrp.2013.09.001.
32. Nourbakhsh F, Namvar AE. Detection of genes involved in biofilm formation in *Staphylococcus aureus* isolates. GMS Hyg Infect Control. 2016;22(11) https://doi.org/10.3205/dgkh000267.
33. Szczuka E, Urbańska K, Pietryka M, Kaznowski A. Biofilm density and detection of biofilm-producing genes in methicillin-resistant *Staphylococcus aureus* strains. Folia Microbiol. 2013;58:47–52 https://doi.org/10.1007/s12223-012-0175-9.
34. Namvar AE, Asghari B, Ezzatifar F, Azizi G, Lari AR. Detection of the intercellular adhesion gene cluster (ica) in clinical *Staphylococcus aureus* isolates. GMS Hyg Infect Control. 2013;29(8) https://doi.org/10.3205/dgkh000203.
35. Peacock S, Moore C, Justice A, Kantazanou M, Story L, Mackie K, et al. Virulent combinations of adhesin and toxin genes in natural populations of *Staphylocccus aureus*. Infect Immun. 2002;70:4987–96.
36. Arciola CR, Campoccia D, Gamberini S, Baldassarri L, Montanaro L. Prevalence of cna, fnbA and fnbB adhesin genes among *Staphylococcus aureus* isolates from orthopedic infections associated to different types of implant. FEMS Microbiol Lett. 2005;246:81–6 https://doi.org/10.1016/j.femsle.2005.03.035.
37. Rahimi F, Katouli M, Karimi S. Biofilm production among methicillin resistant *Staphylococcus aureus* strains isolated from catheterized patients with urinary tract infection. Microb Pathog. 2016;98:69–76 https://doi.org/10.1016/j.micpath.2016.06.031.
38. Zmantar T, Chaieb K, Makni H, Miladi H, Abdallah FB, Mahdouani K, et al. Detection by PCR of adhesins genes and slime production in clinical *Staphylococcus aureus*. J Basic Microbiol. 2018;48:308–14 https://doi.org/10.1002/jobm.20070028.
39. Madani A, Garakani K, Mofrad MRK. Molecular mechanics of *Staphylococcus aureus* adhesin, CNA, and the inhibition of bacterial adhesion by stretching collagen. PLoS One. 2017;12:0179601 https://doi.org/10.1371/journal.pone.0179601.
40. Karlsson A, Arvidson S. Variation in extracellular protease production among clinical isolates of *Staphylococcus aureus* due to different levels of expression of the protease repressor sarA. Infect Immun. 2002;70:4239–46.
41. Pizzaro-Cerda J, Cossart P. Bacterial adhesion and entry into host cells. Cell. 2006;124:715–27 https://doi.org/10.1016/j.cell.2006.02.012.
42. Tang J, Chen J, Li H, Zeng P, Li J. Characterization of adhesin genes, staphylococcal nuclease, hemolysis and biofilm formation among *Staphylococcus aureus* strains isolated from different sources. Foodborne Pathog Dis. 2013;10:757–63 https://doi.org/10.1089/fpd.2012.1474.
43. O'Neill E, Pozzi C, Houston P, Humphreys H, Robinson DA, Loughman A, et al. A novel *Staphylococcus aureus* biofilm phenotype mediated by the fibronectin-binding proteins, FnBPA and FnBPB. J Bacteriol. 2008;190:3835–50 https://doi.org/10.1128/JB.00167-08.
44. Mann EE, Rice KC, Boles BR, Endres JL, Ranjit D, Chandramohan L, et al. Modulation of eDNA release and degradation affects *Staphylococcus aureus* biofilm maturation. PLoS One. 2009;9:e5822 https://doi.org/10.1371/journal.pone.0005822.
45. Saïd-Salim B, Dunman PM, McAleese FM, Macapagal D, Murphy E, McNamara PJ, et al. Global regulation of *Staphylococcus aureus* genes by Rot. J Bacteriol. 2003;185:610–9.

18

Less renal allograft fibrosis with valganciclovir prophylaxis for cytomegalovirus compared to high-dose valacyclovir: a parallel group, open-label, randomized controlled trial

Tomas Reischig[1,2*], Martin Kacer[1,2], Petra Hruba[2,3], Hana Hermanova[4], Ondrej Hes[2,5], Daniel Lysak[2,4], Stanislav Kormunda[2,6] and Mirko Bouda[1,2]

Abstract

Background: Cytomegalovirus (CMV) prophylaxis may prevent CMV indirect effects in renal transplant recipients. This study aimed to compare the efficacy of valganciclovir and valacyclovir prophylaxis for CMV after renal transplantation with the focus on chronic histologic damage within the graft.

Methods: From November 2007 through April 2012, adult renal transplant recipients were randomized, in an open-label, single-center study, at a 1:1 ratio to 3-month prophylaxis with valganciclovir ($n = 60$) or valacyclovir ($n = 59$). The primary endpoint was moderate-to-severe interstitial fibrosis and tubular atrophy assessed by protocol biopsy at 3 years evaluated by a single pathologist blinded to the study group. The analysis was conducted in an intention-to-treat population.

Results: Among the 101 patients who had a protocol biopsy specimen available, the risk of moderate-to-severe interstitial fibrosis and tubular atrophy was significantly lower in those treated with valganciclovir (22% versus 34%; adjusted odds ratio, 0.31; 95% confidence interval, 0.11–0.90; $P = 0.032$ by multivariate logistic regression). The incidence of CMV disease (9% versus 2%; $P = 0.115$) and CMV DNAemia (36% versus 42%; $P = 0.361$) were not different at 3 years.

Conclusions: Valganciclovir prophylaxis, as compared with valacyclovir, was associated with a reduced risk of moderate-to-severe interstitial fibrosis and tubular atrophy in patients after renal transplantation.

Keywords: Cytomegalovirus, Valganciclovir, Prophylaxis, Fibrosis, Renal transplantation

Background

Management of infectious diseases is a critical component of care of solid organ transplant recipients. Both cytomegalovirus (CMV) disease and asymptomatic CMV replication results in increased mortality and graft loss rates [1–5]. These impacts are driven mainly by the cellular and immunological effects of CMV including alloimmune response upregulation by innate immune mechanisms and/or cross-reactivity of CMV-specific T cells with donor MHC-peptide complexes [1, 6–9]. In addition to enhanced graft rejection rates, CMV has been shown to increase the risk of cardiovascular events and other opportunistic infections and is likely to play a role in the development of diabetes and cancer after transplantation [10–13].

Renal allograft fibrosis is the ultimate non-specific histological picture of various allograft injuries [14, 15].

* Correspondence: reischig@fnplzen.cz
[1]Department of Internal Medicine I, Faculty of Medicine in Pilsen, Charles University, Czech Republic and Teaching Hospital, 30460 Pilsen, Czech Republic
[2]Biomedical Centre, Faculty of Medicine in Pilsen, Charles University, 32300 Pilsen, Czech Republic
Full list of author information is available at the end of the article

Moderate-to-severe interstitial fibrosis and tubular atrophy (IFTA) is strong predictor of deteriorated graft survival [16]. The underlying mechanism in the development and progression of fibrosis is activation of the inflammatory cascade with subsequent formation of profibrotic mediators such as TGF-β [14]. Together with donor characteristics, there are a host of post-transplant contributors to IFTA development including inflammation associated with viral infections [14, 15]. Multiple studies have documented upregulation of profibrotic and vasculopathic growth factors in CMV infection, with some studies also reporting a higher incidence of IFTA in patients after previous CMV replication [6, 17–19].

CMV prevention taking the form of prophylaxis or preemptive therapy is recommended [2]. Either strategy results in a reduced incidence of CMV disease and infection, with lower mortality and acute rejection rates as an additional plus with prophylaxis [20–23]. As an alternative to valganciclovir prophylaxis in renal transplant recipients, valacyclovir has also been well documented to be effective [20, 22–24]. Still, in a long-term comparison with valganciclovir-based pre-emptive therapy, valacyclovir prophylaxis was associated with a higher incidence of severe IFTA and inferior graft survival [25].

To establish potential differences between valganciclovir and valacyclovir prophylaxis, we performed a randomized trial (2VAL Study) showing a decrease in the rates of acute rejection with valganciclovir [26]. This article presents the long-term results of the 2VAL Study focused primarily on the incidence of IFTA in late protocol biopsies.

Methods

Patients and interventions

Details of the study design were published previously [26]. In brief, adult renal transplant recipients from a single center were recruited from November 2007 through April 2012. The major exclusion criterion was recipient (R) and donor (D) negative CMV serology (D−/R-). Patients were randomized by the transplant physician using a random-number table, at a 1:1 ratio, to valganciclovir (900 mg daily) or valacyclovir (2 g four times daily) prophylaxis for 3 months. Sequentially numbered sealed envelopes were used for allocation concealment. Polymerase chain reaction (PCR) for CMV DNA from whole blood was performed at predefined time points during the first 12 months [26]. After 12 months, PCR was performed only if clinically required.

The protocol of immunosuppression was described previously [26]. Recipients of grafts from highly marginal donors were treated with basiliximab and low-dose tacrolimus. Polyoma BK virus (BKV) DNAemia was tested every month for the first 6 months, 3 months until 24 months, at 36 months, and if clinically indicated.

Study outcomes and follow-up

The primary endpoint was the incidence of moderate-to-severe IFTA assessed on protocol biopsy at 36 months. Secondary endpoints included intrarenal mRNA expression of profibrotic genes, chronic rejection, CMV DNAemia, CMV disease, biopsy-proven acute rejection, renal function, patient and graft survival (not censored for death), and other infections. In addition, other potential indirect effects of CMV such as cardiovascular events or new-onset diabetes mellitus, malignancy, and routine laboratory parameters were recorded prospectively. All patients remained on follow-up for a minimum of 4 years after transplantation or until death. Patient and graft survival was assessed at 4 years, with other variables at the end of 3 years.

Protocol biopsy sample processing

In patients with functioning grafts, protocol biopsy was performed at 36 months using an 18-gauge needle (biopsy gun). A minimum of two cores were obtained. Tissues for light microscopy were fixed in 4% formaldehyde, embedded in paraffin using routine procedure, and processed as described previously [25]. All biopsies were evaluated according to the Banff classification by a single pathologist blinded to the study group of the patients [27]. Intrarenal mRNA expression analysis was performed as described previously (Additional file 1: Table S1) [4, 25].

Sample size and statistical analysis

We anticipated a 40% incidence of moderate-to-severe IFTA in late protocol biopsy [28]. Based on the association between acute rejection and IFTA [14, 15] and reduction in acute rejection with valacyclovir [23, 24], we assumed a 50% reduction in the relative risk for moderate-to-severe IFTA in the valacyclovir group. It was necessary to enroll at least 82 patients to ensure an 80% power to detect a treatment difference with a type 1 error of 0.05. A minimum of 114 patients was required for the 12-month primary endpoint (acute rejection) assessment [26]. This number was considered sufficient even with the anticipation of patients lost to late protocol biopsy.

Quantitative parametric data were compared using Student's t-test and the Mann-Whitney U-test in non-parametric distribution. Qualitative data were analyzed using the chi-square or Fisher exact test. The risk of moderate-to-severe IFTA in the valganciclovir group compared to valacyclovir was calculated by logistic regression. Because of an imbalance in high-risk donor distribution and related immunosuppression, the odds ratio (OR), and 95% confidence interval (CI) adjusted for calcineurin inhibitor, induction therapy, and advanced chronic histologic damage (moderate-to-severe nephrosclerosis, diabetic nephropathy and/or ≥ 15% of glomerulosclerosis) in donor procurement biopsy were calculated by multivariate logistic regression. The incidence of time dependent variables was calculated using Kaplan-Meier curves, with the log-rank test and the Cox proportional hazard model adjusting for the above variables. Data were analyzed according to the intention-to-treat principle. Statistical calculations were made using SAS software (SAS Institute Inc., Cary, NC). Values of $P < 0.05$ were considered statistically significant.

Results

Study population

Overall, 119 patients were enrolled (Fig. 1), of which number 60 were randomized to valganciclovir prophylaxis and 59 to valacyclovir. The almost double the number of patients treated with basiliximab induction and low-dose tacrolimus protocol, indicated only in high-risk donors, and a detailed analysis of donor procurement biopsies revealed a lower quality of donors in the valganciclovir group (Table 1, Additional file 1: Table S2). The groups did not differ in maintenance immunosuppressive therapy including drug levels and doses in the ensuing years (Additional file 1: Table S3).

Primary endpoint: IFTA in protocol biopsy at 3 years

Protocol biopsy at 36 months with sufficient material was performed in 51 and 50 patients in the valganciclovir and valacyclovir groups, respectively. The main causes for not performing biopsy were death or graft loss. Moderate-to-severe IFTA was less frequent in the valganciclovir group (11 of 51 [22%] versus 17 of 50 [34%]; OR, 0.53; 95% CI, 0.22–1.30; $P = 0.166$ by logistic regression) (Table 2). After adjustment for baseline characteristics, which reflected the higher proportion of high-risk donors in the valganciclovir group, the risk for developing moderate-to-severe IFTA was significantly lower in valganciclovir-treated patients (aOR, 0.31; 95% CI, 0.11–0.90; $P = 0.032$ by multivariate logistic regression). Advanced chronic

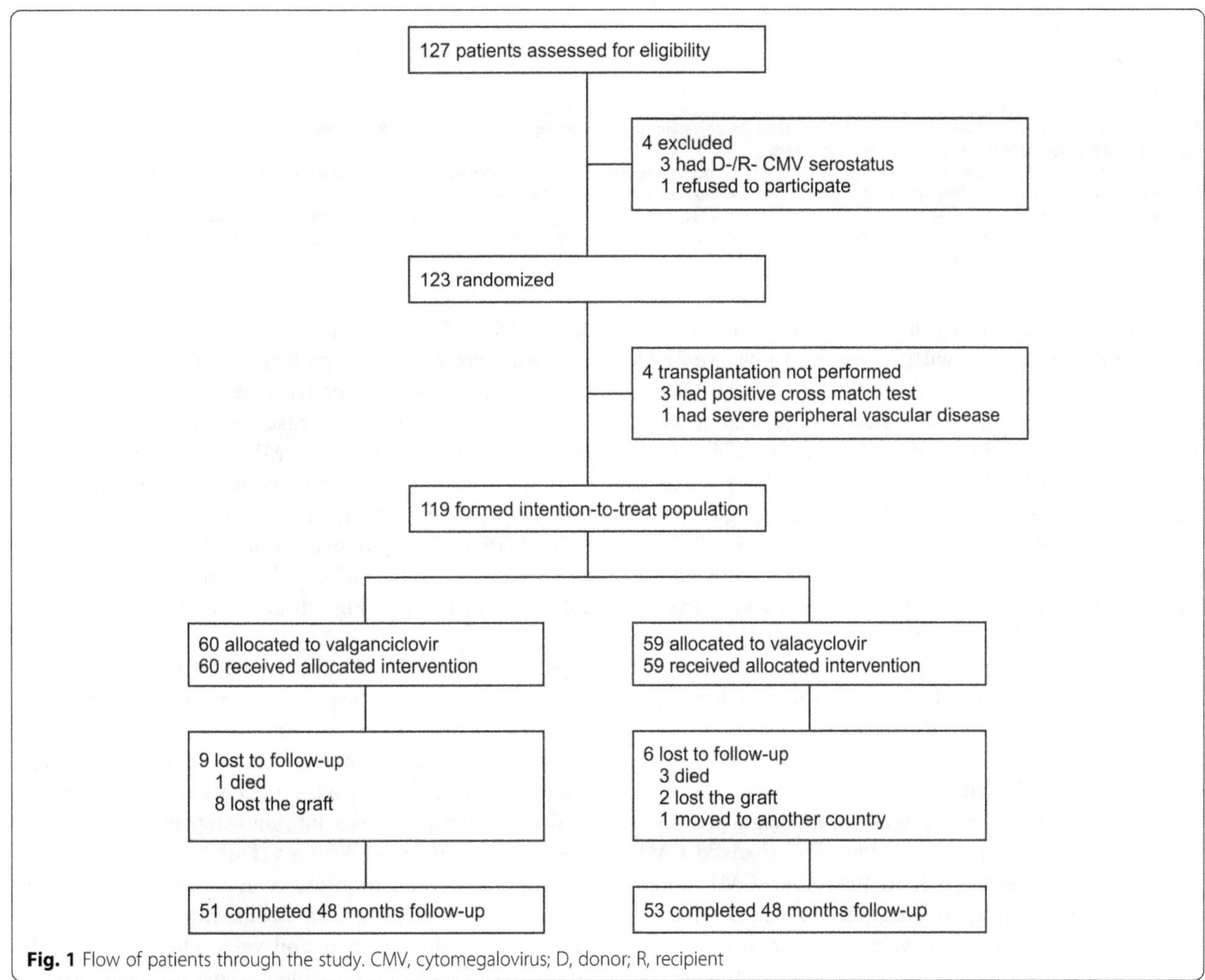

Fig. 1 Flow of patients through the study. CMV, cytomegalovirus; D, donor; R, recipient

Table 1 Patient characteristics of the intention-to-treat population

Characteristic	Valganciclovir (*n* = 60)	Valacyclovir (*n* = 59)	*P* Value
Recipient			
Age (yr)	48 ± 13	50 ± 11	0.224
Gender (male)	47 (78)	37 (63)	0.095
Previous transplantation	9 (15)	7 (12)	0.816
HLA mismatches (n)	3.5 ± 1.2	3.6 ± 1.5	0.508
CMV serostatus			0.289
D+/R-	7 (12)	4 (7)	
D+/R+	44 (73)	49 (83)	
D−/R+	9 (15)	6 (10)	
Donor			
Age (yr)	50 ± 16	49 ± 16	0.702
Donor type (deceased)	57 (95)	54 (92)	0.696
Expanded-criteria donor[a]	34 (57)	32 (54)	0.935
Advanced chronic histologic damage[b]	15 (25)	9 (15)	0.185
Primary immunosuppression[c]			
Cyclosporine + mycophenolate mofetil	25 (42)	35 (59)	0.081
Tacrolimus + mycophenolate mofetil	35 (58)	24 (41)	
No induction therapy	25 (42)	34 (58)	0.119
Basiliximab	26 (43)	14 (24)	0.039
Thymoglobulin	9 (15)	11 (19)	0.775

Data are number of patients (percentage) or mean ± standard deviation. CMV, cytomegalovirus; D, donor; R, recipient

[a]According to the United Network for Organ Sharing criteria

[b]A minimum 1 of the following findings on donor procurement biopsy: moderate-to-severe vascular nephrosclerosis, diabetic nephropathy, and/or ≥ 15% of glomerulosclerosis. Procurement biopsy was performed in 61 selected donors considered to be at increased risk

[c]Low-dose tacrolimus with basiliximab induction was used in recipients of grafts from highly marginal donors (age ≥ 70 years, donors with hypertension or diabetes with impaired renal function or biopsy findings of vascular nephrosclerosis, diabetic nephropathy and/or ≥ 15% of glomerulosclerosis, donors after cardiac death, and dual kidney transplantation)

histologic damage in donor procurement biopsy was significantly associated with moderate-to-severe IFTA (aOR, 7.05; 95% CI, 2.28–21.8; $P < 0.001$). While patients experiencing acute rejection showed a trend toward an increase in moderate-to-severe IFTA (41% versus 23%; aOR, 2.89; 95% CI, 0.88–9.73; $P = 0.087$), the effect of polyoma BKV viremia was negligible (29% versus 27%; aOR, 0.60; 95% CI, 0.18–2.07; $P = 0.422$).

Patients with moderate-to-severe IFTA showed increased intrarenal mRNA expression of a wide range of profibrotic genes (Additional file 1: Table S4). However, univariate unadjusted analysis did not document any significant differences between the valganciclovir and valacyclovir groups (data not shown).

CMV disease and DNAemia

After 12 months, CMV disease was diagnosed in 2 valganciclovir group patients. One case involved CMV syndrome in a D+/R- patient, the other CMV colitis after thymoglobulin administration for acute rejection despite a new course of valganciclovir prophylaxis. The difference was not statistically significant at 36 months (Fig. 2a). After 12 months, CMV DNAemia was present in 5 patients in the valganciclovir group with 3 cases involved a new-onset episode and 2 a recurrent one in contrast to 1 recurrent episode in the valacyclovir group. CMV DNAemia with viral load of ≥1000 copies/mL comprised 3 out of 5 episodes in the valganciclovir group and a single episode in the valacyclovir group. At 36 months, the cumulative incidence of CMV DNAemia was comparable in both groups (Fig. 2b and Table 3).

Rejection, polyomavirus infection, and other outcomes

After 12 months, late acute rejection was detected in 4 and 1 patients in the valganciclovir and valacyclovir groups, respectively. In the valganciclovir group, the event was preceded, in all 4 patients, by their demonstrable noncompliance or immunosuppression reduction due to infectious complications (Fig. 2c).

While, after 12 months, a new-onset episode of polyoma BKV viremia was documented in 4 patients in both the valganciclovir and valacyclovir groups, the cumulative incidence remained – given the differences

Table 2 Histological findings in protocol biopsy at 36 months after transplantation

Characteristic	Valganciclovir ($n = 51$)[a]	Valacyclovir ($n = 50$)[a]	aOR (95% CI)[b]	P Value[c]
Glomeruli per biopsy	10.5 ± 7.6	13.0 ± 6.0		0.004
Arteries per biopsy	1.7 ± 0.9	1.7 ± 1.1		0.903
Moderate-to-severe IFTA[d]	11 (22)	17 (34)	0.31 (0.11–0.90)	0.032
IF/TA (all grades)	21 (41)	24 (48)		0.624
Chronic "ci + ct" score	1.64 ± 1.64	1.82 ± 1.59		0.529
Subclinical rejection	2 (4)	2 (4)		0.624
Borderline changes	7 (14)	3 (6)		0.334
Chronic antibody-mediated rejection	6 (12)	6 (12)		0.786
Chronic T-cell-mediated rejection	2 (4)	1 (2)		0.986
Calcineurin inhibitor toxicity	1 (2)	2 (4)		0.986
Vascular nephrosclerosis	13 (25)	14 (28)		0.952
Glomerulonephritis recurrence	2 (4)	0 (0)		0.484

Data are number of patients (percentage) or mean ± standard deviation. aOR, adjusted odds ratio; CI, confidence interval; IFTA, interstitial fibrosis and tubular atrophy; ci, interstitial fibrosis score; ct, tubular atrophy score

[a]Biopsy not available in valganciclovir: 6 death or graft loss, 1 refused, 2 insufficient material; in valacyclovir: 4 death or graft loss, 1 lost to follow up, 1 technical reason, 3 insufficient material

[b]Adjusted for calcineurin inhibitor, induction therapy, and advanced chronic histologic damage in donor biopsy

[c]Multivariate logistic regression for moderate-to-severe IFTA comparison; chi-squared or Fisher exact test for categorical variables; Mann-Whitney U-test for continuous variables

[d]Grade 2 or more according to the Banff 2013 classification

within the first 12 months – higher with valganciclovir (42% versus 26%; $P = 0.046$ by log-rank test) (Fig. 2d). Likewise, although not significantly different, the incidence of polyomavirus-associated nephropathy (PVAN) was higher in the valganciclovir group (12% versus 4%; $P = 0.098$ by log-rank test). PVAN had an appreciably adverse effect on graft survival (56% versus 91%; $P < 0.001$ by log-rank test) with 3 graft losses directly related to PVAN in valganciclovir-treated patients. The groups did not differ in the incidence of other viral, bacterial, and fungal infections.

At 4 years, patient and graft survival rates were excellent in either group. Regarding the other secondary outcomes, no differences were found between the groups (Table 4).

Discussion

Long-term results of this only randomized study comparing valganciclovir and valacyclovir for CMV prophylaxis in renal transplant recipients published to date demonstrated a lower incidence of moderate-to-severe IFTA at 3 years in patients treated with valganciclovir. This finding was unexpected at study initiation given the promising results of valacyclovir prophylaxis in reducing the risk of rejection in earlier studies [23, 24]. Still, it is fully consistent with the 12-month data of the present study documenting a significant decrease in acute rejection rates with valganciclovir prophylaxis. By contrast, polyoma BKV viremia, whose incidence was increased at 12 months in the valganciclovir group, had no adverse impact on the risk of IFTA [26]. Severe forms of IFTA are associated with a marked increase in the risk of graft failure [14, 16]. The negative effect of IFTA is further enhanced by co-existing graft inflammation or circulating donor-specific anti-HLA antibodies (DSA) [15, 16]. While effective prevention of IFTA from developing is critical for improving transplantation outcomes, it is most difficult because of its multifactorial etiology [14]. Our study has suggested that optimal CMV prevention could be part of a comprehensive strategy to reduce IFTA incidence.

The dominant factors leading to the development and progression of IFTA include nonspecific inflammation and, particularly, inflammation secondary to alloimmune activation. Acute rejection, subclinical rejection including antibody-mediated rejection or the presence of DSA have a strong profibrotic potential and result in the development of severe IFTA with overlapping gene expression profile of biopsies with IFTA and immune-mediated inflammation [15, 29–31]. Because of CMV-associated intragraft inflammation, CMV is a potential risk factor for IFTA regardless of whether the underlying mechanism is heterologous immunity or promotion of local inflammation [6]. Cytomegalovirus significantly increases the risk of acute cellular rejection and, in patients with DSA, it may be involved in the pathogenesis of antibody-mediated rejection [8, 10]. In our study, the reduction of IFTA in patients receiving valganciclovir prophylaxis cannot be explained by different efficacy in CMV prevention. The rates of CMV DNAemia were comparable both in the long-term and early

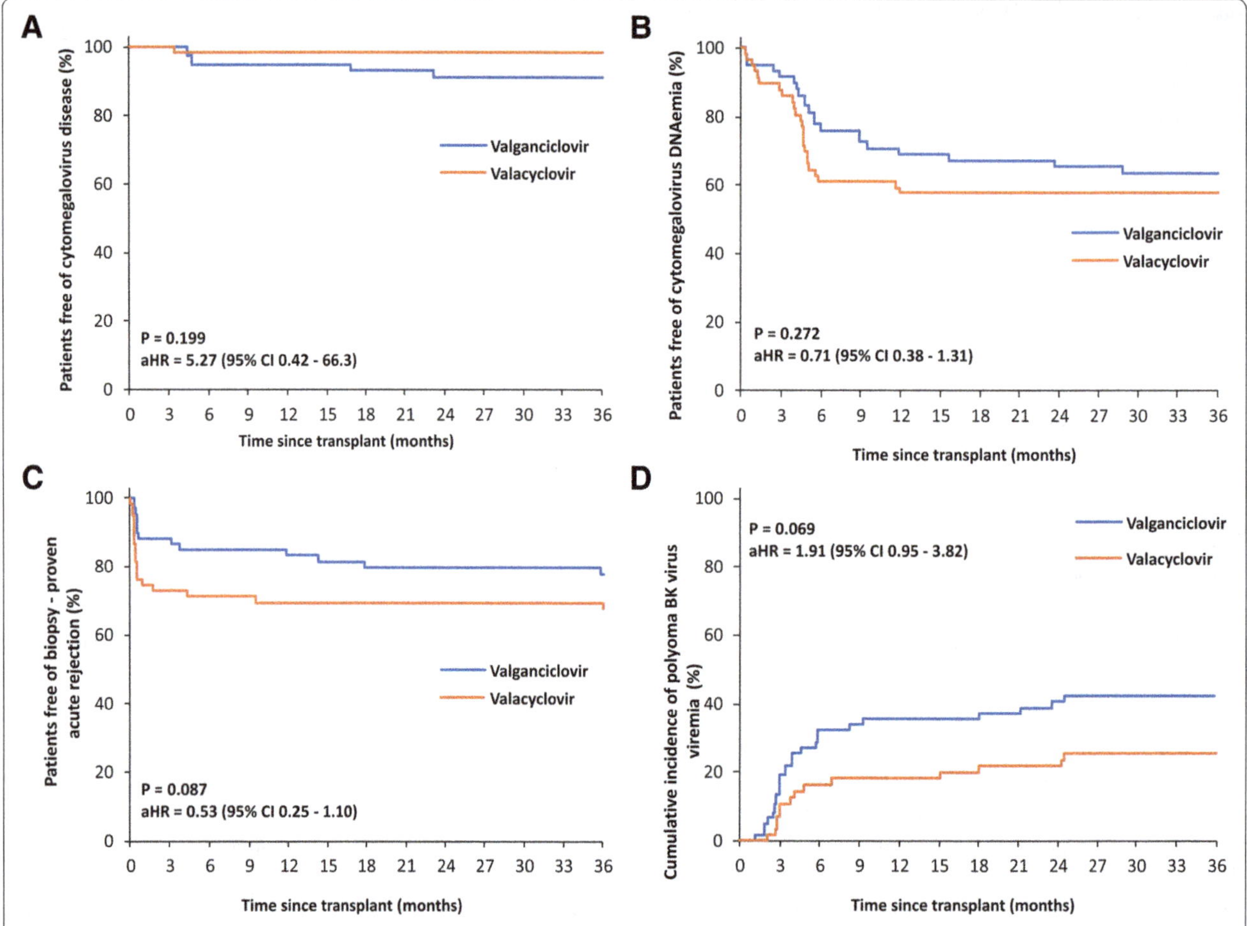

Fig. 2 Kaplan-Meier curves for the cumulative probability of freedom from CMV disease (**a**), CMV DNAemia (**b**), biopsy-proven acute rejection (**c**), and polyoma BK virus viremia (**d**). The Cox proportional hazard model adjusting for calcineurin inhibitor, induction therapy, and advanced chronic histologic damage in donor biopsy. *aHR* adjusted hazard ratio, *CI* confidence interval

period (within 3 months) after transplantation [26]. The most logical cause is the decrease in acute rejection in patients randomized to valganciclovir [26]. Consistent with the above studies, the risk of our patients experiencing acute rejection to develop moderate-to-severe IFTA was almost three times higher. The difference in the incidence of acute rejection occurred in the early post-transplant period. One could speculate that the incidence of subclinical inflammation over the first post-transplant weeks could be also decreased with valganciclovir. While, in our study, the first protocol biopsy was not performed until month 3, recent data suggest a high proportion of inflammation associated mainly with mild IFTA detected by protocol biopsy at 6 weeks [30]. Early subclinical inflammation constitutes a risk factor for IFTA progression [30].

The present study is a second trial documenting inferior outcomes of valacyclovir prophylaxis compared to valganciclovir-based CMV prevention. Compared with preemptive therapy, valacyclovir prophylaxis was associated with a higher incidence of IFTA and profibrotic gene expression [25]. In an animal model, ganciclovir prophylaxis attenuated late renal allograft damage and reduced intragraft immune infiltrates persisting even after prophylaxis discontinuation [32]. A theory explaining the lower rates of acute rejection and subsequent IFTA development with valganciclovir prophylaxis is built on reduced intragraft inflammation through a direct effect of ganciclovir on T-lymphocytes. In studies with healthy volunteers and renal transplant recipients, (val) ganciclovir suppressed T-lymphocyte proliferation and activation by impaired DNA synthesis [33, 34]. Further studies are warranted to confirm the clinical relevance of this theory.

The decrease in IFTA over the 4 years of follow-up did not result in better graft survival in the valganciclovir group. Lower quality donors may have influenced graft survival. While it is likely that follow-up may have been still too short in this respect, an alternative explanation may be an increased incidence of polyoma BKV infection. In our study, BKV viremia was not shown to

Table 3 Details on CMV infection during 36 months

Characteristic	Valganciclovir ($n = 60$)	Valacyclovir ($n = 59$)	P Value
CMV Disease	5 (9)	1 (2)	0.115[a]
CMV Disease by D/R status			
D+/R-	3 (49)	0 (0)	0.125
D+/R+	2 (5)	1 (2)	0.555
D–/R+	0 (0)	0 (0)	–
CMV DNAemia	21 (36)	24 (42)	0.361[a]
CMV DNAemia by D/R status			
D+/R-	4 (64)	2 (50)	0.986
D+/R+	14 (32)	21 (45)	0.180
D–/R+	5 (50)	1 (17)	0.264
Peak viral load (copies/mL)	350 (100–6150)	850 (100–1650)	0.982
Duration of CMV DNAemia (d)	40 (27–78)	31 (15–69)	0.270

Data are number of patients (percentage) or median and interquartile range. CMV, cytomegalovirus; D, donor; R, recipient
[a]CMV Disease: adjusted hazard ratio, 4.96; 95% confidence interval, 0.57–43.1; $P = 0.147$; CMV DNAemia: adjusted hazard ratio, 0.78; 95% confidence interval, 0.43–1.42; $P = 0.418$ by multivariate Cox proportional hazard model after adjustment for calcineurin inhibitor, induction therapy, and advanced chronic histologic damage in donor biopsy

negatively impact the risk of moderate-to-severe IFTA or graft loss, which comes as no surprise since low-viral load BKV viremia was predominantly involved. The risk of graft loss or graft dysfunction is increased with persistent high-viral load BKV viremia or PVAN, where recent data have additionally suggested increased de novo production of DSA [35, 36]. The numerically higher incidence of PVAN in patients treated with valganciclovir prophylaxis requires extra caution. While our study was not powered to detect significant differences in the incidence of PVAN, the rates were clinically not negligible with 3 cases of graft loss directly related to PVAN in the valganciclovir group. Also in a recently published study, full dose valganciclovir prophylaxis resulted in higher rates of PVAN [37]. It is conceivable that valganciclovir had an effect on the BKV-specific cellular immune response making BKV replication more frequent [38, 39].

Several limitations of the study should be mentioned. Despite adequate randomization, there was an imbalance in the proportion of high-risk donors tilted against the valganciclovir group. As expected, tacrolimus-based immunosuppression indicated in at-risk donors and the presence of advanced chronic histologic damage in donor procurement biopsy were strongly associated with moderate-to-severe IFTA. As donor quality is a major risk factor in the development of severe IFTA [14, 16], it was critical to adjust the risk of moderate-to-severe IFTA and other important secondary outcomes for baseline imbalance [40]. Some univariate analyses related to IFTA, and intragraft mRNA gene expression in particular, may have put the valganciclovir group at a disadvantage. Another limitation was the small number of CMV D+/R- patients which does not allow to extrapolate our results to high-risk patients. Generally, the sample size of our study precludes adequate assessment of any potential differences in some secondary outcomes.

Conclusion

Compared with valacyclovir, valganciclovir prophylaxis is associated with lower risk of moderate-to-severe IFTA at

Table 4 Patient and graft survival and other secondary outcomes

Characteristic	Valganciclovir ($n = 60$)	Valacyclovir ($n = 59$)	P Value
Patient survival	59 (98)	56 (95)	0.297
Graft survival	51 (85)	54 (92)	0.287
Estimated GFR[a] (mL/min/1.73 m^2)	54 ± 20	52 ± 19	0.594
Urine protein-to-creatinine ratio (mg/mmol)	23 ± 49	24 ± 43	0.339
Cardiovascular events	15 (25)	14 (24)	0.985
New-onset diabetes or IFG	26 (46)	20 (38)	0.521
Malignancy	6 (10)	2 (3)	0.283

Data are number of patients (percentage) or mean ± standard deviation. GFR, glomerular filtration rate; IFG, impaired fasting glucose
[a]According to the Modification of Diet in Renal Disease 7 formula

3 years after renal transplantation. Further studies are warranted to determine whether the more favorable late histologic findings reported with valganciclovir-based regimens stand out only when compared with high-dose valacyclovir prophylaxis or, possibly, with investigational drugs for CMV prevention such as brincidofovir or letermovir [25, 41, 42].

Abbreviations
aOR: adjusted odds ratio; CI: confidence interval; CMV: cytomegalovirus; D: donor; DSA: donor-specific anti-HLA antibodies; IFTA: interstitial fibrosis and tubular atrophy; PCR: polymerase chain reaction; PVAN: polyomavirus-associated nephropathy; R: recipient

Acknowledgements
The authors thank Lenka Karlikova for her assistance in data collection.

Funding
This work was supported by the National Sustainability Program I [LO1503] provided by the Ministry of Education, Youth and Sports of the Czech Republic, the Charles University Research Fund [Progres Q39], and in part by Institute for Clinical and Experimental Medicine [MZO 00023001].

Authors' contribution
TR wrote the article, designed the study, collected clinical variables, participated in data analysis and interpretation. MK collected clinical variables, participated in data analysis and interpretation, revised the article. PH participated in study design, performed intrarenal gene expression, revised the article. HH performed PCR for CMV DNA, revised the article. OH evaluated kidney graft biopsies, revised the article. DL performed PCR for CMV DNA, revised the article. SK performed statistical analyses, revised the article. MB collected clinical variables, revised the article. All authors read and approved the final manuscript.

Competing interests
The authors declare that they have no competing interests.

Author details
[1]Department of Internal Medicine I, Faculty of Medicine in Pilsen, Charles University, Czech Republic and Teaching Hospital, 30460 Pilsen, Czech Republic. [2]Biomedical Centre, Faculty of Medicine in Pilsen, Charles University, 32300 Pilsen, Czech Republic. [3]Transplant Laboratory, Institute for Clinical and Experimental Medicine, 14021 Prague, Czech Republic. [4]Department of Hemato-oncology, Teaching Hospital, 30460 Pilsen, Czech Republic. [5]Department of Pathology, Faculty of Medicine in Pilsen, Charles University, Czech Republic and Teaching Hospital, 30460 Pilsen, Czech Republic. [6]Division of Information Technologies and Statistics, Faculty of Medicine in Pilsen, Charles University, 32300 Pilsen, Czech Republic.

References
1. Fishman JA. Infection in organ transplantation. Am J Transplant. 2017; 17(4):856–79.
2. Kotton CN, Kumar D, Caliendo AM, Asberg A, Chou S, Danziger-Isakov L, Humar A. Transplantation society international CMVCG: updated international consensus guidelines on the management of cytomegalovirus in solid-organ transplantation. Transplantation. 2013;96(4):333–60.
3. Sagedal S, Hartmann A, Nordal KP, Osnes K, Leivestad T, Foss A, Degre M, Fauchald P, Rollag H. Impact of early cytomegalovirus infection and disease on long-term recipient and kidney graft survival. Kidney Int. 2004;66(1):329–37.
4. Reischig T, Kacer M, Hruba P, Jindra P, Hes O, Lysak D, Bouda M, Viklicky O. The impact of viral load and time to onset of cytomegalovirus replication on long-term graft survival after kidney transplantation. Antivir Ther. 2017; 22(6):503–13.
5. Lollinga WT, Rurenga-Gard L, van Doesum W, van Bergen R, Diepstra A, Vonk JM, Riezebos-Brilman A, Niesters HGM, van Son WJ, van den Born J, et al. High human cytomegalovirus DNAemia early post-transplantation associates with irreversible and progressive loss of renal function - a retrospective study. Transpl Int. 2017;30(8):817–26.
6. Kaminski H, Fishman JA. The cell biology of cytomegalovirus: implications for transplantation. Am J Transplant. 2016;16(8):2254–69.
7. Dzabic M, Rahbar A, Yaiw KC, Naghibi M, Religa P, Fellstrom B, Larsson E, Soderberg-Naucler C. Intragraft cytomegalovirus protein expression is associated with reduced renal allograft survival. Clin Infect Dis. 2011; 53(10):969–76.
8. Bachelet T, Couzi L, Pitard V, Sicard X, Rigothier C, Lepreux S, Moreau JF, Taupin JL, Merville P, Dechanet-Merville J. Cytomegalovirus-responsive gammadelta T cells: novel effector cells in antibody-mediated kidney allograft microcirculation lesions. J Am Soc Nephrol. 2014;25(11):2471–82.
9. Heutinck KM, Yong SL, Tonneijck L, van den Heuvel H, van der Weerd NC, van der Pant KA, Bemelman FJ, Claas FH, Ten Berge IJ. Virus-specific CD8(+) T cells cross-reactive to donor-alloantigen are transiently present in the circulation of kidney transplant recipients infected with CMV and/or EBV. Am J Transplant. 2016;16(5):1480–91.
10. Reischig T, Jindra P, Svecova M, Kormunda S, Opatrny K Jr, Treska V. The impact of cytomegalovirus disease and asymptomatic infection on acute renal allograft rejection. J Clin Virol. 2006;36(2):146–51.
11. Courivaud C, Bamoulid J, Chalopin JM, Gaiffe E, Tiberghien P, Saas P, Ducloux D. Cytomegalovirus exposure and cardiovascular disease in kidney transplant recipients. J Infect Dis. 2013;207(10):1569–75.
12. Hjelmesaeth J, Sagedal S, Hartmann A, Rollag H, Egeland T, Hagen M, Nordal KP, Jenssen T. Asymptomatic cytomegalovirus infection is associated with increased risk of new-onset diabetes mellitus and impaired insulin release after renal transplantation. Diabetologia. 2004;47(9):1550–6.
13. Courivaud C, Bamoulid J, Gaugler B, Roubiou C, Arregui C, Chalopin JM, Borg C, Tiberghien P, Woronoff-Lemsi MC, Saas P, et al. Cytomegalovirus exposure, immune exhaustion and cancer occurrence in renal transplant recipients. Transpl Int. 2012;25(9):948–55.
14. Vanhove T, Goldschmeding R, Kuypers D. Kidney fibrosis: origins and interventions. Transplantation. 2017;101(4):713–26.
15. Gosset C, Viglietti D, Rabant M, Verine J, Aubert O, Glotz D, Legendre C, Taupin JL, Duong Van-Huyen JP, Loupy A, et al. Circulating donor-specific anti-HLA antibodies are a major factor in premature and accelerated allograft fibrosis. Kidney Int. 2017;92(3):729–42.
16. Cosio FG, El Ters M, Cornell LD, Schinstock CA, Stegall MD. Changing kidney allograft histology early Posttransplant: prognostic implications of 1-year protocol biopsies. Am J Transplant. 2016;16(1):194–203.
17. Inkinen K, Soots A, Krogerus L, Loginov R, Bruggeman C, Lautenschlager I. Cytomegalovirus enhance expression of growth factors during the development of chronic allograft nephropathy in rats. Transpl Int. 2005; 18(6):743–9.
18. Reischig T, Jindra P, Hes O, Bouda M, Kormunda S, Treska V. Effect of cytomegalovirus viremia on subclinical rejection or interstitial fibrosis and tubular atrophy in protocol biopsy at 3 months in renal allograft recipients managed by preemptive therapy or antiviral prophylaxis. Transplantation. 2009;87(3):436–44.
19. Smith JM, Corey L, Bittner R, Finn LS, Healey PJ, Davis CL, McDonald RA. Subclinical viremia increases risk for chronic allograft injury in pediatric renal transplantation. J Am Soc Nephrol. 2010;21(9):1579–86.
20. Hodson EM, Ladhani M, Webster AC, Strippoli GF, Craig JC. Antiviral medications for preventing cytomegalovirus disease in solid organ transplant recipients. The Cochrane database of systematic reviews. 2013;2:CD003774.
21. Humar A, Lebranchu Y, Vincenti F, Blumberg EA, Punch JD, Limaye AP, Abramowicz D, Jardine AG, Voulgari AT, Ives J, et al. The efficacy and safety of 200 days valganciclovir cytomegalovirus prophylaxis in high-risk kidney transplant recipients. Am J Transplant. 2010;10(5):1228–37.
22. Reischig T, Jindra P, Mares J, Cechura M, Svecova M, Hes O, Opatrny K Jr, Treska V. Valacyclovir for cytomegalovirus prophylaxis reduces the risk of acute renal allograft rejection. Transplantation. 2005;79(3):317–24.
23. Lowance D, Neumayer HH, Legendre CM, Squifflet JP, Kovarik J, Brennan PJ, Norman D, Mendez R, Keating MR, Coggon GL, et al. Valacyclovir for the prevention of cytomegalovirus disease after renal transplantation. International Valacyclovir cytomegalovirus prophylaxis transplantation study group. N Engl J Med. 1999;340(19):1462–70.

24. Reischig T, Jindra P, Hes O, Svecova M, Klaboch J, Treska V. Valacyclovir prophylaxis versus preemptive valganciclovir therapy to prevent cytomegalovirus disease after renal transplantation. Am J Transplant. 2008;8(1):69–77.
25. Reischig T, Hribova P, Jindra P, Hes O, Bouda M, Treska V, Viklicky O. Long-term outcomes of pre-emptive valganciclovir compared with valacyclovir prophylaxis for prevention of cytomegalovirus in renal transplantation. J Am Soc Nephrol. 2012;23(9):1588–97.
26. Reischig T, Kacer M, Jindra P, Hes O, Lysak D, Bouda M. Randomized trial of valganciclovir versus valacyclovir prophylaxis for prevention of cytomegalovirus in renal transplantation. Clinical journal of the American Society of Nephrology : CJASN. 2015;10(2):294–304.
27. Haas M, Sis B, Racusen LC, Solez K, Glotz D, Colvin RB, Castro MC, David DS, David-Neto E, Bagnasco SM, et al. Banff 2013 meeting report: inclusion of c4d-negative antibody-mediated rejection and antibody-associated arterial lesions. Am J Transplant. 2014;14(2):272–83.
28. Stegall MD, Park WD, Larson TS, Gloor JM, Cornell LD, Sethi S, Dean PG, Prieto M, Amer H, Textor S, et al. The histology of solitary renal allografts at 1 and 5 years after transplantation. Am J Transplant. 2011; 11(4):698–707.
29. El Ters M, Grande JP, Keddis MT, Rodrigo E, Chopra B, Dean PG, Stegall MD, Cosio FG. Kidney allograft survival after acute rejection, the value of follow-up biopsies. Am J Transplant. 2013;13(9):2334–41.
30. Garcia-Carro C, Dorje C, Asberg A, Midtvedt K, Scott H, Reinholt FP, Holdaas H, Seron D, Reisaeter AV. Inflammation in early kidney allograft surveillance biopsies with and without associated Tubulointerstitial chronic damage as a predictor of fibrosis progression and development of De novo donor specific antibodies. Transplantation. 2017;101(6):1410–5.
31. Modena BD, Kurian SM, Gaber LW, Waalen J, Su AI, Gelbart T, Mondala TS, Head SR, Papp S, Heilman R, et al. Gene expression in biopsies of acute rejection and interstitial fibrosis/tubular atrophy reveals highly shared mechanisms that correlate with worse long-term outcomes. Am J Transplant. 2016;16(7):1982–98.
32. Shimamura M, Seleme MC, Guo L, Saunders U, Schoeb TR, George JF, Britt WJ. Ganciclovir prophylaxis improves late murine cytomegalovirus-induced renal allograft damage. Transplantation. 2013;95(1):48–53.
33. Battiwalla M, Wu Y, Bajwa RP, Radovic M, Almyroudis NG, Segal BH, Wallace PK, Nakamura R, Padmanabhan S, Hahn T, et al. Ganciclovir inhibits lymphocyte proliferation by impairing DNA synthesis. Biol Blood Marrow Transplant. 2007;13(7):765–70.
34. Reischig T, Prucha M, Sedlackova L, Lysak D, Jindra P, Bouda M, Matejovic M. Valganciclovir prophylaxis against cytomegalovirus impairs lymphocyte proliferation and activation in renal transplant recipients. Antivir Ther. 2011; 16(8):1227–35.
35. Elfadawy N, Flechner SM, Schold JD, Srinivas TR, Poggio E, Fatica R, Avery R, Mossad SB. Transient versus persistent BK viremia and long-term outcomes after kidney and kidney-pancreas transplantation. Clinical journal of the American Society of Nephrology : CJASN. 2014;9(3):553–61.
36. Sawinski D, Forde KA, Trofe-Clark J, Patel P, Olivera B, Goral S, Bloom RD. Persistent BK viremia does not increase intermediate-term graft loss but is associated with de novo donor-specific antibodies. J Am Soc Nephrol. 2015; 26(4):966–75.
37. Gheith O, Halim MA, Al-Otaibi T, Mansour H, Mosaad A, Atteya HA, Zakaria Z, Said T, Nair P, Nampoory N. Successful cost-effective prevention of cytomegalovirus disease in kidney transplant recipients using low-dose Valganciclovir. Experimental and clinical transplantation : official journal of the Middle East Society for Organ Transplantation. 2017;15(Suppl 1):156–63.
38. Schachtner T, Stein M, Babel N, Reinke P. The loss of BKV-specific immunity from Pretransplantation to Posttransplantation identifies kidney transplant recipients at increased risk of BKV replication. Am J Transplant. 2015;15(8): 2159–69.
39. Schmidt T, Adam C, Hirsch HH, Janssen MW, Wolf M, Dirks J, Kardas P, Ahlenstiel-Grunow T, Pape L, Rohrer T, et al. BK polyomavirus-specific cellular immune responses are age-dependent and strongly correlate with phases of virus replication. Am J Transplant. 2014;14(6):1334–45.
40. Roberts C, Torgerson DJ. Understanding controlled trials: baseline imbalance in randomised controlled trials. BMJ. 1999;319(7203):185.
41. Marty FM, Winston DJ, Rowley SD, Vance E, Papanicolaou GA, Mullane KM, Brundage TM, Robertson AT, Godkin S, Mommeja-Marin H, et al. CMX001 to prevent cytomegalovirus disease in hematopoietic-cell transplantation. N Engl J Med. 2013;369(13):1227–36.
42. Marty FM, Ljungman P, Chemaly RF, Maertens J, Dadwal SS, Duarte RF, Haider S, Ullmann AJ, Katayama Y, Brown J, et al. Letermovir prophylaxis for cytomegalovirus in hematopoietic-cell transplantation. N Engl J Med. 2017; 377(25):2433–44.

19

Pandemic influenza preparedness in the WHO African region: are we ready yet?

Evanson Z. Sambala[1*], Tiwonge Kanyenda[2], Chinwe Juliana Iwu[1,3], Chidozie Declan Iwu[4], Anelisa Jaca[1] and Charles S. Wiysonge[1,5,6]

Abstract

Background: Prior to the 2009 pandemic H1N1, and the unprecedented outbreak of Highly Pathogenic Avian Influenza (HPAI) caused by the H5N1 virus, the World Health Organization (WHO) called upon its Member States to develop preparedness plans in response to a new pandemic in humans. The WHO Member States responded to this call by developing national pandemic plans in accordance with the International Health Regulations (IHR) to strengthen the capabilities of Member States to respond to different pandemic scenarios. In this study, we aim to evaluate the quality of the preparedness plans in the WHO African region since their inception in 2005.

Methods: A standard checklist with 61 binary indicators ("yes" or "no") was used to assess the quality of the preparedness plans. The checklist was categorised across seven thematic areas of preparedness: preparation (16 indicators); coordination and partnership (5 indicators); risk communication (8 indicators); surveillance and monitoring (7 indicators); prevention and containment (10 indicators); case investigation and treatment (10 indicators) and ethical consideration (5 indicators). Four assessors independently scored the plans against the checklist.

Results: Of the 47 countries in the WHO African region, a total of 35 national pandemic plans were evaluated. The composite score for the completeness of the pandemic plans across the 35 countries was 36%. Country-specific scores on each of the thematic indicators for pandemic plan completeness varied, ranging from 5% in Côte d'Ivoire to 79% in South Africa. On average, preparation and risk communication scored 48%, respectively, while coordination and partnership scored the highest with an aggregate score of 49%. Surveillance and monitoring scored 34%, while prevention and containment scored 35%. Case investigation and treatment scored 25%, and ethical consideration scored the lowest of 14% across 35 countries. Overall, our assessment shows that pandemic preparedness plans across the WHO African region are inadequate.

Conclusions: Moving forward, these plans must address the gaps identified in this study and demonstrate clarity in their goals that are achievable through drills, simulations and tabletop exercises.

Keywords: National preparedness plans, Pandemic influenza, Africa, Quality of the plans, Surveillance, Containment, Communication, Ethical framework, Treatment

Background

Pandemic influenza is a rare disease caused by a novel influenza virus, a subtype that has the capability to cause sustained human-to-human transmission and to which the population has no or little immunity [1]. Historically, there have been 31 possible influenza outbreaks since 1580, occurring approximately once every 15 years [2], with 3 occurring in the twentieth century: the outbreaks of 1918, 1957, and 1968. The 1918 pandemic influenza outbreak was the most devastating, causing between 50 and 100 million deaths worldwide [3]. In Africa, the pandemic influenza fatality count was 2.3 million deaths, which is deemed to be underreported [4]. The 1957 and 1968 pandemic influenza in Africa caused about 2–3 million and 1 million excess deaths, respectively [5]. In the twenty-first century, an influenza pandemic occurred in 2009 causing 18,156 deaths globally [6].

* Correspondence: Evanson.Sambala@mrc.ac.za
[1]Cochrane South Africa, South African Medical Research Council, Box 19070, Cape Town, PO 7505, South Africa
Full list of author information is available at the end of the article

The highly pathogenic avian influenza (H5N1) does not usually infect humans, but poses a great threat in spillover from animal to human population, often with fatal outcomes when humans are infected. Between 1990 and 2000, avian virus H5N1 actively circulated uninterrupted among migratory birds and animals in Asia, Europe and Mediterranean, thus giving the prospects for a serious influenza pandemic outbreak in humans [7].

Following these threats and the anticipation of another pandemic, the World Health Organization (WHO) requested Member States to develop preparedness pandemic plans to ensure countries are equipped to mitigate the challenges a pandemic would present. This call was timely, given the limitations of the existing global influenza surveillance and monitoring system to respond, deploy and implement activities to mitigate the impact of an outbreak [8].

In 1999, the WHO published the first guiding principles for pandemic influenza preparedness [8]. These guidelines subsequently underwent revisions in 2005 and 2009, incorporating the practical outbreak response experiences gained from outbreaks of avian H5N1 and 2009 H1N1 influenza [9, 10]. These guidelines provide a framework for organising preparedness and response actions. The WHO recommends that, as Member States develop or update their national plans, they should consider the proposed phases in the context of country-specific needs, priorities and actions.

Based on the WHO resolution issued in April 2005 [11], many countries in Africa drafted their national plans between 2005 and 2007, and subsequently used the plans to respond to the 2009 H1N1 pandemic influenza. However, there is insufficient information on how the preparedness plans were utilized during the 2009 H1N1 pandemic and the lessons that were drawn to improve responses to the next pandemic. Furthermore, since the inception of these plans into action, no study has evaluated the quality of 2009 post pandemic preparedness plans in the WHO African region. The purpose of this present study was to evaluate the completeness of the preparedness plans. We postulated that planning for a pandemic influenza is only as satisfactory as the assumptions on which they are proposed; thus studying them is necessary. Findings from this study will be used to highlight areas of the plans that need strengthening and improvement.

Methods

We searched the electronic databases of the WHO and United Nations (UN) plus grey literature for the availability of the national pandemic influenza preparedness plans from the WHO African region that were published between 2005 and 2017. In instances where the plans were not available online, we contacted the Ministries of Health in the respective countries for their plans. We considered countries that had plans for avian or human influenza, or both. We excluded plans that were not in public domain. Pandemic influenza plans are a blueprint for managing the emergency outbreak and, as such, should be shared with citizens and stakeholders to inform them about their roles and responsibilities in responding to a possible threat [12].

We translated plans written in French into English using google translation software. Where two national plans for a country were available, we read, assessed and treated both the draft and updated version of the plan as a unit. Four assessors (TK, CJI, CDI and AJ) independently read and scored the plans; disagreements or discrepancies that arose during assessment were resolved by a fifth and sixth reviewer (EZS and CSW).

A standard checklist with 61 binary indicators ("yes" or "no") was used to assess the quality of the preparedness pandemic plans. The checklist, shown in Table 1, is grouped across seven thematic areas: preparation (16 indicators); coordination and partnership (5 indicators); risk communication (8 indicators); surveillance and monitoring (7 indicators); prevention and containment (10 indicators); case investigation and treatment (10 indicators) and ethical consideration (5 indicators).

The indicators used to assess the African plans were developed partly from the 20 key indicators on various goals of preparedness recommended by the European Centre for Disease Prevention and Control (ECDC) and WHO Regional Office for Europe [13]. A group of 25 European countries plus Iceland and Norway through a consultative process provided feedback on the content validity of the 20 indicators [13]. Additional indicators specific to the purpose of our study and setting was pulled together by incorporating other recommendations from the WHO guidance on pandemic plan development [13, 14]. The final instrument was validated by pandemic policy planners in 7 select countries with a validity index score of not less than 0.75.

Each plan assessed would score a maximum of 61 points for completeness across the 7 thematic areas of preparedness. We generated descriptive data, such as averages and percent of total, to gauge quality of pandemic preparedness plans. An overall plan score was calculated by assigning 1 or 0 points to each indicator. An indicator score of one is assigned to the plan if denoted by "yes" and zero for "no". The indicator was scored 1 if an item was mentioned in detail or partly described in the plan, while a score of 0 was given if the item assessed was missing or absent in the plan. All the scores were verified before entry in excel by two reviewers (EZS and CDI) prior to analysis.

Table 1 Standardized checklist and scores for 61 indicators grouped across seven categories

INDICATORS		RATIONALE	SCORES	
		Additional assessment guide	Number of countries	
			Yes	No
PREPARATION				
1	Does the country have a national pandemic influenza plan?	Is it publicly available?	35	0
2	Does the national influenza plan target human or avian influenza subtypes?	Human influenza subtype e.g. H1N1 and animal subtype e.g. H5N1	32	3
3	Does the national pandemic influenza plan meet the international (WHO/IHR etc) guidance on preparedness?	Is the plan based on the six phases of planning and response?	22	13
4	Are the responsibilities and actions in the plan defined phase by phase?	This is required for capacity setting, planning and command based on WHO recommendations.	21	14
5	Are there local plans at district and regional level?	See if are there any arrangements in place	9	26
6	Are business continuity plans available across the non-health sectors at national and regional levels? Or are these mentioned in the plans?	Check this among institutions (UN organization and churches etc). Do these plan mention how they will cope with an influenza pandemic and continue to provide other essential health services.	7	28
7	Are the plans flexible?	Does the plan have a severity index or are they able to adjust whether to mild or severe nature of the pandemic?	13	22
8	Do the response and inter-wave planning phases have their own courses of action and budgets which would be implemented?	These tasks should have financial and human resource with a budget provision for a year. Also see question 4	24	11
9	Is the plan sustainable for a longer term?	Influenza funding and development of command structures should not heavily rely on external funding.	0	35
10	Does the plan have a national committee(s) or advisory body in place to oversee preparedness?	Check who drafted the plan and if they were part of the committee.	32	3
11	Does the plan have any assumptions on which the plan is based?	Does the plan mention the expected range of cases and percentage of staff off sick? Check for detailed assumptions and planning principles such as case scenarios that will trigger responses and guide effective implementation of the plan.	14	21
12	Are there a national command and control structure?	This is where data or information is aggregated for the country. The national command centre exercise authority and can designate responsibilities at the local or regional levels.	25	10
13	Are there health services command and control structure?	Check for hospital and clinic plans	8	27
14	Does the pandemic plan regularly and systematically get tested at all levels and across all sectors i.e. national level health sector exercises or drills?	Check if they carry out simulations and tabletop exercises- this is important because it can feedback in the planning as lessons learnt.	8	27
15	Have the legal implications of travel restrictions and other interoperability issues been determined?	Are there any discussions or agreements on a list of issues such as cross-border management and quarantine?	15	20

Table 1 Standardized checklist and scores for 61 indicators grouped across seven categories *(Continued)*

INDICATORS		RATIONALE	SCORES	
		Additional assessment guide	Number of countries	
			Yes	No
16	Do interventions proposed in the plan have exit strategies?	What are the exit options? When should the pandemic be outbreak declared over?	4	31
COORDINATION AND PARTNERSHIPS				
17	Are there any regional or local arrangements in place on how to respond?	Do plans engage local people, families and medical personnel to ensure local services are running smoothly during the pandemic period?	24	11
18	Are there a regional/local planning and coordination structure?	Check for leadership roles and designation of responsibilities among the coordinating structures.	24	11
19	Is the health sector well connected to other sectors such as businesses and civil society?	Private and public partnership necessary to continue providing essential services such as water, energy and safe transport.	12	23
20	Are there joint cooperation and partnership with the neighboring countries on mutually relevant influenza policy areas?	A pandemic outbreak has no borders- check how transborder problems related to pandemic influenza will be resolved or if it is a priority in the plan.	10	25
21	Does the partnership or coordination involve financial and technical support?	This is important for planning continuity purposes and future responses.	16	19
RISK COMMUNICATION				
22	Are they a national communication strategy or is it publicly available?	Has the national communication strategy been published?	22	13
23	Does the national communication strategy sufficiently stress the likely nature or duration of the pandemic, its spread, its peak and decline, nor does it sufficiently inform the public on these issues?	Is the national communication strategy committed to public awareness including communicating the nature, spread, peak and decline of influenza (seasonal and pandemic?	11	24
24	Are there any Information Education and Communication (IEC) material or IEC in place or available?	Check if the plan use or intend to use multi-media communication i.e. newspapers, radio, TV, posters, magazines and social networking sites such as Facebook and Twitter	31	4
25	Are there any definitions of key target groups for specific preventive messages and protection such as health and emergency personnel within the communication plan?	Are there any public hygiene campaigns to highlight the personal public health measures during normal influenza seasons or outbreaks?	23	12
26	Are there effective programmes in place to change public attitudes and perceptions about influenza?	To avoid problems due to poor messages on preventive measures and general hygiene etc.	12	23
27	Are churches or religious groups mentioned in the plan to help communicate preparedness messages?	People are more likely to listen to a religious leaders than from health personnel.	8	27
28	Are there a nation-wide influenza guidance 'intranet' for health authorities respond quickly to an influenza outbreak?	Web reporting systems?	9	26
29	Is information exchanged with stakeholders?	Are conferences, meetings and forums mentioned for information exchange and sharing?	17	18

Table 1 Standardized checklist and scores for 61 indicators grouped across seven categories *(Continued)*

INDICATORS		RATIONALE	SCORES	
		Additional assessment guide	Number of countries	
			Yes	No
SURVEILLANCE AND MONITORING				
30	Are there surveillance systems in place for collecting and sharing of virological and epidemiological data with the WHO and other partners?	Check for Integrated Disease Surveillance Response (IDSR) and check if such data is shared?	18	17
31	Are there a national laboratory or national influenza centre (NIC) or Influenza assessment centres (IAC) for collecting epidemiological data on Influenza Like Illness (ILI) and Severe Acute Respiratory Infections (SARI)	The national laboratory capacity is important to provide timely, high quality, validated routine and diagnostic influenza data. ILI and SARI are indirect measures for influenza- and there are good indicators for pandemic preparedness.	18	17
32	If yes in 31, does the national laboratory have the capacity to perform: Virus isolation? Influenza typing? Influenza s	Check these at the national and administrative regional level.	13	22
33	Are there a PCR machine for testing/sequencing of seasonal and pandemic influenza viruses?	Relevant for monitoring viruses and for estimating additional resources that might be required to tackle pandemic influenza problem.	9	26
34	Are there a national "Early Warning" systems or Event Based Surveillance (EBS)	Are they a computerised hospital system that can readily give age-specific mortality data in real time?	6	29
35	Is the virological and epidemiological data shared with partners/WHO? Are they an influenza web reporting system?	Check if they have a FluNet and FluID reporting systems.	4	31
36	Are they a surveillance working group(s)?	A team of specialized expertise/ epidemiologists to advise on the planning and response etc. See also question 10.	16	19
PREVENTION AND CONTAINMENT				
37	Are non-pharmaceutical intervention plans in place? i.e. closure of schools, ventilators, PPEs, quarantine, isolation, hygiene and sanitation.	Are prevention and cluster control plans in place (i.e. for border and stamping influenza out prior to widespread in the country.	26	9
38	Are pharmaceutical interventions in place? i.e. use of vaccines, antivirals and antibiotics for secondary infections	Check for vaccine strategy if in place?	29	6
39	Are there a procurement strategy of pharmaceutical (vaccines) and non-pharmaceutical products (PPEs)?	Check for political intervention to improve pharmaceutical logistics in acquiring vaccines and other drugs.	17	18
40	Are there contracts and agreements with pharmaceutical companies for the supply of equipment and drugs for influenza preparedness capacity?	Check if there are vaccine and antiviral drug contracts and agreements with the pharmaceutical companies.	2	33
41	Are there a pharmaceutical (vaccine) strategy	If a pandemic vaccine is planned to be used when will the vaccines arrive in health centres? Is it within six months of the start of the pandemic?	12	23
42	Are there accelerated regulatory approvals of influenza vaccines for quick deployment? Or are there a national regulatory capacity in place so that vaccines, diagnostic	Some countries deploying influenza vaccines are required to meet the preconditions for supply of vaccines through the WHO Deployment Initiative.	3	32

Table 1 Standardized checklist and scores for 61 indicators grouped across seven categories *(Continued)*

INDICATORS		RATIONALE	SCORES	
		Additional assessment guide	Number of countries	
			Yes	No
	tests and antiviral medicines for influenza can be deployed quickly?			
43	Are there any additional (surge) capacity to improve responses through training and increasing human resource capacity?	Are there a standardised national educational materials for all health care workers?	21	14
44	Are there effective hospital control policies?	Do hospitals or health centres have their own plans?	5	30
45	Are there plans for recruiting volunteers from local communities?	This is necessary in case of staff absenteeism during the pandemic period.	2	33
46	Are there a reserve list of health professionals?	Necessary in case of staff absenteeism during the pandemic period.	4	31
CASE INVESTIGATION AND TREATMENT				
47	Are there any scientifically-based estimates of the numbers of people likely to be affected by pandemic influenza and needing medical and social care?	These estimates contributes to the planning of resources and for efficient and equitable deployment of vital supplies for pandemic influenza.	8	27
48	Are there a list of critical information that is needed early in a pandemic (e.g. attack rates by age and locality, strain type, likely antiviral sensitivity, response to antivirals and public health measures, etc)?	What is the proportion of the population that may need treatment i.e. target groups for prophylaxis?	9	26
49	Are there criteria for the types and amounts of antivirals to be used?	Does the plan have priorities on the types of antivirals or drug combinations?	18	17
50	Are there a local distribution channel to deliver these antivirals and vaccines?	Hotlines e.g. telephone lines for requests and local influenza centres to deliver.	13	22
51	Are there any consideration of mechanisms to monitor the usefulness of vaccines, effectiveness, side-effects and resistance of antivirals through real time surveillance?	Necessary for efficient and timely decision-making	8	27
52	Are border screenings in place and will the cases be followed-up?	Contact tracing e.g. interviewing patient cases and carrying out surveys for possible sources?	15	20
53	Are isolation or quarantine rooms provided at the port of entry?	Rooms to hold suspected cases.	16	19
54	Are there a national annual seasonal influenza vaccination programme in place?	Necessary if countries will be able to vaccinate timely during the pandemic period.	0	35
55	If yes it is achieving > 75% uptake in over 65 s and increasing uptake in occupational and clinical risk groups?	Vaccinating the elderly and at risk adults, for example, is unlikely to establish indirect protective effects because these groups represent a small percentage of the population among whom the virus spreads.	0	35
56	Are there vaccine uptake figures or are these published annually?	If the vaccine uptakes are low, are there plans in educating the public on attitudes and perceptions?	0	35

Table 1 Standardized checklist and scores for 61 indicators grouped across seven categories *(Continued)*

INDICATORS		RATIONALE	SCORES	
		Additional assessment guide	Number of countries	
			Yes	No
ETHICAL CONSIDERATIONS				
57	Is there an ethical framework in place?	Necessary to avoid ethical problems that might arise	1	34
58	Are there any ethical consideration for appropriate use of quarantine procedures, treatment of patients with vaccines and antiviral drugs?	Are there priority setting and equitable access to therapeutic and prophylactic measures? What are the core governmental responsibilities on this?	4	31
59	During implementation of the plan, are there consideration to balance public health and human rights?	During a pandemic influenza emergency, policymakers experience tension and disputes, and that they struggle to balance public health decisions between what is best for the individual and society as a whole.	6	29
60	Are there evidence base for public health measures on which decisions will be based or are based?	Check in the plans if policymakers use science	6	29
61	Are there transparency, public engagement and social mobilization in the plan?	Is there a list that shows the beneficiaries for the interventions or how the beneficiaries were selected as eligible candidates for the interventions or limited resources?	7	28

Results

Of the 47 countries in the WHO African region, 35 national pandemic plans were retrieved for assessment in this study (Table 2). We could not find plans for 12 countries- either they were not publicly available or we could not access them from the Ministry of Health in these countries upon request.

Of the plans reviewed, 60% were initially developed between 2006 (Table 2) in response to specific threats posed by the continuing spread of the avian influenza (H5N1) virus. Figure 1 shows composite scores of preparedness plans by country. The composite score for the completeness of the pandemic plans was 36% across the 35 countries. Country-specific scores on each of the thematic indicators for pandemic plan completeness varied, ranging from 5% in Côte d'Ivoire to 79% in South Africa (Fig. 1). Overall, our assessment shows that pandemic plans across the WHO African region remain inadequate, with no details on ethical considerations, case investigation and treatment. Nigeria was the only country that scored 60% across all the thematic areas of preparedness.

Figure 2 shows completeness of the preparedness plans of countries by thematic area. On average, preparation and risk communication scored 48%, respectively, while coordination and partnership scored highest with an aggregate score of 49%. Surveillance and monitoring scored 34%, while prevention and containment scored 35%. Case investigation and treatment scored 25% and ethical consideration scored the lowest of 14% across 35 countries.

Table 1 shows the scores of the assessment indicators for all thematic areas. Of the countries that had a plan available online, 33 countries planned against both human and avian influenza subtypes. Three plans- those from Algeria, Chad and Cote d'Ivoire- specifically focused on the planning for and response to avian influenza subtypes. 22 of 35 plans followed the WHO guidance on six phases of planning and response. 14 countries cited hypothetical scenarios on which the plan is based, for example, when doses of vaccines and antivirals need to be acquired to treat patients. There were 9 plans with planning initiatives at the district and regional levels, and 7 plans mentioned that they had business continuity plans across the non-health sector. We found 13 plans to be flexible with regards to the ability to quickly adjust to the severity of the pandemic. 24 countries had a budget provision for each course of action, however, all the plans were heavily dependent on external funding with no sustainable budget for their preparedness. Maximum funding for some countries, such as the Democratic Republic of Congo, was only 3 years. All but 3 countries- Algeria, Cabo Verde and Central African Republic- mentioned having a national committee or advisory body to oversee preparedness. Eight plans tested their planning for and responses through exercises and drills at the national level. There were 25 plans that had a national command and control structure, where influenza data or epidemiological information is aggregated and shared

Table 2 Country pandemic plans assessed, year of development and last updated

	Country	Year		Country	Year
1	Algeria	2009	19	Madagascar	2006
2	Benin	2006/2009	20	Malawi	2006
3	Botswana	2005	21	Mali	2006
4	Burkina Faso	2005	22	Mauritania	2006
5	Cameroon	2006	23	Mauritius	2006
6	Cabo Verde	2006	24	Mozambique	2006
7	Central African Republic (the)	2006	25	Namibia	2005
8	Chad	2006	26	Niger (the)	2006
9	Comoros (the)	2006	27	Nigeria	2007
10	Côte d'Ivoire	2009	28	Rwanda	2006
11	Democratic Republic of the Congo (the)	2006	29	Senegal	2005/2009
12	Gabon	2007	30	Seychelles	2007
13	Gambia (the)	2006/2009	31	Sierra Leone	2005/2009
14	Ghana	2005/2009	32	South Africa	2006/2017
15	Guinea	2006/2009	33	Swaziland	2006
16	Kenya	2005	34	Uganda	2006
17	Lesotho	2006	35	United Republic of Tanzania (the)	2007
18	Liberia	2009			

with regional and district levels. Hospital plans were available in 8 plans and only 4 countries had planned for exit strategies after the pandemic.

Coordination and partnership indicators showed that 24 plans engaged local people, families and medical personnel to ensure local services run smoothly during the pandemic. Another 24 plans had a functional local or regional coordination structure. 12 countries had a private and public partnership to offer essential services such as the delivery of health, safety and energy. Ten national plans had a joint co-operation and partnership with a neighbouring

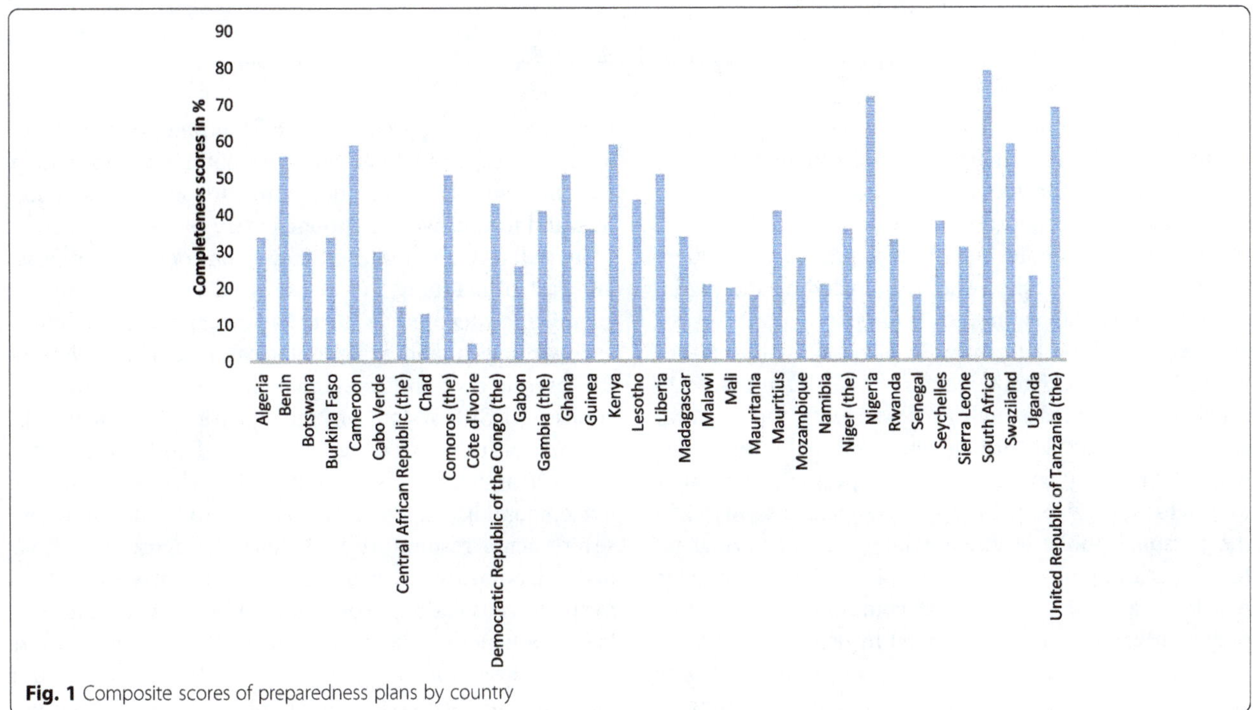

Fig. 1 Composite scores of preparedness plans by country

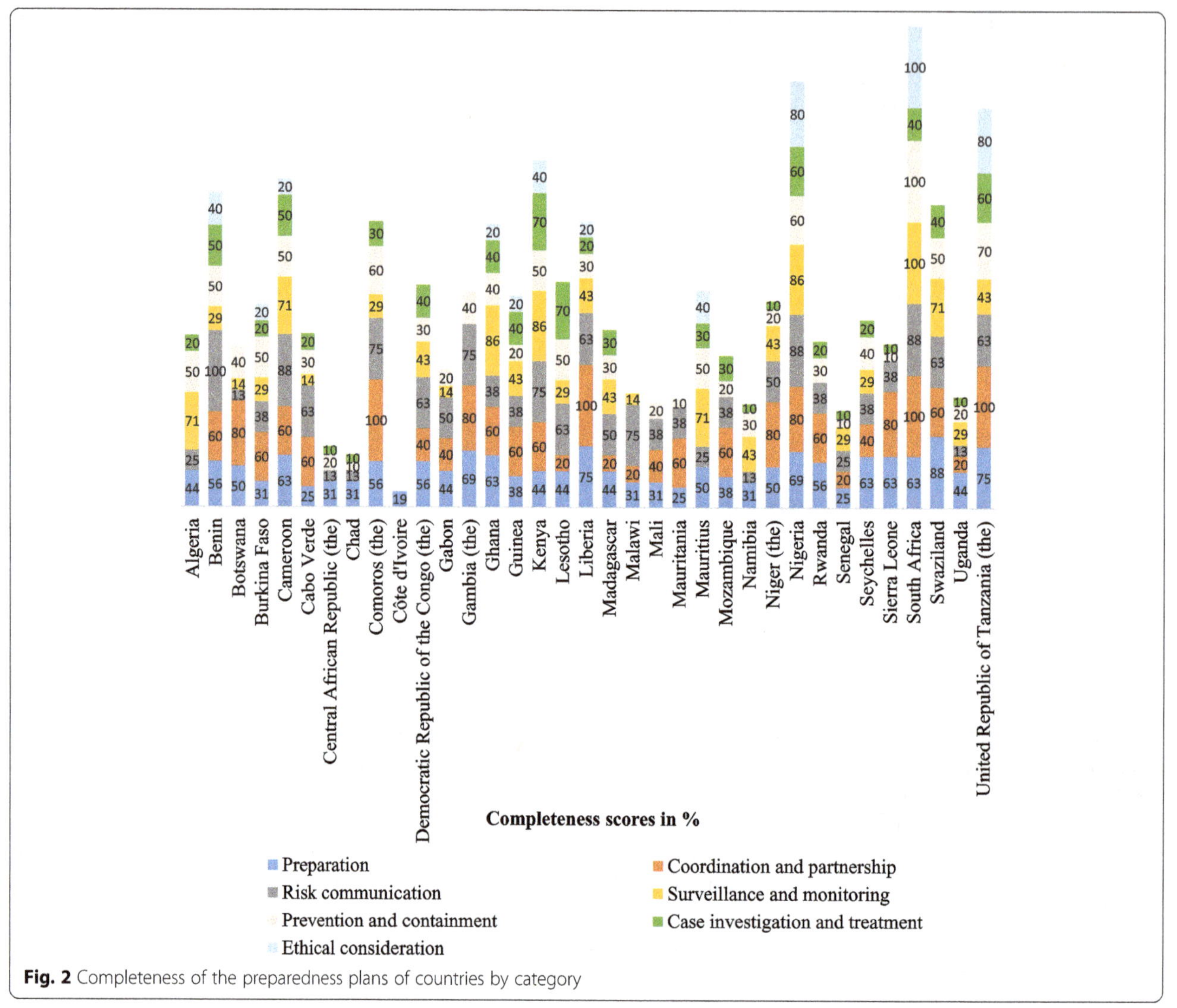

Fig. 2 Completeness of the preparedness plans of countries by category

country on mutually relevant influenza policy. 16 countries held partnership and coordination that involved financial and technical support.

The risk communication indicator showed that 22 plans had a communication strategy and 11 plans mentioned the role of public awareness, including sharing information on the nature, transmission patterns, peak and decline of the influenza. 31 plans had Information, Education and Communication (IEC) materials published in multi-media such as newspapers, radio, television and social networking sites on the internet. 23 plans defined key target groups for specific preventative messages, such as public hygiene campaigns to highlight the personal public health measures during normal influenza seasons or outbreaks. 12 plans planned to avoid problems arising due to poor communication around preventative measures and general hygiene. Only 8 plans mentioned churches or religious groups to assist with communicating messages on preparedness. 9 countries had web reporting systems, such as intranet or FluNet, to speed up responses to an influenza outbreak. Information exchange among stakeholders through conferences, meetings and forums were mentioned by 17 plans.

Surveillance and monitoring are considered an important part of planning, yet 17 plans failed to mention the surveillance techniques of collecting and sharing influenza virological and epidemiological data. This is despite the presence of the integrated disease surveillance response (IDSR) system in many African countries. In these countries, there was no national influenza centre (NIC) or influenza assessment centres (IAC) for collecting epidemiological data on influenza-like illnesses and severe acute respiratory infections. Amongst those that had a laboratory, 13 countries had the capacity to perform virus isolation, typing and subtyping. 9 countries had a polymerase chain reaction (PCR) machine to test and monitor influenza circulation. Only six plans had a computerised hospital system as an early warning system that can readily give real-time data on influenza outbreaks. Epidemiological and virological data was shared with the WHO and other partners by 4 countries-Algeria, Ghana, Kenya and South Africa. There were 16 plans that mentioned having a surveillance working group to give advice on surveillance and monitoring.

As part of prevention and containment of influenza, 26 countries planned for non-pharmaceutical interventions, such as closure of schools, use of ventilators, use of personal protective equipment, quarantine, isolation, hygiene and sanitation. In terms of pharmaceutical interventions, 29 plans mentioned strategies that would use vaccines, antivirals and antibiotics for treatment of secondary infections. With regards to detailed assessment of the pharmaceutical strategy, we found that 12 plans had a vaccine strategy, while 17 plans had a procurement strategy for either pharmaceutical or non-pharmaceuticals products. Only 2 plans, those from the United Republic of Tanzania and South Africa, had advanced contracts and agreements with pharmaceutical companies in place for the supply of equipment and drugs for influenza treatment. 3 plans, those from the United Republic of Tanzania, Swaziland and South Africa, had in place accelerated regulatory approval of influenza products for quick deployment. Additional surge capacity to improve responses through training and human resources was available in 21 of the plans. The hospital plans were available in 5 plans and 2 plans (Algeria and South Africa) mentioned the need for recruiting volunteers from the local community. In terms of human resource, 4 plans suggested recruitment of staff from a reserve list of health professionals.

In the category of case investigation and treatment, 8 plans had science based influenza planning assumptions for efficient and equitable deployment of vital supplies against influenza. As part of planning, 9 plans included critical information such as attack rates by age and locality, strain type, antiviral sensitivity or who to target for prophylaxis. 18 plans mentioned the criteria and types of antivirals to use in an event of an outbreak. The most commonly mentioned antivirals were zanamivir and oseltamivir. About 13 plans mentioned that they will deliver these antivirals through local distribution channels, including the use of telephone line and local influenza centres. Mechanisms to monitor the effectiveness, side effects and resistance of vaccines or antivirals were considered in 8 plans through real time surveillance. Plans to screen cases at the borders and follow up cases were indicated in 15 plans, while isolation or the provision of rooms at the border entry were only mentioned in 16 plans. No plan reported the intention to vaccinate seasonally (i.e. achieving > 75 uptake in the elderly population), nor published any vaccination figures despite indicating that they will vaccinate its population.

Ethical consideration was inadequately reported in most plans, with only 1 plan (South Africa) having completely reported to have an ethical framework in place. 4 plans considered an ethically appropriate use of quarantine procedures, fair allocation of treatment and limited resources such as vaccines. 6 plans considered how to balance between public health and human rights interests if they came into conflict. 7 of the plans indicated the need for transparency in decision making, for example, how eligible beneficiaries would be selected to receive scarce interventions.

Discussion

Preparing for a response towards a pandemic extends beyond the development of the plan to include an implementation plan that lays out how the goals of the plan match available resources, tasks and responsibilities, to meet the needs of the population affected by the pandemic outcomes. Preparedness plans are crucial to build frameworks for emergency response, thereby providing countries with the opportunity to plan, strategise and mobilise human and capital resources before a pandemic occurs. Adequate and thorough plans ensure that countries can respond immediately when a pandemic is declared.

While our study showed that the majority of the African countries have a plan (74%), the majority of these plans are inadequate, with many tasks necessary to address pandemic threats of the twenty-first century remains unmet. This finding corresponds to studies that evaluated preparedness plans and responses to the 2009 H1N1 pandemic in Ghana and Malawi, where such plans were found to be weak and unable to elicit the most desired responses during the pandemic [15, 16]. The findings of this study also concur with an evaluation done by Ortu et al. (2008), who reported that the plans lacked operational clarity and focus of the planning objectives [17].

Our findings indicate that the majority of plans have not been updated over time, despite the lessons offered by the 2009 H1N1 pandemic. Our findings also show that only 7 of the assessed countries in Africa updated or revised their plans periodically to incorporate the changing circumstances and lessons gathered from the 2009 pandemic. For instance, South Africa is one of the countries with consistent updates to its plan, with a recently developed five-year national influenza policy and strategic plan outlining a comprehensive approach to influenza prevention and control [18]. A plan needs to be a living document, periodically adapted as new information on the influenza becomes available and thus ready to provide a guide to the protocols, procedures, and division of responsibilities in emergency response [12].

Results of our study also suggest that many countries did not consider the proposed phases of preparedness to respond more efficiently to the influenza pandemic. This is despite the fact that the WHO has provided an up-to-date evidence-based guidance to support countries to develop and revise pandemic preparedness plans. Recently, the WHO published an updated pandemic influenza preparedness checklist to help Members States build capacity for pandemic response [14]. However, our review highlights how many countries in the WHO African region are yet to incorporate these guidelines despite the need to improve existing plans.

Our study also shows that many countries do not have business continuity plans across the non-health sector at the subnational level. An influenza pandemic is an unpredictable event that can create a major management crisis of unprecedented scale and cost. High absence of workers from duty could drastically interrupt the functioning of critical infrastructure, such as services essential to health, technology and communication networks, economic wellbeing, safety and security. Due to the disruptive nature of the pandemic to social services and the economy, development of business continuity plans embedded within the national plan is critical for an effective country response that minimizes the financial consequences on all businesses of all sizes and types [19].

In our study, we observed that only a few national plans engaged with specific sectors, such as education, hospitals, industry and local community. It is useful for plans to make meaningful arrangements at the local level, because this is where the burden of the disease occurs and is largely felt. In addition, in the aftermath of the pandemic, the local level is where the plans can continue to be implemented. Interestingly, apart from local coordination, we found that few countries had joint cooperation and partnership from non-health sector in preparedness, thus making interoperability and integration of planning efforts and services impossible. The purpose of planning and involving cooperation and partnership at all levels is to support and promptly restore key routines and functions prone to disruptions in our societies. Even a well-designed and motivated plan without partnerships will fall short in managing the crisis, and will struggle to guide recovery effectively if it does not extend responsibilities and command across local government, stakeholders and international partners.

Although surveillance is considered one of the most crucial planning activities, in this study we found that half of the plans did not incorporate the techniques of collecting virological and epidemiological data for the early detection of the virus causing an epidemic. The majority of the surveillance plans in place were weak. The role of surveillance techniques and systems is to send early signals of an imminent influenza outbreak in the human and animal population, and yield knowledge for treatment, prevention and control of influenza [20]. For many plans, it was impossible to fulfill these tasks in the absence of laboratories and equipment, such as PCR machines to perform virus typing and subtyping. According to the IHRs, all countries are mandated to monitor and rapidly report disease outbreaks that pose a threat to other countries [11]. Apart from alerting respective countries about the nature of the influenza virus in circulation, understanding disease virology can be useful for vaccine production. However, without the necessary tools to conduct surveillance, public health interventions to reduce influenza pandemic are jeopardized.

An interesting finding from this study was that 26 countries proposed to use non-pharmaceutical interventions (case isolation, restricting children's visits to hospitals, workplace closure etc.), while nearly all indicated the use of pharmaceutical interventions i.e. vaccines, antivirals and antibiotics for treatment of secondary infections. Although vaccines are a primary strategy for preventing and mitigating influenza outbreaks, many plans do not specify whether vaccines will be acquired on time. Since influenza viruses change overtime due to the antigenic shifts and drifts, it is difficult to produce an appropriate and effective influenza vaccine for unknown subtypes [20].

As such, during the first few months of a pandemic influenza, vaccination will not be a primary intervention strategy. The time during which there are no vaccines, combined approaches of non-pharmaceutical interventions can minimize morbidity and mortality due to influenza pandemic. There is no point in making arrangements to use vaccines (including other treatments products and materials) when these products will not be available or are unlikely to be supplied within a useful time frame to mitigate the disease. If specific arrangements are proposed, then plans should take into account both the limitations and the capabilities of the responses.

Most importantly, although often forgotten in the majority of the preparedness plans is the need for ethical considerations. Our study indicates that, with the exception of one plan (South Africa), no other plans reported having an ethical framework in place. There is an expectation that during a pandemic influenza outbreak, ethical issues will arise due to conflicting interests between civil liberties (i.e. violation of human rights) and population health (i.e. greatest good for the greatest number) [20]. In the absence of an ethical plan, it is difficult to respond appropriately to ethical dilemmas and this can constitute a threat to preparedness and response. We propose that all countries develop an ethical framework that can be used to address ethical problems such as these of rationing limited vaccines or failure by health care-workers to work on the bedside during the pandemic.

Our study has several limitations. Our analysis was based on pandemic plans that are freely available online and thus it is possible that some of these plans would have been updated and the revised versions of the plans not yet published. Our study may therefore be a misrepresentation of the preparedness. We were only able to assess written materials in the protocols, yet crisis preparedness extends beyond these documents to include the ability to perform within the means using the necessary and available tools and infrastructure. Thus, we are not suggesting that countries that scored high in the completeness scores for preparedness will do the same in real crisis situations. However, for country preparedness to be truly effective at preventing and responding to influenza, plans must be created and drills and exercises conducted to ensure they prevent and address influenza pandemic. Another limitation involved the process of scoring the plans without a weighting scale, which may have introduced bias especially among those indicators that fell between 1 and 0. A further methodological limitation involved scoring the same plan twice i.e. the initial draft and updated version. As such, countries with more than one national plan may have been more likely to achieve a higher score, thus skewing the scores for those plans. Finally, we used google translation software to translate French plans into English and thus some words may have been lost in translation. Most importantly, we excluded one French written plan (Togo) from the analysis because the format of the plan made it unable to be translated.

Conclusion

Based on our assessment of the plans, we found preparedness plans to be weak therefore, these plans must address the gaps identified in this study. We recommend improving the overall goals in preparedness and these are achievable through drills, simulations and tabletop exercises.

Abbreviations

EBS: Event based surveillance; ECDC: European centre for disease prevention and control; H: Hemagglutinin; HPAI: Highly pathogenic avian influenza; IAC: Influenza assessment centres; IDSR: Integrated disease surveillance response; IEC: Information, education and communication; IHR: International health regulations; ILI: Influenza like illness; N: Neuraminidase; NIC: National influenza centre; PCR: Polymerase chain reaction; SARI: Severe acute respiratory infections; WHO: World Health Organization

Acknowledgements

The authors would like to thank Dr. Sara Cooper for proof reading the article and Ms. Lindi Mathebula for making the graphs visible.

Funding

We did not receive funding for this study.

Authors' contributions

EZS conceived the study. EZS, AJ, CDI, TK, CJI and CSW collected the data and performed the analysis. EZS wrote the manuscript and all the authors contributed to shaping of the argument of the article, and participated in the manuscript writing. All the authors read and approved the final manuscript.

Competing interests

The authors declare that they have no competing interests.

Author details

[1]Cochrane South Africa, South African Medical Research Council, Box 19070, Cape Town, PO 7505, South Africa. [2]Vaccines for Africa Initiative, Division of Medical Microbiology and Institute of Infectious Disease and Molecular Medicine, University of Cape Town, Cape Town, South Africa. [3]Division of Health Systems and Public Health, Department of Global Health, Faculty of Medicine and Health Sciences, Stellenbosch University, Cape Town, South Africa. [4]Department of Biochemistry and Microbiology, University of Fort Hare, Alice, South Africa. [5]Division of Epidemiology and Biostatistics, School of Public Health and Family Medicine, University of Cape Town, Cape Town, South Africa. [6]Centre for Evidence-Based Health Care, Division of Epidemiology and Biostatistics, Department of Global Health, Faculty of Medicine and Health Sciences, Stellenbosch University, Cape Town, South Africa.

References

1. Sleman SS. How influenza a causes "epidemics and pandemics" among the population: novel targets for anti-influenza molecules. Biom Biostat Int J. 2018;7(5):452–5. https://doi.org/10.15406/bbij.2018.07.00246.
2. Tognotti E. Influenza pandemics: A historical retrospect. The Journal of Infection in Developing Countries. 2009;3(05):331–4.
3. Taubenberger JK, Morens DM. 1918 influenza: the mother of all pandemics. Emerg Infect Dis. 2006;12(1):15–22.
4. Johnson NP, Mueller J. Updating the accounts: global mortality of the 1918-1920" Spanish" influenza pandemic. Bull Hist Med. 2002;76(1):105–15.
5. Nicholson KG, Wood JM, Wood JM, Zambon M. Influenza. Lancet. 2003; 362(9397):1733–45.
6. World Health Organization (WHO). Pandemic (H1N1) 2009 - update 112 [updated May 23, 2010]. Available from: http://www.who.int/csr/don/2010_08_06/en/
7. Peiris JS, de Jong MD, Guan Y. Avian influenza virus (H5N1): a threat to human health. Clin Microbiol Rev. 2007;20(2):243–67.
8. World Health Organization (WHO). Influenza Pandemic Plan - The role of WHO and Guidelines for National and Regional Planning, Geneva, Switzerland, 1999. Available from: http://www.who.int/iris/handle/10665/66155.
9. World Health Organization (WHO). WHO global influenza preparedness plan: the role of WHO and recommendations for national measures before and during pandemics. 2005. Available from: http://www.who.int/csr/resources/publications/influenza/WHO_CDS_CSR_GIP_2005_5.pdf.
10. World Health Organization (WHO). Global Influenza Programme: Pandemic influenza preparedness and response: a WHO guidance document: World Health Organization; 2009.
11. World Health Organization (WHO). International health regulations (2005). In: World Health Organization; 2008.
12. Alexander D: Disaster and emergency planning for preparedness, response, and recovery. In Edited by Anonymous Oxford University Press; 2015.
13. European Centre for Disease Prev Control (ECDP). Guide to revision of national pandemic influenza preparedness plans - Lessons learned from the 2009 A(H1N1) pandemic. Stockholm: ECDC; 2017. Available from: [https://ecdc.europa.eu/sites/portal/files/documents/Guide-to-pandemic-preparedness-revised.pdf].
14. World Health Organization: Essential steps for developing or updating a national pandemic influenza preparedness plan 2018.
15. Sambala EZ, Manderson L. Anticipation and response: pandemic influenza in Malawi. 2009 Global health action. 2017;10(1):1341225.
16. Sambala EZ, Manderson L. Policy perspectives on post pandemic influenza vaccination in Ghana and Malawi. BMC Public Health. 2017;17(1):227.
17. Ortu G, Mounier-Jack S, Coker R. Pandemic influenza preparedness in Africa is a profound challenge for an already distressed region: analysis of national preparedness plans. Health Policy Plan. 2008;23(3):161–9.

20

Feasibility of the string test for tuberculosis diagnosis in children between 4 and 14 years old

Karla T. Tafur[1*], Julia Coit[2], Segundo R. Leon[2], Cynthia Pinedo[1], Silvia S. Chiang[3,4], Carmen Contreras[1], Roger Calderon[1], Milagros J. Mendoza[1], Leonid Lecca[1,2] and Molly F. Franke[2]

Abstract

Background: The enteric string test can be used to obtain a specimen for microbiological confirmation of tuberculosis in children, but it is not widely used for this. The aim of this analysis to evaluate this approach in children with tuberculosis symptoms.

Methods: We conducted a cross-sectional study to assess children's ability to complete the test (feasibility), and self-reported pain (tolerability). We examined caregivers' and children's willingness to repeat the procedure (acceptability) and described the diagnostic yield of cultures for diagnostic tools. We stratified estimates by age and compared metrics to those derived for gastric aspirate (GA).

Results: Among 148 children who attempted the string test, 34% successfully swallowed the capsule. Feasibility was higher among children aged 11–14 than in children 4–10 years (83% vs 22% respectively, $p < 0.0001$). The string test was better tolerated than GA in both age groups; however, guardians and older children reported higher rates of willingness to repeat GA than the string test (86% vs. 58% in children; 100% vs. 83% in guardians). In 9 children with a positive sputum culture, 6 had a positive string culture. The one children with a positive gastric aspirate culture also had a positive string culture.

Conclusion: Although the string test was generally tolerable and accepted by children and caregivers; feasibility in young children was low. Reducing the capsule size may improve test success rates in younger children.

Keywords: Pediatric, Peru, Tolerability, Feasibility, Gastric aspirate

Background

The World Health Organization (WHO) estimated that one million of the 10 million cases of tuberculosis (TB) worldwide in 2017 occurred in children < 15 years of age [1]. This is likely an underestimate given that TB is notoriously difficult to diagnose in children. The WHO guidelines for diagnosing TB in children indicate evaluation of the child's TB contact history and exposure, a test of infection (tuberculin skin test, interferon gamma release assay), chest radiograph, and bacteriological confirmation by culture [2]. As noted by Chiang, et al. [3] there are serious limitations to each step in the diagnostic process. Bacteriologic confirmation of pulmonary TB is the most certain method for determining disease status, but this test depends on sputum, which is difficult to collect in young children who are often unable to expectorate spontaneously [3]. The alternative sample type for bacteriologic confirmation of *Mycobacterium tuberculosis* in children who cannot produce sputum is gastric aspirate; however, the procedure to obtain this sample is invasive and it is not broadly available in resource-constrained settings due to a limited number of health providers trained in the procedure and/or a lack adequate space within primary health facilities [4–9]. Furthermore, the paucibacillary nature of TB in children decreases the sensitivity of acid-fast smear microscopy, mycobacterial culture and nucleic acid amplification tests, all of which often are negative in children with clinically diagnosed TB disease [10, 11].

* Correspondence: ktafur_ses@pih.org
[1]Socios En Salud Sucursal Perú, Av. Túpac Amaru 4480, Comas, Lima, Peru
Full list of author information is available at the end of the article

The enteric string test, typically used to diagnose intestinal parasites, consists of ingestion of a small, dissolvable gelatin capsule containing a string that absorbs stomach fluids [12]. Because the string could also absorb sputum that has been swallowed, it has been proposed as a technique for obtaining lower respiratory specimens for tuberculosis testing in children. Several studies in adults have found that string samples have a diagnostic yield that is roughly similar to induced sputum [13–15]. The handful of studies in children have reported that > 80% could swallow the capsule and complete the test [4, 16, 17]; though this rate may vary by the child's age, with the youngest children least able to swallow the capsule [13]. Among children who complete the test, diagnostic yield is comparable to sputum or gastric aspirate [13, 18]. In spite of its perceived simplicity and promise, the string test has not been widely adopted.

To respond to the need for a noninvasive clinical sample for routine TB diagnosis that is easily collected from children, we examined the feasibility and diagnostic effectiveness of the string test in children with suspected pulmonary TB in Lima, Peru.

Methods

Study population

The study population consisted of children in Lima, Peru who were consecutively enrolled in a larger pediatric TB diagnostic study, which aimed to identify sample types other than sputum that could be used for pediatric TB diagnosis. Children were less than 15 years old, had a history of contact with an adult with pulmonary TB and met at least one of the following criteria for inclusion in pediatric TB diagnostic studies, as defined by an expert panel [19]: persistent, unremitting, and unexplained cough for > 2 weeks, unexplained weight loss, unexplained fever for > 1 week, or unexplained fatigue or lethargy. Based on prior studies that found that the string test performed well in children as young as four years [16], we requested a string specimen from children four years of age and older. This analysis included all children that attempted the string test between May 2015 and December 2016.

Standard of care for pediatric TB diagnosis in Peru

All children received the standard of care for pediatric TB diagnosis as defined by Peru Ministry of Health (MoH) guidelines [20]. Children provided two lower respiratory specimens and underwent chest X-ray, a tuberculin skin test (TST) and a physical examination by a MoH pediatric pulmonologist. Sputum induction and gastric aspiration were performed when was necessary. To preserve the viability of *Mycobacterium tuberculosis* for culture, we neutralized gastric aspirate samples at the time of collection by adding a few drops of sodium bicarbonate until the pH reached to between 6.8 and 7.2. All collected samples were then transported using cold chain (2 to 8 °C) to the laboratory for acid-fast smear microscopy and TB culture.

String test procedure

Children were asked to swallow a nylon string coiled inside of a dissolvable, weighted gelatin capsule. Following an approximately eight-hour fast, a trained study nurse attached the proximal end of the string to the child's cheek with tape and placed the capsule on the back of the child's tongue. The child was asked to swallow the capsule with a glass of water. The string remained in situ for up to four hours of intragastric downtime. Drinking water was permitted if children complained of a dry or scratchy throat. The study team provided children with coloring books, puzzles, and electronic tablets with games while they waited to avoid potential agitation of the string. A study nurse removed the string by holding the proximal end and pulling it out of the stomach with a gentle tug, ensuring it made no contact with the tongue or other external surfaces. Using sterile scissors, the string was cut 10 cm from the distal end of the string that had been inside the stomach. The cut section was placed in a phosphate buffered saline solution with a Ph among 6.8 to 7.2 and transported at room temperature to the study laboratory within four hours of collection. All collected samples were then transported using cold chain (2 to 8 °C) to the laboratory for TB culture.

The capsules used in the study were manufactured locally in Peru. Capsule size and string lengths were determined based on participant age, the reference height of children from anthropometric tables developed by the Peru MoH, and estimates of the distance from mouth to stomach developed by Beckstrand et al. [21]. Encapsulated strings were designed with the following specifications: 1.6 cm-long capsules containing 50 cm of coiled string for children < 7 years old, 1.8 cm-long capsules containing 60 cm of coiled string for children 8–10 years old, and 2.2 cm-long capsules containing 70 cm of coiled string for children > 10 years old. All capsules were 0.5 cm in diameter.

Culture procedures

String, sputum, and gastric aspirate samples were centrifuged at 3000 rpm (rpm); the pellet was then decontaminated with NALC-NaOH and neutralized with phosphate buffer. We performed culture using BACTEC MGIT 960 (Becton Dickinson, Franklin Lakes, NJ) on each sample type, following the manufacturer's recommendations [22].

Data collection

We collected demographic, epidemiologic, laboratory and clinical data via interviews with children and caregivers and clinical chart abstraction. Clinical data included signs and symptoms of TB and results of TST, chest x-ray, and clinical evaluation for TB disease.

Through surveys administered to children and guardians, we evaluated acceptability and tolerability of the string and gastric aspirate procedures. These surveys were first implemented five months after the study began and, therefore, only children and guardians enrolling in or after November 2015 completed these surveys.

Feasibility

We assessed the feasibility of the string test by the percentage of children who successfully swallowed the string capsule. We classified a child as having had an unsuccessful test if s/he could not swallow the capsule or hold it down.

Acceptability

We assessed acceptability in two ways. First, we asked guardians and children who attempted the string test and/or gastric aspiration how comfortable they felt with the procedure while it was underway and once it was over. For gastric aspiration, this was assessed for the first sample collected. Then, following completion of each procedure, we asked children and guardians to report whether they would be willing to repeat it.

Tolerability

We evaluated tolerability among children who completed the string test using the Wong-Baker FACES® Pain Rating Scale [23, 24]. Children were asked to indicate with which of six cartoon facial expressions they most identified during and after the procedures. Response choices were 'Doesn't hurt', 'Hurts a little', 'Hurts a bit more', 'Hurts more', 'Hurts a lot', and 'Hurts worst' (Fig. 1).

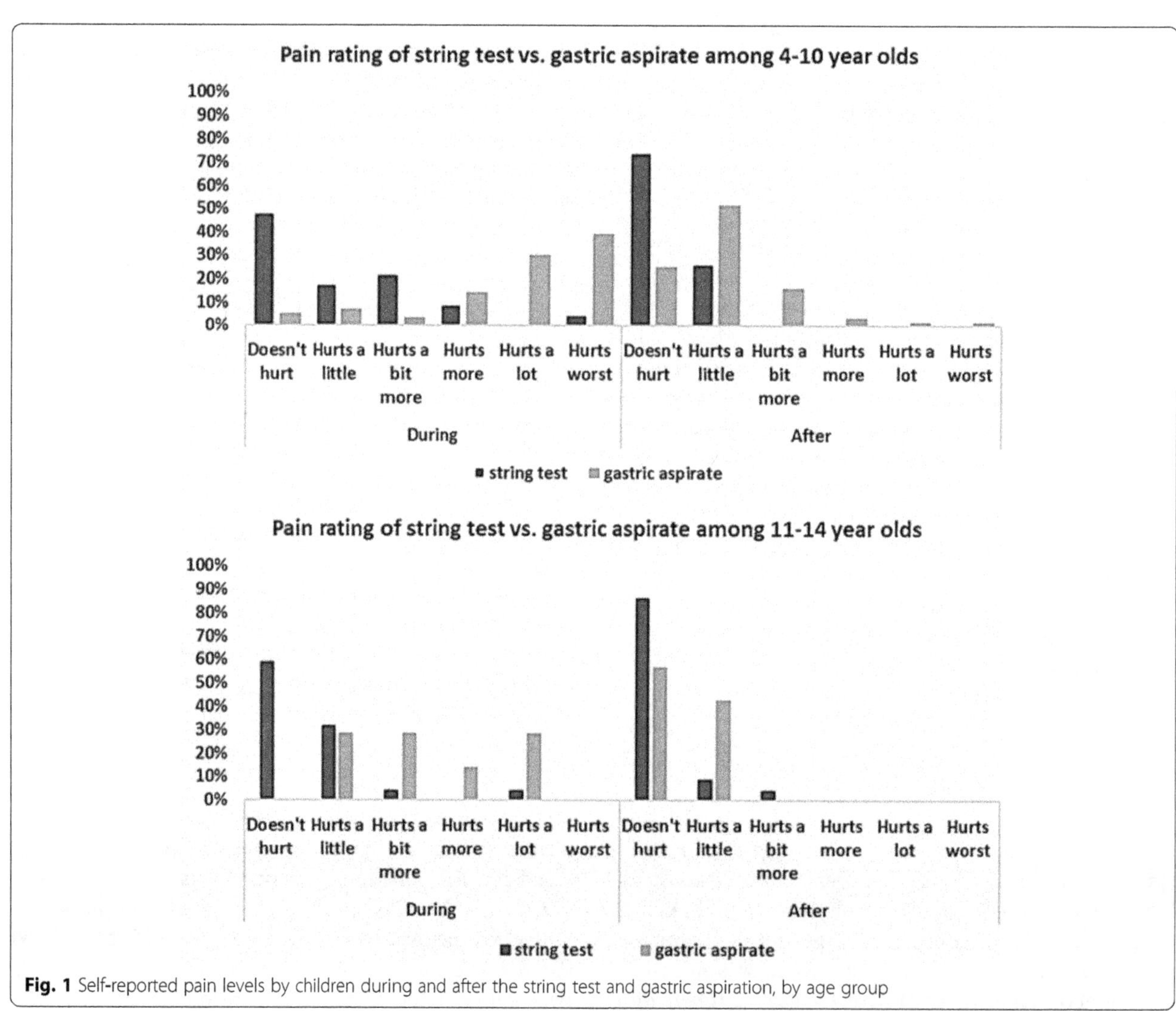

Fig. 1 Self-reported pain levels by children during and after the string test and gastric aspiration, by age group

Diagnostic effectiveness

To assess diagnostic effectiveness, we compared culture results from string test samples to those from cultures conducted on gastric aspirate and sputum.

Statistical methods

Feasibility

We calculated the percentage of children who successfully completed the string test among those who attempted it and compared success rates across age groups (4–10 and 11–14 year olds) using Chi-squared tests.

Acceptability

We compared the percentage of participants willing to repeat the string test and gastric aspiration using the Rao-Scott Chi-squared test. These methods accounts for repeated measures among participants who completed assessments for both sample types. We stratified percentages by participant type (child or adult) and child age group (4–10 or 11–14 years). Participants responding that they 'Definitely agree,' 'Probably agree,' or 'Only agree if absolutely necessary' to repeat the test were classified as 'Willing.' Those responding 'Unlikely agree,' 'Don't agree,' or 'Will not repeat procedure' were classified as 'Unwilling.'

We replicated these analyses for comfort level during and after the string and gastric aspirate procedures as reported by guardians. Responses of 'Very comfortable,' 'Comfortable,' or 'Slightly comfortable,' with a test were classified as 'Comfortable.' Responses of 'Slightly uncomfortable,' 'Uncomfortable,' or 'Very uncomfortable' were classified as 'Uncomfortable.'

Tolerability

We describe the reported pain levels using Wong-Baker FACES® Pain Rating Scale [23] and graphed frequency of responses for the string and gastric aspirate procedures, stratifying responses by age group.

Diagnostic effectiveness

We reported the frequency of culture positivity for each sample type, stratified by age group.

Data were analyzed data using SPSS version 22.0 (IBM, Armonk, New York, USA) and Microsoft Excel™ (Microsoft Corporation, Seattle, WA).

Results

We included 148 children (median age: 8.2 years, IQR: 5.5–10.0 years) in whom the string test was attempted. Table 1 provides descriptive statistics for the children and Table 2 shows an overview of study enrollment and procedures. Over half of children (54%) were under seven years old, and no child had known HIV-infection. Nearly all participants provided at least one sputum or gastric aspirate sample ($n = 146$, 99%) with 57% ($n = 82$) providing sputum (74 spontaneous and 8 induced samples, two children provided one of each), and 51% ($n = 75$) providing gastric aspirates. Thirty-two children were diagnosed with TB by a pediatric pulmonologist, of whom 12 (38%) had bacteriologic confirmation of TB by culture of sputum or gastric aspirate.

Feasibility

Of the 148 children, 50 (34%) successfully swallowed the capsule. More children in the 11–14 year age group were able to swallow the capsule as compared to children in the 4–10 year age group (83% vs 22% respectively, $p < 0.0001$). Among the 72 children that could not produce a spontaneous sputum sample, 13/66 children in the 4–10 group (20%) and 6/6 children in 11–14 group (100%) successfully completed the string test.

Acceptability among children and guardians

Table 3 shows that 39% of children aged 4 to 10 years old were willing to repeat the string test, while 21% were willing to repeat gastric aspiration ($p = 0.017$). In contrast, guardians of younger children were more often willing to have their child repeat gastric aspiration as compared to the string test (96% vs 81%, $p = 0.005$). Children 11 to 14 years old and their guardians were more likely to report willingness to repeat the gastric aspirate procedure as compared to the string test (86% vs. 58% in children; $p = 0.182$, 100% vs. 83% in guardians). While more caregivers reported comfort during the string test than during the gastric aspirate procedure, nearly all caregivers reported comfort with both the string test and gastric aspiration after they were completed (Table 3).

Tolerability

Figure 1 shows that nearly all younger children (95%) reported at least some pain during the gastric aspirate procedure and 39% reported the highest level ('hurts worst'). In contrast, during the string test, only 52% reported pain and 4% reported the highest level. All older children (100%) reported at least some pain during the gastric aspiration whereas only 41% reported any pain during the string test.

Diagnostic effectiveness

Table 4 shows culture positivity by sample type by age group in children with a successful string test. Among children with both a string and gastric aspirate sample, culture positivity was 5% for both sample types. Among the 34 children with both a string and sputum sample (either spontaneously expectorated or induced), 9 had a positive sputum culture, of which six were positive by string culture. All six of the positive cultures from string

Table 1 Characteristics of 148 children (ages 4 to 14 years) who attempted the string test

Characteristics	4–10 years old *N* = 119 (80%)		11–14 years old *N* = 29 (20%)		TOTAL *N* = 148	
	n	%	n	%	n	%
Female sex	55	46	15	52	70	47
Clinical symptoms (last 4 weeks)						
Cough	117	98	28	97	145	98
Productive cough (among those with cough)*	88	74	19	66	107	72
Hemoptysis	5	4	3	10	8	5
Chest pain	33	28	10	34	43	29
Fever	37	31	11	38	48	32
Dyspnea	34	29	8	28	42	28
Loss of appetite	50	42	11	38	61	41
Night sweats	33	28	7	24	40	27
Vomiting	24	20	6	21	30	20
Sore or itchy throat	56	47	10	34	66	45
Pain with swallowing	26	22	6	21	32	22
Hoarseness	35	29	5	17	40	27
Positive tuberculin skin test (TST) ($n = 133$) **	53	48	14	61	67	45
Exposure to an adult with positive sputum smear test	109	92	26	90	135	91
Provided a spontaneous sputum sample	53†	45	21‡	72	74	50
Provided an induced sputum sample	5	4	3‡	10	9	6
Provided a gastric aspirate sample	68†	57	7	24	75	51
Result of evaluation for TB disease ($n = 147$)						
Clinically diagnosed TB without culture confirmation	19	16	1	3	20	14
Culture-confirmed TB	4	3	8	28	12	8
Not TB	95	81	20	69	115	78

*Percent with productive cough was calculated among those with cough
**Percentages for TST results were based on available results: $N = 110$ for 4–10 year olds, $N = 23$ for 11–14 year olds
†Seven children provided one spontaneous and one gastric aspirate sputum sample
‡Two children provided one spontaneous and one induced sputum sample

were among children 11–14 years old. Among the 21 children with both a string and gastric aspirate sample, one children had a positive gastric aspirate culture and a positive string culture. Every child with a positive string culture also had a positive culture by sputum or gastric aspirate.

Discussion

This study demonstrated that the string test, although generally tolerable and accepted by children and their caregivers, was not reliably feasible, especially among younger children. This is the group least likely to be able to produce a spontaneous sputum sample and therefore, in greatest need of an alternative sample type. There were no positive string cultures in this group. We did not observe increased bacteriological detection when using the string test as compared to conventional sample types. Among children who were able to produce a sputum sample (either spontaneously or through induction), we found that culture positivity for the string test was lower than sputum (6 of 9 children with positive sputum cultures, had positive string cultures). The single gastric aspirate sample in our study that was positive by culture was also positive by string.

Most children in the 4–10 year-old age group (78%) were not able to swallow the capsule. In contrast, older children were generally able to swallow the capsule and successfully complete the test. String test success rates were higher (> 80%) in other studies with a similar median age [4, 16, 17]; though these studies also found the string test to be least successful in young children. Had gastric aspirate and sputum induction not been available in our setting, the string test would have resulted in a sample for culturing in 13 (20%) children 4–10 and 6 (100%) children 11–14 who would not have otherwise had one because they could not produce a spontaneous sputum sample.

Table 2 Data collection for 148 children who attempted the string test (ages 4 to 14 years) and their guardians

	n/N	%
At least 1 upper respiratory sample collected	146/148	99%
Gastric aspirate	75/148	51%
Sputum (spontaneous and or induced)	82/148	55%
Successful string test	50/148	34%
Enrolled after survey implementation (November 2015)	124/148	84%
String test attempted		
Caregiver comfort after string test or attempt	111/124	90%
Caregiver willingness to repeat the string test	112/124	90%
Child willingness to repeat the test	112/124	90%
Children: Wong Baker FACES® scale after string test or attempt	114/124	92%
String capsule swallowed	50/124	40%
Caregiver comfort during procedure	43/50	86%
Children: Wong Baker FACES® scale during the procedure	45/50	90%
Gastric aspirate collected	63/75	84%
Caregiver comfort during procedure	63/63	100%
Caregiver comfort after procedure	63/63	100%
Caregiver willingness to repeat the test	63/63	100%
Child willingness to repeat the test	63/63	100%
Wong Baker FACES® scale during the procedure	63/63	100%
Wong Baker FACES® scale after the procedure	63/63	100%

Our capsule sizes for children < 10 years were the same size or smaller than the pediatric Entero-Test (HDC Corporation, San Jose, CA), which was used in previous studies [4, 17] or adapted from Entero-test [18]. Smaller capsules and additional interventions to facilitate pill swallowing [25] could improve string test feasibility. One potential explanation for differential string test success across settings relates to pill taking familiarity. For example, one third of children that participated in the study conducted in Uganda by Nansumba, et al. [4] were living with HIV, and therefore may have been more accustomed to swallowing pills.

For the diagnosis of pediatric TB in primary health centers, the string test may have advantages over gastric aspiration, which requires more supplies, experienced, well-trained personnel and an adequate environment in which to perform the procedure. Both methods require overnight fasting. Notably, older children and guardians of children in both age groups were more likely to report willingness to repeat gastric aspiration than to repeat the string test. Study nurses reported that many guardians praised the brevity of gastric aspiration as compared to the long duration of the string test, which could be disruptive to daily activities. While gastric aspirate takes an average of 20 min and is completed in one attempt, the string test requires up to 4 h of intragastric downtime. Although one study in adults suggested that intragastric downtime could be reduced to one hour without a loss in diagnostic yield, it is unknown to what extent these findings apply to children, who are more likely to have paucibacillary disease [26]. Though longer, most children reported that the string test was relatively painless, as compared to the gastric aspirate.

We compared the diagnostic yield from a single string sample to the yield from up two sputum and/or gastric aspirate samples. An additional string sample may have improved detection relative to sputum; however, given that the string test would be most valuable in children unable to produce sputum, we do not perceive this as a major study limitation. A second limitation is the small sample number of children with culture-confirmed TB, which precluded us from formally testing the diagnostic yield of the string sample relative to conventional respiratory samples.

Table 3 Acceptability of string test and gastric aspirate procedures among children and their guardians

	4–10 years old					11–14 years old				
	String test		Gastric aspirate		*p*-value	String test		Gastric aspirate		*p*-value
	n/N	%	n/N	%		n/N	%	n/N	%	
Guardian reported comfort with the procedure:										
During	24/25	96	35/56	63	0.001	21/21	100	4/7	57	**
After	83/88	94	53/56	95	0.925	23/24	96	7/7	100	**
Willing to repeat the procedure:										
Child	34/88	39	12/56	21	0.017	15/26	58	6/7	86	0.182
Parent	71/88	81	54/56	96	0.005	20/24	83	7/7	100	**

***Clustered p-value could not be calculated due to a cell count of zero*

Table 4 *Mycobacterium tuberculosis* culture positivity by sample type among 50 children with a successful string test

Sample type	4–10 years old		11–14 years old		Total	
	N = 26		*N* = 24		*N* = 50	
	n/N	%	n/N	%	n/N	%
String vs. Gastric Aspirate						
String test	0/ 14	0	1/7	14	1/21	5
Gastric aspirate	0/14	0	1/7	14	1/21*	5
String vs. Sputum						
String test	0/ 15	0	6/19	32	6/34	18
Spontaneous sputum	1/13	8	7/18*	41	8/31	26
Induced sputum	0/2	0	1/2*	50	1/4*	25

**Children with multiple respiratory sample types (spontaneous sputum, induced sputum, gastric aspirate) are included in the denominator of each sample type; therefore, the denominator is greater than the number of children. In the 11–14 age group: one child provided one spontaneous and one induced sputum sample, both culture negative. Another child in this group provided one gastric aspirate and one induced sputum; both culture positive*

Conclusions

Our findings reinforce those from a small body of literature examining the string test as a diagnostic specimen for children with suspected TB. The string test is a well-tolerated and acceptable alternative sample type for diagnosing TB in children among those who are able to swallow the capsule. In contexts where gastric aspirate is not available, it may be an acceptable substitute; however, the sample and case detection yield may be small to moderate.

Abbreviations

GA: Gastric aspirate; HIV: Human Immunodeficiency Virus; MoH: Ministry of Health; rpm: Revolutions per minute; TB: Tuberculosis; TST: Tuberculin Skin Test; WHO: World Health Organization

Acknowledgements

The authors wish to thank all the children and guardians who participated in this study. We also thank the health authorities and nurses of the primary health centers (Lima jurisdiction) who performed gastric aspiration and facilitated the string test in their facilities; and field personnel of Socios En Salud who participated in the execution of the study.

Funding

The study was funded by National Institute of Health Grant N° 5U19AI109755-02. Karla T Tafur is a Fogarty fellow supported by Fogarty Grant (N° D43TW009379).

Author's contributions

KT led the statistical analysis and data interpretation and wrote the first draft. JC analyzed the data, interpreted it and contributed to writing and editing. SL contributed to writing and editing of manuscript. CC, MM, CP, SC, LL and RC contributed to design and implementation of the study. MF conceptualized and designed the study and contributed to writing and editing. All authors critically reviewed the manuscript and approved the final version.

Competing interests

The authors declare that they have no competing interests.

Author details

[1]Socios En Salud Sucursal Perú, Av. Túpac Amaru 4480, Comas, Lima, Peru. [2]Department of Global Health and Social Medicine, Harvard Medical School, Boston, MA, USA. [3]Department of Pediatrics, Alpert Medical School of Brown University, Providence, RI, USA. [4]Center for International Health Research. Rhode Island Hospital, Providence, RI, USA.

References

1. WHO. Global Tuberculosis Report 2018. Switzerland: World Health Organization; 2018.
2. WHO. Guidance for national tubeculosis programmes on the managment of tuberculosis in children. Switzerland: World Health Organization; 2014.
3. Chiang SS, Swanson DS, Starke JR. New diagnostics for childhood tuberculosis. Infect Dis Clin N Am. 2015;29(3):477–502.
4. Nansumba M, Kumbakumba E, Orikiriza P, Muller Y, Nackers F, Debeaudrap P, et al. Detection yield and tolerability of string test for diagnosis of childhood intrathoracic tuberculosis. Pediatr Infect Dis J. 2016;35(2):146–51.
5. Mukherjee A, Singh S, Lodha R, Singh V, Hesseling AC, Grewal HM, et al. Ambulatory gastric lavages provide better yields of Mycobacterium tuberculosis than induced sputum in children with intrathoracic tuberculosis. Pediatr Infect Dis J. 2013;32(12):1313–7.
6. Zar HJ, Hanslo D, Apolles P, Swingler G, Hussey G. Induced sputum versus gastric lavage for microbiological confirmation of pulmonary tuberculosis in infants and young children: a prospective study. Lancet. 2005;365(9454): 130–4.
7. Perez-Velez CM, Marais BJ. Tuberculosis in children. N Engl J Med. 2012; 367(4):348–61.
8. Bates M, O'Grady J, Maeurer M, Tembo J, Chilukutu L, Chabala C, et al. Assessment of the Xpert MTB/RIF assay for diagnosis of tuberculosis with gastric lavage aspirates in children in sub-Saharan Africa: a prospective descriptive study. Lancet Infect Dis. 2013;13(1):36–42.
9. Reid MJ, Saito S, Fayorsey R, Carter RJ, Abrams EJ. Assessing capacity for diagnosing tuberculosis in children in sub-Saharan African HIV care settings. Int J Tuberc Lung Dis. 2012;16(7):924–7.
10. Starke JR. Pediatric tuberculosis: time for a new approach. Tuberculosis (Edinb). 2003;83(1–3):208–12.
11. Perez-Velez CM, Roya-Pabon CL, Marais BJ. A systematic approach to diagnosing intra-thoracic tuberculosis in children. J Inf Secur. 2017;74(Suppl 1):S74–83.
12. Korman SH. The duodenal string test. A simple multipurpose diagnostic tool in clinical pediatrics. Am J Dis Child. 1990;144(7):803–5.
13. Atwine D, Nansumba M, Orikiriza P, Riera M, Nackers F, Kamara N, et al. Intra-gastric string test: an effective tool for diagnosing tuberculosis in adults unable to produce sputum. Int J Tuberc Lung Dis. 2015;19(5):558–64.
14. Vargas D, García L, Gilman RH, Evans C, Ticona E, Navincopa M, et al. Diagnosis of sputum-scarce HIV-associated pulmonary tuberculosis in Lima, Peru. Lancet. 2005;365(9454):150–2.
15. Lora MH, Reimer-McAtee MJ, Gilman RH, Lozano D, Saravia R, Pajuelo M, et al. Evaluation of microscopic observation drug susceptibility (MODS) and the string test for rapid diagnosis of pulmonary tuberculosis in HIV/AIDS patients in Bolivia. BMC Infect Dis. 2015;15:222.
16. Chow F, Espiritu N, Gilman RH, Gutierrez R, Lopez S, Escombe AR, et al. La cuerda dulce-a tolerability and acceptability study of a novel approach to specimen collection for diagnosis of paediatric pulmonary tuberculosis. BMC Infect Dis. 2006;6:67.
17. Marcy O, Ung V, Goyet S, Borand L, Msellati P, Tejiokem M, et al. Performance of Xpert MTB/RIF and alternative specimen collection methods for the diagnosis of tuberculosis in HIV-infected children. Clin Infect Dis. 2016;62(9):1161–8.
18. Imperiale BR, Nieves C, Mancino B, Sanjurjo M, Tártara S, Di Giulio Á, et al. String test: a new tool for tuberculosis diagnosis and drug-resistance detection in children. Int J Mycobacteriol. 2018;7(2):162–6.
19. Cuevas LE, Browning R, Bossuyt P, Casenghi M, Cotton MF, Cruz AT, et al. Evaluation of tuberculosis diagnostics in children: 2. Methodological issues for conducting and reporting research evaluations of tuberculosis diagnostics for intrathoracic tuberculosis in children. Consensus from an expert panel. J Infect Dis. 2012;205(Suppl 2):S209–15.

20. MINSA. Norma técnica de la salud para el control de la Tuberculosis. Peru: Ministerio de Salud; 2013.
21. Beckstrand J, Cirgin Ellett ML, McDaniel A. Predicting internal distance to the stomach for positioning nasogastric and orogastric feeding tubes in children. J Adv Nurs. 2007;59(3):274–89.
22. Rüsch-Gerdes S, Pfyffer GE, Casal M, Chadwick M, Siddiqi S. Multicenter laboratory validation of the BACTEC MGIT 960 technique for testing susceptibilities of Mycobacterium tuberculosis to classical second-line drugs and newer antimicrobials. J Clin Microbiol. 2006;44(3):688–92.
23. Foundation W-BF. Wong-Baker FACES ® Pain Rating Scale: Whaley & Wong's Nursing Care of Infants and Children . © Elsevier Inc.; 2016 [Available from: http://wongbakerfaces.org/. Accessed 8 Oct 2018.
24. Hockenberry MJ, Wilson D, Rodgers CC. Wong's Essentials of Pediatr Nurs. 10th ed. St.Louis: ELSEVIER; 2017.
25. Patel A, Jacobsen L, Jhaveri R, Bradford KK. Effectiveness of pediatric pill swallowing interventions: a systematic review. Pediatrics. 2015;135(5):883–9.
26. Bae WH, Salas A, Brady MF, Coronel J, Colombo CG, Castro B, et al. Reducing the string test intra-gastric downtime for detection of Mycobacterium tuberculosis. Int J Tuberc Lung Dis. 2008;12(12):1436–40.

21

Evaluation of Influenza A H1N1 infection and antiviral utilization in a tertiary care hospital

Talita Rantin Belucci[1,2*], Alexandre R. Marra[2,3], Michael B. Edmond[3,4], João Renato Rebello Pinho[5,8], Paula Kiyomi Onaga Yokota[2], Ana Carolina Cintra Nunes Mafra[6,7] and Oscar Fernando Pavão dos Santos[2]

Abstract

Background: Influenza A H1N1 infections carry a significant mortality risk. This study describes inpatients with suspected and confirmed Influenza A H1N1 infection who were prescribed oseltamivir, the risk factors associated with infection, the association between infection and mortality, and the factors associated with in-hospital mortality in infected patients.

Methods: This study was a matched case-control study of hospitalized patients who underwent real-time polymerase chain reaction testing for Influenza A H1N1 and were treated with oseltamivir from 2009 to 2015 in a tertiary care hospital. Cases (patients with positive Influenza A H1N1 testing) were matched 1:1 to controls (patients with negative test results).

Results: A total of 1405 inpatients who underwent PCR testing and received treatment with oseltamivir were identified in our study and 157 patients confirmed Influenza A H1N1. Almost one third of patients with Influenza A H1N1 were diagnosed in the pandemic period. There was no difference in mortality between cases and controls. Immunocompromised status, requirement of vasoactive drugs, mechanical ventilation, acute hemodialysis, albumin administration, surgical procedures and thoracic procedures and length of stay were associated with increased risk of death in Influenza A H1N1 infected patients.

Conclusions: We found no increased risk of mortality for patients with proven Influenza A H1N1 when compared to similar patients without confirmed Influenza.

Keywords: Influenza a H1N1, Oseltamivir, Hospitalized patients

Background

According to the World Health Organization (WHO), during the Influenza A H1N1 pandemic 59 million people were infected, resulting in 265,000 hospitalizations and 12,000 deaths in the United States. This virus has high transmissibility, a short incubation period, and high rates of morbidity and mortality [1].

The goal of this study is to describe inpatients treated with oseltamivir and suspected and confirmed Influenza A H1N1 infection, the associated factors with infection, the association between infection and mortality, and the factors associated with in-hospital mortality in patients with confirmed Influenza A H1N1.

* Correspondence: talita.belucci@hotmail.com
[1]Hospital Israelita Albert Einstein, São Paulo, Brazil
[2]Division of Medical Practice, Hospital Israelita Albert Einstein, Avenida Albert Einstein, 627 – bloco A1, 1° andar, Morumbi, São Paulo 05651-901, Brazil
Full list of author information is available at the end of the article

Methods

This study was conducted in a tertiary care, private hospital in São Paulo, Brazil with 629 beds and approximately 194,000 patient-days yearly and approved by the Institutional Review Board and Ethics Committee of Hospital Israelita Albert Einstein and informed consent was not required.

A retrospective study was conducted from January 2009 to December 2015.

This study describes inpatients treated with oseltamivir who had suspected or confirmed Influenza A H1N1 infection and were tested for Influenza A H1N1 by real-time polymerase chain reaction (RT-PCR). The primary reason for hospitalization was not necessarily Influenza. This study also describes the factors associated with infection, the association between infection and mortality and the factors associated with in-hospital mortality in patients with confirmed Influenza A H1N1.

A matched (1:1) case-control study was performed to analyze the factors associated with infection and in-hospital mortality, comparing patients who would have similar illness severity during hospitalization and thus isolate the impact of the infection on the outcome of in-hospital mortality. Cases were defined as patients with Influenza A H1N1 confirmed by RT-PCR, and controls had a negative result for Influenza A (H1N1 and H3N2) and Influenza B and were treated with oseltamivir for up to four days. All patients in the matched case-controls study were tested both for Influenza A H1N1 and Influenza A H3N2, but only 31.6% (444/1.405) were tested for Influenza B. Patients excluded were those under 18 years of age and those in whom the length of stay exceeded 365 days. The criteria of length of stay was based on the long-term hospitalized patients.

The data abstracted from the electronic medical record included demographics and clinical data, Influenza RT-PCR assay results, oseltamivir treatment (duration, frequency and dose), outcome status (death was defined as in-hospital mortality), and underlying conditions (lung disease, cardiovascular disease, neurological and neuro-developmental conditions, blood disorders, diabetes mellitus, kidney disease, liver disease, immunosuppression (e.g., HIV, cancer or chronic treatment with corticosteroids), and pregnancy or post-partum state [up to two weeks after childbirth]). We also collected possible indicators of complications during hospitalization (which may or may not be associated with H1N1 infection): data on intensive care unit (ICU) admission, transfusions, use of mechanical ventilation, acute hemodialysis, use of vasopressor drugs, albumin and antibiotic administration, surgical procedures, or thoracic procedures (e.g., pulmonary biopsy or segmentectomy, tracheostomy).

Patients were not followed up after hospital discharge. Antiviral therapy was prescribed according to the institutional protocol [2], with oseltamivir initiated empirically based on clinical presentation or after a positive PCR test. The empiric therapy for Influenza is based on the symptoms, such as fever, cough, sore throat, runny and/or stuffy nose, muscle or body aches, headaches, and fatigue, as well as for patients at high risk for developing Influenza- related complications. This includes age $\geq$ 60 years, patients of any age with certain chronic medical conditions (such as cardiovascular disease, lung disease, diabetes mellitus, kidney disease, liver disease, neurological and neuro-developmental conditions, and immunocompromised states), and pregnant women or post-partum state [1, 2].

Statistical analysis

Descriptive analysis was performed using the median and inter-quartile range (IQR) for continuous variables and absolute frequencies and percentages for categorical variables. Simple associations were analyzed using logistic models and odds ratio were determined. The level of significance was set at 0.05.

For matching cases and controls we used the Matching package [3], which weighs all variables involved in order to have a balanced final pairing. Cases and controls were matched on factors impacting mortality: age, ICU admission, surgical procedure, use of vasoactive drugs, use of mechanical ventilation, albumin administration, and blood or platelet transfusion. After matching, the logistic model predicting death was adjusted by means of generalized estimation equations, with the Geepack package [4]. We used R software version 3.4.1.

Results

Of 1,405 inpatients who underwent PCR testing and received treatment with oseltamivir, 1051 (74.8%) were PCR negative. Twenty-two patients were positive for Influenza B, 175 positive for Influenza A H3N2, and 157 positive for Influenza A H1N1. Of the uninfected patients, 642 received oseltamivir treatment up to four days and 157 of those were matched as controls. For the 157 controls, 32 (20.4%) underwent Influenza B testing and were also negative for Influenza B (Fig. 1).

When considering the entire period of the study, 19.2% of the requests for PCR tests combined with oseltamivir prescriptions occurred during the period of the pandemic, with the majority (60.7%) occurring between 2013 and 2015. These occurred in older patients (55.1% $\geq$ 60 years), 49.9% males, 1.9% pregnant or post-partum state, 8.1% immunocompromised, 23.7% with diabetes mellitus, 24.3% with lung disease, 1.2% with liver disease, 6.0% with kidney disease, 46.8% with cardiovascular disease and 6.8% with neurological and neuro-developmental conditions (Additional file 1: Table S1). The primary diagnosis was a disease of the respiratory system in 66.6% of hospitalizations (Additional file 1: Table S1).

Of the 157 Influenza A H1N1 cases, 49.7% (78/157) were diagnosed in the pandemic period. In 85.4% (134/157) of the patients with Influenza A H1N1 infection, the daily dosage of oseltamivir was 150 mg and 92.4% (145/157) were treated for 5–10 days (Table 1).

From 2013, the number of hospitalizations increased, especially in the uninfected group (666/1051) (Table 1). Infected patients were 2.86 fold more likely to be immunocompromised ($P = 0.033$) and one-third less likely to

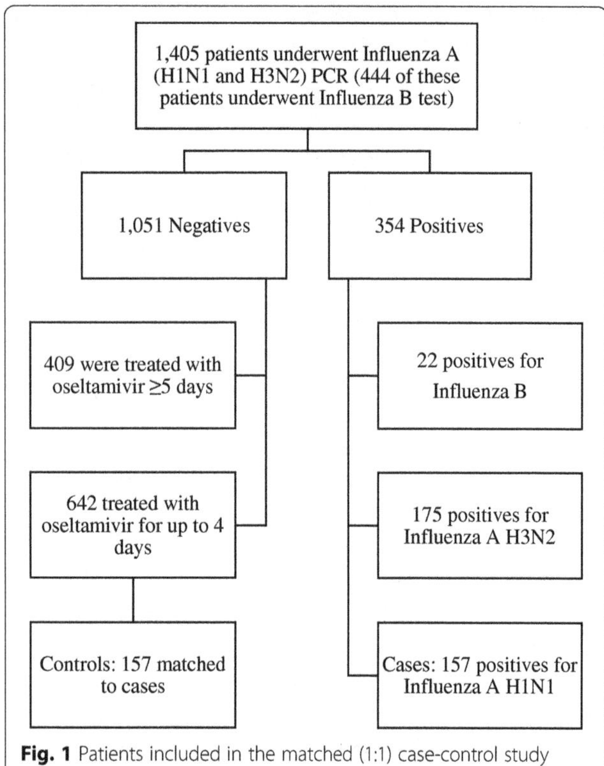

Fig. 1 Patients included in the matched (1:1) case-control study

receive antibacterial therapy ($P = 0.005$) when compared to similar patients without confirmed Influenza (Table 2).

Table 2 also shows for those patients with Influenza A H1N1 infection, 86% (135/157) were also treated with antibacterials. The median of length of stay was 5 days, and 39.5% (62/157) of the patients were admitted to the

Table 1 Characteristics of inpatients with suspected Influenza ($N = 1208$)

Variable	Influenza status	
	Infected ($n = 157$)	Uninfected ($n = 1051$)
Period – *n* (%)		
2009 (Pandemic period)	78 (49.7)	185 (17.6)
2010 to 2012	12 (7.7)	200 (19.0)
2013 to 2015	67 (42.7)	666 (63.4)
Oseltamivir daily dosage – *n* (%)		
75 mg	–	2 (0.2)
150 mg	134 (85.4)	925 (88.0)
300 mg	23 (14.6)	124 (11.8)
Oseltamivir treatment duration (days) – *n* (%)		
< 5 days	–	642 (61.1)
5 to 10 days	145 (92.4)	405 (38.5)
> 10 days	12 (7.6)	4 (0.4)

Category variables presented by absolute and relative frequencies. Numerical variables presented by median and inter-quartile range

ICU. Eight patients (5.1%) required acute hemodialysis and six patients (3.8%) underwent a thoracic procedure (lung biopsy, lung segmentectomy, thoracostomy with closed drainage, drainage of chest wall hematoma, or tracheostomy).

Of patients with Influenza A H1N1, 5.1% died. Independent factors associated with mortality were requirement for vasoactive drugs (OR = 17.13, IC 95%: 5.28–55.59, $P < 0.001$), and length of stay (OR = 1.03, IC 95%: 1.01–1.06, $P = 0.010$), and when controlling for these two factors, infection with Influenza A H1N1 was not an independent predictor of mortality (OR = 0.45, CI 95%: 0.15–1.35, $P = 0.154$) (Table 3).

When considering only the 157 patients with Influenza A H1N1 infection, the associated factors with death were: immunocompromised state ($P = 0.019$), requirement for vasoactive drugs ($P < 0.001$), mechanical ventilation ($P < 0.001$), acute hemodialysis ($P = 0.024$), surgical procedure ($P < 0.001$), thoracic surgery ($P < 0.001$), albumin administration ($P < 0.001$), and length of stay ($P < 0.001$) (Table 4).

Discussion

We observed a high proportion of negative PCRs among patients treated with oseltamivir because the treatment was administered empirically based on symptoms. The recommendation is to initiate the treatment with oseltamivir within 48 h of Influenza symptom onset [5], especially in critically ill patients, in order to reduce symptom duration, complications such as pneumonia, and possibly death [6]. However, empiric therapy leads to uninfected patients receiving treatment and testing modalities other than PCR often have low sensitivity and specificity [7, 8].

This study considered the RT-PCR test as a gold standard, but other tests, such Influenza A and B by immunofluorescence, Influenza A serology, Influenza B serology, Rapid Influenza A and B diagnostic test, screening for respiratory virus (Influenza A and B) by immunofluorescence, viral culture (Influenza A and B), may have been conducted during the study period.

In our study, surgical procedures and thoracic procedures were associated with an increased risk of death in Influenza A H1N1 patients, but we did not find others studies that analyzed surgical procedures in inpatients with Influenza A H1N1 infection.

More than 80% of the patients with Influenza A H1N1 in our study were treated with antibacterials, which in some cases was due to pneumonia complicating Influenza. In our study it was not possible to identify if the patients had pneumonia, but in a large cohort study [9] 31% of the patients with Influenza A H1N1 infection were diagnosed with bacterial pneumonia.

We observed that the number of hospitalizations increased substantially from 2013 onward. This rise can be explained by the fact that in that period a viral panel

Table 2 Patients profile and associated factors with H1N1 infection based on matched case-control study ($n = 314$)

Variable	Influenza status		OR (95% CI)	*P* value
	Infected ($n = 157$)	Uninfected ($n = 157$)		
Characteristics of patients				
Male	85 (54.1)	83 (52.9)	1.05 (0.68–1.64)	0.821
Age (> 60 years old)	37 (23.6)	58 (36.9)	–	–
Cardiovascular disease	54 (34.4)	49 (31.2)	1.16 (0.72–1.85)	0.548
Lung disease	31 (19.7)	42 (26.8)	0.67 (0.39–1.14)	0.143
Diabetes mellitus	28 (17.8)	28 (17.8)	1.00 (0.56–1.79)	1.000
Pregnant or post-partum state	11 (7.0)	4 (2.5)	2.88 (0.96–10.58)	0.075
Immunocompromised	16 (10.2)	6 (3.8)	2.86 (1.14–8.15)	0.033
Kidney disease	11 (7.0)	6 (3.8)	1.90 (0.70–5.63)	0.219
Liver disease	1 (0.6)	3 (1.9)	0.329 (0.016–2.602)	0.338
Neurological and neuro-developmental conditions	8 (5.1)	11 (7.0)	0.71 (0.27–1.81)	0.479
Hospitalization characteristics				
Antibacterial therapy (intravenous or oral)	135 (86.0)	150 (95.5)	0.29 (0.11–0.66)	0.005
ICU stay	62 (39.5)	74 (47.1)	0.73 (0.47–1.14)	0.172
Mechanical ventilation	17 (10.8)	17 (10.8)	–	–
Acute hemodialysis	8 (5.1)	0 (0.0)	–	–
Vasoactive drugs	20 (12.7)	20 (12.7)	–	–
Red blood cell or platelet transfusion	4 (2.5)	4 (2.5)	–	–
Surgical procedure	15 (9.6)	15 (9.6)	–	–
Thoracic procedure	6 (3.8)	0 (0.0)	–	–
Albumin administration	23 (14.6)	24 (15.3)	–	–
Length of stay (days)	5.00 [3.00; 8.00]	5.00 [3.00, 10.00]	1.00 (0.98–1.01)	0.680
In–hospital death	8 (5.1)	14 (8.9)	0.55 (0.21–1.32)	0.190

Category variables presented by absolute and relative frequencies. Numerical variables presented by median and inter-quartile range. Odds ratio (OR), confidence interval (95% CI) and *p* value obtained by simple logistic regression

performed by PCR method was introduced in the hospital's testing routine, and beyond Influenza A H1N1, the panel could also identify Influenza A H3N2 and Influenza B. That is why the information on Influenza B is not available for all patients in the study. From 2013 to 2015, the most prevalent Influenza virus in the Southeast region of Brazil, (where the hospital is located) was Influenza A H3N2 [10–12].

In the matched case-controls study results, there was no difference in mortality between patients with and without Influenza infection. However, it should be noted that all patients were treated with oseltamivir. This finding reinforces the need for treatment within 48 h of symptom onset, even in those patients who are not at high risk of developing Influenza–related complications [1, 5].

Table 3 Independent predictors of death in inpatients with suspected Influenza A H1N1 ($n = 314$)

Variable	OR (95% CI)	*P* value
Influenza A H1N1 infection	0.45 (0.15; 1.35)	0.154
Administration of vasoactive drugs	17.13 (5.28; 55.59)	< 0.001
Length of stay (days)	1.03 (1.01; 1.06)	0.010

OR odds ratio. CI: 95% confidence interval

In our study, only 8 (5.1%) patients with Influenza A H1N1 infection died. Immunocompromised states were associated with mortality in patients with Influenza A H1N1 infection in our study and in a Spanish study in which 25% (68/274) of immunocompromised inpatients with Influenza A H1N1 infection died [13]. A study performed in immunosuppressed patients with Influenza A H1N1 admitted to the ICU concluded that this population has a poor outcome and the use of corticosteroids is strongly discouraged [14].

Patients that require vasoactive drugs and mechanical ventilation were also at increased risk of death from Influenza A H1N1 infection. In the same Spanish study, 78.7% (214/274) Influenza A H1N1 infected patients requiring vasoactive drugs and 92.2% (249/274) requiring mechanical ventilation also died [13]. The median length

Table 4 Univariate predictors of death in patients with confirmed Influenza A H1N1 infection ($n = 157$)

Variable	Discharge ($n = 149$)	Death ($n = 8$)	OR (95% CI)	*P* value
Male gender	79 (53.0)	6 (75.0)	2.66 (0.59; 18.55)	0.240
Age (> 60 years old)	35 (23.5)	2 (25.0)	1.09 (0.15; 4.96)	0.922
Immunocompromised status	13 (8.7)	3 (37.5)	6.28 (1.18; 28.72)	0.019
Diabetes mellitus	25 (16.8)	3 (37.5)	2.98 (0.58; 12.94)	0.153
Kidney disease	9 (6.0)	2 (25.0)	5.19 (0.69; 26.60)	0.063
Cardiovascular disease	50 (33.6)	4 (50.0)	1.98 (0.45; 8.69)	0.348
Hospitalization characteristics				
Vasoactive drugs	14 (9.4)	6 (75.0)	28.93 (6.04; 210.94)	< 0.001
Mechanical ventilation	12 (8.1)	5 (62.5)	19.03 (4.18; 102.52)	< 0.001
Acute hemodialysis	6 (4.0)	2 (25.0)	7.94 (1.02; 44.30)	0.024
Surgical procedure	10 (6.7)	5 (62.5)	23.17 (5.00; 127.25)	< 0.001
Thoracic surgery	3 (2.0)	3 (37.5)	29.20 (4.49; 199.40)	< 0.001
Albumin administration	17 (11.4)	6 (75.0)	23.29 (4.93; 168.04)	< 0.001
Length of stay (days)	5 [3, 7]	38 [11.5, 53.75]	1.07 (1.03; 1.11)	< 0.001

Category variables presented by absolute and relative frequencies. Numerical variables presented by median and inter-quartile range. *OR* odds ratio. *95% CI* 95% confidence interval

of stay for inpatients who died in our study was much higher than that observed in this same study (13 days) [13].

Another Spanish study found that chronic conditions were an independent risk factor for mortality [15]; we noted a similar trend in our study that was not statistically significant.

Our study has some limitations, primarily that it is single center and retrospective. The retrospective nature of the study made it impossible to identify the exact cause of pneumonia. We also cannot attribute the cause of death to Influenza infection. Our study evaluated only patients tested by PCR and were treated with oseltamivir. The patients were not followed after discharge, so it was only possible to identify in-hospital deaths. It was also not possible to check the patient's vaccination status.

Conclusion

In conclusion, the profiles of the infected and uninfected patients were very similar and there was no difference in mortality. The only risk factor associated with death in infected patients was an immunocompromised state.

Abbreviations

CI: Confidence intervals; ICU: Intensive care unit; IQR: Inter-quartile range; OR: Odds ratios; RT-PCR: Real-time polymerase chain reaction; WHO: World Health Organization

Acknowledgements

We gratefully acknowledge the healthcare workers that cared for H1N1 Influenza patients at Hospital Israelita Albert Einstein, São Paulo, Brazil.

Funding

No funding was obtained for this study.

Authors' contributions

TRB, JRRP, PKOY participated in the data collected. TRB, ARM, ACCNM, OFPS participated in the data analysis. TRB, ARM, MBE, OFPS participated in the design and coordination. TRB, ARM, MBE, JRRP, PKOY, ACCNM, OFPS helped to draft the manuscript and to provide critical review to the manuscript. All authors read and approved the final manuscript.

Competing interests

The authors declare that they have no competing interests. This research received no specific grant from any funding agency in the public, commercial, or non-for-profit sectors.

Author details

[1]Hospital Israelita Albert Einstein, São Paulo, Brazil. [2]Division of Medical Practice, Hospital Israelita Albert Einstein, Avenida Albert Einstein, 627 – bloco A1, 1° andar, Morumbi, São Paulo 05651-901, Brazil. [3]Office of Clinical Quality, Safety and Performance Improvement, University of Iowa Hospitals and Clinics, Iowa City, IA, USA. [4]Division of Infectious Diseases, Department of Internal Medicine, University of Iowa Carver College of Medicine, Iowa City, IA, USA. [5]Clinical Laboratory, Hospital Israelita Albert Einstein, São Paulo, Brazil. [6]Statistics Department, Instituto Israelita de Ensino e Pesquisa Albert Einstein, Hospital Israelita Albert Einstein, São Paulo, Brazil. [7]Núcleo de Indicadores e Sistemas de Informações, Hospital Israelita Albert Einstein, São Paulo, Brazil. [8]LIM 03/07, Faculdade de Medicina da USP, São Paulo, Brazil.

References

1. Writing Committee of the WHO Consultation on Clinical Aspects of Pandemic (H1N1) 2009 Influenza. Clinical aspects of pandemic 2009 influenza a (H1N1) virus infection. N Engl J Med. 2010;362(18):1708–19 Review. Erratum in: N Engl J Med 2010 May 27;362(21):2039.
2. Hospital Israelita Albert Einstein Síndrome gripal – diretrizes para diagnóstico e tratamento [institucional protocol]. [2014 Feb 10; updated 2015 Apr 25; Pires EM].
3. Sekhon JS. Multivariate and propensity score matching software with automated balance optimization: the matching package for R. J Stat Softw. 2011;42(7):1–52.
4. Halekoh U, Højsgaard S, Yan J. The R package geepack for generalized estimating equations. J Stat Softw. 2006;15(2):1–11.
5. Rewar S, Mirdha D, Treatment RP. Prevention of pandemic H1N1 influenza. Ann Glob Health. 2015;81:645–53.

6. Coleman BL, Hassan K. Pre-and post-pandemic trends in antiviral use in hospitalized patients with laboratory – confirmed influenza: 2004/05 – 2013/14, Toronto, Canada. Antivir Res. 2017;140:158–63.
7. McGeer AJ. Diagnostic testing or empirical therapy for patients hospitalized with suspected influenza: what to do? Clin Infect Dis. 2009;48:S14–9.
8. Zazueta-García R, Canizalez-Roman A, Flores-Villaseñor H, Martínez-Garcia J, Llausas-Vargas A, León-Sicairos N. Effectiveness of two rapid influenza tests in comparison to reverse transcription–PCR for influenza a diagnosis. J Infect Dev Ctries. 2014;8:331–8.
9. Shah SN, Greenber JA, McNulty MC, Gregg KS, Riddell J, Mangino JE, et al. Severe influenza in 33 US hospitals, 2013 – 2014: complications and risk factors for death in 507 patients. Infect Control Hosp Epidemiol. 2015; 36:1251–60.
10. Brazil. Ministério da Saúde. Secretaria de Vigilância em Saúde. Influenza: monitoramento até a semana epidemiológica 52 de 2013 [Internet]. Brasília (DF); [201-?] [cited in 2014 May 22]. (Boletim epidemiológico) Available from: http://portalarquivos.saude.gov.br/images/pdf/2014/maio/22/boletim-influenza-se52de2013-220514.pdf
11. Brazil. Ministério da Saúde. Secretaria de Vigilância em Saúde. Influenza: monitoramento até a semana epidemiológica 28 de 2014 [Internet]. Brasília (DF); [201-?] [cited in 2014 May 22]. (Boletim epidemiológico) Available from: http://portalarquivos2.saude.gov.br/images/pdf/2014/julho/22/Boletim-Epidemiol%2D%2Dgico-Influenza-SE28.pdf
12. Brazil. Ministério da Saúde. Secretaria de Vigilância em Saúde. Influenza: monitoramento até a semana epidemiológica 25 de 2015 [Internet]. Brasília (DF); [201-?] [cited in 2015 Jul 25]. (Boletim epidemiológico) Available from: http://portalarquivos2.saude.gov.br/images/pdf/2015/julho/07/Boletim-Epidemiol%2D%2Dgico-Influenza-SE25-2015%2D%2D2-.pdf
13. Álvarez-Lerma F, Marín-Corral J, Vilà C, Masclans JR, Loeches IM, et al. Characteristics of patients with hospital – acquired influenza a (H1N1) pdm09 virus admitted to the intensive care unit. J Hosp Infect. 2017;95:200–6.
14. Garnacho-Monteiro J, León-Moya C, Gutiérrez-Pizarraya A, Arenzana-Seisdedos A, Vidaur L, et al. Clinical characteristics, evolution, and treatment-related risk factors for mortality among immunosuppressed patients with influenza a (H1N1) virus admitted to the; intensive care unit. J Crit Care. 2018;48:172–7.
15. Rodríguez-Rieiro C, Carrasco-Garrido P, Hernández-Barrera V, Andrés A, Jimenez-Trujillo I, et al. Pandemic influenza hospitalization in Spain (2009): incidence, in-hospital mortality, comorbidities and costs. Human Vaccines & Immunotherapeutics. 2012;8:443–7.

The efficacy of paritaprevir/ritonavir/ombitasvir +dasabuvir and ledipasvir/sofosbuvir is comparable in patients who failed interferon-based treatment with first generation protease inhibitors - a multicenter cohort study

Ewa Janczewska[1*], Dorota Zarębska-Michaluk[2], Hanna Berak[3], Anna Piekarska[4], Andrzej Gietka[5], Dorota Dybowska[6], Włodzimierz Mazur[7], Teresa Belica-Wdowik[8], Witold Dobracki[9], Magdalena Tudrujek-Zdunek[10], Zbigniew Deroń[11], Iwona Buczyńska[12], Marek Sitko[13], Agnieszka Czauż-Andrzejuk[14], Beata Lorenc[15], Jolanta Białkowska-Warzecha[16], Jolanta Citko[17], Łukasz Laurans[18], Jerzy Jaroszewicz[19], Łukasz Socha[18], Olga Tronina[20], Brygida Adamek[1], Andrzej Horban[21], Waldemar Halota[6], Barbara Baka-Ćwierz[8], Krzysztof Tomasiewicz[10], Krzysztof Simon[12], Aleksander Garlicki[13], Marta Wawrzynowicz-Syczewska[18] and Robert Flisiak[14]

Abstract

Background: According to the EASL and AASLD guidelines, the recommended treatment for patients who failed to achieve a sustained virologic response (SVR) on prior interferon-based triple therapy with protease inhibitors (PI), is a combination of sofosbuvir and NS5A inhibitors. Polish national recommendations also allow the use of paritaprevir/ritonavir/ombitasvir+dasasbuvir±ribavirin (PrODR) in this group of patients. The aim of the study was to evaluate the efficacy and safety of PrODR vs. ledipasvir/sofosbuvir±RBV (LSR) in PI-experienced patients in real-life setting.

Methods: Our analysis included patients registered in the nationwide, investigators initiated, multicentre EpiTer-2 database.

Among 4530 patients registered, 335 with genotype 1 (93% 1b) were previously treated with IFN-based regimens with PIs: 127 with boceprevir (BOC), 208 with telaprevir (TVR).

Patients with advanced fibrosis (F3/F4) were significantly predominant (BOC 28.4%/61.4%, TVR 18.8%/64.4%, respectively). Subjects were assigned to IFN-free retreatment as follows: BOC - 64 (50.4%) PrODR and 63 (49.6%) LSR; TVR- 103 (49.5%) PrODR and 105 (50.5%) LSR.

(Continued on next page)

* Correspondence: e.janczewska@poczta.fm
[1]Department of Basic Medical Sciences, School of Public Health in Bytom, Medical University of Silesia, ID Clinic, Janowska 19, 41-400 Mysłowice, Bytom, Poland
Full list of author information is available at the end of the article

(Continued from previous page)

Results: SVR rates were comparable for particular groups: BOC → PrODR- 100%; BOC → LSR - 98%; TVR → PrODR - 97%; TVR → LSR - 96% (intent-to treat analysis-ITT) and BOC → PrODR→100%; BOC → LSR - 99%; TVR → PrODR - 99%; TVR → LSR - 98% (modified intent-to treat analysis-mITT).

Both treatment regimens had a favourable safety profile. Adverse events (AEs) were generally mild or moderate in severity. Three deaths were reported. The treatment was stopped due to AEs in five patients (three treated with PrODR and two with LSR).

Conclusion: Efficacy and safety of treatment with PrODR and LSR is comparable in BOC or TVR-experienced patients.

Keywords: Chronic hepatitis C, Liver cirrhosis, Protease inhibitors, Retreatment, Sustained virologic response

Background

Progress achieved in recent years in the treatment of patients with viral hepatitis C has enabled elimination of hepatitis C virus (HCV) infection in most patients. This progress has been achieved through the use of drugs that produce a direct antiviral action (direct-acting antivirals-DAAs). These therapies are highly effective even in patients with advanced fibrosis, as well as hepatic insufficiency. Effective therapy inhibits progression of the disease, often leading to a fibrosis regression [1–4].

The efficacy of DAA-based therapies can be reduced by the presence of substitutions causing drug resistance (resistance-associated substitutions-RASs) [5–7]. Such substitutions can occur in patients untreated previously; however, their occurrence is more often associated with ineffective antiviral therapy, which involved DAAs with a low genetic barrier, for example first-generation protease inhibitors (PI) such as boceprevir (BOC) or telaprevir (TVR).

These drugs were the first DAAs used with pegylated interferon (PegIFN) and ribavirin (RBV) in antiviral therapies for patients infected with HCV genotype 1.

In the following years, drugs belonging to other classes and having other mechanism of action disrupting the process of HCV replication were introduced: polymerase inhibitors and non-structural protein 5A (NS5A) inhibitors. The combined use of drugs belonging to 2 or 3 therapeutic groups allowed the development of effective and safe interferon-free regimens.

In patients who had already undergone ineffective BOC or TVR triple therapy, there was a risk of reduced efficacy of subsequent IFN-free therapies in which one of the components was a protease inhibitor due to the RASs generated during the first use of these drugs.

According to the guidelines of the European Association for the Study of the Liver (EASL), and the American Association for the Study of the Liver Diseases (AASLD), the re-use of first-generation protease inhibitors is not recommended in patients who do not respond to these drugs in the past [8, 9].

Recommended therapeutic regimens were combinations of polymerase and NS5A inhibitors: ledipasvir/sofosbuvir or daclatasvir+sofosbuvir [8, 9]. These recommendations were based on the randomized clinical trials findings [10–13]. Moreover, in this patient group, the EASL recommendations provide for ribavirin addition to the DAAs to improve efficacy and reduce potential resistance [8].

In Poland, the first and for some time the only therapy composed of DAAs was paritaprevir/ ritonavir/ombitasvir ± dasabuvir ± ribavirin (PrODR), not mentioned in the above guidelines as recommended for patients after PI treatment failure.

Initially, this drug combination was used in the early access program, in patients with advanced fibrosis, the majority of whom underwent ineffective prior IFN-based treatment (AMBER study) [14]. Among the patients included in this cohort were those who failed triple therapies involving boceprevir or telaprevir. However, the number of these patients was small. High efficacy observed in this group were considered in the recommendations of the Polish Group of HCV Experts [15] and caused inclusion of PrODR along with ledipasvir/sofosbuvir ±RBV (LSR) and sofosbuvir + daclatasvir (SOF + DCV), to be used in patients with a history of prior BOC + PegIFN +RBV or TVR + PegIFN+RBV regimens.

In 2015, PrODR and LSR became available (reimbursed) for Polish patients, whereas SOF + DCV combination was not accepted for reimbursement in Poland.

The purpose of this study was to evaluate in the real-life setting the efficacy and safety of PrODR versus LSR in patients who failed prior triple IFN-based therapies with first generation protease inhibitors.

Material and methods

Study population

On the investigators' initiative, a national EpiTer-2 database of patients receiving antiviral treatment due to HCV infection in Poland was established in 2016 based on regimens available within the therapeutic program of the National Health Fund. Twenty-two hepatology centres applied for participation in the project. Treatment efficacy and safety data were collected in the EpiTer-2 web database.

Demographic data of the patients, information related to HCV genotype, stage of fibrosis, liver function parameters (Child-Turcotte-Pugh and MELD scores), prior antiviral therapy, concomitant diseases and drugs used in relation thereto, HBV and/or HIV coinfections were collected in the database.

Hepatic fibrosis was evaluated by liver biopsy based on the METAVIR or Scheuer scoring system, transient elastography (TE) using the FibroScan (Echosens, Paris) device or the real-time shear wave elastography (SWE) using the Aixplorer (Supersonic, Aix-en-Provence) device. Among BOC-experienced patients: liver biopsy was performed in 31 (24.4%), TE in 73 (57.5%), and SWE in 23 (18.1%) patients, and in the TVR group: biopsy was performed in 44 (21.2%), TE in 138 (66.3%), and SWE in 26 (12.5%) patients.

HCV RNA was monitored prior to and after the treatment (end of treatment virologic response: EOT-VR), and then after at least 12-week follow-up period (sustained virologic response -SVR). Two assays were used to measure HCV RNA, depending on local practices at the testing site: Roche COBAS TaqMan with a lower limit of quantification (LLOQ) of 15 IU/mL or Abbott RealTime with an LLOQ of 12 IU/mL.

Adverse events (AEs) observed during the treatment and follow-up period were reported as well. Criteria for assessing AEs as serious were: resulting in death, life-threatening, requiring hospitalisation or prolongation of existing hospitalization, resulting in persistent or significant disability, or congenital anomaly or birth defect.

In 2016 and 2017 up to now, a total of 4530 patients were registered in the EpiTer-2 database, including 335 patients having failed prior triple-drug regimens with boceprevir or telaprevir, retreated with interferon-free regimens PrOD and LSR, being the subject of this study.

Baseline characteristics of the patients are presented in Table 1. Sex, age, and BMI distribution were similar for both BOC- and TVR-experienced groups of patients. Notably, patients with GT1b prevailed significantly in both groups, which is typical for Polish population [16]. Patients with cirrhosis (F4) and advanced fibrosis (F3) were predominant, while only few patients showed severe liver impairment symptoms (Child-Turcotte-Pugh B or C) at the beginning of the therapy or decompensation in the previous history. The percentage of patients with confirmed oesophageal varices was similar in both subgroups.

The choice of the drug, dosage and length of treatment regimen (12 vs. 24 weeks, addition of ribavirin) was made by the treating physicians based on the applicable product characteristics and recommendations of Polish Group of HCV Experts [15, 17]. All patients qualified for class B or C of Child-Turcotte-Pugh scoring system received LSR.

Statistical analysis

Data are presented as absolute numbers (%) or mean ± standard deviation. No sample size was planned. All patients who started the treatment were included in the analysis, and efficacy analyses were performed on an intent-to-treat (ITT) basis (missing virological measurements were imputed as treatment failures) and modified intent-to-treat (mITT) basis, which excludes patients with missing data of sustained virologic response (at least 12 weeks after treatment completion). The proportion of patients who achieved SVR was calculated. The significance of difference was calculated by use of Chi-square or Fischer's exact test where appropriate. P values of < 0.05 were considered to be statistically significant.

Statistical analyses were performed with STATISTICA12.0 (Statsoft, Tulsa, OK, USA).

Results

This study focuses on the analysis of the data from the EpiTer-2 database concerning 335 patients having failed prior triple, IFN-based regimens with boceprevir or telaprevir. Patients previously treated with telaprevir containing regimen prevailed (62%) in the cohort (Table 1).

Patients with relapse of infection following prior antiviral treatment prevailed in BOC subgroup, while those with non-response prevailed in TVR subgroup. There were no patients with HIV coinfection or active HBV coinfection. Only a few patients had a history of hepatocellular carcinoma (one in BOC and four in the TVR subgroup). Moreover, in both subgroups, there were patients who began treatment after liver transplantation (one in BOC and five in the TVR subgroup).

A majority of patients from both subgroups had concomitant diseases, most often hypertension and diabetes. BOC patients (63.8%) and 67.8% of TVR patients were taking additional drugs due to these diseases.

Different dosage regimens of PrODR or LSR were applied in this therapy depending on the current guidelines. Among 127 BOC patients 64 (50.4%) were being treated using one of the PrODR (BOC➔PrODR), while 63 (49.6%) patients with LSR regimens (BOC➔LSR). In the TVR subgroup, 103 (49.5%) patients received PrODR (TVR➔PrODR) and 105 (50.5%) patients received LSR (TVR➔LSR). Distribution of these regimens among studied population is summarized in Table 2.

Treatment efficacy

Figure 1 presents the treatment course and the reasons of discontinuation.

In both groups, a majority of patients completed the full course of treatment scheduled and only five patients (1.5%) had to interrupt it due to adverse events (AEs). All patients, whose treatment was discontinued, reached SVR despite the reduced duration of treatment. Only

Table 1 Baseline Characteristics of 335 Patients Included in the Study

Parameter	Boceprevir-experienced	Telaprevir-experienced
Number of patients, n (%)	127 (38%)	208 (62%)
Gender: females/males, n (%)	63 (49.6%)/65 (50.4%)	95 (45.7%)/ 113 (54.3%)
Age (years) mean ± SD; min-max	55.4 ± 10.9; 23–74	60.3 ± 10.7; 27–78
BMI mean ± SD; min-max	27.4 ± 4.99; 19–38	27.6 ± 4.11; 19–44
HCV Genotype: n (%)		
1b	120 (94.5%)	191 (91.8%)
1a	5 (3.9%)	9 (4.3%)
1	2 (1.6%)	8 (3.9%)
Fibrosis, n (%)		
F4	78 (61.4%)	134 (64.4%)
F3	36 (28.4%)	39 (18.8%)
F2	9 (7.1%)	19 (9.1%)
F1	4 (3.1%)	16 (7.7%)
Child-Turcotte-Pugh, n (%)		
A	123 (96.9%)	201 (96.6%)
B	4 (3.1%)	5 (2.4%)
C	0 (0%)	2 (1%)
Response to previous treatment with PI+PegIFN+RBV, n (%)		
Non-response	45 (35.4%)	83 (39.9%)
Relapse	48 (37.8%)	66 (31.7%)
Discontinuation	17 (13.4%)	37 (17.8%)
Unknown	17 (13.4%)	22 (10.6%)
History of hepatic decompensation, n (%)	9 (7.1%)	11 (5.3%)
Ascites	9 (7.1%)	9 (4.3%)
Encephalopathy	0 (0%)	2 (1%)
Documented oesophageal varices, n (%)	21 (16.5%)	47 (22.6%)
History of hepatocellular carcinoma, n (%)	1 (0.8%)	4 (1.9%)
HBV coinfection, n (%)		
HBsAg positive	4 (3.1%)	0 (0%)
HBV DNA positive	0 (0%)	0 (0%)
Anti-HBc positive	11 (8.7%)	17 (8.2%)
HIV coinfection, n (%)	0 (0%)	0 (0%)
History of liver transplantation, n (%)	1 (0.8%)	5 (2.4%)
Comorbidities, n (%)		
Any comorbidity	87 (68.5%)	142 (68.3%)
Hypertension	48 (37.8%)	82 (39.4%)
Diabetes	17 (13.4%)	34 (16.3%)
Renal insufficiency	1 (0.8%)	2 (1%)
Autoimmune diseases	2 (1.6%)	2 (1%)
Non-HCC tumours	1 (0.8%)	0 (0%)
Other	21 (16.5%)	46 (22.1%)
Concomitant medications, n (%)	81 (63.8%)	141 (67.8%)

one BOC and two TVR patients (non-responders) failed to achieve SVR among the total number of 14 patients in whom HCV RNA was detectable at the end of the treatment (EOT).

The remaining subjects achieved SVR despite a positive result at the EOT. This phenomenon, specific for DAA regimens, was not observed during interferon-based therapies.

On the other hand, despite of undetectable HCV RNA at the EOT, 3 patients relapsed. Two patients from BOC and three from TVR group were lost to follow-up and evaluation of SVR was not possible.

As shown in Fig. 2, end of treatment virologic response (EOT-VR) and SVR evaluated in the ITT analysis was insignificantly lower in TVR groups.

In the mITT evaluation in BOC group, SVR was 99% for BOC→LSR and 100% for BOC→PrODR, while in TVR group it was 98% for TVR→LSR and 99% for TVR→PrODR.

Therefore, we can assume that both drugs are highly effective irrespective of the first-generation protease inhibitor which was used in the primary treatment.

Treatment safety

The most important adverse events (AEs) that occurred during the treatment and in the follow-up period are summarized in Table 3.

These were observed in 52 patients of BOC group and in 99 patients of TVR group. Severity was generally mild or moderate. Fatigue, headache, and anaemia prevailed,

Table 2 Current Treatment Regimens

Treatment regimen	Boceprevir-experienced	Telaprevir-experienced
LDV/SOF, n (%)	*n* = 63	*n* = 105
LDV/SOF 12 weeks	11 (8.7%)	26 (12.5%)
LDV/SOF 24 weeks	6 (4.7%)	9 (4.3%)
LDV/SOF + RBV 12 weeks	41 (32.3%)	63 (30.3%)
LDV/SOF + RBV 24 weeks	5 (3.9%)	7 (3.4%)
PrOD, n (%)	*n* = 64	*n* = 103
PrOD 12 weeks	29 (22.8%)	42 (20.2%)
PrOD+RBV 12 weeks	33 (26%)	56 (26.9%)
PrOD+RBV 24 weeks	2 (1.6%)	5 (2.4%)

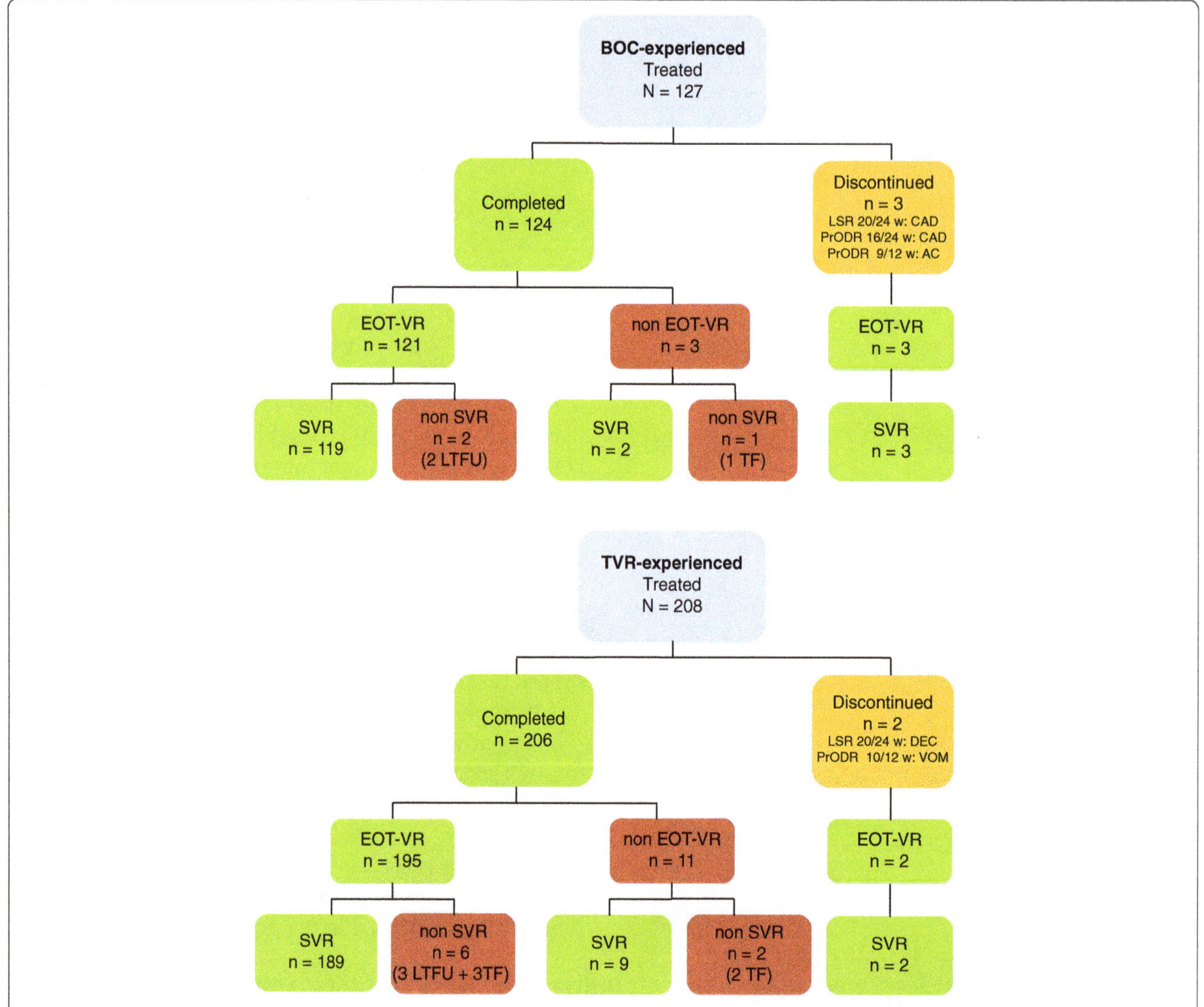

Fig. 1 Patients' disposition and reasons for discontinuation. *EOT-VR* end of treatment virologic response, *SVR* sustained virologic response, *LTFU* lost to follow-up, *TF* treatment failure, *DEC* hepatic decompensation, *CAD* exacerbation of pre-existing coronary arterial disease, *AC* acute cholecystitis, VOM-vomiting

which mainly occurred in the patients treated with therapeutic regimens containing ribavirin. Treatment discontinuation due to AE occurred in three patients of the BOC group and two patients of the TVR group (Fig. 1).

According to the treating physicians' evaluation, AEs leading to discontinuation of the treatment in BOC group, were not associated with the DAA applied, while persistent vomiting in one TVR patient was probably associated with PrODR.

The second case (decompensation) was probably associated with the baseline stage of the disease rather than antiviral treatment. It occurred in a patient with a history of hepatic insufficiency treated with LSR.

Serious adverse events (SAEs) occurred in two patients from BOC group. One of them, being treated with PrODR, underwent cholecystectomy due to acute cholecystitis, which entailed discontinuation of the treatment on the 9th week. Another patient was diagnosed with cholangiocarcinoma after completing treatment with LSR and died on the 20th week of the follow-up period.

In TVR group, two patients treated with LSR died of cancer during the follow-up period (hepatocellular carcinoma and pancreatic cancer). Both patients had undetectable HCV RNA 12 weeks after the treatment end. Portal vein thrombosis was detected in one patient treated with PrOD in the course of the treatment. This patient also achieved SVR.

All SAEs were assessed as irrelevant to the antiviral treatment and at least SVR12 was confirmed in all of these patients.

Discussion

The introduction of interferon-free therapy regimens had a beneficial effect in patients with chronic hepatitis

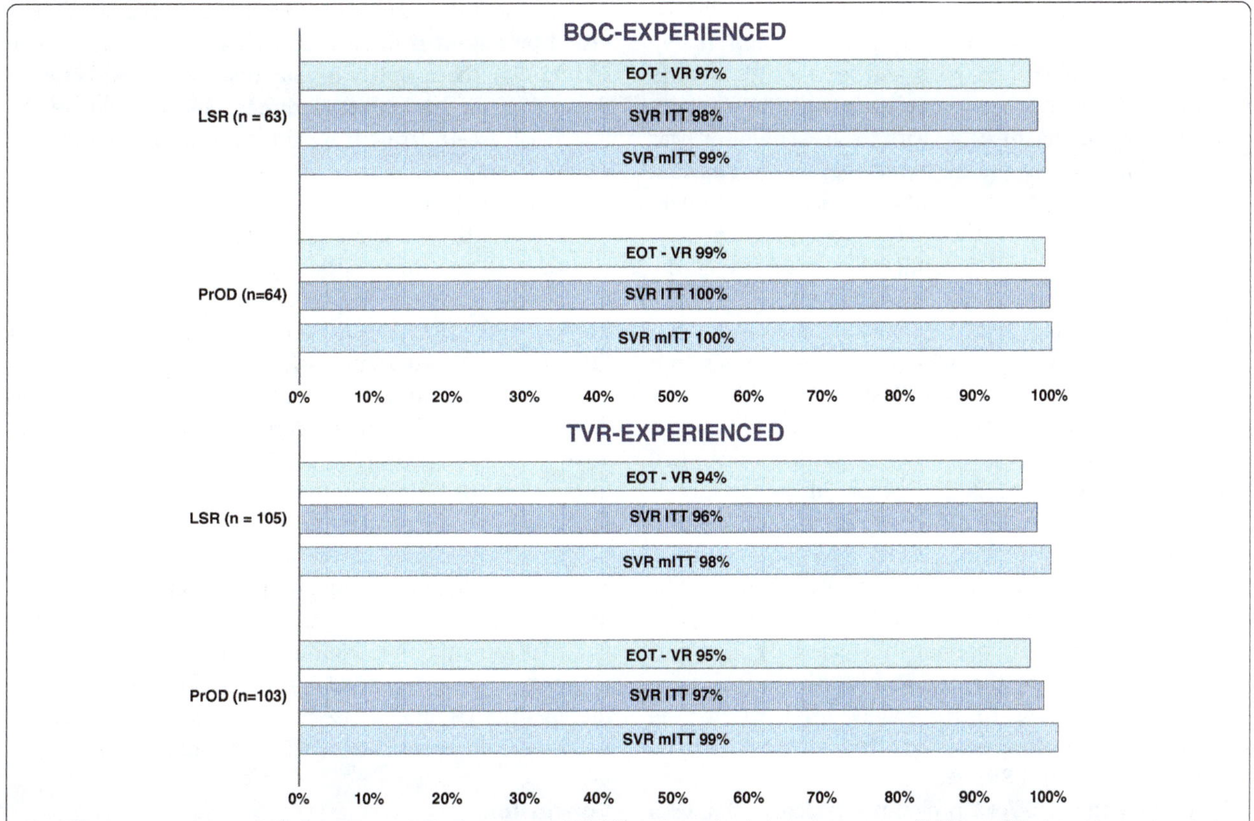

Fig. 2 Treatment outcome. End of treatment virologic response (EOT-VR) and sustained virologic response (SVR) rate; ITT—intent-to-treat analysis, which included all patients receiving at least 1 dose of the treatment, mITT—modified ITT analysis, which excluded patients with missing data of sustained virologic response (at least 12 weeks after treatment completion)

C. These regimens have become highly effective and safe, irrespective of the severity of liver disease.

In the interferon era, prior treatment failure was an important factor restricting efficacy of subsequent antiviral therapies [18–20]. Introduction of triple-drug regimens significantly increased chances for recovery only in patients with mild to moderate fibrosis, treatment naïve or relapsers after PegIFN+RBV therapy. Patients with cirrhosis and/or lack of virologic response to prior therapy showed significantly worse response to the interferon-based treatment, which included first generation PIs [21–25].

Breakthrough was only made through the use of interferon-free therapies. As specified in the introduction, international hepatology societies recommend the use of LSR or SOF + DVC after failed triple-drug

Table 3 Adverse Events

Parameter	Boceprevir-experienced		Telaprevir-experienced	
	LDV/SOF (*n* = 63)	PrOD (*n* = 64)	LDV/SOF (*n* = 105)	PrOD (*n* = 103)
Patients with at least one AE, n (%)	24 (38.1%)	28 (43,8%)	44 (41.9%)	45 (43.7%)
RBV-containing regimen	18 (28.6%)	19 (29.7%)	31 (29.5%)	33 (32%)
Most common AEs (> 5%), n (%)				
Fatigue	15 (23.8%)	17 (26.6%)	27 (25.7%)	30 (29.1%)
Anaemia	9 (14.3%)	13 (20.3%)	15 (14.3%)	22 (21.4%)
Headache	8 (12.7%)	11 (17.2%)	10 (9.5%)	12 (11.7%)
Nausea	4 (6.3%)	4 (6.3%)	7 (6.7%)	8 (7.8%)
Serious AEs, n (%)	1 (1.6%)	1 (1.6%)	2 (1.9%)	1 (1%)
Deaths	1 (1.6%)	0 (0%)	2 (1.9%)	0 (0%)

therapies. Other available drugs (simeprevir+SOF, PrOD) were not recommended for this patient group [8, 9]. However, daily clinical practice and local conditions do not always enable rigorous compliance with these guidelines. Combinations of SOF with NS5A inhibitor was not available in Poland until November 2015. The first interferon-free drug which could be used was PrODR, initially available under the early-access program and, beginning from July 2015, under the program of the National Health Fund.

Due to the urgent need to apply the therapy to numerous queuing patients with advanced fibrosis and cirrhosis, they were given an accessible drug, which was considered a rescue therapy. The first group of patients (AMBER cohort) also included 16 patients who had failed triple treatment with boceprevir or telaprevir [14]. SVR was achieved in all these patients. Taking into account these encouraging results and local realities, the Polish Group of HCV Experts included this therapeutic regimen in its recommendations as acceptable for use in the patients previously treated by PIs. This drug was approved by the national health insurance institution and started to be widely used within the framework of the drug program, first as the only drug and then along with LSR.

Therefore, the Epi-Ter2 program enabled to gather a vast group of patients treated with the PrODR regimen seldom used in other countries.

Description of small patient groups can be mostly found in the literature, e.g. only 7 patients after PI treatment, who received PrODR therapy, were included in the Italian VIRONET-C cohort [26].

A large German cohort involving a total of 1017 patients treated by PrODR [27], included 72 patients treated previously with TVR or BOC. A Spanish cohort consisting of 1567 patients included only 49 patients treated by PrODR [28]. In the aforementioned cohorts, most of the patients with the history of PI therapy, received LSR. Therefore, our patient group is one of the largest, in which efficacy of PrODR in patients after first generation PI treatment was evaluated.

In our study, we demonstrated that PrODR regimens are as effective in this patient group as LSR, including patients with advanced liver disease irrespective of prior treatment failure.

Initial concerns were not substantiated that first-generation PI treatment would be associated with selection of RASs significantly reducing efficacy of subsequent therapies. Any probable RAS faded, and wild virus type begins dominating within the period of a year after the end of the PI therapy. Whereas, RASs in NS5A region characterized by higher durability had a demonstrable influence on subsequent treatment efficacy, which proved to be a significant problem [29–31].

The baseline presence of RAS in our patients was not tested because it is not a routine examination in real-life setting. For the majority of patients, the period between the end of the triple drug treatment and the start of the interferon-free treatment was longer than 12 months.

Both therapy types were characterized by a favourable safety profile, including cirrhosis patients.

The strength of our study is a large group of patients treated with the therapeutic regimen, which is relatively infrequently used in the patients after PI in Western Europe and USA. Results of our study confirm that PrODR can be used successfully and equivalently with other accessible drugs in patients with compensated liver disease. This can be particularly relevant for countries where the full scope of the interferon-free therapies is unavailable, or administrative restrictions in the choice of drugs exist.

The limitation may be the use of different therapeutic regimens in individual subgroups of patients (duration of treatment, addition of RBV) which results from the fact that the study was conducted in real-life conditions, without a predetermined protocol. However, all the therapeutic regimens, used according to the current label, were characterized by very high efficacy.

Conclusion

In the future, as availability increases, novel, pangenotypic DAAs will surely start dominating. However, as long as an access to these newest drugs is limited, the drugs of the previous generation will remain in widespread use.

The results of our study may be useful in the daily clinical practice, proving that the patients after failed IFN-based triple therapies containing PI, can be cured using both PrODR and LSR regimens with comparable efficacy and safety.

Abbreviations

AASLD: American European Association for the Study of the Liver Diseases; AE: Adverse Adverse event; BOC: BoceprevirBoceprevir; DAAs: DirectDirect-acting antivirals; DCV: DaclatasvirDaclatasvir; EASL: European Association for the Study of the Liver; EOT-VR: End End of treatment virologic response; HBV: Hepatitis Hepatitis B virus; HCV: Hepatitis Hepatitis C virus; HIV: Human Human immunodeficiency virus; ITT: IntentIntent-to treat analysis; LSR: LedipasvirLedipasvir/sofosbuvir ± RBV; mITT: modified intent-to treat analysis; NS5A: NonNon-structural protein 5A; PegIFN: Pegylated Pegylated interferon; PI: Protease Protease inhibitor; PrODR: ParitaprevirParitaprevir/ritonavir/ombitasvir+dasasbuvir ±ribavirin; RASs: ResistanceResistance-associated substitutions; RBV: RibavirinRibavirin; SAE: Serious Serious adverse events; SOF: SofosbuvirSofosbuvir; SVR: Sustained Sustained virologic response; SWE: Shear Shear wave elastography; TE: Transient Transient elastography; TVR: TelaprevirTelaprevir

Acknowledgements

Data contained in the manuscript were presented as the poster at the International Liver Congress, 2018 in Paris.

Funding

This is an investigators-initiated study, conducted in routine clinical practice setting. No funding was received.

Authors' contributions

Conceptualization: EJ, RF. Data analysis: EJ. Patients care, investigation and data collection: EJ, DZM, HB, AP, AG, DD, WM, TBW, WD, MTZ, ZD, IB, MS, ACA, BL, JBW, JC, ŁL, JJ, ŁS, OT, AB, AH, WH, BBC, KT, KS, AG, MWS, R. Writing original draft: EJ. Writing, review and editing: all authors. All authors have read and approved the manuscript.

Competing interests

EJ has received research grants and/or fees for lectures, advisory boards, scientific consultancies from Abbvie, Allergan, Bristol Meyer Squibb, Gilead Sciences, Janssen Cilag, MSD, Vertex, Tobira. AP has received research grants and/or fees for lectures, advisory boards, scientific consultancies from: AbbVie, Gilead, Merck, Roche. WM has received research grants and/or fees for lectures, advisory boards, scientific consultancies from: AbbVie, BMS, Gilead, Janssen, Merck, Roche. TBM has received research grants and fees for scientific consultancies for: AbbVie, Gilead. WD has received fees for scientific consultancies from: AbbVie, Gilead. ACA has received research grants from: AbbVie, Merck. JJ has received research grants and/or fees for lectures, advisory boards, scientific consultancies from: AbbVie, BMS, Gilead, Merz, Roche. ŁS has received fees for scientific consultancies from BMS. BA has received research grants from BMS and fees for scientific consultancies from Roche, AbbVie, BMS, Gilead, MSD. WH has received research grants and/or fees for lectures, advisory boards, scientific consultancies from: AbbVie, BMS, Gilead, Janssen, Merck, Roche. BBC has received research grants and/or fees for lectures, scientific consultancies from: AbbVie, Gilead, Roche. KT has received research grants and/or fees for lectures, advisory boards, scientific consultancies from: AbbVie, Alfa Wasserman, BMS, Gilead, Janssen, Merck, Roche. KS has received research grants and/or fees for lectures, advisory boards, scientific consultancies from: AbbVie, Gilead, BMS, Merck, Janssen, Alfa-Wassermann, Baxter, Bayer, Roche Allergan, EISAI, Gilead, Intercept, Tobira, Pfizer.

AG has received research grants and/or fees for lectures, advisory boards, scientific consultancies from: AbbVie, Bristol-Myers Squibb, Gilead, GlaxoSmithKline, Janssen, Roche, Sanofi Pasteur, Amgen, Pfizer. MWS has received fees for lectures, scientific consultancies from: Gilead, AbbVie, Merck. RF has received research grants and/or fees for lectures, advisory boards, scientific consultancies from: AbbVie, Alfa Wasserman, BMS, Gilead, Janssen, Merck, Roche, Shionogi. DZM, HB, DD, MTZ, ZD, IB, MS, BL, JBW, JC, ŁL, OT, AH, AG declare no competing interest.

Author details

[1]Department of Basic Medical Sciences, School of Public Health in Bytom, Medical University of Silesia, ID Clinic, Janowska 19, 41-400 Mysłowice, Bytom, Poland. [2]Department of Infectious Diseases, Wojewódzki Szpital Zespolony, Kielce, Poland. [3]Hospital of Infectious Diseases, Warszawa, Poland. [4]Department of Infectious Diseases and Hepatology, Medical University of Łódź, Łódź, Poland. [5]Department of Internal Medicine and Hepatology, Central Clinical Hospital of the MSWiA, Warszawa, Poland. [6]Department of Infectious Diseases and Hepatology, Faculty of Medicine, Collegium Medicum Bydgoszcz, Nicolaus Copernicus University Toruń, Bydgoszcz, Poland. [7]Department of Infectious Diseases, Infectious Hepatology and Acquired Immunodeficiency, Medical University of Silesia in Katowice, Chorzów, Poland. [8]Regional Center for Diagnosis and Treatment of Viral Hepatitis and Hepatology, John Paul II Hospital, Kraków, Poland. [9]MED-FIX Medical Center, Wrocław, Poland. [10]Department of Infectious Diseases, Medical University of Lublin, Lublin, Poland. [11]Ward of Infectious Diseases and Hepatology, Biegański Regional Specialist Hospital, Łódź, Poland. [12]Department of Infectious Diseases and Hepatology, Wrocław Medical University, Wrocław, Poland. [13]Department of Infectious and Tropical Diseases, Collegium Medicum, Jagiellonian University, Kraków, Poland. [14]Department of Infectious Diseases and Hepatology, Medical University of Białystok, Białystok, Poland. [15]Pomeranian Center of Infectious Diseases, Department of Infectious Diseases, Medical University of Gdansk, Gdansk, Poland. [16]Department of Infectious and Liver Diseases, Medical University of Łódź, Łódź, Poland. [17]Medical Practice of Infections, Regional Hospital, Olsztyn, Poland. [18]Department of Infectious Diseases, Hepatology and Liver Transplantation, Pomeranian Medical University, Szczecin, Poland. [19]Department of Infectious Diseases and Hepatology, Medical University of Silesia in Katowice, Bytom, Poland. [20]Department of Transplantation Medicine, Nephrology, and Internal Diseases, Medical University of Warsaw, Warszawa, Poland. [21]Warsaw Medical University & Hospital of Infectious Diseases Warszawa, Warszawa, Poland.

References

1. Kobayashi N, Iijima H, Tada T, Kumada T, Yoshida M, Aoki T, et al. Changes in liver stiffness and steatosis among patients with hepatitis C virus infection who received direct-acting antiviral therapy and achieved sustained virological response. Eur J Gastroenterol Hepatol. 2018;30:546–51. https://doi.org/10.1097/MEG.0000000000001106.
2. Tada T, Kumada T, Toyoda H, Sone Y, Takeshima K, Ogawa S, et al. Viral eradication reduces both liver stiffness and steatosis in patients with chronic hepatitis C virus infection who received direct-acting anti-viral therapy. Aliment Pharmacol Ther. 2018;47:1012–22. https://doi.org/10.1111/apt.14554.
3. Trivedi HD, Lin SC, TY Lau D. Noninvasive Assessment of Fibrosis Regression in Hepatitis C Virus Sustained Virologic Responders. Gastroenterol Hepatol. 2017;13:587–95.
4. Kozbial K, Moser S, Al-Zoairy R, Schwarzer R, Datz C, Stauber R, et al. Follow-up of sustained virological responders with hepatitis C and advanced liver disease after interferon/ribavirin-free treatment. Liver Int. 2017. https://doi.org/10.1111/liv.13629.
5. Bartlett SR, Grebely J, Eltahla AA, Reeves JD, Howe AYM, Miller V, et al. Sequencing of hepatitis C virus for detection of resistance to direct-acting antiviral therapy: a systematic review. Hepatol Commun. 2017;22(1):379–90. https://doi.org/10.1002/hep4.1050.
6. Kjellin M, Wesslén T, Löfblad E, Lennerstrand J, Lannergård A. The effect of the first-generation HCV-protease inhibitors boceprevir and telaprevir and the relation to baseline NS3 resistance mutations in genotype 1: experience from a small Swedish cohort. Ups J Med Sci. 2018;123:50–6. https://doi.org/10.1080/03009734.2018.1441928.
7. Wang GP, Terrault N, Reeves JD, Liu L, Li E, Zhao L, et al. Prevalence and impact of baseline resistance-associated substitutions on the efficacy of ledipasvir/sofosbuvir or simeprevir/sofosbuvir against GT1 HCV infection. Sci Rep. 2018;8:3199. https://doi.org/10.1038/s41598-018-21303-2.
8. European Association for the Study of the Liver. EASL Recommendations on Treatment of Hepatitis C. 2015. J Hepatol. 2015;63:199–236.
9. Hepatitis C Guidance. AASLD-IDSA recommendations for testing, managing, and treating adults infected with hepatitis C virus. HEPATOLOGY. 2015;62(3): 932–54.
10. Afdhal N, Reddy KR, Nelson DR, Lawitz E, Gordon SC, Schiff E, et al. Ledipasvir and sofosbuvir for previously treated HCV genotype 1 infection. N Engl J Med. 2014;370(16):1483–93. https://doi.org/10.1056/NEJMoa1316366.
11. Bourlière M, Bronowicki JP, de Ledinghen V, Hézode C, Zoulim F, Mathurin P, et al. Ledipasvir-sofosbuvir with or without ribavirin to treat patients with HCV genotype 1 infection and cirrhosis non-responsive to previous protease-inhibitor therapy: a randomised, double-blind, phase 2 trial (SIRIUS). Lancet Infect Dis. 2015;15:397–404. https://doi.org/10.1016/S1473-3099(15)70050-2.
12. Lawitz E, Poordad FF, Pang PS, Hyland RH, Ding X, Mo H, et al. Sofosbuvir and ledipasvir fixed-dose combination with and without ribavirin in treatment-naive and previously treated patients with genotype 1 hepatitis C virus infection (LONESTAR): an open-label, randomised, phase 2 trial. Lancet. 2014;383(9916):515–23. https://doi.org/10.1016/S0140-6736(13)62121-2.
13. Sulkowski MS, Gardiner DF, Rodriguez-Torres M, Reddy KR, Hassanein T, Jacobson I, et al. Daclatasvir plus sofosbuvir for previously treated or untreated chronic HCV infection. N Engl J Med. 2014;370:211–21. https://doi.org/10.1056/NEJMoa1306218.
14. Flisiak R, Janczewska E, Wawrzynowicz-Syczewska M, Jaroszewicz J, Zarębska-Michaluk D, Nazzal K, et al. Real-world effectiveness and safety of ombitasvir/paritaprevir/ritonavir ± dasabuvir ± ribavirin in hepatitis C: AMBER study. Aliment Pharmacol Ther. 2016;44(9):946–56. https://doi.org/10.1111/apt.13790.
15. Halota W, Flisiak R, Boroń-Kaczmarska A, Juszczyk J, Małkowski P, Pawłowska M, et al. Recommendations for the treatment of hepatitis C issued by the polish group of HCV experts – 2016. Clin Exp Hepatol. 2016;2:27–33. https://doi.org/10.5114/ceh.2016.59099.
16. Flisiak R, Pogorzelska J, Berak H, Horban A, Orłowska I, Simon K, et al. Prevalence of HCV genotypes in Poland - the EpiTer study. Clin Exp Hepatol. 2016;2:144–8. https://doi.org/10.5114/ceh.2016.63871.
17. Halota W, Flisiak R, Juszczyk J, Małkowski P, Pawłowska M, Simon K, et al. Recommendations for the treatment of hepatitis C in 2017. Clin Exp Hepatol. 2017;3(2):47–55 https://doi.org/10.5114/ceh.2017.67782.

18. Gonçales FL Jr, Moma CA, Vigani AG, Ngerami AF, Gonçales ES, Tozzo R, et al. Retreatment of hepatitis C patients with pegylated interferon combined with ribavirin in non-responders to interferon plus ribavirin. Is it different in real life. BMC Infect Dis. 2010;10:212. https://doi.org/10.1186/1471-2334-10-212.
19. Oze T, Hiramatsu N, Yakushijin T, Mochizuki K, Oshita M, Hagiwara H, et al. Efficacy of re-treatment with pegylated interferon plus ribavirin combination therapy for patients with chronic hepatitis C in Japan. J Gastroenterol. 2011; 46:1031–7. https://doi.org/10.1007/s00535-011-0409-7.
20. Berg T, von Wagner M, Nasser S, Sarrazin C, Heintges T, Gerlach T, et al. Extended treatment duration for hepatitis C virus type 1: comparing 48 versus 72 weeks of peginterferon- alfa-2a plus ribavirin. Gastroenterology. 2006;130(4):1086–97.
21. Jacobson I, McHutchison J, Dusheiko G, Di Bisceglie AM, Reddy KR, Bzowej NH, et al. Telaprevir for previously untreated chronic hepatitis C virus infection. N Engl J Med. 2011;364:2405–16.
22. Poordad F, McCone J Jr, Bacon BR, Bruno S, Manns MP, Sulkowski MS, et al. Boceprevir for untreated chronic HCV genotype 1 infection. N Engl J Med. 2011;364(13):1195–206.
23. Zeuzem S, Andreone P, Pol S, Lawitz E, Diago M, Roberts S, et al. Telaprevir for retreatment of HCV infection. N Engl J Med. 2011;364(25):2417–28.
24. Bacon BR, Gordon SC, Lawitz E, Marcellin P, Vierling JM, Zeuzem S, et al. Boceprevir for previously treated chronic HCV genotype 1 infection. N Engl J Med. 2011;364(13):1207–17.
25. Reddy KR, Zeuzem S, Zoulim F, Weiland O, Horban A, Stanciu C, et al. Simeprevir versus telaprevir with peginterferon and ribavirin in previous null or partial responders with chronic hepatitis C virus genotype 1 infection (ATTAIN): a randomised, double-blind, non-inferiority phase 3 trial. Lancet Infect Dis. 2015;15:27–35. https://doi.org/10.1016/S1473-3099(14)71002-3 Erratum in: Lancet Infect Dis. 2016 Apr;16(4):404.
26. Cento V, Barbaliscia S, Lenci I, Ruggiero T, Magni CF, Paolucci S, et al. Optimal efficacy of interferon-free HCV retreatment after protease inhibitor failure in real life. Clin Microbiol Infect. 2017;23:777.e1–4. https://doi.org/10.1016/j.cmi.2017.04.005.
27. Welzel TM, Hinrichsen H, Sarrazin C, Buggisch P, Baumgarten A, Christensen S, et al. Real-world experience with the all-oral, interferon-free regimen of ombitasvir/paritaprevir/ritonavir and dasabuvir for the treatment of chronic hepatitis C virus infection in the German hepatitis C registry. J Viral Hepat. 2017;24:840–9.
28. Calleja JL, Crespo J, Rincón D, Ruiz-Antorán B, Fernandez I, Perelló C, et al. Effectiveness, safety and clinical outcomes of direct-acting antiviral therapy in HCVgenotype 1 infection: results from a Spanish real-world cohort. J Hepatol. 2017;66:1138–48. https://doi.org/10.1016/j.jhep.2017.01.028.
29. Dietz J, Susser S, Vermehren J, Peiffer KH, Grammatikos G, Berger A, et al. Patterns of Resistance-Associated Substitutions in Patients With Chronic HCV Infection Following Treatment With Direct-Acting Antivirals. Gastroenterology. 2018;154(4):976–988.e4. https://doi.org/10.1053/j.gastro.2017.11.007.
30. Di Maio VC, Cento V, Lenci I, Aragri M, Rossi P, Barbaliscia S, et al. Multiclass HCV resistance to direct-acting antiviral failure in real-life patients advocates for tailored second-line therapies. Liver Int. 2017;37: 514–28. https://doi.org/10.1111/liv.13327.
31. Kozuka R, Hai H, Motoyama H, Fujii H, Uchida-Kobayashi S, Morikawa H, et al. The presence of multiple NS5A RASs is associated with the outcome of sofosbuvir and ledipasvir therapy in NS5A inhibitor-naïve patients with chronic HCV genotype 1b infection in a real-world cohort. J Viral Hepat. 2017. https://doi.org/10.1111/jvh.12850.

23

Antimicrobial susceptibilities of specific syndromes created with organ-specific weighted incidence antibiograms (OSWIA) in patients with intra-abdominal infections

Lianxin Liu[1*] and Yuxing Ni[2*]

Abstract

Background: The aim was to evaluate the value of organ-specific weighted incidence antibiogram (OSWIA) percentages for bacterial susceptibilities of Gram-negative bacteria (GNB) collected from intra-abdominal infections (IAIs) during SMART 2010–2014.

Methods: We retrospectively calculated the OSWIA percentages that would have been adequately covered by 12 common antimicrobials based on the bacterial compositions found in the appendix, peritoneum, colon, liver, gall bladder and pancreas.

Results: The ESBL positive rates were 65.7% for *Escherichia coli*, 36.2% for *Klebsiella pneumoniae*, 42.9% for *Proteus mirabilis* and 33.1% for *Klebsiella oxytoca. Escherichia coli* were mainly found in the appendix (76.8%), but less so in the liver (32.4%). *Klebsiella pneumoniae* constituted 45.2% of the total liver pathogenic bacteria and 15.2–20.8% were found in 4 other organs, except the colon and appendix (< 10%). The percentages of *Pseudomonas aeruginosa* infections were higher in the gall bladder, intra-abdominal abscesses, pancreas and colon (10.2–13.2%) and least (5.4%) in the appendix. The susceptibilities of hospital acquired (HA) and community acquired (CA) IAI isolates from appendix, gall bladder and liver showed ≥80% susceptibilities to amikacin (AMK), imipenem (IPM), piperacillin-tazobactam (TZP) and ertapenem (ETP), while the susceptibility of isolates in abscesses and peritoneal fluid showed ≥80% susceptibility only to amikacin (AMK) and imipenem (IPM). In colon CA IAI isolates susceptibilities did not reach 80% for AMK and ETP, and in pancreatic IAIs susceptibilities of HA GNBs did not reach 80% to AMK, TZP and ETP, and CA GNBs to IMP and ETP. In addition, besides circa 80% susceptibility of HA and CA IAI isolates from appendix to cefoxitin (FOX), IAI isolates from all other organs had susceptibilities between 7.6 and 67.9% to all cephalosporins tested, 28.3–75.2% to fluoroquinolones and 7.6–51.0% to ampicillin-sulbactam (SAM), whether they were obtained from CA or HA infections.

Conclusion: The calculated OSWIA susceptibilities were specific for different organs in abdominal infections.

Keywords: SMART, Intra-abdominal infection, Gram-negative bacteria, Antibiotics, Organ-specific weighted incidence antibiogram (OSWIA), Organ-specific susceptibility

* Correspondence: liulianxin@medmail.com.cn; yuxing_ni@126.com
[1]Department of Hepatobiliary Surgery, the First Affiliated Hospital of Harbin Medical University. Key Laboratory of Hepatosplenic Surgery, Ministry of Education, No. 23 Youzheng Street, Harbin 150001, China
[2]Department of Hospital Infection Control, Rui Jin Hospital, Shanghai Jiao Tong University School of Medicine, No. 197 Rui-Jin 2nd Road, Shanghai 200025, China

Background

The massive over prescribing of antimicrobial agents has led to dramatic changes in clinical susceptibilities to antibiotics and multidrug-resistant (MDR) infection has been proven to be one of the major causes of mortality, especially those patients with IAIs [1, 2]. Mortality rates associated with secondary peritonitis and severe sepsis or septic shock average approximately 30%. [3, 4]

In 2012, Tabah et al. conducted a prospective, multicentre non-representative cohort study in 162 intensive care units (ICUs) in 24 countries, and showed that MDR and pan-drug-resistance (PDR) was increased in Europe, and Gram-negative bacterial infections were especially associated with an increased 28-day mortality [5]. Lack of effective initial empirical antimicrobial treatment within 24 h increases mortality significantly compared with appropriate antimicrobial treatment (63.0–65.2% vs 30.6–42.0%) [6, 7]. It has also been noted that effective empirical treatment needs to be supported by epidemiological studies and antimicrobial susceptibility data about the prevalence of local pathogenic bacteria. However, traditional epidemiological studies are limited to the description of the broad bacterial distributions and variable drug susceptibilities in individual hospitals, while detailed organ-specific data are usually lacking. Recently, Herbert et al. (2012) developed a novel method of displaying microbiology data to support early empirical antimicrobial treatments, which they termed the weighted-incidence syndromic combination antibiogram (WISCA). It classifies patients by syndrome and determines, for each patient with a given syndrome, whether a particular treatment regimen (one or more drugs) would have covered all the organisms recovered from their infections [8]. These data are calculated by dividing the number of the patients treated with a particular antimicrobial drug by the total number of patients. In the present study we created OSWIAs, which estimated the probability of organ specific isolates being susceptible to particular antibiotics.

Using data from the SMART study, we analyzed organ specific antimicrobial susceptibilities of Gram-negative bacteria in abdominal infections via OSWIA determinations in order to explore the practicability of this protocol and to assess its potential benefits in clinical practice in China.

Materials and methods

The Human Research Ethics Committee of Peking Union Medical College Hospital approved this study and waived the need for consent (Ethics Approval Number: SK238). Patient data were collected from a total of 21 hospitals in 16 Chinese cities from 2010 to 2014 and according to the SMART protocol each participating hospital provided at least 100 consecutive aerobic and facultative Gram-negative bacilli from patients with IAIs excluding duplicate isolates.

Isolates (8066) of Gram-negative aerobic bacteria and other pathogenic bacteria were obtained from different infected abdominal organs, including fermentative and non-fermentative bacteria in the appendix, peritoneum, colon, liver, gall bladder and pancreas from 2012 to 2014. All duplicate isolates (the same genus and species from the same patient) were excluded. Isolates collected within 48 h of hospitalization were categorized as community acquired (CA) IAIs, and those collected after 48 h were categorized as hospital acquired (HA) IAIs. The majority of intra-abdominal specimens were obtained during surgery, though some paracentesis specimens were also collected.

Bacterial identification and antimicrobial susceptibility testing

Bacteria were identified by standard methods used in the participating clinical microbiology laboratories and all organisms were deemed clinically significant according to local criteria. All isolates were sent to the central clinical microbiology laboratory of Peking Union Medical College Hospital for re-identification using MALDI-TOF MS (Vitek MS, BioMérieux, France).

To assess antimicrobial susceptibilities, minimum inhibitory concentrations (MICs) were determined with dehydrated MicroScan broth micro dilution panels (Siemens Medical Solutions Diagnostics, West Sacramento, CA, USA), according to the guidelines of the 2012 Clinical and Laboratory Standards Institute (CLSI) [9]. Susceptibility interpretations were based on the CLSI M100-S23 clinical breakpoints [10], and the ATCC 25922 strain of *Escherichia coli* (*E. coli*), the ATCC 27853 strain of *Pseudomonas aeruginosa* (*P. aeruginosa*), and the ATCC 700603 strain of *Klebsiella pneumoniae* (*K. pneumoniae*) were used as reference strains in each set of MIC tests for quality control. The antibiotics tested were the aminoglycoside amikacin (AMK), the carbapenems ertapenem (ETP) and imipenem (IPM), the cephamycins cefoxitin (FOX), ceftazidime (CAZ), cefepime (FEP), cefotaxime (CTX) and ceftriaxone (CRO), the fluoroquinolones levofloxacin (LVX) and ciprofloxacin (CIP) as well as the broad spectrum penicillins combined with β-lactamase inhibitors ampicillin-sulbactam (SAM) and piperacillin-tazobactam (TZP).

Phenotypic identification of extended-spectrum β-lactamase (ESBL) positive bacteria were carried out by CLSI recommended methods [10]. If MICs were ≥ 2 μg/mL for cefotaxime or ceftazidime, the MICs of cefotaxime or ceftazidime plus clavulanic acid (4 μg/mL) were determined and ESBL production was defined as a ≥ 8-fold decrease of MICs for cefotaxime or ceftazidime plus clavulanic acid.

Organ-specific weighted incidence antibiogram (OSWIA) calculation

We evaluated the data retrospectively and analyzed the pathogenic bacteria distribution in various abdominal organs. OSWIAs were calculated using the following equation: Weighted susceptibility of a certain antimicrobial drug in a certain organ = antimicrobial susceptibility of A × the constituent ratio of A in the organ + antimicrobial susceptibility of B × the constituent ratio of B in the organ + antimicrobial susceptibility of C × the constituent ratio of C in the organ + (where A, B, C represent the pathogenic bacteria in a certain organ).

Statistical analysis

The susceptibility of all Gram-negative isolates combined was calculated using breakpoints appropriate for each species and assuming 0% susceptibility for species with no breakpoints for any given drug. The 95% confidence intervals (CIs) were calculated using the adjusted Wald method; linear trends of ESBL rates in different years were assessed for statistical significance using the Cochran-Armitage test and comparison of ESBL rates were assessed using a chi-squared test. *P*-values < 0.05 were considered to be statistically significant.

Results

Distribution of gram-negative enteric bacteria from 2010 to 2014

The majority if IAI isolates included *E. coli*, with 3764 strains in total (46.7%), of which 2472 (65.7%) were ESBL-producing strains, followed by *K. pneumoniae* with 1486 strains in total (18.4%) of which 538 (36.2%) were ESBL-producing strains. Other major pathogenic bacteria included 804 strains of *P. aeruginosa* (10.0%) and 558 strains of *Acinetobacter baumannii* (*A. baumannii*) (6.9%), which both belong to the non-fermentative bacteria group, as well as 410 strains of *Enterobacter cloacae (E. cloacae)* (5.1%). The rest of the pathogenic bacteria comprised < 2% of the total. The majority of non-fermentative GNBs was isolated from HA IAIs (Table 1). A total of 61 other strains were rarely isolated and detailed information is listed in Additional file 1: Table S1.

Table 1 Distribution of pathogenic Gram-negative bacteria responsible for IAIs (2010–2014)

Organism	Sum (%)
Fermentative bacteria	
Escherichia coli	3764 (46.7%)
ESBL-producing strains (of % *E. coli*)	2.472 (65.7%)
Klebsiella pneumoniae	1.486 (18.4%)
ESBL-producing strains (of % *K. pneumoniae*)	538 (36.2%)
Enterobacter cloacae	410 (5.1%)
Proteus mirabilis	147 (1.8%)
ESBL-producing strains (of % *P. mirabilis*)	63 (42.9%)
Enterobacter aerogenes	138 (1.7%)
Citrobacter freundii	138 (1.7%)
Klebsiella oxytoca	124 (1.5%)
ESBL-producing strains (of % *K. oxytoca*)	41 (33.1%)
Morganella morganii	93 (1.2%)
Serratia marcescens	53 (0.7%)
Aeromonas hydrophila	35 (0.4%)
Proteus vulgaris	22 (0.3%)
Citrobacter braakii	21 (0.3%)
Citrobacter koseri	17 (0.2%)
Non-Fermentative bacteria	
Pseudomonas aeruginosa	804 (10.0%)
HA	636 (79.1)
CA	162 (20.1)
Acinetobacter baumannii	558 (6.9%)
HA	451 (80.8)
CA	101 (18.1)
Stenotrophomonas maltophilia	86 (1.1%)
HA	66 (76.7)
CA	20 (23.3)
Other[a]	170 (2.1%)
Total	8066

[a]Other includes < 0.2% of *Enterobacteriaceae* or < 1.1% of non-fermentative bacterial strains isolated from the IAIs ($n = 61$)

Comparison of the pathogenic distribution of abdominal infections in different organs (2010–2014)

In Figure 1, we show the pathogenic distribution of Gram-negative bacteria in some infected organs in the abdomen, including 2510 strains from the gall bladder (31.1%), 2078 strains from peritoneal fluid (25.8%), 1444 strains from abdominal abscesses (17.9%), and the remainder from the appendix (405 strains), colon (174 strains), liver (553 strains) and pancreas (256 strains), respectively.

The majority of the abdominal pathogenic bacteria included fermentative bacteria comprising *E. coli*, *K. pneumoniae*, and the non-fermentative bacteria *A. baumannii* and *P. aeruginosa*. The highest percentage of *E. coli* was found in the appendix (76.8%) and the least percentage in the liver (32.4%). *K. pneumoniae* accounted for 45.2% of the total pathogenic bacteria in the liver and moderate fractions (15.2–20.8%) in the gall bladder, peritoneal fluid, abscesses and pancreas, but only 7.7% in the appendix and 5.7% in the colon. *P. aeruginosa* was one of the major pathogens found in the gall bladder (11.5%), abscesses (10.2%), pancreas (12.2%) and colon (13.2%). The highest

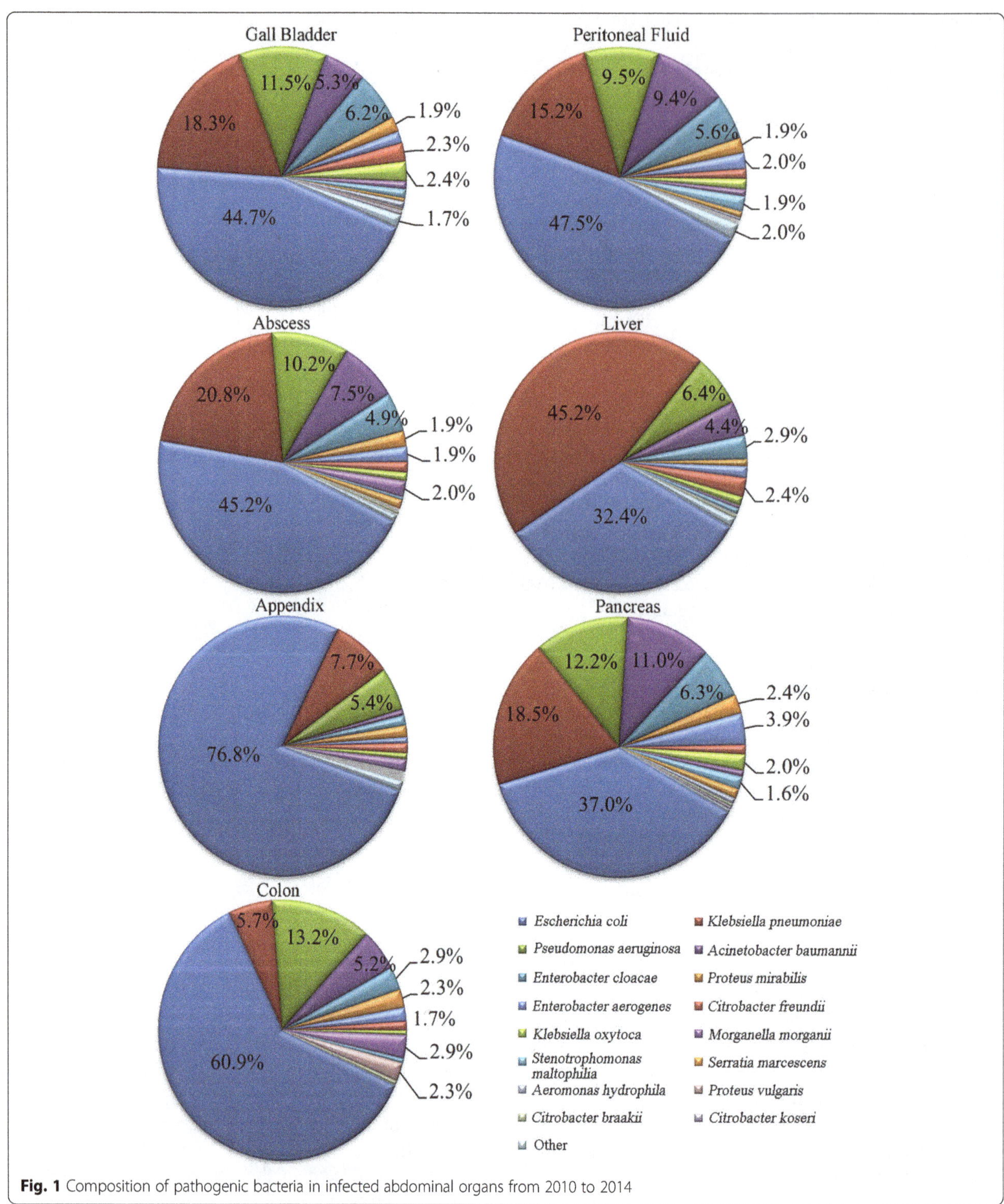

Fig. 1 Composition of pathogenic bacteria in infected abdominal organs from 2010 to 2014

percentage of *A. baumannii* was found in the pancreas (11.0%) and the least percentage in the appendix (≤ 1%) (Fig. 1).

Non-fermentative GNBs accounted for 12.5% of liver and 6.7% of appendix infections, whereas the percentages in other organs were 18.8–25.8%. More non-fermentative bacteria were found in HA compared to CA infections in all abdominal organs except the appendix. In pancreas infections, the ESBL producing rates of *Enterobacteriaceae* were slightly higher in HA compared to CA IAIs, but in the liver the GNB rate was almost double. There were obvious differences between *Enterobacteriaceae* ESBL producing rates within the organs, being highest in the colon followed by the pancreas and peritoneal fluid infections (Table 2).

Antimicrobial susceptibilities of specific syndromes determined by OSWIAs in IAIs.

Next, we calculated the OSWIAs (Fig. 2). Additionally, apart from the liver, all other organs presented with a typical "stair-step" shape, with only AMK, IPM, TZP and ETP susceptibilities being ≥80%; the rest of the antibiotics had activity far below this level. The highest susceptibility rates to AMK, IMP, TZP and ETP were found in he appendix and differences between HA and CA IAI susceptibilities were more pronounced in the colon, peritoneal fluid and pancreas, being higher in CA derived strains from peritoneal fluid and pancreas but less in CA strains isolated from colon infections. Apart from susceptibility of appendix isolates to FOX, IAI isolates from all other organs were susceptible (18–74.5% to all cephalosporins tested including cefoxitin, whether they were obtained from CA or HA infections, suggesting a high prevalence of ESBL production. Susceptibilities to fluoroquinolones were 28.3–75.2% and to SAM 7.6–51.0% (Fig. 2).

Discussion

A timely worldwide multi-center cross-sectional study showed that abdominal infections constituted 19.6% of infected patients in ICUs. The mortality of patients was higher than those with other infections (29.4% vs 24.4%, $P < 0.001$). Nearly all patients were treated with antibiotics (98.1%), but the results of microbial culture were obtained in only about two-thirds of patients [11]. The common use of empirical antimicrobial drugs needs to refer to local epidemiological studies and antimicrobial susceptibility data [12]. Traditional epidemiological studies are conducted in a "bacteria-antibiotics" mode, which first describes the isolated local bacteria strains, then reports the corresponding drug susceptibilities. In 2012, Herbert et al. proposed that WISCAs could determine the likelihood that a specific regimen can effectively treat all organisms in a patient with a specific syndrome after microbial and clinical data analysis [8]. This method is based on significant differences in the distribution of pathogenic bacteria sites, which is usually lacking in traditional microbial/epidemiological studies; thus, the patients cannot be treated precisely.

In addition, OSIWA estimates for empirical therapies of IAIs might serve as an initial hint for the choice of antibiotics when other information is not available, since bacterial strain identification and antibiograms requires some time to produce the data, particularly for IAIs.

SMART is a global multi-center abdominal infection program that mainly monitors Gram-negative bacteria and their susceptibility to antibiotics. The data showed that *Enterobacteriaceae* were still the major strains found in abdominal infections (2010–2014) in China, the most common types being *E. coli* and *K. pneumoniae*, which is in agreement with a previous study [13].

Other non-fermentative bacteria include *P. aeruginosa* and *A. baumannii*, which accounted for 10.0 and 6.9% of pathogens, respectively. *A. baumannii* were not commonly detected in general abdominal infections, but its distribution rate was high in certain organs such as the pancreas. According to our analyses, the composition of pathogenic Gram-negative bacteria isolated from the abdominal cavity is different, based on the isolation sites. For example, Gram-negative *E. coli* bacteria from the appendix accounted for 76.8%, but was distributed < 40% in the liver and pancreas. *K. pneumoniae* accounted for 45.2% of the total pathogenic bacteria in the liver but < 6% in the colon, which is in line with previous reports that liver infections caused by *K. pneumoniae* are increasing [14, 15].

Therefore, the distribution of pathogenic bacteria in different abdominal organs should be considered in empirical therapy. We further analyzed comprehensive antimicrobial susceptibilities using the OSWIA algorithm,

Table 2 HA and CA IAI isolate distributions of *Enterobacteriaceae* and non-fermenting GNBs in the indicated organs

	Non-fermenting GNBs[a] N (%)		*Enterobacteriaceae* N (%)				
	HA	CA	HA		CA		Total
				ESBL+ (% of HA)		ESBL+ (% of CA)	
Gall bladder[b]	390 (15.5)	84 (3.4)	1593 (63.5)	701 (44.0)	438 (17.5)	162 (37.0)	2510
Peritoneal fluid[c]	375 (18.1)	82 (4.0)	1184 (57.0)	635 (53.6)	415 (20.0)	196 (47.2)	2078
Abscess[d]	225 (15.6)	46 (3.2)	891 (61.7)	434 (48.7)	281 (19.5)	133 (47.3)	1444
Liver	59 (10.7)	10 (1.8)	378 (68.4)	153 (40.5)	106 (19.2)	23 (21.7)	553
Appendix	11 (2.7)	16 (4.0)	146 (36.1)	72 (49.3)	232 (57.3)	101 (43.5)	405
Pancreas	55 (21.5)	11 (4.3)	155 (60.6)	86 (55.5)	35 (13.7)	21 (60)	256
Colon	23 (13.2)	10 (5.8)	122 (70.1)	81 (66.4)	19 (10.9)	12 (63.2)	174

[a]There was no ESBL+ isolates in non-fermenting GNBs
[b]There were 5 unidentified isolates in the *Enterobacteriaceae*
[c]There were 9 unidentified isolates in non-fermenting GNB and 13 not identified isolates in the *Enterobacteriaceae*
[d]There was 1 unidentified isolate in the *Enterobacteriaceae*

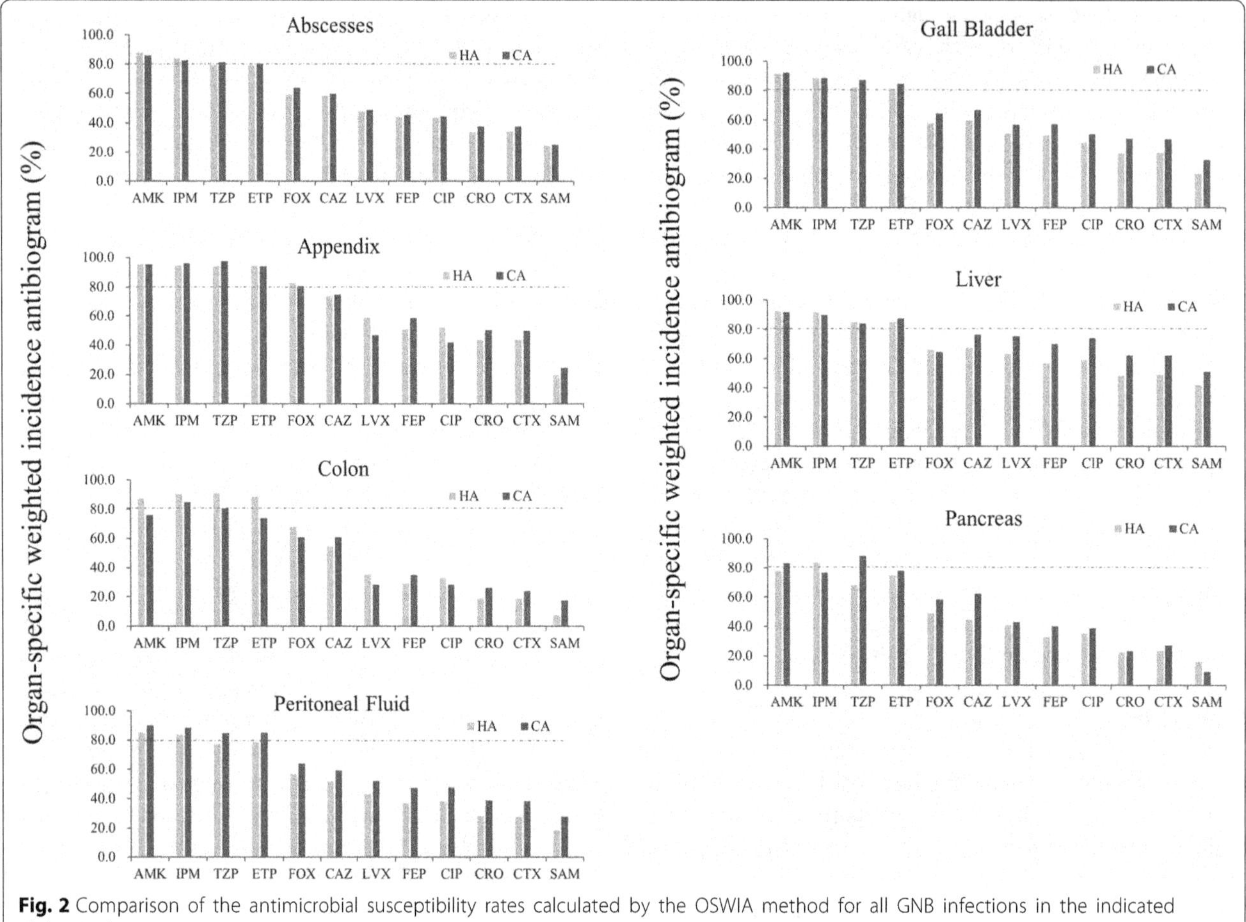

Fig. 2 Comparison of the antimicrobial susceptibility rates calculated by the OSWIA method for all GNB infections in the indicated abdominal organs

which is calculated according to the susceptibility of each bacterium to a specific drug times the sum of the total proportion of the bacterium present in a specific infection. We found that OSWIA closely matched the clinical data: compared with pancreatitis and other infection sites, appendicitis had a higher overall antimicrobial susceptibility. Additionally, the susceptibility rates for liver and gall bladder infections was somewhere in between, but it should be noted that the therapeutic effects of antimicrobial drugs can be highly variable when treating different infected organs.

Let's consider OSWIA > 80% as the initial gold standard. For example, the OSWIA of FOX is around 80% in the appendix, but was < 70% in the other 5 organs examined. Thus, it would only be appropriate for the treatment of specific infections in the appendix. Piperacillin/tazobactam (TZP) is recommended to treat many infections, but OSWIA was only 68.3% in HA pancreas infections, which is inappropriate for empirical treatment. Additionally, we found that apart from liver infections, the weighted susceptibility for each abdominal organ presented as a typical "stair-step" shape, with some of drugs such as ertapenem, amikacin, imipenem and piperacillin/tazobactam being > 80%, and the rest far below this level. The weighted susceptibilities of ertapenem, amikacin, imipenem and piperacillin/tazobactam were highest in all organs, which is in line with another study on Chinese IAIs [13].

ESBL rates of *Enterobacteriaceae* essentially differed between organs (Table 2), which were reflected in the low susceptibility rates to cephalosporins of colon, pancreas and peritoneal fluid isolates (Fig. 2). The high proportion of ESBL-producing strains in the pathogens of the studied organs certainly indicate a high risk for Chinese IAI patients becoming infected with an ESBL producing bacterial strain.

We analyzed the epidemiological data of antimicrobial susceptibilities using an "organ–bacteria–susceptibility" approach, but still a large number of clinical factors could not be included in the analysis, including the drug concentrations at the infection sites and the physical condition of individual patients.

Moreover, drawbacks in our data analysis have been noted. First, a classification based on infected organs reduced the sample size in each group, which decreased the reliability of the statistical analysis, and Gram-negative anaerobes and Gram-positive bacteria were not included. Second, because of the limited strain numbers in each year, we combined data from several years, which might not reflect the actual situation in each year. Yearly OSWIA analysis with sufficient samples should be conducted in large hospitals, as a complement to the traditional model of "bacteria-susceptibility" to support appropriate regimen selection of antibiotics for empirical therapy.

Conclusions

There are significant variations in the distributions of bacteria in different abdominal organs, with various antimicrobial organ-specific susceptibilities. OSWIA may be used as a complement to the traditional model of "bacteria–susceptibility", and aid appropriate regimen selection of antibiotics for empirical therapy, particularly for CA IAIs. However, further studies will need to be conducted to validate the correlations between OSWIA, and the cure and survival rates of patients.

Abbreviations

ETP: (ertapenem); AMK: (amikacin); IPM: (imipenem); TZP: (piperacillin/tazobactam); FOX: (cefoxitin); CAZ: (ceftazidime); LVX: (levofloxacin); FEP: (cefepime); CIP: (ciprofloxacin); CRO: (ceftriaxone); CTX: (cefotaxime); SAM: (ampicillin/sulbactam)

Acknowledgments

Merck Sharp & Dohme (MSD; Whitehouse Station, NJ, US) provided funds to support this study.

Funding

None.

Authors' contributions

Both of the authors listed have read and approved the manuscript. The authors were solely responsible for the conception and performance of the study and for writing the manuscript. Medical writing and editorial assistance was provided by Shanghai BIOMED Science Technology (Shanghai, China) through funding provided by MSD China. The authors were solely responsible for the conception and performance of the study and for the contents and the writing of this manuscript.

Competing interests

The authors declare that they have no competing interests.

References

1. Paterson DL, Rossi F, Baquero F, Hsueh PR, Woods GL, Satishchandran V, Snyder TA, Harvey CM, Teppler H, Dinubile MJ, et al. In vitro susceptibilities of aerobic and facultative gram-negative bacilli isolated from patients with intra-abdominal infections worldwide: the 2003 study for monitoring antimicrobial resistance trends (SMART). J Antimicrob Chemother. 2005; 55(6):965–73.
2. Superti SV, Augusti G, Zavascki AP. Risk factors for and mortality of extended-spectrum-beta-lactamase-producing Klebsiella pneumoniae and Escherichia coli nosocomial bloodstream infections. Rev Inst Med Trop Sao Paulo. 2009;51(4):211–6.
3. Sartelli M. A focus on intra-abdominal infections. World J Emerg Surg. 2010;5:9.
4. Weigelt JA. Empiric treatment options in the management of complicated intra-abdominal infections. Cleve Clin J Med. 2007;74(Suppl 4):S29–37.
5. Tabah A, Koulenti D, Laupland K, Misset B, Valles J, Bruzzi de Carvalho F, Paiva JA, Cakar N, Ma X, Eggimann P, et al. Characteristics and determinants of outcome of hospital-acquired bloodstream infections in intensive care units: the EUROBACT international cohort study. Intensive Care Med. 2012; 38(12):1930–45.
6. Garnacho-Montero J, Garcia-Garmendia JL, Barrero-Almodovar A, Jimenez-Jimenez FJ, Perez-Paredes C, Ortiz-Leyba C. Impact of adequate empirical antibiotic therapy on the outcome of patients admitted to the intensive care unit with sepsis. Crit Care Med. 2003;31(12):2742–51.
7. Valles J, Rello J, Ochagavia A, Garnacho J, Alcala MA. Community-acquired bloodstream infection in critically ill adult patients: impact of shock and inappropriate antibiotic therapy on survival. Chest. 2003;123(5):1615–24.
8. Hebert C, Ridgway J, Vekhter B, Brown EC, Weber SG, Robicsek A. Demonstration of the weighted-incidence syndromic combination antibiogram: an empiric prescribing decision aid. Infect Control Hosp Epidemiol. 2012;33(4):381–8.
9. CLSI: Methods for Dilution Antimicrobial Susceptibility Tests for Bacteria That Grow Aerobically; Approved Standards. 9th ed. Document M07-A: Clinical and Laboratory Standards Institute, Wayne, Penn.; 2012.
10. CLSI: Performance standards for antimicrobial susceptibility testing; twenty-third informational supplement. Document M100-S23 clinical and laboratory standards institute, Wayne, Penn.; 2013.
11. De Waele J, Lipman J, Sakr Y, Marshall JC, Vanhems P, Barrera Groba C, Leone M, Vincent JL, Investigators EI. Abdominal infections in the intensive care unit: characteristics, treatment and determinants of outcome. BMC Infect Dis. 2014;14:420.
12. Zhang S, Huang W. Epidemiological study of community- and hospital-acquired intraabdominal infections. Chin J Traumatol. 2015;18(2):84–9.
13. Zhang H, Yang Q, Liao K, Ni Y, Yu Y, Hu B, Sun Z, Huang W, Wang Y, Wu A, et al. Update of incidence and antimicrobial susceptibility trends of Escherichia coli and Klebsiella pneumoniae isolates from Chinese intra-abdominal infection patients. BMC Infect Dis. 2017;17(1):776.
14. Liu Y, Wang JY, Jiang W. An increasing prominent disease of Klebsiella pneumoniae liver abscess: etiology, diagnosis, and treatment. Gastroenterol Res Pract. 2013;2013:258514.
15. Siu LK, Yeh KM, Lin JC, Fung CP, Chang FY. Klebsiella pneumoniae liver abscess: a new invasive syndrome. Lancet Infect Dis. 2012;12(11):881–7.

24

A prospective cohort study to evaluate immunosuppressive cytokines as predictors of viral persistence and progression to pre-malignant lesion in the cervix in women infected with HR-HPV: study protocol

K. Torres-Poveda[1,2*], M. Bahena-Román[1], K. Delgado-Romero[3] and V. Madrid-Marina[1]

Abstract

Background: Cervical cancer (CC) is caused by a persistent infection of high-risk human papillomavirus (HR-HPV). While most HPV infections are transient, persistent HPV infections are a significant health problem in Mexico. With an estimated HPV prevalence of 10% among women in reproductive age, approximately 25% of these women present at least a positive result in triage test, which according to previous studies is expected to be confirmed as positive CIN-2/3. The immune system has a key role in the natural history of HPV infection; alterations in the cellular immune response are responsible for the failure to eliminate HPV. The objective of this project is to assess the prognostic value of detecting immune markers (IL-10, IL-4, TGFβ1, IFNγ, IL-6, and TNFα), the expression of HPV-HR E6/E7 proteins, and the viral load at the cervical level with respect to the persistence or clearance of HR-HPV infection, and the regression or progression of a cervical premalignant lesion.

Methods: A dynamic cohort study is being conducted in women with colposcopic, cytological, and histopathological results negative for squamous intraepithelial lesion (SIL) in the cervix and a positive HPV test; the subjects will be followed-up for 5 years, period from which 3 years have already elapsed, with yearly studies (colposcopy, cytology, and histopathology diagnosis, along with molecular HPV test, quantification of viral load and of IL-10, IL-4, TGFβ1, INFγ, IL-6, and TNFα levels, along with the expression of the HR-HPV E6/E7 proteins in the cervix as a viral marker. The outcome will be categorized as viral persistence or clearance; and as SIL persistence, progression, or regression. Binomial and/or multinomial regression models adjusted for potential confounders will be used, associating the relative risk of the outcome with the immune and viral markers evaluated.

Discussion: This research will generate knowledge about immune markers with predictive value for the persistence and clearance of HPV, which will improve the triage of positive HPV women and thus reduce the economic burden for the Mexican health system imposed by the management of high-grade SIL and CC cases, which are still detected in late stages.

Keywords: HPV, Viral persistence, Cytokines, Cohort, Mexico

* Correspondence: kjtorres@insp.mx
[1]Chronic Infectious Diseases and Cancer Division, Center for Research on Infectious Diseases, Instituto Nacional de Salud Pública (INSP), Cuernavaca, Morelos, Mexico
[2]CONACYT-INSP, Cuernavaca, Morelos, Mexico
Full list of author information is available at the end of the article

Background

Cervical cancer (CC) is caused by a persistent infection by high-risk human papilloma virus (HR-HPV). The prevalence and estimated role of different HPV genotypes in the development of cervix premalignant lesions and CC has been described in several meta-analyses [1, 2]. In one of the first prospective studies on the prevalence of oncogenic HPV, a concordant pattern relating HPV prevalence with younger age, viral elimination, and the reduction of exposure to new types of HPV was reported [3]. Viral prevalence is the product of incidence (acquisition of new infections) and duration (persistence). Factors that could favor a higher HPV prevalence include age, female or male sexual behavior, increased detection of HPV infection, changes in the cervicovaginal epithelium due to age or related to the menopause, and age-related immune senescence, which leads to the reactivation of latent infections and thus to an apparent increase in the detection of new infection cases [3].

A persistent HR-HPV infection has been considered as a prerequisite for CC development [4]. In most studies, viral persistence is defined as the detection of the same HPV type or the same type-group in two consecutive visits; however, the inter-visit period ranges from 4 months to 5–7 years [3, 5–7]. Thus, some studies suggest restricting the analysis to incidental infections, taking into account the duration of the infection instead of the number of positive tests [5, 8]. An agreement on the definition of viral persistence would facilitate making comparisons of the results in studies of this type and would provide a guide to define the endpoints to be evaluated in clinical trials of HPV vaccines and to make recommendations to improve the CC screening policies.

The reasons why some HPV infections are cleared whilst others persist, increasing the high risk of squamous intraepithelial lesions (SIL), are still under study. The mechanistic explanation of HPV elimination relies on specific immunological reactions, where competent cellular and humoral responses are both required [9]. The immune system plays a key role in the natural history of HPV infection; alterations in the cellular immune response are responsible for the failure to eliminate HPV [10]. On the other hand, immune tolerance has been reported to favor viral persistence and progression to cancer [11].

Highlighting the relevance of acquired immunity in women with HPV infection, a higher SIL incidence has been observed in immunocompromised patients [12]. While an impaired cellular immunity hinders the clearance of HPV infection, 2% of HR-HPV infections persist in apparently immunocompetent individuals [13].

Many molecular alterations in those women who progress to CC have been described, the most common being immunosuppression produced by Th2 (IL-4, IL-6, IL-10) and Th3 (TGFβ1) cytokines [14, 15]. Patients with HPV-associated neoplasia showing a Th1 cytokine profile had a better clinical outcome compared to those patients exhibiting a Th2 profile [12]. CC progression has been associated with an undesirable Th1- to Th2-cytokine type shift induced by two E7-derived epitopes and an increase in IL-10 expression [16].

The role of IL-10 and TGFβ1 in the immunosuppression observed in cervix SIL and CC patients has been described [17–19]. IL-10 is a potent immunosuppressive cytokine that favored viral persistence in a model of persistent cytomegalovirus infection [20]. HPV regulates the expression of these cytokines, and both the HPV-16-derived E6 and E7 proteins have been reported to increase the expression of TGFβ1, while the HPV-derived E2 protein regulates the expression of IL-10 [17, 21].

Some genetic risk determinants of persisting HPV infection have been defined [22], including polymorphisms in genes controlling effector T cell responses [13]. Most association studies for CC around the world evaluate single nucleotide polymorphisms (SNPs) in candidate genes involved in oncogenesis and the cellular immune response, since there is much evidence of viral evasion to the immune response in patients with persistent HPV infection and CC [19, 23, 24].

Several studies have reported an association between CC and polymorphisms in the promoter region of IL-10, IL-4, IL-6, and TGFβ1, showing an increased expression of these cytokines in the cervix; based on this evidence, a genetic immune profile (Th2-Th3) was postulated as underlying the susceptibility to CC [25]. However, this profile was defined in cross-sectional studies, and a cohort study is required to determine whether this genetic profile actually favors viral persistence.

Previous studies on HPV persistence evaluating the immune response were made after viral persistence was established, so it was not possible to determine whether immune dysregulation leads to HPV persistence or vice versa. Therefore, follow-up studies such as the one proposed in this protocol are required to address the question on whether the persistence of HPV infection is the cause or the consequence of immune dysregulation. On the other hand, immunological predictors are much needed to identify women with potential for viral persistence and progression to SIL, alleviating the current overload in diagnosis and treatment services, improving thus the CC prevention strategy.

Methods/design

Objectives

The general objective of this project is to assess the prognostic value of detecting immune markers (IL-10, IL-4, TGFβ1, IFNγ, IL-6, and TNFα) at the systemic and cervical levels, either coupled or not with the expression of HR-HPV E6/E7 proteins and viral load in the cervix, with respect to the persistence or clearance of HPV infection and to the incidence, regression, or progression of SIL in cervix.

To achieve this, a baseline study will be conducted, and risk groups will be generated by determining the frequency of HPV genotypes. The levels of the immune biomarkers IL-10, IL-4, TGFβ1, IFNγ, IL-6, and TNFα; the levels of the oncoproteins E6 and E7; and the viral load at the level of cervix, will also be determined.

For the follow-up of the cohort, changes in the levels of the immune biomarkers IL-10, IL-4, TGFβ1, IFNγ, IL-6, TNFα, the oncoproteins E6 and E7, and the viral load will be determined in the cervix of the subjects at fixed times. The number of new cases of persistence and viral clearance, along with the incidence of cervix SIL regression or progression will be determined.

To assess the final event of the cohort, the relative risk for possible persistence and viral clearance adjusted by confounders with respect to high levels of each immune biomarker in the cervix will be estimated, as well as with respect to high levels of the proteins E6 and E7, and to viral load at the cervical level.

The relative risk adjusted for possible confounders of incidence, regression or progression of SIL in cervix with respect to high levels of each immune biomarker in the cervix will also be evaluated, as well as with respect to high levels of the proteins E6 and E7 and to viral load at the cervical level. Finally, the interaction between cervical levels of each immune marker and the viral load, and its association with HPV persistence, will be evaluated.

Design and population

A prospective, dynamic cohort study will be conducted on women attending the Women's Health Care Center—CAPASAM of the Health Services of the State of Morelos, Mexico, after an abnormal result in cytology studies recently issued by a referring health center.

Inclusion and exclusion criteria

All women attending the CAPASAM are eligible for recruitment if they: (1) are 30 years-old or older; (2) have resided for 5 years or more in Morelos; (3) agree to participate in the study, sign an informed consent form, complete a questionnaire, and donate blood and cervix exudate samples; (3) have a negative diagnosis for chronic inflammatory or autoimmune diseases at the beginning of the study and during follow-up, and a negative pregnancy status; (4) received no previous anti-HPV vaccination, nor immunosuppressive treatment within 6 months before their inclusion in the cohort; and (5) provide at least a telephone number to be contacted. Those individuals for whom follow-up is impossible and those who decide to stop participating in the study at any time will be excluded.

Recruitment

Recruitment started in September 2015, and it is planned to continue until 2020. A unique study identification number is assigned to each woman. This number identifies and tracks the questionnaires and biological samples collected during the study to make them reversibly anonymized. This procedure is fundamental to link the collected information, ensure confidentiality, and protect personal data in accordance to Mexican laws.

Sample size

Assuming a power of 90% and a confidence level of 95%, a sample size of the risk groups to be followed-up in the cohort with an estimated loss of 20% during the follow-up period was calculated, taking into account the mean serum levels (pg/mL) and the respective standard deviation for each cytokine to be evaluated as immune marker, obtained in a previous cross-sectional study in HPV-positive patients with no SIL and HPV-positive women with SIL in cervix [25]. Thus, the inclusion of 200 HPV-positive women was determined as necessary. Calculations were performed with Stata v. 14.0 (StataCorp, College Station, TX, USA).

Sampling and follow-up

All included subjects will be evaluated and followed-up for 5 years (Fig. 1). At the baseline (sampling 1), a structured questionnaire will be given to each subject and the information in each questionnaire will be entered in a database. The software Stata v.14.2 will be used for this. From each participant who has signed the informed consent form and completed the questionnaire, a blood sample will be taken by a healthcare professional, using EDTA-containing Vacutainer tubes (7 mL) and serum-separator Vacutainer tubes (4 mL) (Becton Dickinson, BD Franklin Lakes, NJ, USA). A CAPASAM-ascribed colposcopic gynecologist will take three exudate samples from the endocervical canal; the first sample will be collected by applying an ophthalmic sponge for 30 s, removing the device from the patient, and immediately placing it in a cryovial and into liquid nitrogen to measure cytokine levels in the cervix; approximately 10 min later, a second sample will be taken with an exfoliative brush (cytobrush) and placed in a tube with preservation medium to measure the expression levels of the HPV oncoproteins E6 and E7; finally, a third sample will be taken using the ThinPrep HOLOGIC vial for automated HPV genotyping.

In addition, the gynecologist will make a colposcopic diagnosis at the consultation time, will take a sample for a cytology or Papanicolaou study, and will send it for

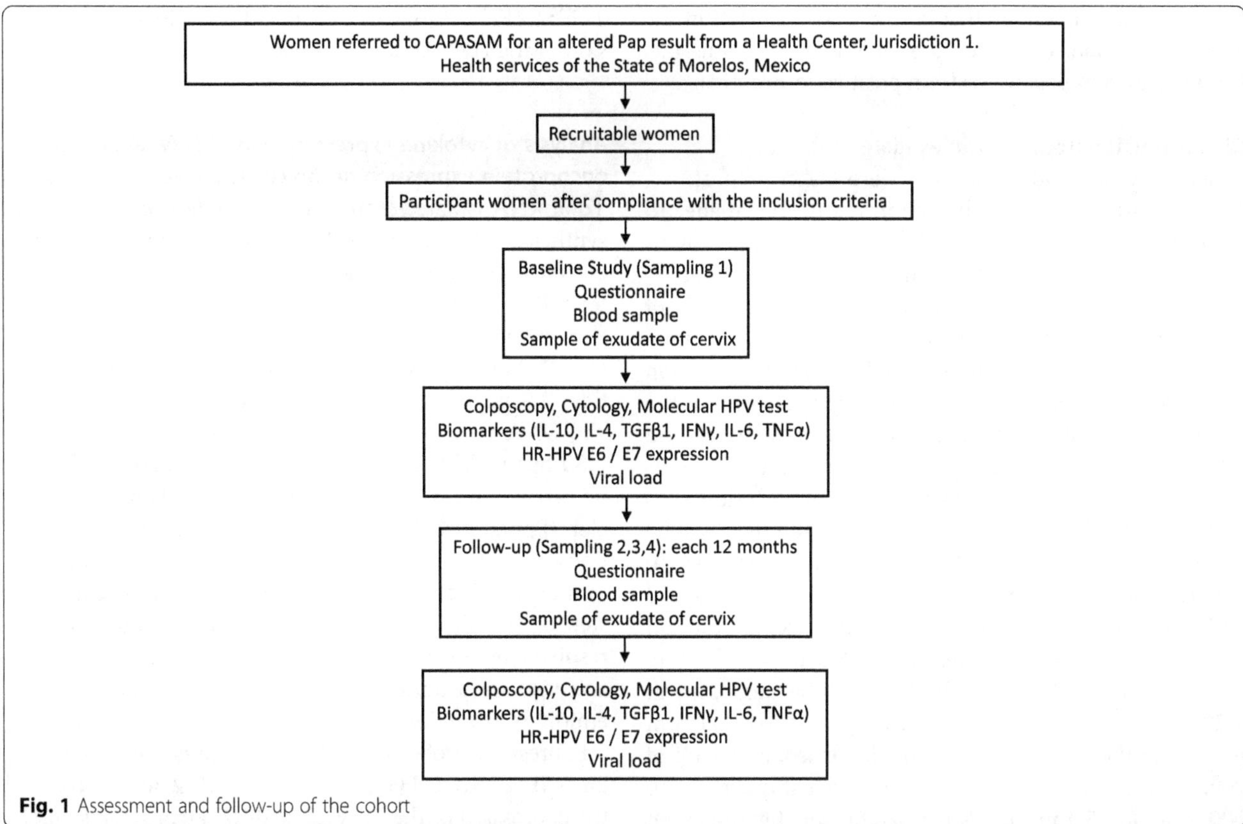

Fig. 1 Assessment and follow-up of the cohort

pathological analysis to the CAPASAM Pathology Unit. Any potential risk and discomfort during sampling are clearly described in the informed consent form. Four follow-up samplings will be performed, one every 12 months through the five-year study. For follow-up samplings, the patients will be contacted by telephone and invited to attend the CAPASAM to perform each programmed blood and cervix exudate sampling. Additionally, variables of the gynecological-obstetric history and sexual behavior that may have changed over time, such as marital status and number of sexual partners, will be recorded.

Variables

Dependent variables

HPV persistence, understood as the detection of the same HPV genotype in two or more consecutive intervals.

Viral clearance, understood as the negative detection of the same genotype in a consecutive interval, following a positive sample (first negative PCR result after an incidental infection).

SIL persistence: histopathological diagnosis of (low- or high-grade) SIL after a first SIL diagnosis. Persistence of the same lesion in two or more successive liquid cytologic studies.

SIL regression: histopathological diagnosis for SIL negative after a first (low- or high-grade) SIL diagnosis. Regression of the lesion in two or more successive cytologic studies and subsequent healing.

Progression of (low- or high-grade) SIL: histopathological diagnosis of high-grade SIL or cancer in situ after a first diagnosis of SIL (low- and high-grade, respectively).

Main independent variable: levels at the cervix of the immune biomarkers IL-10, IL-4, TGFβ1, IFNγ, IL-6, and TNFα, expressed in pg/mL.

Other independent variables

Expression levels of the proteins E6 and E7 in the cervix, reported in terms of expression over the endogenous glyceraldehyde-3-phosphate dehydrogenase (GAPDH) gene. Viral load in cervix, reported as the number of viral copies. Age, number of sexual partners, age at menarche, age at start of active sex life, socioeconomic level, parity, smoking (years, number of cigarettes per day, whether the habit is old or current, previous years of tobacco use), hormonal contraception (years of duration, current situation), viral genotype, history of other sexually transmitted infections (STIs), conservative clinical treatment for previous SIL and duration of an incidental HPV infection, understood as the time elapsed from the onset of incidental infection in the cohort until its elimination, assuming that both events occurred in the inter-visit period, observed as a shift in HPV status (i.e. from negative to positive or from positive to negative).

DNA extraction from cervical exudate

When cervical exudate samples were taken with an exfoliative brush (cytobrush), efforts will be made to recover most of the cells in the brush; the supernatant will be centrifuged at 5000 rpm for 3 min. Cells recovered from the cytobrush will be added with 400 μL of lysis solution. After incubating at 65 °C for 5 min, 600 μL of chloroform will be added, mixed by inversion five times, and centrifuged at 10 000 rpm for 4 min; the upper phase will be transferred to a new tube, and 800 μL per sample of freshly prepared precipitation solution (80 μL of concentrated precipitation solution plus 720 μL of sterilized water) will be added; the tube will be mixed by inversion for 40 s and centrifuged at 10 000 rpm for 4 min; the supernatant will be discarded and the DNA tablet will be dissolved in NaCl solution and homogenized 3–4 times; then, 300 μL of absolute ethanol will be added and the tube will be incubated at – 20 °C for 10–20 min and centrifuged at 10 000 rpm for 4 min; the supernatant will be discarded, and 1 ml of 70% ethanol will be added; after centrifuging at 10 000 rpm for 5 min, the supernatant will be discarded and the DNA pellet will be dissolved in 50 μL of sterile water. When cervical exudate samples were taken with the Merocel ophthalmic sponge, the extraction will be performed according to a previously described protocol [26]. DNA concentration and purity will be assessed in a Thermo Scientific NanoDropTM 1000 Spectrophotometer (260/280) and the integrity of the DNA will be determined by electrophoresis in 0.8% agarose gels.

RNA extraction from cervical exudate

Per 6×10^6 cells or 50–100 mg of sample, 1 ml of Trizol will be added. The sample will be homogenized and incubated for 5 min at room temperature. Then, 200 μL of chloroform per milliliter of Trizol will be added, mixed, and incubated for 2–3 min at room temperature. The tube will be centrifuged at 12 000 rpm for 15 min at 8 °C or 10 min at 4 °C. The upper phase, containing RNA, will be transferred to a tube; 500 μL of isopropanol will be added, mixed, and incubated at – 20 °C for 15 min; after centrifuging at 12 000 rpm for 10 min at 4 °C, the supernatant will be removed. The RNA pack will be washed with 1 mL of 75% ethanol, mixed and centrifuged at 10 000 rpm for 7 min at 4 °C; the supernatant will be discarded, and the tablet will be resuspended in 20 μL of RNase- and DNase-free water. Then, the sample will be incubated at 65 °C for 10 min, and RNA will be quantified and stored at – 80 °C until used for real time RT-PCR assays to analyze the expression of the cytokines IL-10, IL-4, TGFβ1, IFNγ, IL-6, and TNFα, and to evaluate the expression of the HPV E6 and E7 oncoproteins.

Analysis of cytokine expression and of HPV E6 and E7 oncoprotein expression at the cervical level

Total RNA isolated from cervical exudate will be used to synthesize cDNA; this will be performed in the presence of 200 U of reverse M-MLV transcriptase and 2.5 μg of total RNA under standard conditions. PCR will be carried out in a reaction volume of 25 μL containing 1 μL of cDNA, dNTPs 0.2 mM, 15 pmol of each oligonucleotide, 2.5 μL of reaction buffer and 1 U of recombinant Taq DNA polymerase. The constitutive gene of GAPDH (250 bp) will be used to verify DNA integrity. PCR will be carried out in a Mastercycler PCR gradient thermocycler (Eppendorf, Germany) under the following conditions: 5 min at 94 °C, 35 one-minute cycles at 94 °C, 1 min at 60 °C, and 1 min at 72 °C, with a final extension step of 10 min at 72 °C. Amplification products will be resolved by electrophoresis in a 6% polyacrylamide gel and visualized under ultraviolet light after staining with ethidium bromide.

Expression probes to analyze the expression of the cytokines IL-10, IL-4, TGFβ1, IFNγ, IL-6, IL-2, and TNFα and the expression of the HPV E6 and E7 oncoproteins will be obtained from Applied Biosystems for real-time PCR analysis. The HPRT1 (hypoxanthine phosphoribosyl transferase) gene will be used to normalize the amount of mRNA in each sample to analyze IL-10, IL-4, TGFβ1, IFNγ, IL-6, and TNFα. The GAPDH gene will be used to normalize the amount of mRNA in each sample to analyze the expression of the HPV E6 and E7 oncoproteins.

Real-time PCR will be performed by adding 2 μL of each cDNA sample to a final reaction volume of 10 μL, containing 5 μL of Master Mix for expression, 0.4 μL of probe, and 2.6 μL of molecular grade, DNase-free water. Amplification cycles will be carried out in an Applied Biosystems VIA-VII equipment (Foster City) under the following conditions: 10 min at 94 °C, 40 one-minute cycles at 94 °C, 1 min at 54 °C, and 1.5 min at 72 °C, with a final extension step of 15 min at 72 °C. The level of mRNA expression for the genes under study will be calculated by relative quantification with the comparative Ct method (2-ΔCt) and plotted as expression relative units of each gene relative to the endogenous gene (HPRT-1 or GAPDH) and to the group of comparison. All samples will be analyzed in duplicate.

Cytokine evaluation in cervical secretions

The levels of IL-10, IL-4, TGFβ1, IFNγ, IL-6, and TNFα will be determined by the Luminex Multiplex assay, according to a previously described protocol [27].

HPV detection and genotyping in cervical exudate samples

Samples taken in ThinPrep (Pap test) vials from each subject who agreed to participate in the cohort study will be stored at 4 °C until use for HPV genotyping by the automated Cobas HPV Test. The Cobas 4800 is a fully automated real-time PCR system that separately detects HR-HPV-16 and -18 genotypes in addition to ten other high-risk genotypes (31, 33, 35, 39, 45, 51, 52, 56, 58, 59) and two of "probable high risk" (66 and 68). The procedure will be performed according to Roche Diagnostic's instructions.

Viral load quantification

Viral load in the cervix will be evaluated with the Seegene HPV 28 Anyplex system, using DNA extracted from cervix exudate from each patient. This will allow us to confirm HPV diagnosis and at the same time to estimate the viral load by genotype in each patient.

Data collection and statistical analysis

A descriptive analysis of the sociodemographic and gynecological-obstetric characteristics, familial history of cancer, and lifestyle-related variables in the population under study will be performed. The questionnaire will include, among other variables: sociodemographic characteristics such as age, marital status, religion, education level, smoking habit (years, number of cigarettes per day, whether the habit is old or current, previous years of tobacco use), and socioeconomic level; for this variable, an index (low, medium, and high tertiles) will be constructed using the analysis of main components for the population included in the cohort, with information on household floor materials and availability of tap water, washing machine, refrigerator, television, radio and stove; gynecological-obstetric traits such as the number of sexual partners, regular partners (defined as sexual activity with that person for at least 6 months), age at menarche, age at start of active sex life, parity, hormonal contraception (years of duration, current situation), history of sexually transmitted diseases, condom use, genital hygiene, previous HPV infection, previous local treatment for a cervical lesion, and familial history of cancer, including type of cancer and consanguinity.

For continuous variables, expressed as a mean ± standard deviation, the Kruskal-Wallis test will be used. For categorical variables, expressed as a percentage, the chi-square test will be used. Results will be regarded as statistically significant for $P < 0.05$. All data will be analyzed with STATA v.14 for Windows. Missing data will be addressed by using Maximum likelihood, multiple imputation, and inverse probability weighting and analyzed via multilevel mixed-effects linear regression models.

To evaluate the levels of the immune biomarkers IL-10, IL-4, TGFβ1, IFNγ, IL-6, and TNFα and the expression levels of the proteins E6 and E7 in the cervix, the non-parametric Mann-Whitney U test will be used. A curve of diagnostic performance (ROC-receiver operating characteristic) will be plotted to obtain the cut-off point of greater discrimination with respect to the variable of evolution (viral persistence, viral clearance, SIL incidence, SIL persistence, SIL progression. Once obtained, the sensitivity, specificity, positive predictive value, and negative predictive value for the cut-off points of each variable will be calculated. With respect to viral load, the Wilcoxon rank sum test will be used to measure the difference in median viral load for each HPV type, according to the infection status (HPV persistence or HPV clearance). All possible 2-way interactions between cervical levels of each immune marker and the viral load, and its association with HPV persistence, will be evaluated by adding multiplicative terms in the multivariate logistic models.

The incidence and cumulative incidence rate of each outcome (HPV persistence, HPV clearance, SIL incidence, SIL persistence, SIL progression) will be determined, adjusting for changing levels of the immune biomarkers IL-10, IL-4, TGFβ1, IFNγ, IL-6, and TNFα and the expression levels of E6 and E7 in the cervix.

To assess the association of viral persistence or clearance, SIL incidence, regression, or progression with cervical levels of the immune biomarkers IL-10, IL-4, TGFβ1, IFNγ, IL-6, and TNF, as well as with E6 and E7 expression levels and with cervical viral load, a Cox regression analysis will be performed, adjusting for the co-variables age, number of sexual partners, age at menarche, age at start of active sex life, parity, smoking, hormonal contraception, history of other STIs, conservative clinical treatment, viral genotype, co-infection with two or more HPV genotypes, and duration of incidental HPV infections. The viral load will be included in the analysis as the maximum viral load reached during an incidental infection for each viral group. The endpoints for the analysis will be persistence or viral clearance and SIL incidence, regression, or progression.

The Kaplan-Meier method will be used to estimate the median duration of infection for most HPV types and for each previously defined viral group. Infections will be considered as persistent when their duration is longer than the median duration of the infection. A longitudinal approach will be applied to cluster all possible triplets of consecutive visits per individual, to compare the results of this measure of persistence with that obtained by using the traditional persistence definition (i.e. two consecutive positive samples).

To evaluate the association of persistent infection with the risk to develop cervical intraepithelial neoplasm

(CIN) grade-1 or grade-2/3, a Cox regression analysis will be performed, adjusting for cofactors relevant to the infection, like smoking and co-infection, along with the levels of the immune biomarkers IL-10, IL-4, TGFβ1, IFNγ, IL-6, and TNFα, the expression levels of E6 and E7 and the viral load in the cervix, and co-infection with two or more HPV genotypes. The endpoints for the analysis will be the histopathological diagnosis of CIN 1, CIN 2, CIN 3, or carcinoma in situ.

According to the results of HPV genotyping, type-specific viral clearance rates in single and multiple infections will be compared with the stratified log-rank test. This test will also determine the probability of viral clearance among HPV variants. The effect of co-infection by HPV genotype on incidence rates for CIN 1 and CIN 2/3 in women with simple and multiple infections will be assessed by the Cochran Mantel-Haenszel test stratified by age, the result of cytologic studies, and HPV type.

Discussion

The worldwide prevalence of HPV infection in women without cervix abnormalities is 11–12%, with the highest rates reported in sub-Saharan Africa (24%), Eastern Europe (21%), and Latin America (16%). The two most frequent viral types are HPV-16 (3.2%) and HPV-18 (1.4%). Prevalence increases in women with cervical pathology in direct proportion to the severity of the lesion, approaching to 90% in women with CIN 3 and invasive cancer [28, 29]. Most HPV infections are transient and intermittent. The immune system plays an important role in the natural history of HPV infections, since most high-risk HPV infections (90%) [30], as well as most low-grade intraepithelial lesions (75%) are eliminated [31, 32]. However, if the infection with a high-risk HPV type persists, viral genes can interfere with the cellular control mechanisms and trigger neoplastic changes, which eventually could progress to an invasive carcinoma [33].

The natural history of CC has been established by several prospective cohort studies, and the factors involved in the regression, persistence, and progression of cervical lesions are well known [9]. The outcome of HPV infections follow a well-characterized pattern where a dynamic balance is set between incidental infections and virus clearance. A rapid accumulation of incidental infections once sex activity starts (women younger than 20 years of age) is followed by a shift in this balance after the subjects are 25 years old, to favor virus clearance. This explains the steadily declining age-specific prevalence of HPV infections until menopause [9].

However, various aspects of the dynamics of HPV infection are still poorly understood [34, 35]. In particular, the mechanisms of virus clearance are controversial [35]. The importance of HPV clearance and persistence has been recognized for some years, and the number of studies addressing these issues has increased substantially [9]. The clearance of HPV infection is usually attributed to an effective immune response, and the observation of longer clearance times in immunocompromised individuals further corroborates this assumption [36, 37].

A wide variety of variables have been explored as potential co-determinants and/or predictors of HPV clearance; however, this is a yet largely unexplored area [9]. The likelihood of an HPV infection to become persistent and progress into invasive CC should be seen as the result of the combined effect of certain viral- (HPV genotype) and host-dependent features (the immune status of the subject) [12].

Direct evidence linking host immunologic responses to the risk of HPV persistence is sparse. The few studies that have been published to date have been modest in size. Therefore, it is not surprising that the results have been mixed. While some studies have suggested that the immune response to HPV is associated to viral clearance, others have concluded otherwise [9]. Further studies on host immunologic factors associated with HPV persistence in well-characterized, larger studies are clearly needed [22].

Given that a persistent infection by HR-HPV may be regarded as an intermediate phenotype and is a reliable predictor of CC, this study is expected to have a scientific impact since it will establish the prognostic value of detecting immune markers (IL-10, IL-4, TGFβ1, IFNγ, IL-6, and TNFα), the expression of HR-HPV E6/E7 proteins, and the cervical viral load with respect to the persistence or clearance of HPV infection and the incidence, regression, or progression of SIL in cervix, which can be evaluated at the population level and used to monitor and prevent the progression of this intermediate phenotype to CC.

The immune markers with potential predictive value for HPV persistence or clearance studied in this project will improve the triage of positive HPV women and thus reduce the costs imposed by the management of high-grade premalignant lesions and CC, which are still detected in later, advanced stages.

Although measuring viral persistence has a prognostic value and is useful to understand the natural history of HPV infection and SIL, it is necessary to study additional viral variables to improve risk assessment. In this study, we propose to evaluate the expression of E6 and E7 and the viral load at the cervical level. HPV viral load has been reported as an auxiliary marker of persistent HPV infection; since the biological behavior of the various HPV types differ, the predictive value for viral persistence of the HPV DNA load can also vary among HPV types [38]. Therefore, the relationship of the type-specific HPV viral load with the clearance or persistence of HPV infection and the incidence, regression, or progression of SIL will also be explored in this study.

The limitations of this research project are those inherent to a cohort study; for instance, losses in follow-up could arise as this project develops, since patients can leave the study either due to a lack of interest or a change of residence; likewise, additional losses in follow-up may occur due to pregnancy or a disease compromising the immune response of the patients being monitored. A second limitation is the possibility of information biases, since although the interview will be conducted by qualified personnel, the patients may not remember accurately the information required for the study.

Abbreviations

CC: Cervical cancer; CIN: Cervical intraepithelial neoplasm; GAPDH: Glyceraldehyde-3-phosphate dehydrogenase; HPRT1: Hypoxanthine phosphoribosyl transferase; HR-HPV: High-risk human papilloma virus; IFNγ: Interferon-gamma; IL-10: Interleukin 10; IL-4: Interleukin 4; IL-6: Interleukin 6; RT-PCR: *Reverse-transcription* polymerase chain reaction; SIL: Squamous intraepithelial lesions; SNPs: Single nucleotide polymorphisms; STIs: Sexually transmitted infections; TGFβ1: Transforming growth factor beta 1; Th: T helper cells; TNFα: Tumor necrosis factor alpha

Acknowledgements

The authors would like to express their appreciation to Maribel Almonte Pacheco, Rolando Herrero (Prevention and Implementation Group, International Agency for Research on Cancer), and Aurelio Cruz (Instituto Nacional de Salud–INSP, Center for Population Health Research–CISP) for their advice and their valuable contributions to this protocol.

Funding

The government agency that granted funding for the study was the National Council of Science and Technology of Mexico (CONACYT) from the Health Fund in the SSA / IMSS / ISSSTE Call for Applications 2014-1-233538 and did not participate in any of the activities of study design, collection, analysis and interpretation of the data and in the drafting of the manuscript. This work was also supported by CONACYT Fund E0013 APOYO COMPLEMENTARIO CÁTEDRAS-2014-01-245520. K. Torres-Poveda is a CONACyT Research Fellow at the Instituto Nacional de Salud Pública (INSP), Cuernavaca, Morelos, Mexico.

Authors' contributions

Author contributions were as follows: TPK conceived the study, participated in its design and coordination, and drafted the manuscript. BRM participated in the design and coordination of the study, DRK participated in the design and coordination of the study, and VMM participated in the design of the study and helped to draft the manuscript. All authors read and approved the final manuscript.

Competing interests

The authors declare that they have no competing interests.

Author details

[1]Chronic Infectious Diseases and Cancer Division, Center for Research on Infectious Diseases, Instituto Nacional de Salud Pública (INSP), Cuernavaca, Morelos, Mexico. [2]CONACYT-INSP, Cuernavaca, Morelos, Mexico. [3]Centro de Atención para la Salud de la Mujer (CAPASAM) (Center for Women's Health), Health Services of the State of Morelos, Cuernavaca, Mexico.

References

1. Smith JS, Lindsay L, Hoots B, Keys J, Franceschi S, Winer R, et al. Human papillomavirus type distribution in invasive cervical cancer and high-grade cervical lesions: a meta-analysis update. Int J Cancer. 2007;121:621–32.
2. Insinga RP, Liaw KL, Johnson LG, Madeleine MM. A systematic review of the prevalence and attribution of human papillomavirus types among cervical, vaginal, and vulvar precancers and cancers in the United States. Cancer Epidemiol Biomark Prev. 2008;17:1611–22.
3. Castle PE, Schiffman M, Herrero R, Hildesheim A, Rodriguez AC, Bratti MC, et al. A prospective study of age trends in cervical human papillomavirus acquisition and persistence in Guanacaste, Costa Rica. J Infect Dis. 2005; 191(11):1808–16.
4. Bosch FX, Burchell AN, Schiffman M, Giuliano AR, de Sanjose S, Bruni L, et al. Epidemiology and natural history of human papillomavirus infections and type-specific implications in cervical neoplasia. Vaccine. 2008;6(Suppl 10):K1–K16.
5. Muñoz N, Hernandez-Suarez G, Méndez F, Molano M, Posso H, Moreno V, et al. Persistence of HPV infection and risk of high-grade cervical intraepithelial neoplasia in a cohort of Colombian women. Br J Cancer. 2009;100(7):1184–90.
6. Miranda PM, Silva NN, Pitol BC, Silva ID, Lima-Filho JL, Carvalho RF, et al. Persistence or clearance of human papillomavirus infections in women in Ouro Preto, Brazil. Biomed Res Int. 2013;2013:578276.
7. Jalil EM, Bastos FI, Melli PP, Duarte G, Simoes RT, Yamamoto AY, et al. HPV clearance in postpartum period of HIV-positive and negative women: a prospective follow-up study. BMC Infect Dis. 2013;13:564.
8. Woodman CB, Collins S, Winter H, Bailey A, Ellis J, Prior P, et al. Natural history of cervical human papillomavirus infection in young women: a longitudinal cohort study. Lancet. 2001;357(9271):1831–6.
9. Syrjänen K. Mechanisms and predictors of high-risk human papillomavirus (HPV) clearance in the uterine cervix. Eur J Gynaecol Oncol. 2007;28(5):337–51.
10. Song SH, Lee JK, Lee NW, Saw HS, Kang JS, Lee KW. Interferon-γ (IFN-γ): a possible prognostic marker for clearance of high-risk human papillomavirus (HPV). Gynecol Oncol. 2008;108:543–8.
11. Einstein KH, Schiller JT, Viscidi RP, Strickler HD, Coursaget P, Tan T, et al. Clinician's guide to human papillomavirus immunology: knowns and unknowns. Lancet Infect Dis. 2009;9:347–56.
12. Conesa-Zamora P. Immune responses against virus and tumor in cervical carcinogenesis: treatment strategies for avoiding the HPV-induced immune escape. Gynecol Oncol. 2013;131(2):480–8.
13. Frazer IH. Interaction of human papillomaviruses with the host immune system: a well evolved relationship. Virology. 2009;384(2):410–4.
14. Ovestad IT, Gudlaugsson E, Skaland I, Malpica A, Kruse AJ, Janssen EA, et al. Local immune response in the microenvironment of CIN2-3 with and without spontaneous regression. Mod Pathol. 2010;23:1231–40.
15. Feng Q, Wei H, Morihara J, Stern J, Yu M, Kiviat N, et al. Th2 type inflammation promotes the gradual progression of HPV-infected cervical cells to cervical carcinoma. Gynecol Oncol. 2012;127(2):412–9.
16. Woo YL, van den Hende M, Sterling JC, Coleman N, Crawford RA, Kwappenberg KM, et al. A prospective study on the natural course of low-grade squamous intraepithelial lesions and the presence of HPV16 E2-, E6- and E7-specific T-cell responses. Int J Cancer. 2010;126:133–41.
17. Peralta-Zaragoza O, Bermúdez-Morales V, Gutiérrez-Xicotencatl L, Alcocer-González J, Recillas-Targa F, Madrid-Marina V. Human papilomavirus-16 E6 and E7 proteins induce activation of human TGF-β1 basal promoter in epithelial cells throughout a Sp1 recognition sequence. Viral Immunol. 2006;19(3):468–80.
18. Bermúdez-Morales VH, Burguete AI, Gutierrez ML, Alcocer-González JM, Madrid-Marina V. Correlation between IL-10 expression and human papillomavirus infection in cervical cancer. A mechanism for immune response escape. Cancer Investig. 2008;26:1037–43.
19. Torres-Poveda K, Bahena-Román M, Madrid-González C, Burguete-García AI, Bermúdez-Morales VH, Peralta-Zaragoza O, et al. Role of IL-10 and TGF-β1 in local immunosuppression in HPV-associated cervical neoplasia. World J Clin Oncol. 2014;5(4):753–63.
20. Brooks DG, Trifilo MJ, Edelmann KH, Teyton L, McGavern DB, Oldstone MB. Interleukin-10 determines viral clearance or persistence in vivo. Nat Med. 2006;12(11):1301–9.
21. Bermúdez-Morales VH, Peralta-Zaragoza O, Moreno J, Alcocer-González JM, Madrid-Marina V. IL-10 expression is regulated by HPV E2 protein in cervical cancer cells. Mol Med Rep. 2011;4:369–75.

22. Garcia-Pineres AJ, Hildesheim A, Herrero R, Trivett M, Williams M, Atmetlla I, et al. Persistent human papillomavirus infection is associated with a generalized decrease in immune responsiveness in older women. Cancer Res. 2006;66:11070–6.
23. Stanley MA, Sterling JC. Host responses to infection with human papillomavirus. Curr Probl Dermatol. 2014;45:58–74.
24. Martínez-Nava GA, Fernández-Niño JA, Madrid-Marina V, Torres-Poveda K. Polymorphisms associated with cervical cancer: systematic review and metaanalysis. Cervical Cancer genetic susceptibility: a systematic review and meta-analyses of recent evidence. PLoS One. 2016;11(7):e0157344.
25. Torres-Poveda K, Burguete-García AI, Bahena-Román M, Méndez-Martínez R, Zurita-Díaz MA, López-Estrada G, et al. Risk allelic load in Th2 and Th3 cytokines genes as biomarker of susceptibility to HPV-16 positive cervical cancer: a case control study. BMC Cancer. 2016;16(1):330.
26. Castle PE, Rodriguez AC, Bowman FP, Herrero R, Schiffman M, Bratti MC, et al. Comparison of ophthalmic sponges for measurements of immune markers from cervical secretions. Clin Diagn Lab Immunol. 2004;11(2):399–405.
27. Koshiol J, Sklavos M, Wentzensen N, Kemp T, Schiffman M, Dunn ST, et al. Evaluation of a multiplex panel of immune-related markers in cervical secretions: a methodologic study. Int J Cancer. 2014;134(2):411–25.
28. Forman D, de Martel C, Lacey CJ, Soerjomataram I, Lortet-Tieulent J, Bruni L, et al. Global burden of human papillomavirus and related diseases. Vaccine. 2012;30(Suppl 5):F12–23.
29. Bruni L, Diaz M, Castellsagué X, Ferrer E, Bosch FX, de Sanjosé S. Cervical human papillomavirus prevalence in 5 continents: meta-analysis of 1 million women with normal cytological findings. J Infect Dis. 2010;202(12):1789–99.
30. Rodríguez AC, Schiffman M, Herrero R, Wacholder S, Hildesheim A, Castle PE, et al. Rapid clearance of human papillomavirus and implications for clinical focus on persistent infections. J Natl Cancer Inst. 2008;100(7):513–7.
31. Jit M, Gay N, Soldan K, Hong Choi Y, Edmunds WJ. Estimating progression rates for human papillomavirus infection from epidemiological data. Med Decis Mak. 2010;30(1):84–98.
32. Insinga RP, Perez G, Wheeler CM, Koutsky LA, Garland SM, Leodolter S, et al. Incident cervical HPV infections in young women: transition probabilities for CIN and infection clearance. Cancer Epidemiol Biomark Prev. 2011;20:287–96.
33. Rodríguez AC, Schiffman M, Herrero R, Hildesheim A, Bratti C, Sherman ME, et al. Longitudinal study of human papillomavirus persistence and cervical intraepithelial neoplasia grade 2/3: critical role of duration of infection. J Natl Cancer Inst. 2010;102(5):315–24.
34. Woodman CB, Collins SI, Young LS. The natural history of cervical HPV infection: unresolved issues. Nat Rev Cancer. 2007;7(1):11–22.
35. Vargas-Parada L. Pathology: three questions. Nature. 2012;488(7413):S14–5.
36. Ahdieh L, Klein RS, Burk R, Cu-Uvin S, Schuman P, Duerr A, et al. Prevalence, incidence, and type-specific persistence of human papillomavirus in human immunodeficiency virus (HIV)-positive and HIV negative women. J Infect Dis. 2001;184(6):682–90.
37. Ryser MD, Myers ER, Durrett R. HPV clearance and the neglected role of stochasticity. PLoS Comput Biol. 2015;11(3):e1004113.
38. Ramanakumar AV, Goncalves O, Richardson H, Tellier P, Ferenczy A, Coutlée F, et al. Human papillomavirus (HPV) types 16, 18, 31, 45 DNA loads and HPV-16 integration in persistent and transient infections in young women. BMC Infect Dis. 2010;10:326.

25

Study protocol of the iMPaCT project: a longitudinal cohort study assessing psychological determinants, sexual behaviour and chlamydia (re)infections in heterosexual STI clinic visitors

Daphne A. van Wees[1*], Janneke C. M. Heijne[1], Titia Heijman[2], Karlijn C. J. G. Kampman[3], Karin Westra[4], Anne de Vries[5], Mirjam E. E. Kretzschmar[1,6] and Chantal den Daas[1,7]

Abstract

Background: *Chlamydia trachomatis* (chlamydia), the most commonly reported sexually transmitted infection (STI) in the Netherlands, can lead to severe reproductive complications. Reasons for the sustained chlamydia prevalence in young individuals, even in countries with chlamydia screening programs, might be the asymptomatic nature of chlamydia infections, and high reinfection rates after treatment. When individuals are unaware of their infection, preventive behaviour or health-care seeking behaviour mostly depends on psychological determinants, such as risk perception. Furthermore, behaviour change after a diagnosis might be vital to reduce reinfection rates. This makes the incorporation of psychological determinants and behaviour change in mathematical models estimating the impact of interventions on chlamydia transmission especially important. Therefore, quantitative real-life data to inform these models is needed.

Methods: A longitudinal cohort study will be conducted to explore the link between psychological and behavioural determinants and chlamydia (re)infection among heterosexual STI clinic visitors aged 18–24 years. Participants will be recruited at the STI clinics of the public health services of Amsterdam, Hollands Noorden, Kennemerland, and Twente. Participants are enrolled for a year, and questionnaires are administrated at four time points: baseline (before an STI consultation), three-week, six-month and at one-year follow-up. To be able to link psychological and behavioural determinants to (re)infections, participants will be tested for chlamydia at enrolment and at six-month follow-up. Data from the longitudinal cohort study will be used to develop mathematical models for curable STI incorporating these determinants to be able to better estimate the impact of interventions.

Discussion: This study will provide insights into the link between psychological and behavioural determinants, including short-term and long-term changes after diagnosis, and chlamydia (re)infections. Our mathematical model, informed by data from the longitudinal cohort study, will be able to estimate the impact of interventions on chlamydia prevalence, and identify and prioritise successful interventions for the future. These interventions could be implemented at STI clinics tailored to psychological and behavioural characteristics of individuals.

Keywords: Chlamydia trachomatis, Sexually transmitted diseases, Reinfection, Psychological determinants, Sexual behaviour, Behaviour change, STI clinic, Mathematical model

* Correspondence: daphne.van.wees@rivm.nl
[1]Centre for Infectious Disease Control, National Institute for Public Health and the Environment, Bilthoven, The Netherlands
Full list of author information is available at the end of the article

Background

Chlamydia trachomatis (chlamydia) is the most commonly diagnosed bacterial STI among young heterosexual men and women in many western countries, including the Netherlands with up to 55,000 diagnosed infections in STI clinics nationally each year [1]. Control of this infection is of public health importance, because it can cause severe reproductive complications, including pelvic inflammatory disease (PID), ectopic pregnancy and tubal subfertility [2–5]. However, it is unclear why the prevalence of chlamydia remains unchanged even in countries with chlamydia screening programs, such as England, Australia, Canada, and the United States [6].

A difficulty in controlling chlamydia transmission is that most infections are asymptomatic [7]. Since people are unaware of their infection, initiation of preventive behaviours (i.e., condom use), or health-care seeking behaviour (i.e., chlamydia testing), mostly depends on psychological determinants, such as risk perception, self-efficacy or attitudes regarding condom use [8–11]. Previous studies have mainly focussed on identifying behavioural risk factors for chlamydia infection [12–15], while understanding how psychological determinants influences such behaviour might be more informative for the development of effective interventions [10]. For example, an increased number of sexual partners has previously been identified as a risk factor for chlamydia infection [12, 14], but having many sexual partners might not necessarily be risky if people would realistically perceive their risk for acquiring a STI and take the necessary steps to protect themselves. Therefore, studying the link between psychological determinants and behaviour and relating these to chlamydia infections might increase our understanding of chlamydia transmission. For instance, many young people tend to underestimate their personal risk of acquiring chlamydia [8, 16], which could have a negative effect on their condom use and testing uptake [8, 10, 17].

Another reason for the sustained chlamydia prevalence might be high reinfection rates after treatment or natural clearance [15, 18–20].To reduce the risk of reinfections, behaviour change (i.e., more consistent condom use) might be essential [21, 22]. Several studies have shown that individuals who were diagnosed with an STI were more likely to change into less risky sexual behaviour after they received the test results than individuals who tested negative [21, 23–27], but the influence of STI test results on underlying psychological determinants are not known. Behaviour change might be dependent on a number of psychological determinants, such as risk perception, perceived norms, perceived susceptibility, self-efficacy, knowledge, intentions, and attitudes regarding condom use [8–11, 17]. For example, while increased perceived risk of STI as a result of a positive diagnosis might induce behaviour change, receiving negative test results could lead to a false sense of security in high-risk individuals, and changing their risky sexual behaviour after the STI test may be deemed unnecessary [24]. However, regardless of the diagnosis, fear experienced before receiving the STI test results [17], might provide enough motivation to increase condom use. Quantitative longitudinal data is needed to explore the interplay between psychological and behavioural determinants after diagnosis and over time.

Longitudinal data on psychological and behavioural determinants could be used to investigate the impact of interventions aimed at reducing chlamydia (re)infections in mathematical models. Mathematical models are a tool for understanding the transmission of infectious diseases and establish a scientific basis for decision-making [28]. Predictions of the impact of interventions on prevalence arising from these models can be used to inform national health policies [29, 30]. However, psychological determinants are hardly ever incorporated in mathematical models describing STI transmission, and many models do not take into account that behaviour can change over time. Incorporating psychological determinants and behavioural change might improve the estimation of the impact of interventions on chlamydia prevalence in mathematical models. It may also increase our understanding on how to control chlamydia transmission more effectively, for example by identifying core risk groups that contribute most to transmission.

To explore the link between (changes in) psychological and behavioural determinants, and chlamydia (re)infection, a study called 'Mathematical models incorporating Psychological determinants: control of Chlamydia Transmission' (iMPaCT) was initiated. A longitudinal cohort study will be conducted among individuals testing for chlamydia at the STI clinic. Individual data on (re)infection rates, psychological determinants, and behaviour will be collected at different points in time to link these to chlamydia (re)infections and to study changes over time. These changes include short-term changes after a diagnosis, and long-term changes (1 year after a diagnosis at baseline). Mathematical models will be developed incorporating psychological and behavioural determinants using data from the longitudinal study. We will explore how incorporating these variables, including short- and long-term changes, influence chlamydia prevalence estimations from models.

Methods

Study aim

The aim of the iMPaCT study is to explore the link between psychological and behavioural determinants, and chlamydia (re)infection among heterosexuals aged

18-24 years visiting STI clinics. The following aims will be addressed:

1. To identify predictors of chlamydia infection;

- What demographic, psychological, and behavioural determinants are associated with chlamydia infection?

2. To investigate short-term and long-term changes (or stability) in psychological determinants and sexual behaviour over time;

- What is the influence of a chlamydia test result (positive or negative) on psychological determinants and subsequent sexual behaviour?
- Regarding these determinants, does change (or stability) in psychological and/or behavioural determinants affect the probability of reinfection?
- How do psychological and behavioural determinants change over time during 1 year of follow-up?

3. To explore the influence of psychological determinants on the predicted impact of intervention measures to reduce chlamydia transmission by mathematical models;
4. To explore the influence of changes in psychological determinants and sexual behaviour on the predicted impact of intervention measures to reduce chlamydia transmission by mathematical models.

Design

A longitudinal cohort study will be conducted among young heterosexual STI clinic visitors in the Netherlands.

Setting

Participants will be recruited from STI clinics of the Public Health Services (GGD) of Amsterdam, Kennemerland, Hollands Noorden, and Twente. In 2015, these STI clinics tested around 20,000 heterosexual men and women under the age of 25 for chlamydia according to the national registry. The majority of this group was female, ≥ 20 years old, and Dutch, and approximately 15% tested positive for chlamydia [31].

Study population

Heterosexual men and women aged 18 to 24 years visiting the STI clinic of the GGD Amsterdam, Kennemerland, Hollands Noorden, or Twente are eligible to participate. All enrolled individuals will be invited for follow-up data collection moments, irrespective of their test result at baseline. Individuals, who are not living in the Netherlands, are not able to read or speak Dutch, commercial sex workers, men who have sex with men (including men who have sex with both men and women), and women who have sex with women, will be excluded from participation in this study. Women who have sex with both men and women will only be excluded if their last three partners were women.

Recruitment

Participants will be recruited during the process of making an appointment at the STI clinic. To fit the study into the daily flow of the STI clinics, two different procedures will be applied. At the GGD Amsterdam, Kennemerland, and Hollands Noorden, individuals who are eligible to participate will be invited during the process of making an appointment online. Individuals will receive information about iMPaCT when they confirm their appointment. At the GGD Twente, the receptionist will invite individuals who are eligible to participate when they are making an appointment by telephone, and send them an email with information about iMPaCT. Recruitment is expected to take approximately 6 to 8 months.

Inclusion and follow-up

Participants will be enrolled for 1 year, and data on (re)-infection rates, psychological determinants, and behaviour will be collected at four different points in time to link these to chlamydia (re)infections and study changes (or stability) in psychological determinants and sexual behaviour over time. Data collection will occur at the following time points: at baseline, three-week follow-up, six-month follow-up and at one-year follow-up (Fig. 1).

At baseline, individuals eligible to participate will be invited during the process of making an appointment at the STI clinic. If an individual agrees to participate, an online questionnaire (the questionnaire is described in more detail below) will be administered, which starts after participants gave informed consent. Subsequently, participants are tested for chlamydia at the STI clinic. During the consultation at the STI clinic, the participants will receive information on prevention of STI and motivational-interviewing based counselling from the nurses. Since this might have an effect on psychological and behavioural determinants [32] and possibly lead to biased answers, participants will complete the baseline questionnaire before the consultation. Therefore, participants have approximately 1 to 2 weeks to fill out the questionnaire, between making their appointment and their STI clinic visit. Individuals who agree to participate will receive an email, as a reminder, with information about iMPaCT and a web link, which will guide them directly to the online questionnaire. Participants, who completed the questionnaire after their consultation at the STI clinic, will be excluded.

The participants will receive the chlamydia test results within 2 weeks of the STI clinic visit. Approximately 1

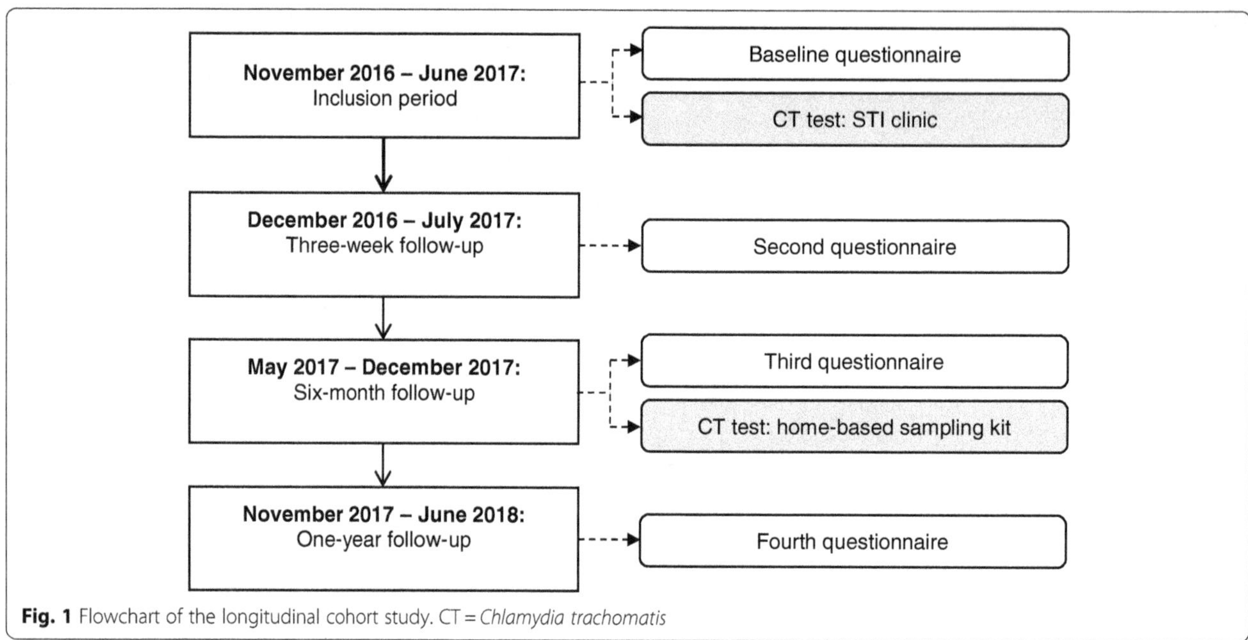

Fig. 1 Flowchart of the longitudinal cohort study. CT = *Chlamydia trachomatis*

week after the communication of the test results (three to 4 weeks after the STI clinic visit), all participants who completed the baseline questionnaire will be invited via email to fill out the second questionnaire online. Participants, who have not finished the second questionnaire, will receive two reminders by email: 1 week and 2 weeks after the invitation for the second questionnaire.

The third data collection moment will take place 6 months after baseline, because reinfections usually occur within 6 months after the initial infection [15, 18, 33, 34]. Firstly, all participants who completed the baseline questionnaire will be invited via email to fill out an online questionnaire. Additionally, all participants will be invited for a retest, irrespective of the test result at baseline. They will receive a self-swab test-kit at their home address or another preferred address, as specified in the third questionnaire, in a plain package fitting letterboxes. In this package, the participants will find simple instructions about the type of sample that they need to provide (urogenital test only, urine sample for men and vaginal swab for women) and how to collect these samples. Subsequently, the participants mail the testing-kits directly to the laboratory for chlamydia and gonorrhoea testing. The results will be communicated within three working days after the arrival of their material in the laboratory, via email with a link to a secured webpage, where the participants can download the results of their test with the login data attached in the email. Participants, who have not finished the online questionnaire, will receive two reminders by email: 1 week and 2 weeks after the invitation for the third questionnaire. Participants, who have completed the online questionnaire, but who have not mailed the test-kit to the laboratory, will receive two reminders by email: 2 weeks and 4 weeks after the test-kits are sent. The number of reminders for the retest will be the same as the number of reminders for the questionnaires, but the reminders will be spread further apart due to the possibility of delays in the logistics of the retest. Participants, who test positive, will be advised to make an appointment with their GP or at the STI clinic for appropriate treatment. A letter for the GP or STI clinic with information about the iMPaCT study, and a copy of the laboratory results will be provided.

Finally, 1 year after baseline, all participants who completed the baseline questionnaire will be invited via email to fill out the fourth online questionnaire. Participants, who have not finished the online questionnaire, will receive two reminders by email: 1 week and 2 weeks after the invitation for the fourth questionnaire. After completing the last questionnaire, irrespective of completing the three-week and six-month follow-up questionnaires, participants will receive a gift voucher with a value of €5 within a week (by mail).

Demographic and consultation information

National STI surveillance data will be used to complement the information gathered in the questionnaires. This surveillance data includes routinely registered data of all consultations from all STI clinics in the Netherlands, such as demographic information (i.e. age, sex, ethnicity and level of education), previous testing behaviour, previous STI diagnosis, reason for testing (i.e., notified by chlamydia-positive partner, symptoms), several behavioural determinants and STI test results. In the surveillance data, each STI clinic visitor has an anonymous identification (ID) number. This ID number will automatically be incorporated in the web link to the questionnaire, which enables linkage of the surveillance data to the questionnaire. To identify chlamydia reinfections before the retest at six-month follow-up, information on STI clinic visits between baseline and six-month follow-up of the participants will also be extracted from the national STI surveillance data using this ID number, including the reason for their visit and the test result.

Laboratory testing

The chlamydia-test performed at baseline is routine practice of the consultation at the STI clinic, using nucleic acid amplification tests (NAAT) to detect chlamydia, such as Transcription-mediated amplification (TMA) or polymerase chain reaction (PCR). Six months after baseline, all participants will be invited for a retest, irrespective of the test result at baseline. Home-based sampling and returning test kits to a laboratory by mail can be used to test for STI, such as chlamydia and gonorrhoea [18, 35–39]. The testing-kits can be mailed directly to the laboratory using the pre-paid return envelope provided. All samples will be tested for chlamydia and gonorrhoea using NAAT/PCR, with respectively a sensitivity of 97.0 and 99.3% and specificity of 98.9 and 99.3% [38].

Defining chlamydia (re)infection

Chlamydia infection at baseline will be defined as confirmed positive NAAT-results for *Chlamydia trachomatis* at any anatomic location (urogenital, anorectal, pharyngeal) at the STI clinic. Chlamydia reinfection will be defined as confirmed positive NAAT-result for *Chlamydia trachomatis* based on either the samples provided by the participants at six-month follow-up through the self-swab testing kit (urogenital only) and/or a test at the STI clinic between baseline and six-month follow-up at any anatomic location (urogenital, anorectal, pharyngeal).

Questionnaires

We have conducted a pilot survey in May 2016 among 296 heterosexuals aged 16–34 to evaluate the conciseness and the comprehensibility of the online questionnaire using factor and reliability analysis and comments from the respondents. People were recruited via social media and at a vocational school in Amersfoort, the Netherlands. The duration of the questionnaires in the iMPaCT study was estimated based on the results from this pilot survey; the questionnaire at baseline will take about 10–15 min and the other questionnaires will take less than 10 min. All questionnaires will be sent via Formdesk [40], a tool to create and manage online forms. Each participant has an anonymous study ID number, which will be used to link the questionnaire data from Formdesk to the information in the national STI surveillance data.

The baseline questionnaire has two parts: one part on psychological determinants, and one part on sexual behaviour. Psychological determinants included in the questionnaires that might play a role in acquiring STI are; risk perception [41–45], impulsiveness [46–50], intentions regarding condom use [11, 51], attitudes regarding prevention of chlamydia [52, 53], health goals [9, 51], knowledge [11], stigma [54–56], shame [54–56], anxiety [54–56], self-efficacy [43, 57], social support [11], peer norms [11] and self-esteem [58]. These determinants were included in the questionnaire based on associations in the literature with sexual risk behaviour, testing-behaviour, and behavioural change. Answers to these questions are measured on a 5-point Likert scale.

The questions about sexual behaviour are based on several validated questionnaires, including questionnaires from previous STI studies [11, 59–61], and the UK NATSAL [13]. Participants will be asked about the number of sex partners, age at sexual debut, condom use, and we will pose detailed questions on the last three partners, including begin and end of the partnership, condom use, sex frequency, type of sex, and partner characteristics.

The follow-up questionnaires will be the same as the baseline questionnaire, with a few additional questions. To explore short-term effects of diagnoses (and if applicable treatment) on possible changes in psychological and sexual behaviour determinants, the questionnaire at three-week follow-up will include the same questions on psychological determinants and sexual behaviour as the baseline questionnaire. For participants who test positive at baseline, questions are added about partner notification in the week following treatment. In the questionnaire at six-month and one-year follow-up, questions will be added about visits to the STI clinic between baseline and six-month follow-up and between six-month follow-up and one-year follow-up, including test results, treatment, and reasons for the visit(s).

Expected response

Based on the number of consultations at the STI clinics of the public health services in Twente, Hollands Noorden, Kennemerland and Amsterdam in the last 6 months of 2015 in the national registry, around 10,000 heterosexual STI clinic visitors will meet the inclusion criteria during 6 months of recruitment (40% men and 60% women). Table 1 shows the expected response for each data collection moment by STI clinic. The response rate at baseline is expected to be low, because recruitment at baseline is internet-mediated (passive recruitment) and there will be no face-to-face interaction with potential participants [62, 63]. We aim to include 2000 people at baseline (20% response rate), of which 800 are men and 1200 are women, based on the distribution of heterosexual male and female visitors at the STI clinics [31]. We

Table 1 Expected number of participants per STI clinic at each follow-up moment

STI clinic	Expected number of participants					
	Baseline (men/women)	Baseline Ct+	Three-week	Six-month	Six-month Ct+	One-year
Twente	400 (160/240)	60	320	193	31	120
Hollands Noorden	400 (160/240)	60	320	193	31	120
Kennemerland	400 (160/240)	60	320	193	31	120
Amsterdam	800 (320/480)	120	640	385	62	240
Total	2000 (800/1200)	300	1600	964	155	600

Abbreviations: *Ct+* chlamydia positive

expect 15% of the participants at baseline to test positive ($N = 300$) [31].

The response rates at the follow-up moments are expected to be higher than at baseline, because the participants will receive personal invitations by email instead of the impersonal baseline invitation addressed to all the STI clinic visitors who were eligible to participate. However, the response rates might decline over time [30]. At three-week follow-up, a response rate of 80% ($N = 1600$) is expected (this includes sending reminders) [30]. All participants will be contacted by email again at the six-month follow-up, also participants who did not respond to the three-week follow-up. The participation rate at six-month follow-up among people who tested chlamydia positive at baseline is expected to be around 66% [18], and the participation rate is likely to be lower for individuals who tested chlamydia negative at baseline [24] and is expected to be around 45%. Therefore, approximately 1000 participants will be tested for chlamydia at six-month follow-up. We expect 15% of the participants that were chlamydia negative (Ct-) at baseline and 20% of the participants that were chlamydia positive (Ct+) at baseline to test positive at six-month follow-up ($N = 155$) [31, 33, 34]. All participants who completed the baseline questionnaire will be contacted again at the one-year follow-up, also participants who did not respond to the three-week follow-up and/or the six-month follow-up, and we expect a response rate of 30% ($N = 600$). Participants can choose to leave the study at any time for any reason. If participants formally withdraw from the study by email, they will not be invited for follow-up data collection.

Sample size and power calculations

To explore if the study population will be large enough to detect differences in psychological and behavioural determinants between baseline and six-month follow-up with adequate statistical power, sample size and statistical power calculations were performed in Stata version 13.0 [64]. Firstly, sample size calculations for at least 80% power were performed for the participants who tested positive (Ct+) and participants who tested negative for chlamydia at baseline (Ct-), assuming a type I error (α) of 0.05, 34% loss to follow-up after 6 months in the Ct + group, and 55% loss to follow-up after 6 months in the Ct- group (based on the expected response rates described above). Secondly, power calculations were performed with the expected sample size of 2000 participants at baseline, assuming 15% chlamydia positivity ($n = 300$) [31].

The sample size and power calculations for sexual behaviour were calculated with condom use as an example. Soetens et al., (2015) [26] found that condom use 1 year after the chlamydia test at baseline increased in the Ct + group and decreased in the Ct- group. Based on these results, the percentage of participants in our study using a condom with the last sexual contact was assumed to increase in individuals after a Ct + baseline test and decrease in individuals after a Ct- baseline test. The sample size and power for sexual behaviour were calculated for three different scenarios: 10 (scenario 1), 15 (scenario 2), or 20 (scenario 3) percent change at six-months follow-up (Table 2).

This is, to our knowledge, the first study assessing changes in psychological determinants after diagnosis of chlamydia or over a longer period of time. Therefore, no literature is available to inform possible changes in psychological determinants in our sample size calculations. The sample size and power calculations for the psychological determinants were calculated with risk perception as an example, but this can also be generalised to other psychological determinants. Research has shown that people chronically underestimate their personal risk of acquiring chlamydia [8]. Tailored risk information (i.e. after a consultation at the STI clinic) might increase an individual's perceived risk for STI [65]. Furthermore, individuals with previous STI diagnoses are more likely to report higher perceived risk for STI than those with no previous STI diagnoses [66, 67]. Therefore, we hypothesized that risk perception, which will be assessed in the questionnaire as the estimated personal risk of chlamydia on a scale from 0 to 100, might increase in individuals after a Ct + baseline test and decrease in individuals after a Ct- baseline test. The sample size and power for the psychological determinants were calculated with the same hypothesized percent change as for sexual behaviour (Table 2).

Table 2 Sample size and power calculations for different scenarios

	Change (%)	Sample size needed at baseline (80% power)		Expected power with sample size $n = 2000$ at baseline	
		Ct+	Ct-	Ct + (n = 300)	Ct- (n = 1700)
Scenario 1	10%	470	611	60%	> 99%
Scenario 2	15%	220	286	91%	> 99%
Scenario 3	20%	129	167	> 99%	> 99%

Sample size and power calculations to detect a change in psychological determinants or sexual behaviour at six-month follow-up with at least 80% power, assuming 34% loss to follow-up in the chlamydia positives (Ct+) and 55% loss to follow-up in the chlamydia negatives (Ct-)
Abbreviations: *Ct+* chlamydia positive, *Ct-* chlamydia negative

The expected sample size of 2000 participants will be large enough to detect a change of 10–20% in psychological determinants and behavioural with adequate statistical power (power > 80%). The expected sample size of 300 in the Ct + group is too small for detecting 10% change (scenario 1) for ≥70% power, but the expected sample size is sufficient for detecting ≥15% change (scenario 2 and 3), which might be more likely in this group [26].

Statistical analyses

The main analysis will include all participants who completed the baseline questionnaire, irrespective of their test result. Possible response bias will be explored in a (non-)response study using anonymised national STI surveillance data of all individuals eligible to participate who visited the STI clinic in the inclusion period. Demographic characteristics, sexual behaviour, and STI consultation information will be compared between participants who completed the baseline questionnaire, and all the STI clinic visitors who were invited to participate, but did not complete or start the baseline questionnaire. The participants who completed the baseline questionnaire will be identified in the surveillance data, using the previously described ID number incorporated in the web link to the questionnaire.

We expect only few missing values in the completed baseline questionnaires, because each question has to be answered before the next question appears. Furthermore, data consistency checks will be incorporated in the online questionnaire. Missing values in variables extracted from the national STI surveillance data or in the second, third and last questionnaire due to loss to follow-up will be included as a separate category if more than 5% is missing.

Baseline characteristics of the study population will be presented, using summary statistics, including means, standard deviations, medians and ranges for continuous variables and frequency distributions for binary and categorical variables. To identify predictors of participation in the (non-)response study, and to identify predictors of chlamydia (re)infection, univariable and multivariable logistic regression analysis will be performed. In the univariable analysis, variables significantly associated with the outcome (participation or chlamydia (re)infection) will be included in the multivariable models. Multivariable models will be constructed using a backward elimination procedure. Statistical significance will be defined as a p-value ≤0.1, and odds ratios and 95% confidence intervals of each predictor variable will be reported. Covariates based on a priori hypotheses will be examined as potential confounder or effect modifiers in the models.

To identify distinct risk groups for chlamydia (re)infection, based on the results of the multivariable logistic regression analysis, we will use latent class analysis for multivariable categorical data. In this analysis, underlying dimensions (latent classes) of the dependent variables can be inferred based on patterns in the observed data. The latent classes arising from this analysis could be combinations of several measured psychological, behavioural and demographic variables. Covariates that are independent of the outcome, but might influence the latent classes will be included in the analysis. The number of latent classes will be determined by increasing the number of classes until the best fitting model has been found, using the Bayesian Information Criterion (BIC) to assess the goodness of fit. The latent classes can be used to define distinct sexual risk profiles, which can be implemented in future mathematical models.

To explore changes in psychological determinants and sexual behaviour over time using data from the three-week, six-month, and one-year follow-up moments, and to identify risk profiles for chlamydia reinfection, we will use latent transition analysis, which is an extension of the latent class analysis described above. In this analysis, movement from one latent class to another over time can be determined. Similar to the latent class model, the BIC will be used to assess how well the latent transition model fits the observed data. The estimated transition probabilities can be implemented in future mathematical models of the transmission of chlamydia, which might enable us to better capture the complexity of sexual behaviour.

Mathematical model

The mathematical model will be a pair compartmental model representing a heterosexual population of men and women aged 18–24 years. Chlamydia will be described with a susceptible-infected-susceptible (SIS) structure. The infection parameters for chlamydia are reasonably well established and will be used from the available literature. The transmission rate per sex act will be calibrated to the positivity rate found at baseline. The model population will be subdivided into risk groups according to the risk classes identified in the latent class model (based on psychological and behavioural determinants from the baseline questionnaire).

Behavioural change after a diagnosis and in time will be incorporated by moving people from one risk group to another based on the latent transition model. First, we will explore the influence of a diagnosis on short-term changes of psychological and behavioural determinants in the model. This data will be based on differences between the baseline, three-week, and the six-month follow-up questionnaires. Second, we will theoretically explore the effect of long-term behaviour change on the impact of intervention measures, using the questionnaire data at one-year follow-up.

Discussion

The iMPaCT study will provide insights into the link between psychological determinants and sexual behaviour, behavioural change, and chlamydia (re)infections. We propose that incorporating these determinants in mathematical models will improve the impact assessment of interventions aimed at reducing chlamydia transmission. Chlamydia interventions that have been applied in practice have mainly focused on increasing testing uptake, and previous mathematical modelling studies have shown that, depending on the coverage of chlamydia testing in the general population, testing and treatment could be an effective strategy to reduce chlamydia prevalence, [30, 68, 69]. However, empirical studies have established that the coverage of chlamydia testing has not been high enough to observe a significant reduction in the population prevalence of chlamydia [13, 61, 70]. Therefore, a paradigm shift is needed to control chlamydia transmission more effectively. For example, interventions could be focused on increasing testing uptake among core risk groups based on psychological and behavioural characteristics to prevent reinfection after a diagnosis. Our mathematical model informed by the data of the cohort study will be able to estimate the impact of such interventions on chlamydia prevalence, and identify and prioritise successful interventions for specific risk groups, which might lead to more efficient ways to control chlamydia transmission. Subsequently, these interventions could be implemented at STI clinics tailored to psychological and behavioural characteristics of individuals.

Strengths

This is the first longitudinal cohort study investigating short-term and long-term changes in psychological determinants and sexual behaviour after chlamydia diagnosis. The prospective study design of this study with repeated measurements, namely the follow-up questionnaires and the retest, and the combination of an extensive selection of psychological determinants will expand our knowledge of risk factors for (re)infection. Another strength of this study is the combination of two data sources: longitudinal questionnaire data on psychological determinants and sexual behaviour, and national STI surveillance data on demographics, previous testing behaviour, and laboratory confirmed STI diagnosis. Therefore, we are able to obtain extensive knowledge with a relatively concise questionnaire, because questions on demographics, previous testing behaviour, STI diagnosis and other variables that are available in the national STI surveillance could be omitted in the online questionnaire.

The pilot survey, which has been conducted a few months before the start of iMPaCT study, enabled us to improve the comprehensibility of the questionnaire. This, in combination with sending reminder emails and offering incentives (gift voucher, free home-based sampling kit), might lead to higher response and completion rates [71]. Furthermore, the psychometric evaluation of the pilot survey and the advantages of using online questionnaires, such as programmed warning alerts to prevent incorrect answers (i.e., number of partners last 6 months can't be higher than the number of partners in the last year), ensured optimal reliability and validity of the longitudinal questionnaire data.

Finally, most mathematical models for infectious disease transmission incorporating behaviour change are entirely theoretical and lack validation with empirical data [72]. Our mathematical model will be informed by real-life data on behaviour change, which might result in more realistic model estimations and the opportunity to validate the model outcomes. The model outcomes could be directly translated into to advice for public health policy makers about effective intervention measures.

Limitations

First, the questionnaire data is self-reported, which could lead to reporting bias, such as under- or over-reporting of sexual behaviour. Although sexual behaviour in the national STI surveillance data is also self-reported, and thus prone to bias, sexual behaviour in the surveillance data will be matched to sexual behaviour as reported in the questionnaire to check for consistency. Furthermore, being notified for an STI or having STI-related symptoms might affect answers in the questionnaire [54, 67] and this will be taken into account in the statistical analyses. Response bias may also occur, and we will assess this in a (non-)response study by extracting the iMPaCT participants from the national STI surveillance data, and compare demographics, sexual behaviour, and STI consultation information between the participants and all eligible STI clinic visitors who were invited to participate, but did not complete or start the baseline questionnaire. We will use this (non-)response study to estimate the generalizability of the iMPaCT study population with reference to all young heterosexual STI clinic visitors and to guide the interpretation of the results. The iMPaCT study population is not likely to be representative of the general population, as STI clinic visitors tend to be more high-risk compared to the general population. However, this group potentially benefits the most from improved interventions. Thus, in this study we will gather detailed information for exactly the group of interest.

Previous longitudinal chlamydia studies have shown that response rates decline over time and our study will most likely not be an exception [18, 30]. To minimize loss to follow-up, free home-based sampling kits and promised monetary incentives will be used to encourage participation rates at six-month and one-year follow-up. The samples size and power calculations, taking loss to follow-up into account, showed that through recruitment at multiple STI clinics in different regions of the Netherlands, a sufficiently large and nationally representative group of STI clinic visitors can be approached for participation in the iMPaCT study.

It is likely that periods of high and low risk behaviour alternate during individual sexual careers [73], such as a period of high risk sexual behaviour after separating from a long standing partnership. Therefore, the timing of the follow-up data collection moments is crucial. For example, it could be argued that the period between the follow-up questionnaire after 3 weeks and baseline is too short to detect changes in sexual behaviour, and the questionnaires 6 months and 1 year after baseline might not be long-term enough to capture changes in people's behaviour that are not necessarily offset by an event such as a diagnosis. However, we speculate that the effect of a positive STI diagnosis on psychological determinants, such as intentions and attitudes regarding condom use, might be strongest in the first few days after receiving the test results. Furthermore, the optimal timing of testing for reinfections is not known, and the recommended timing of retesting across different countries ranges between 3 to 12 months [74, 75]. Therefore, participants will be invited for the retest 6 months after the baseline chlamydia test combined with a questionnaire, and after the same length of time (6 months after the retest), the participants will be invited to fill out the last questionnaire at one-year follow up.

Abbreviations

BIC: Bayesian information criterion; Ct: *Chlamydia trachomatis*; GGD: Public health services (in Dutch: Gemeentelijke Gezondheids Dienst);
ID: Identification number; NAAT: Nucleic acid amplification test; NATSAL: The national survey of sexual attitudes and lifestyles; PCR: Polymerase chain reaction; PID: Pelvic inflammatory disease; STI: Sexually transmitted infection; TMA: Transcription-mediated amplification

Acknowledgements

We are grateful to the staff at the STI clinics of Amsterdam, Kennemerland, Hollands Noorden, Twente, who are involved in the recruitment and data collection of participants, and Marlous Ratten and Klazien Visser from Soapoli-online, who are involved in the coordination of laboratory testing of the home-based sampling kits at six-month follow-up. We also thank the staff at the STI department at the National Institute for Public Health and the Environment, especially Birgit van Benthem.

Funding

This project is funded by the Strategic Programme (SPR) of the National Institute for Public Health and the Environment (RIVM) (project number S/113004/01/IP). The funders had no role in study design, data collection and analysis, decision to publish, or preparation of the manuscript.

Authors' contributions

CdD, JH, and DvW coordinate the study and drafted the manuscript. MK has been involved with optimising the study design. TH, KK, KW, and AdV are involved with the coordination of the iMPaCT study recruitment at the STI clinics of Amsterdam, Twente, Hollands Noorden and Kennemerland. All authors reviewed the manuscript and approved the final version for publication.

Authors' information

Not applicable.

Competing interests

The authors declare that they have no competing interests.

Author details

[1]Centre for Infectious Disease Control, National Institute for Public Health and the Environment, Bilthoven, The Netherlands. [2]Public Health Service Amsterdam, Amsterdam, The Netherlands. [3]Public Health Service Twente, Enschede, The Netherlands. [4]Public Health Service Hollands Noorden, Alkmaar, The Netherlands. [5]Public Health Service Kennemerland, Haarlem, The Netherlands. [6]Julius Centre for Health Sciences and Primary Care, University Medical Centre Utrecht, Utrecht, The Netherlands. [7]Department of Interdisciplinary Social Science, Faculty of Social and Behavioural Sciences, Utrecht University, Utrecht, The Netherlands.

References

1. Visser M, Van Aar F, van Oeffelen AAM, Van den Broek IVF, Op de Coul ELM, Hofstraat SHI, et al. Sexually transmitted infections including HIV, in the Netherlands in 2016. Bilthoven: Centre for Infectious Disease Control, National Institute for Public Health and the Environment (RIVM); 2017. Available from: http://www.rivm.nl/Documenten_en_publicaties/Wetenschappelijk/Rapporten/2017/Juni/Sexually_transmitted_infections_including_HIV_in_the_Netherlands_in_2016
2. Davies B, Turner KME, Frølund M, Ward H, May MT, Rasmussen S, et al. Risk of reproductive complications following chlamydia testing: a population-based retrospective cohort study in Denmark. Lancet Infect Dis. 2016;16(9):1057–64. https://doi.org/10.1016/S1473-3099(16)30092-5.
3. Haggerty CL, Gottlieb SL, Taylor BD, Low N, Xu F, Ness RB. Risk of sequelae after chlamydia trachomatis genital infection in women. J Infect Dis. 2010;201(Suppl 2):S134–55. https://doi.org/10.1086/652395.
4. Holmes KK, Sparling PF, Stamm WE, Piot P, Wasserheit JN, Corey L, et al. Sexually transmitted diseases. 4th ed. New York: McGraw-Hill; 2008.
5. Reekie J, Donovan B, Guy R, Hocking JS, Kaldor JM, Mak DB, et al. Risk of pelvic inflammatory disease in relation to chlamydia and gonorrhea testing, repeat testing, and positivity: a population-based cohort study. Clin Infect Dis. 2017. https://doi.org/10.1093/cid/cix769.
6. Unemo M, Bradshaw CS, Hocking JS, de Vries HJC, Francis SC, Mabey D, et al. Sexually transmitted infections: challenges ahead. Lancet Infect Dis. 2017;17(8):e235–79. https://doi.org/10.1016/S1473-3099(17)30310-9.
7. Gottlieb SL, Martin DH, Xu F, Byrne GI, Brunham RC. Summary: the natural history and immunobiology of chlamydia trachomatis genital infection and implications for chlamydia control. J Infect Dis. 2010;201(Suppl 2):S190–204. https://doi.org/10.1086/652401.

8. Abel G, Brunton C. Young people's use of condoms and their perceived vulnerability to sexually transmitted infections. Aust N Z J Public Health. 2005;29(3):254–60. https://doi.org/10.1111/j.1467-842X.2005.tb00764.x.
9. den Daas C, Häfner M, de Wit J. The impact of long-term health goals on sexual risk decisions in impulsive and reflective cognitive states. Arch Sex Behav. 2014;43(4):659–67. https://doi.org/10.1007/s10508-013-0183-0.
10. Ten Hoor GA, Ruiter RAC, van Bergen JEAM, Hoebe CJPA, Dukers-Muijrers NHTM, Kok G. Predictors of chlamydia trachomatis testing: perceived norms, susceptibility, changes in partner status, and underestimation of own risk. BMC Public Health. 2016;16(1):55. https://doi.org/10.1186/s12889-016-2689-6.
11. Wolfers ME, Kok G, Mackenbach JP, de Zwart O. Correlates of STI testing among vocational school students in the Netherlands. BMC Public Health. 2010;10:725. https://doi.org/10.1186/1471-2458-10-725.
12. Harder E, Thomsen LT, Frederiksen K, Munk C, Iftner T, van den Brule A, et al. Risk factors for incident and redetected chlamydia trachomatis infection in women: results of a population-based cohort study. Sex Transm Dis. 2016;43(2):113–9. https://doi.org/10.1097/OLQ.0000000000000394.
13. Sonnenberg P, Clifton S, Beddows S, Field N, Soldan K, Tanton C, et al. Prevalence, risk factors, and uptake of interventions for sexually transmitted infections in Britain: findings from the National Surveys of sexual attitudes and lifestyles (Natsal). Lancet. 2013;382(9907):1795–806. https://doi.org/10.1016/S0140-6736(13)61947-9.
14. Velicko I, Ploner A, Sparen P, Marions L, Herrmann B, Kuhlmann-Berenzon S. Sexual and testing behaviour associated with chlamydia trachomatis infection: a cohort study in an STI clinic in Sweden. BMJ Open. 2016;6(8): e011312. https://doi.org/10.1136/bmjopen-2016-011312.
15. Walker J, Tabrizi SN, Fairley CK, Chen MY, Bradshaw CS, Twin J, et al. Chlamydia trachomatis incidence and re-infection among young women--behavioural and microbiological characteristics. PLoS One. 2012;7(5):e37778. https://doi.org/10.1371/journal.pone.0037778.
16. Samkange-Zeeb F, Pottgen S, Zeeb H. Higher risk perception of HIV than of chlamydia and HPV among secondary school students in two German cities. PLoS One. 2013;8(4):e61636. https://doi.org/10.1371/journal.pone.0061636.
17. Wolfers ME, de Zwart O, Kok G. Adolescents in the Netherlands underestimate risk for sexually transmitted infections and deny the need for sexually transmitted infection testing. AIDS Patient Care STDs. 2011;25(5): 311–9. https://doi.org/10.1089/apc.2010.0186.
18. Gotz HM, van den Broek IV, Hoebe CJ, Brouwers EE, Pars LL, Fennema JS, et al. High yield of reinfections by home-based automatic rescreening of chlamydia positives in a large-scale register-based screening programme and determinants of repeat infections. Sex Transm Infect. 2013;89(1):63–9. https://doi.org/10.1136/sextrans-2011-050455.
19. Heijne JC, Herzog SA, Althaus CL, Low N, Kretzschmar M. Case and partnership reproduction numbers for a curable sexually transmitted infection. J Theor Biol. 2013;331:38–47. https://doi.org/10.1016/j.jtbi.2013.04.010.
20. LaMontagne D, Baster K, Emmett L, Nichols T, Randall S, McLean L, et al. Incidence and reinfection rates of genital chlamydial infection among women aged 16-24 years attending general practice, family planning and genitourinary medicine clinics in England: a prospective cohort study by the chlamydia recall study advisory group. Sex Transm Infect. 2007;83(4):292–303. https://doi.org/10.1136/sti.2006.022053.
21. Fortenberry JD, Brizendine EJ, Katz BP, Orr DP. Post-treatment sexual and prevention behaviours of adolescents with sexually transmitted infections. Sex Transm Infect. 2002;78(5):365–8. https://doi.org/10.1136/sti.78.5.365.
22. Ward DJ, Rowe B, Pattison H, Taylor RS, Radcliffe KW. Reducing the risk of sexually transmitted infections in genitourinary medicine clinic patients: a systematic review and meta-analysis of behavioural interventions. Sex Transm Infect. 2005;81(5):386–93. https://doi.org/10.1136/sti.2004.013714.
23. Crosby RA, DiClemente RJ, Wingood GM, Salazar LF, Rose E, Levine D, et al. Associations between sexually transmitted disease diagnosis and subsequent sexual risk and sexually transmitted disease incidence among adolescents. Sex Transm Dis. 2004;31(4):205–8. https://doi.org/10.1097/01.OLQ.0000114940.07793.20.
24. Nielsen A, Marrone G, De Costa A. Chlamydia trachomatis among youth-testing behaviour and incidence of repeat testing in Stockholm County, Sweden 2010-2012. PLoS One. 2016;11(9):e0163597. https://doi.org/10.1371/journal.pone.0163597.
25. Reed JL, Simendinger L, Griffeth S, Kim HG, Huppert JS. Point-of-care testing for sexually transmitted infections increases awareness and short-term abstinence in adolescent women. J Adolesc Health. 2010;46(3):270–7. https://doi.org/10.1016/j.jadohealth.2009.08.003.
26. Soetens LC, van Benthem BHB, Op de Coul EL. Chlamydia test results were associated with sexual risk behavior change among participants of the chlamydia screening implementation in the Netherlands. Sex Transm Dis. 2015;42(3):109–14. https://doi.org/10.1097/OLQ.0000000000000234.
27. Sznitman SR, Carey MP, Vanable PA, DiClemente RJ, Brown LK, Valois RF, et al. The impact of community-based sexually transmitted infection screening results on sexual risk behaviors of African American adolescents. J Adolesc Health. 2010;47(1):12–9. https://doi.org/10.1016/j.jadohealth.2009.12.024.
28. Garnett GP, Cousens S, Hallett TB, Steketee R, Walker N. Mathematical models in the evaluation of health programmes. Lancet. 2011;378(9790): 515–25. https://doi.org/10.1016/S0140-6736(10)61505-X.
29. Kretzschmar MEE, Turner KM, Barton PM, Edmunds WJ, Low N. Predicting the population impact of chlamydia screening programmes: comparative mathematical modelling study. Sex Transm Infect. 2009;85(5):359–66. https://doi.org/10.1136/sti.2009.036251.
30. Schmid BV, Over EAB, van den Broek IVF, op de Coul ELM, JEAM v B, JSA F, et al. Effects of population based screening for Chlamydia infections in the Netherlands limited by declining participation rates. PloS One. 2013;8(3): e58674. https://doi.org/10.1371/journal.pone.0058674.
31. van den Broek IVF, Van Aar F, van Oeffelen AAM, Op de Coul ELM, Woestenberg PJ, Heijne JCM, et al. Sexually Transmitted Infections in the Netherlands in 2015. Bilthoven: Centre for Infectious Disease Control, National Institute for Public Health and the Environment (RIVM); 2016. Available from: http://www.rivm.nl/Documenten_en_publicaties/Wetenschappelijk/Rapporten/2016/juni/Sexually_transmitted_infections_in_the_Netherlands_in_2015
32. Kuyper L, de Wit J, Heijman T, Fennema H, van Bergen JEAM, Vanwesenbeeck I. Influencing risk behavior of sexually transmitted infection clinic visitors: efficacy of a new methodology of motivational preventive counseling. AIDS Patient Care STDs. 2009;23(6):423–31. https://doi.org/10.1089/apc.2008.0144.
33. Geisler WM, Lensing SY, Press CG, Hook EW 3rd. Spontaneous resolution of genital chlamydia trachomatis infection in women and protection from reinfection. J Infect Dis. 2013;207(12):1850–6. https://doi.org/10.1093/infdis/jit094.
34. Kampman CIG, Koedijk FDH, Driessen-Hulshof HCM, Hautvast JLA, Van den Broek IVF. Retesting young STI clinic visitors with urogenital chlamydia trachomatis infection in the Netherlands; response to a text message reminder and reinfection rates: a prospective study with historical controls. Sex Transm Infect. 2015;92(2):124–9. https://doi.org/10.1136/sextrans-2015-052115.
35. Götz HM, Bom RJ, Wolfers ME, Fennema J, van den Broek IV, Speksnijder AG, et al. Use of Chlamydia trachomatis high-resolution typing: an extended case study to distinguish recurrent or persistent infection from new infection. Sex Transm Infect. 2013;90(2):155–60. https://doi.org/10.1136/sextrans-2013-051218.
36. Mollers M, Scherpenisse M, van der Klis FR, King AJ, van Rossum TG, van Logchem EM, et al. Prevalence of genital HPV infections and HPV serology in adolescent girls, prior to vaccination. Cancer Epidemiol. 2012;36(6):519–24. https://doi.org/10.1016/j.canep.2012.07.006.
37. van Bergen JEAM, Fennema JSA, van den Broek IVF, Brouwers EEHG, de Feijter EM, Hoebe CJPA, et al. Rationale, design, and results of the first screening round of a comprehensive, register-based, chlamydia screening implementation programme in the Netherlands. BMC Infect Dis. 2010;10(1): 293. https://doi.org/10.1186/1471-2334-10-293.
38. van den Broek IVF, Sukel B, Bos H, and den Daas C. Evaluation of online providers of STI self-tests in the Netherlands [in Dutch]. Bilthoven, the Netherlands: RIVM 2016. Available from: http://www.rivm.nl/Documenten_en_publicaties/Wetenschappelijk/Rapporten/2016/september/Evaluatie_van_het_aanbod_van_online_aanbieders_van_soa_zelftesten_in_Nederland.
39. Vriend HJ, Boot HJ, van der Sande MA. Type-specific human papillomavirus infections among young heterosexual male and female STI clinic attendees. Sex Transm Dis. 2012;39(1):72–8. https://doi.org/10.1097/OLQ.0b013e318235b3b0.
40. Formdesk. Formdesk Innovero Software Solutions B.V. Wassenaar, The Netherlands. 2017.
41. Blais AR, Weber EU. A domain-specific risk-taking (DOSPERT) scale for adult populations. Judgm Decis Mak. 2006;1(1):33–47.
42. Carey MP, Carey KB, Weinhardt LS, Gordon CM. Behavioral risk for HIV infection among adults with a severe and persistent mental illness: patterns and psychological antecedents. Community Ment Health J. 1997;33(2):133–42. https://doi.org/10.1023/A:1022423417304.
43. de Graaf H, Meijer S, Poelman J, Vanwesenbeeck I. Seks onder je 25e: Seksuele gezondheid van jongeren in Nederland anno 2005 [In Dutch]. Delft: Eburon Uitgeverij BV; 2005.

44. Dew AF, Henley TB. Reconsidering unique invulnerability in the context of sexual behavior. J Gend Cult Health. 1999;4(4):307–13.
45. van der Velde FW, Hooykaas C, van der Pligt J. Risk perception and behavior: pessimism, realism, and optimism about AIDS-related health behavior. Psychol Health. 1992;6(1–2):23–38. https://doi.org/10.1080/08870449208402018.
46. Cyders MA, Littlefield AK, Coffey S, Karyadi KA. Examination of a short English version of the UPPS-P impulsive behavior scale. Addict Behav. 2014; 39(9):1372–6. https://doi.org/10.1016/j.addbeh.2014.02.013.
47. Cyders MA, Smith GT, Spillane NS, Fischer S, Annus AM, Peterson C. Integration of impulsivity and positive mood to predict risky behavior: development and validation of a measure of positive urgency. Psychol Assess. 2007;19(1):107–18. https://doi.org/10.1037/1040-3590.19.1.107.
48. Dewitte S, Schouwenburg HC. Procrastination, temptations, and incentives: the struggle between the present and the future in procrastinators and the punctual. Eur J Personal. 2002;16(6):469–89. https://doi.org/10.1002/per.461.
49. Lynam DR, Smith GT, Whiteside SP, Cyders MA. The UPPS-P: Assessing five personality pathways to impulsive behavior. West Lafayette: Purdue University; 2006.
50. Whiteside SP, Lynam DR. The five factor model and impulsivity: using a structural model of personality to understand impulsivity. Personal Individ Differ. 2001;30(4):669–89. https://doi.org/10.1016/s0191-8869(00)00064-7.
51. Fishbein M, Ajzen I. Predicting and changing behavior: the reasoned action approach. New York: Taylor & Francis; 2011.
52. Crandall CS, Moriarty D. Physical illness stigma and social rejection. Br J Soc Psychol. 1995;34(Pt 1):67. https://doi.org/10.1111/j.2044-8309.1995.tb01049.x.
53. Penke L. Revised sociosexual orientation inventory. Handbook of sexuality-related measures. 3rd Ed. Edinburgh: Taylor & Francis; 2011. p. 622–5.
54. Cunningham SD, Kerrigan D, Pillay KB, Ellen JM. Understanding the role of perceived severity in STD-related care-seeking delays. J Adolesc Health. 2005;37(1):69–74. https://doi.org/10.1016/j.jadohealth.2004.07.018.
55. Cunningham SD, Kerrigan DL, Jennings JM, Ellen JM. Relationships between perceived STD-related stigma, STD-related shame and STD screening among a household sample of adolescents. Perspect Sex Reprod Health. 2009;41(4):225–30.
56. Cunningham SD, Tschann J, Gurvey JE, Fortenberry JD, Ellen JM. Attitudes about sexual disclosure and perceptions of stigma and shame. Sex Transm Infect. 2002;78(5):334–8. https://doi.org/10.1136/sti.78.5.334.
57. Barkley TW, Burns JL. Factor analysis of the condom use self-efficacy scale among multicultural college students. Health Educ Res. 2000;15(4):485–9. https://doi.org/10.1093/her/15.4.485.
58. Robins RW, Hendin HM, Trzesniewski KH. Measuring global self-esteem: construct validation of a single-item measure and the Rosenberg self-esteem scale. Personal Soc Psychol Bull. 2001;27(2):151–61. https://doi.org/10.1177/0146167201272002.
59. Mollema L, De Melker H, Hahné S, Van Weert J, Berbers G, and Van Der Klis F. PIENTER 2-project: second research project on the protection against infectious diseases offered by the national immunization programme in the Netherlands. 2010. Available from: http://www.rivm.nl/Documenten_en_publicaties/Wetenschappelijk/Rapporten/2010/maart/PIENTER_2_project_second_research_project_on_the_protection_against_infectious_diseases_offered_by_the_national_immunization_programme_in_the_Netherlands.
60. van den Broek IVF. Chlamydia screening implementation Netherlands: impact evaluation and cost effectiveness. RIVM: Bilthoven; 2012. Available from: http://www.rivm.nl/en/Documents_and_publications/Scientific/Reports/2012/juli/Chlamydia_Screening_Implementation_Netherlands_impact_evaluation_and_cost_effectiveness
61. van den Broek IVF, van Bergen JE, Brouwers EE, Fennema JS, Gotz HM, Hoebe CJ, et al. Effectiveness of yearly register-based screening for chlamydia in the Netherlands: controlled trial with randomised stepped wedge implementation. BMJ. 2012;345:e4316. https://doi.org/10.1136/bmj.e4316.
62. Estabrooks P, You W, Hedrick V, Reinholt M, Dohm E, Zoellner J. A pragmatic examination of active and passive recruitment methods to improve the reach of community lifestyle programs: the talking health trial. Int J Behav Nutr Phys Act. 2017;14(1):7. https://doi.org/10.1186/s12966-017-0462-6.
63. Sauermann H, Roach M. Increasing web survey response rates in innovation research: an experimental study of static and dynamic contact design features. Res Policy. 2013;42(1):273–86. https://doi.org/10.1016/j.respol.2012.05.003.
64. StataCorp. Stata Statistical Software: Release 13. College Station, Austin, Texas: StataCorp LP; 2013.
65. Mevissen FEF, Meertens RM, Ruiter RAC, Mares M. Chlamydia prevention by influencing risk perceptions. Edited by Mihai mares. Rijeka: InTech; 2012.
66. Ethier KA, Kershaw TS, Niccolai LM, Lewis JB, Ickovics JR. Adolescent women underestimate their susceptibility to sexually transmitted infections. Sex Transm Infect. 2003;79(5):408–11. https://doi.org/10.1136/sti.79.5.408.
67. Ford CA, Jaccard J, Millstein SG, Bardsley PE, Miller WC. Perceived risk of chlamydial and gonococcal infection among sexually experienced young adults in the United States. Perspect Sex Reprod Health. 2004;36(6):258–64. https://doi.org/10.1363/psrh.36.258.04.
68. Herzog SA, Heijne JC, Scott P, Althaus CL, Low N. Direct and indirect effects of screening for chlamydia trachomatis on the prevention of pelvic inflammatory disease: a mathematical modeling study. Epidemiology. 2013; 24(6):854–62. https://doi.org/10.1097/EDE.0b013e31829e110e.
69. Regan DG, Wilson DP, Hocking JS. Coverage is the key for effective screening of chlamydia trachomatis in Australia. J Infect Dis. 2008;198(3): 349–58. https://doi.org/10.1086/589883.
70. Datta SD, Torrone E, Kruszon-Moran D, Berman S, Johnson R, Satterwhite CL, et al. Chlamydia trachomatis trends in the United States among persons 14 to 39 years of age, 1999-2008. Sex Transm Dis. 2012;39(2):92–6. https://doi.org/10.1097/OLQ.0b013e31823e2ff7.
71. Rolstad S, Adler J, Rydén A. Response burden and questionnaire length: is shorter better? A review and meta-analysis. Value Health. 2011;14(8):1101–8. https://doi.org/10.1016/j.jval.2011.06.003.
72. Verelst F, Willem L, Beutels P. Behavioural change models for infectious disease transmission: a systematic review (2010-2015). J R Soc Interface. 2016;13(125):20160820. https://doi.org/10.1098/rsif.2016.0820.
73. Pines HA, Gorbach PM, Weiss RE, Shoptaw S, Landovitz RJ, Javanbakht M, et al. Sexual risk trajectories among MSM in the United States: implications for pre-exposure prophylaxis delivery. JAIDS. 2014;65(5):579–86. https://doi.org/10.1097/QAI.0000000000000101.
74. Heijne JCM, Herzog SA, Althaus CL, Tao G, Kent CK, Low N. Insights into the timing of repeated testing after treatment for chlamydia trachomatis: data and modelling study. Sex Transm Infect. 2013;89(1):57–62. https://doi.org/10.1136/sextrans-2011-050468.
75. Hosenfeld CB, Workowski KA, Berman S, Zaidi A, Dyson J, Mosure D, et al. Repeat infection with chlamydia and gonorrhea among females: a systematic review of the literature. Sex Transm Dis. 2009;36(8):478–89. https://doi.org/10.1097/OLQ.0b013e3181a2a933.

26

Chronic hepatitis B genotype E in African migrants: response to nucleos(t)ide treatment in real clinical practice

José Ángel Cuenca-Gómez[1*], Ana Belén Lozano-Serrano[1], María Teresa Cabezas-Fernández[1], Manuel Jesús Soriano-Pérez[1], José Vázquez-Villegas[2], Matías Estévez-Escobar[3], Isabel Cabeza-Barrera[1] and Joaquín Salas-Coronas[1]

Abstract

Background: Hepatitis B virus (HBV) genotype E is a poorly studied genotype that almost exclusively occurs in African people. It seems to harbour intrinsic potential oncogenic activity and virological characteristics of immune scape but a paucity of information is available on clinical and virological characteristic of HBV genotype E-infected patients as well as on the efficacy of anti-HBV drugs for such patients. The increasing flow of migrants from high endemic HBV sub-Saharan Africa, where genotype E is the predominant one, to Western countries makes improving such knowledge critical in order to deliver proper medical care.

Methods: Prospective observational study of naïve patients of sub-Saharan origin treated for chronic HBV genotype E infection at a Tropical Medicine clinic sited in Spain from February 2004 to January 2018. The aim of the study was to describe the response of chronic HBV genotype E infection to nucleos(t)ide analogues (NA), entecavir or tenofovir, in real clinical practice.

Results: During the study period, 2209 sub-Saharan patients were assisted at our Tropical Medicine Unit and 609 (27.6%) had chronic HBV (CHB) infection. Genotype information was available for 55 naïve patients initiating treatment with NA (entecavir or tenofovir), 43 (84.3%) of them being genotype E, although 15 were excluded because they did not meet study inclusion criteria. Thus, a total of 28 CHB genotype E patients were included and followed for 24 months at least. Twenty-one patients were in HBeAg-negative chronic hepatitis phase and 7 patients in HBeAg-positive chronic hepatitis phase. After one year of treatment, among those with good adherence, 89.4% (17/19) of the HBeAg-negative patients and 80% of the HBeAg-positive ones had undetectable viral loads. Response rates reached 100% in both groups after 15–18 months of follow-up. Out of the 7 HBeAg-positive patients, 6 (85.7%) presented HBeAg loss in a median time of 31.8 months. Neither serious adverse effects nor hepatocarcinoma cases happened during the study period.

Conclusions: HBV genotype may influence disease progression and antiviral response. Our study provides precious information on the efficacy and safety of NA treatment for CHB genotype E infection, a fairly unknown genotype with and increasing epidemiological impact.

Keywords: Hepatitis B, Genotype E, Tenofovir, Entecavir, African migrants

* Correspondence: jacuencag@gmail.com
[1]Tropical Medicine Unit, Hospital de Poniente, Carretera de Almerimar s/n, PD: 07400 Almería, El Ejido, Spain
Full list of author information is available at the end of the article

Background

Hepatitis B virus (HBV) chronic infection is a very prevalent disease worldwide. It is estimated that more than 240 million people are infected and that around 686,000 people annually die from complications of this disease, including liver cirrhosis and hepatocarcinoma [1].The vast majority of them live in low- and middle-income regions such as sub-Saharan Africa, where roughly more than 50 million people are infected.

Hepatitis B could be considered, in some parts of the world, a neglected disease for a number of reasons [2]:the major burden of morbidity and mortality from HBV is borne by tropical and subtropical countries; HBV infection is a silent disease leading to a large pool of undiagnosed infection; it disproportionately affects populations living in poverty; it causes stigma and discrimination; lack of public/media representation because HBV is "eclipsed" by higher profile infections such as HIV or malaria; lack of existing investment and development of infrastructure through which to provide education, prevention, diagnosis, and treatment; poor-quality data contributing to misinformation about epidemiology and risk factors and lack of assessment regarding feasibility of interventions; and, finally, lack of major dedicated funding agencies. As a result, mortality due to viral hepatitis (HBV and HCV) is increasing while mortality from other diseases such as HIV and malaria has declined [3].

To date, 10 genotypes (A-J) and more than 40 sub-genotypes have been identified for HBV. The distribution of HBV genotypes differs throughout the world [4]: genotypes A and D are the most prevalent in Europe; D in Asia; B, D and G in North America; F in South America; and E in sub-Saharan Africa, comprising up to 70% of all African HBV-infected patients.

HBV genotype may influence disease progression and antiviral response [5] and there are numerous studies related to such aspects: evolution of the disease according to genotype or risk of chronicity [6–9]; percentage of HBeAg or HBsAg loss [10, 11]; HBV DNA levels [12–15]; risk of progression of liver disease [16, 17] and risk of hepatocellular carcinoma [18–20]; and response to treatment [21–25]. However, most studies are performed on genotypes A, B, C, and D.

Although it seems to harbour intrinsic potential oncogenic activity and virological characteristics of immune scape [26], there is limited literature on the natural course of HBV genotype E chronic infection, and even fewer studies addressing its response to antiviral treatment.

A search in PUBMED with the commands "hepatitis B" AND "genotype E", without any type of filter, retrieved 141 articles. Of these, only 10 [12, 27–35] (7.1%) describe genotype E response to treatment in a variety of distinct scenarios: HIV-HBV co-infected patients [27–30], rescue after lamivudine failure [31], adefovir phase III clinical trials including a total of 6 genotype E patients [12]; response to interferon [33, 34] and a follow-up study of HBsAg decline in entecavir-responding patients [32]. Finally, one retrospective study addresses HBV genotypes E-H response to antiviral therapy in naïve mono-infected patients but includes just 6 genotype E patients treated with nucleos(t)ide analogues [35]. Current international guidelines do not consider either patients with HBV-genotype E chronic hepatitis [36].

HBV genotype E almost exclusively occurs in African people but due to the significant migratory flow from sub-Saharan countries that has occurred in Europe in recent years, an increasing number of patients with chronic HBV hepatitis are been treated and followed up [37]. In some studies, more than 80% of these patients had a genotype E [38]. A better knowledge of the evolution of CHB genotype E infection and its response to treatment is of great importance when making recommendations that could differ from those issued for other genotypes, in order to deliver proper medical care.

Our Tropical Medicine Unit (TMU) belongs to the Hospital of Poniente, sited in the province of Almeria, in Southern Spain. It serves a population of about 270,000 people, of which around 30% are immigrants, with a high proportion of people coming from West African countries. Chronic hepatitis B is one of the most prevalent infectious diseases among immigrant patients, especially among those of sub-Saharan origin [39].

The aim of this study is to analyze the response to treatment with NA (entecavir or tenofovir) in sub-Saharan patients with CHB genotype E infection in real world practice.

Methods

Study design

Prospective observational study intended to describe virological outcome of naïve African patients with CHB genotype E infection treated with NA in real clinical practice.

Study population and data collection

The study was carried out at the TMU of the Hospital of Poniente from February 2004 to January 2018. The following inclusion criteria were followed: i) CHB genotype E infection; ii) absence of coinfection with human immunodeficiency, hepatitis C or hepatitis D viruses, and absence of any other liver disease, such as autoimmune hepatitis; iii) individual follow-up for at least 24 months.

Decision to start HBV treatment was based on current recommendations of the European Association for the Study of Liver on force at the time [40, 41]. The choice of starting treatment with tenofovir or entecavir was at the discretion of the physician responsible for the patient, except in the presence of impaired renal function, where entecavir was used. On the contrary, all women of reproductive age were treated with tenofovir. Treatment with INF/PEG-INF was not considered because, although the available information is truly scarce, a recent study has shown poor response to interferon-based treatment in patients with chronic HBV genotype E infection [34], and also because of a less favourable tolerability-security profile as compared to NA treatment, specially for the migrant population, often conditioned by language barrier, infectious co-morbidities and poor socio-economic status.

For each included patient, laboratory and imaging data were prospectively registered. Data were analysed anonymously.

Laboratory data

Serum samples were evaluated for the presence of HBsAg, anti-HBc and anti-HBs. When HBsAg was detected, HBeAg and anti-HBe were determined. Patients with HBsAg and anti-HBe positivity, viral load under 2000 IU/mL, and persistently normal transaminase levels were defined as inactive chronic carriers. The remaining patients with HBsAg positivity were classified either as HBeAg-positive chronic hepatitis (HBeAg-positive, anti-HBe-negative), or HBeAg-negative chronic hepatitis (HBeAg-negative, anti-HBe-positive), following the criteria of the European Association for the Study of the Liver on force [40, 41]. In HBsAg-positive patients, the quantification of HBV-DNA was performed by real-time PCR (COBAS Amplipre / CobasTaqman-Roche Diagnostics), with a limit of detection of 10 IU/ml. HBV genotype was determined by partial amplification and sequencing of the HBsAg coding gene.

Follow-up

Visits were scheduled every 3 months, during the first year and afterwards. Viral load was programmed to be determined at months 3, 6 and 12 months, and every 6 months from there on. The evolution of alanine aminotransferase (ALT) and HBV-DNA viral load were analysed. Normal ALT was defined as ≤30 IU/L in men and ≤ 19 IU/L in women [42]; and undetectable viral load as HBV-DNA < 10 IU/mL.

As an actual clinical practice study, determination of HBV viral load was adapted to whenever patients came to the clinic, trying to roughly follow the aforementioned scheme. For those visits with no viral load available, it was assumed that it was detectable if it was detectable at the previous and subsequent visits (± 3 months), and undetectable if it was so at the previous and subsequent ones (± 3 months).

All patients underwent a liver ultrasound before treatment and every 6 months thereafter. An ultrasound-guided liver biopsy was performed in those patients presenting any medical reason for. METAVIR classification was used for classification of liver fibrosis and activity grade [43].

To evaluate adherence to treatment, clinical interview at every scheduled visit to the clinic and verification of patients' drug withdrawal from the hospital pharmacy were used. To assess the safety of the treatment, urine sediment and dipstick analysis, glomerular filtration and plasma phosphorus level were measured at each visit.

Statistical analysis

A descriptive statistical analysis was performed where continuous variables were expressed as medians and interquartile ranges (IQR), and categorical variables were described using a table of frequencies and proportions. STATA version 12 was the statistical program used to analyse the data.

Literature review

To analyse the relevance of genotype E in the literature, a bibliographic search was carried out in PUBMED using the commands "hepatitis B" AND "genotype E", without any type of filter.

Results

During the study period, a total of 2209 sub-Saharan patients were assisted at the TMU; 609 (27.6%) of them presented CHB infection: 370 (60.7%) were classified as inactive chronic carriers, 181 (29.7%) were in a chronic HBeAg-negative phase, and 58 (9.5%) in a chronic HBeAg-positive phase. Treatment was initiated in 72 patients; genotype information was available in 55 of them: 43 (84.3%) genotype E, 6 genotype A, and 2 genotype D. Finally, out of the 43 patients with genotype E, 15 were excluded because they did not meet the inclusion criteria of the study. Thus, a total of 28 patients were included.

Demographic data

Out of the 28 patients, 24 (85.7%) were men and the median age was 31.5 years (IQR 8). Median length of stay in Spain was 54 months (IQR 49). The countries of origin were Mali (7 patients), Guinea-Bissau (7 patients), Senegal (5 patients), Guinea-Conakry (3 patients), Ghana (3 patients), and Gambia, Nigeria and Burkina Faso (1 patient each).

Hepatitis B laboratory data results

Twenty-one patients were in HBeAg-negative chronic hepatitis phase and 7 patients in HBeAg-positive chronic hepatitis phase; 26 patients (92.9%) presented abnormal elevated ALT measurements before starting treatment. Median ALT in HBeAg-negative patients was 64.5 IU/L (IQR 119), and 84 IU/L (IQR 61) in HBeAg-positive patients. One hundred per cent of patients had detectable viral load at the time of treatment initiation. Median viral load at the start of treatment for HBeAg-negative patients was 5.28 logIU/mL (IQR 6.26), and 7.23 logIU/mL (IQR 5.23) for HBeAg-positive patients. Baseline characteristics at the start of treatment are described in Table 1.

Ultrasound and biopsy findings

Hepatic ultrasonography was abnormal (showing signs of chronic liver disease) in 5 patients (17.9%). Hepatic biopsy was performed in 10 patients: 3 had stage A1F1, 3 patients A1F2, 1 patient A2F1, 1 patient A2F2, 1 patient A3F2, and 1 patient A3F3, as for METAVIR classification.

Treatment outcome and follow-up

Treatment with tenofovir 245 mg/day was initiated in 24 patients (17 HBeAg-negative and 7 HBeAg-positive), and with entecavir 0.5 mg/day in 4 patients (all of them HBeAg-negative).

During the first year of follow up, 93% of patients had good adherence, attending to scheduled visits regularly and showing good treatment compliance. This figure almost reached 100% during the second year.

For the analysis of the evolution of ALT levels and viral load, only those patients who showed good adherence to the treatment were selected (20 HBeAg-negative patients and 6 HBeAg-positive). The proportions of compliant patients with normal ALT or undetectable viral load in each visit are shown in Figs. 1 and 2. After two years of treatment, 66.7% of HBeAg-positive patients and 45% of HBeAg-negative ones had normalized transaminases. ALT figures may have been influenced by the fact that two patients were coinfected by *S. mansoni* and one patient had a fatty liver. After one year of treatment, 89.4% (17/19) of HBeAg-negative compliant patients had an undetectable viral load, rising to 100% at month 15. In the case of HBeAg-positive compliant patients, 80% had an undetectable viral load after one year of treatment, and 100% at 18 months.

Of the 7 HBeAg-positive patients, 6 (85.7%) presented HBeAg loss (5 with anti-HBe seroconversion) in a mean time of 31.8 months. No HBsAg loss happened during follow-up in any patient. No cases of hepatocarcinoma were detected during the study period.

There were not any serious adverse reactions during the whole follow-up period. Only 6 cases of mild and self–limited hypophosphatemia were detected in tenofovir treated patients, none of them requiring discontinuation of the drug. None of the tenofovir treated patients presented evidence of impaired renal function.

Table 1 Baseline characteristics at the start of treatment

	HBeAg-positive	HBeAg-negative
Number of patients: N (%)	7 (25%)	21 (75%)
Age (years)[a]	24 (8)	33 (7)
Male sex: N (%)	5 (71.4%)	19 (90.5%)
Mean length of stay in Spain (months)[a]	11 (72)	69 (28)
Co-morbidities	None	Coinfection with *S. mansoni* (2 patients) Fatty liver (1 patient)
ALT (IU/L)[a]	84 (61)	64.5 (119)
AST (IU/L)[a]	62 (26)	56.5 (93)
GGT (IU/L)[a]	30 (41)	48.5 (34)
ALP (IU/L)[a]	104 (66)	92 (35)
Total bilirubin (mg/dL)[a]	0.4 (0.2)	0.66 (0.93)
Platelets $\times 10^3$ μL[a]	204 (97)	168.5 (111)
Prothrombin time (%)[a]	78 (18)	90.5 (20.3)
Alpha-fetoprotein (ng/mL)[a]	4.6 (3.6)	2.5 (1.4)
HBV-DNA (log IU/mL)[a]	7.23 (5.23)	5.28 (6.26)
FIB- 4 score[a]	0.8 (1.8)	1.5 (0.9)
APRI score[a]	0.9 (1.2)	1 (1.7)
Chosen treatment	Tenofovir (7 patients)	Tenofovir (17 patients) Entecavir (4 patients)

[a]Values are median and (IQR). *ALT* Alanine aminotransferase, *AST* Aspartate aminotransferase, *GGT* Gamma-glutamyl transferase, *ALP* Alkaline phosphatase. FIB-4 score: Fibrosis-4 score. APRI score: AST to Platelet Ratio Index

Discussion

With the data we provide, we can state that treatment with nucleos(t)ide analogues in sub-Saharan patients with CHB genotype E infection have at least as favorable results as the ones reported for other genotypes, in terms of virological response rates, normalization of transaminases, and loss of HBeAg.

These finding are relevant because sub-Saharan people are one of the populations with the highest prevalence of HBV infection of the world, and genotype E in particular is highly endemic in most of sub-Saharan Africa. Even though HBV genotype E horizontal transmission is also possible, among the migrant population coming from sub-Saharan Africa the infection is most frequently acquired vertically at birth or during the first years of life as a consequence of traditional medicine practices and tribal scarifications [44]. This fact means that, although our patients were fairly young (mean age 31.5 years), HBV infection has probably been present for all that long.

There are many studies relating to chronic hepatitis B infection in recent years but a paucity of information is available on the clinical and virological characteristics of HBV genotype E-infected patients as well as on the efficacy of anti-HBV drugs. Epidemiological studies have suggested the carcinogenic potential of genotype E, and in fact, African regions in which genotype E is endemic are characterized by a higher incidence of hepatocellular carcinoma. Although the mechanisms underlying this

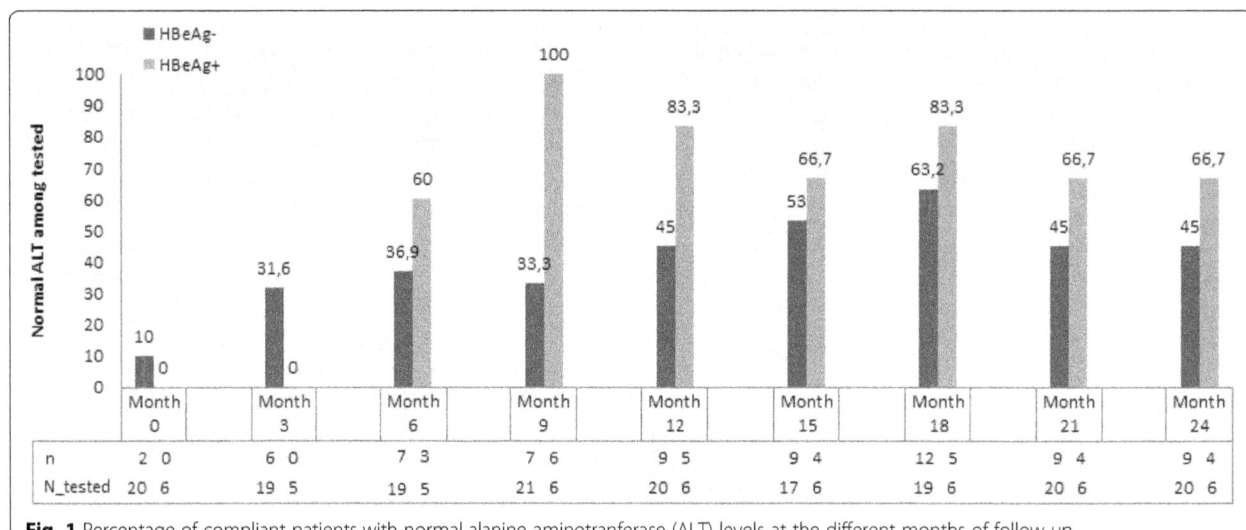

	Month 0	Month 3	Month 6	Month 9	Month 12	Month 15	Month 18	Month 21	Month 24
HBeAg- (%)	10	31,6	36,9	33,3	45	53	63,2	45	45
HBeAg+ (%)	0	0	60	100	83,3	66,7	83,3	66,7	66,7
n	2 0	6 0	7 3	7 6	9 5	9 4	12 5	9 4	9 4
N_tested	20 6	19 5	19 5	21 6	20 6	17 6	19 6	20 6	20 6

Fig. 1 Percentage of compliant patients with normal alanine aminotranferase (ALT) levels at the different months of follow-up

hypothetic oncogenic potential have not yet been clarified, they could be related to immune escape phenomena [26] as well as to other possible variables involved, such as HIV co-infection, dietary iron overload or aflatoxins consumption [45].

As there is a growing migration movement from these African regions to western countries [46], dealing with migrant patients with hepatitis B genotype E is becoming more frequent in western hepatology clinics and hospitals. Out of the actual clinical practice studies, only the studies by Marcellin [47] et al. and Boglione et al. [32, 34] include a considerable number of sub-Saharan patients, although in Marcellin's study no genotype information is available.

HBV genotype may influence antiviral response, but the main studies that analyze the role of HBV genotype in the treatment with NA mostly deal with genotypes A, B, C and D [5, 48]. The importance of our work is that, to our knowledge, is the first prospective clinical practice study truly exploring the virological response to NA therapy in CHB genotype E patients.

There is one clinical practice study about treatment of CHB genotype E patients with NA [32], but it is focused in the decrease of HBsAg titles. In this work, the authors conclude that the decrease of HBsAg titles is smaller in the 34 patients infected by genotype E as compared to patients infected by genotypes A or D, although the analysis only included those patients who had achieved previously virological response (HBV-DNA undetectable after 24 weeks of therapy), and the meaning of HBsAg-title changes in this setting is still unclear. Another study with genotype E-infected patients, also conducted by Boglione et al. [34], explores the response to interferon therapy finding very low rates of response;

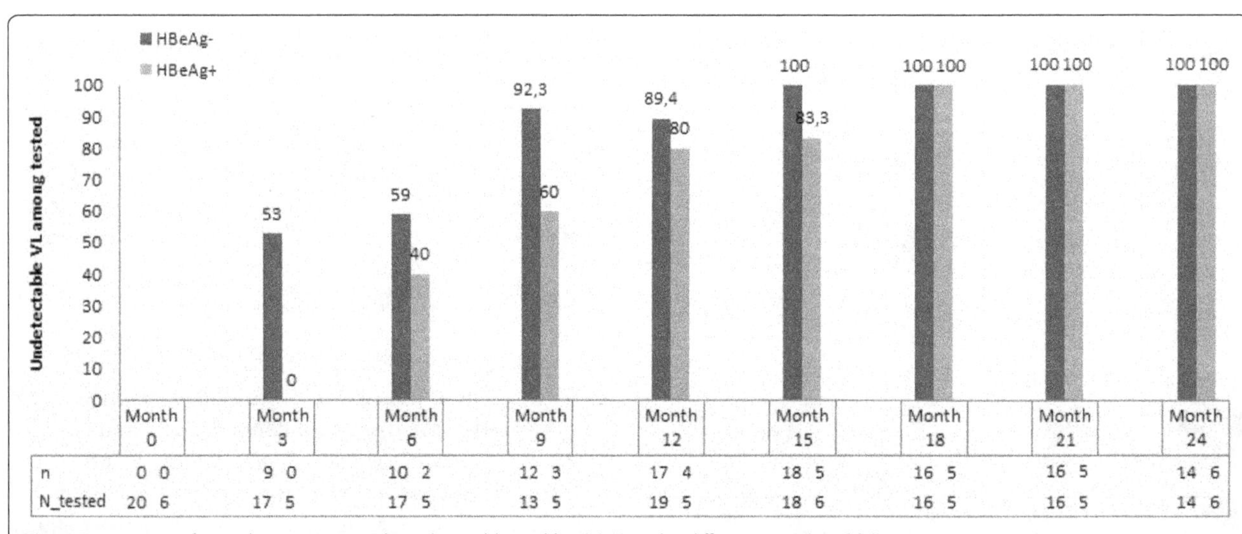

	Month 0	Month 3	Month 6	Month 9	Month 12	Month 15	Month 18	Month 21	Month 24
HBeAg- (%)		53	59	92,3	89,4	100	100	100	100
HBeAg+ (%)		0	40	60	80	83,3	100	100	100
n	0 0	9 0	10 2	12 3	17 4	18 5	16 5	16 5	14 6
N_tested	20 6	17 5	17 5	13 5	19 5	18 6	16 5	16 5	14 6

Fig. 2 Percentage of compliant patients with undetectable viral load (VL) at the different months of follow-up

10 patients were rescued with entecavir after failing interferon treatment and virological response was achieved in 60% of them after a follow-up median of 5.2 months. There is also one retrospective study that addresses HBV genotypes E-H response to antiviral therapy in naïve mono-infected patients, but includes just 6 genotype E patients treated with nucleos(t)ide analogues [35]. Current international guidelines do not yet mention patients with HBV-genotype E chronic hepatitis [36].

Finally, a handful of articles deal with CHB genotype E patients and NA treatment in different clinical scenarios, like HIV-HBV co-infected patients [27–30], rescue after lamivudine failure [31], and the phase III studies of adefovir dipivoxil reported by Westland et al. [12] where 6 patients with genotype E were included.

In our study we have included 28 treatment-naive patients and have observed that at 12 months of treatment with NA, 89.4% of HBeAg-negative and 80% of HBeAg-positive patients negativize the viral load. This proportion increases to 100% in both groups at month 18. In other studies conducted in real clinical practice with chronic hepatitis B patients, overall viral load negativization rates at 12 months in patients treated with tenofovir ranged from 59.2 to 91.9% [24, 25, 47, 49–51]; and with entecavir, from 41 to 89.4% [21–23, 51–62]. These differences between the studies are possibly due to the diverse populations studied in each case, the different sensitivity of the PCR used to detect viral load, and to the fact that, in many studies, patients previously treated with other treatments for HBV are included. None of these studies do, however, mention HBV genotyping.

Table 2 compares those other studies that do analyze the response to treatment, as ALT normalization and viral load undetectability, according to HBV genotype. Among the few available studies, it stands out one conducted by Ono et al. [22], where genotype C predominates (70.9%), and the proportion of patients with undetectable viral load after one year of treatment is 88%, similar to that of our work. In the study of Zoutendijk [23], where genotype D predominates in non-cirrhotic patients (49%), 68% of patients have undetectable viral load after one year. Due to the relatively small number of patients included in these studies, no clear conclusions can be drawn about a faster response to treatment in patients with one genotype or another. Although these data may suggest that patients with genotypes C and E respond faster to treatment with nucleos(t)ide analogues than those with genotype D.

Regarding normalization of transaminase levels, in the present study rates were 42.1 and 85.7% after one year in HBeAg–negative and HBeAg-positive patients respectively. These percentages reached 55.6% in HBeAg-negative and 100% in HBeAg-positive patients at 18 months of follow up. In other studies of actual clinical practice, the percentage of patients with normal transaminases at 12 months ranged from 34.6–95.5% [21–25, 47, 49–53, 56–60, 62]. These discrepant results may be explained by the different cutoff points taken for normal ALT in the different studies, and by the different stages of hepatopathy of the included patients, since in some cases they include patients with established cirrhosis and even with hepatocarcinoma.

HBeAg loss occurred in 85.7% of patients in a median time of 31.8 months. Seroconversion rate during the first year was 12.5%. Although there are few HBeAg-positive patients in our study, these results are similar to those found in other published works where these rates oscillate between 8 and 16% [22, 24, 53, 55, 61].These studies also show that HBeAg-loss rates increase significantly after more than 3 years of treatment. In these works, like in ours, no HBsAg loss is observed.

It should be noted the high adherence to treatment observed in our study: 86.7% in the first year and almost 100% in the second year. Among migrants this may be especially striking, since many are the reasons that hamper their compliance and follow-up (labour mobility, visits to their home countries, barriers to access to health care systems, etc.). The reasons for such good adherence are probably related to the collaboration of mediators and community health agents, the use of cost-free drugs, and the lack of barriers to access to the public health care system, either primary or specialized care, as is established in Andalusia, our administrative region.

The main limitation of this study is that the number of patients is not very high, although figures are according to the scarce published studies that describe the response to treatment of genotype E chronic hepatitis B patients, either with interferon or with nucleos(t)ide analogues [12, 32, 34, 35]. It would have also been interesting to compare patients with genotype E with other patients of similar origin and socioeconomic circumstances but with different genotypes. In relation to this last aspect, the number of African migrants that we deal with harbouring other genotypes is so low that does not allow valid comparisons. One last limitation is that therapeutic drug monitoring and HBsAg quantification were not available in our hospital, even though the role of the last one during therapy with oral NA is still debatable.

Nevertheless, studies like ours, that shed light on the response of CHB to different antiviral treatments depending on the genotype, are relevant. This is especially true in the case of relatively unknown genotypes like genotype E, a genotype associated to immune scape mutations [26] and whose epidemiological impact is steadily increasing in the Western world due to migration from Africa. Improving our knowledge on CHB genotype E infection and its response to treatment is critical to issue proper and specific recommendations. In addition, although access to NA in Africa is currently difficult, all evidence gathered is useful with a view to future

Table 2 Studies on actual clinical practice using entecavir or tenofovir where HBV genotype and virological response information is available

	No. of patients	Drug	Race	Genotype	HBeAg-negative, %	Months of follow-up (Median)	Undetectable DNA, %	ALT normal, %	AgHBe loss %
Lampertico 2011	**418**	Entecavir	–	D (90%)	83	60	100 (HBeAg+) 99 (HBeAg-)	90 (36 months)	55
Ono 2012	**474**	Entecavir	–	A (2.5%) B (14.1%) C (70.9%)	53	28	88 (12 months) 96 (48 months)	83 (12 months) 93 (48 months)	16 (12 months) 38 (48 months)
Zoutendijk 2013	**372**	Entecavir	48% White 27% Asian 25% Others	A (9.4%) B (6.7%) C (10%) D (36%)	58	20	68 (12 months) 93 (36 months)	78 (Total at the end of treatment))	17
Kim 2015	**151**	Tenofovir	100% Asian	C (100%)	39.1	13	64.2 (12 months)	97.7 (12 months)	12 (6 months) 15.2 (12 months)
Lovett 2017	**92 (55 naive)**	Tenofovir	83.7% Asian 7.6% White 4.3% African 4.4% Others	A (3.3%) B (7.6%) C (14.1%) D (3.3%)	65.5	24	59.2 (12 months) 89.3 (36 months)	86% (Total at the end of treatment)	16.7 (36 months)

strategies for the treatment and prevention of this disease in the countries of origin. May our work then be considered a small and humble contribution to HBV infection clinical care research.

Conclusions

As shown in this real practice study, treatment with nucleos(t)ide analogues is safe and effective in sub-Saharan migrants with CHB genotype E infection. However, direct comparison studies seem to be necessary to conclude whether there are significant differences in the response to treatment when compared to other HBV genotypes.

Migration is altering geographical distribution of HBV genotypes around the world making considering the clinical and epidemiological implications of less known HBV genotypes, such as genotype E, critical in order to provide proper tailored care.

In our setting, where health care and antiviral drugs are cost-free and available with no barriers, high rates of adherence to treatment can be achieved. But these results could also be transferable to low- and middle-income African populations if therapy with such drugs were to be generally available in the future, contributing to research into a neglected disease that affects a large part of the population living in the poorest regions of the world.

Abbreviations

ALP: Alkaline phosphatase; ALT: Alanine aminotransferase; anti-HBc: Hepatitis B core antibody; anti-HBe: Hepatitis B envelope antibody; anti-HBs: Hepatitis B surface antibody; AST: Aspartate aminotransferase; CHB: Chronic Hepatitis B; CI: Confidence interval; GGT: Gammaglutamyl transferase; HBeAg: Hepatitis B envelope antigen; HBsAg: Hepatitis B surface antigen; HBV: Hepatitis B virus; HCV: Hepatitis C virus; HIV: Human immunodeficiency virus; INF/PEG-INF: Interferon/pegylated-interferon; IQR: Interquartile range;
NA: Nucleos(t)ide analogues; PCR: Polymerase chain reaction; SD: Standard deviation; TMU: Tropical Medicine Unit

Acknowledgements

The authors thank Mª Carmen Olvera Porcel, technician in Research Methodology and Biostatistics from FIBAO, for providing invaluable support for the statistical analysis of the data.

Funding

This study has been funded by RICET (Red de Investigación Cooperativa en Enfermedades Tropicales, -Cooperative Investigation Network for Tropical Diseases-; Exp. N.: RD16/0027/0013), Instituto de Salud Carlos III, and cofinanced by the European Regional Development Fund of the European Union.
This study has been conducted within the activities developed by the research group PAIDI CTS 582 of the regional Ministry of Gender, Health and Social Policy of the Government of Andalusia, RICET and CEMyRI (Center for the Study of Migration and Intercultural Relations of the University of Almeria, Spain).

Authors' contributions

Conceptualization and study design: JSC, JACG MTCF, MEE. Investigation: JSC, MTCF, MEE, JACG. Project collaboration: JSC, JACG, MTCF, MEE, ABLS, JVV, MJSP, ICB. Supervision: JSC, JVV, MJSP. Writing - original draft: JACG, JSC, ABLS. Writing - review & editing: JSC, JACG, MTCF, MEE, ABLS, JVV, MJSP, ICB. All authors read and approved the final manuscript.

Competing interests

JSC participated on one advisory board for Gilead Sciences and received travel grants from Gilead Sciences and Bristol-Myers Squibb. ABLS participated on advisory boards for Bristol-Myers Squibb, and reports travel funding, educational grants and speaker fees from GlaxoSmithKline (ViiV Healthcare), Gilead Sciences, Tibotec (Janssen) Therapeutics, Abbie, Merck Sharp and Dohme, BoehringerIngelheim, Roche Pharma, Pfizer, and Bristol-Myers Squibb. JACG, MJSP and JVV received travel grants from Gilead Sciences. MEE received speaker fees and/or travel funding from Gilead Sciences, Bristol-Myers Squibb, Abbie, Merck Sharp and Dohme. All other authors declare no competing interests.

Author details

[1]Tropical Medicine Unit, Hospital de Poniente, Carretera de Almerimar s/n, PD: 07400 Almería, El Ejido, Spain. [2]Tropical Medicine Unit, Distrito Poniente, Almería, Spain. [3]Digestive Service, Hospital de Poniente, Almería, El Ejido, Spain.

References

1. WHO. Hepatitis B: WHO; 2018 [cited 2018 10-08-2018]. Available from: http://www.who.int/mediacentre/factsheets/fs204/es/.
2. O'Hara GA, McNaughton AL, Maponga T, Jooste P, Ocama P, Chilengi R, et al. Hepatitis B virus infection as a neglected tropical disease. PLoS Negl Trop Dis. 2017;11(10):e0005842.
3. WHO. Global hepatitis report, 2017. In: WHO; 2017.
4. Shi W, Zhang Z, Ling C, Zheng W, Zhu C, Carr MJ, et al. Hepatitis B virus subgenotyping: history, effects of recombination, misclassifications, and corrections Infection, genetics and evolution. Journal of molecular epidemiology and evolutionary genetics in infectious diseases. 2013;16:355–61.
5. Rajoriya N, Combet C, Zoulim F, Janssen HLA. How viral genetic variants and genotypes influence disease and treatment outcome of chronic hepatitis B. time for an individualised approach? J Hepatol. 2017;67(6):1281–97.
6. Zhang HW, Yin JH, Li YT, Li CZ, Ren H, Gu CY, et al. Risk factors for acute hepatitis B and its progression to chronic hepatitis in Shanghai, China. Gut. 2008;57(12):1713–20.
7. Mayerat C, Mantegani A, Frei PC. Does hepatitis B virus (HBV) genotype influence the clinical outcome of HBV infection? J Viral Hepat. 1999;6(4):299–304.
8. Kobayashi M, Arase Y, Ikeda K, Tsubota A, Suzuki Y, Saitoh S, et al. Clinical characteristics of patients infected with hepatitis B virus genotypes a, B, and C. J Gastroenterol. 2002;37(1):35–9.
9. Suzuki Y, Kobayashi M, Ikeda K, Suzuki F, Arfase Y, Akuta N, et al. Persistence of acute infection with hepatitis B virus genotype a and treatment in Japan. J Med Virol. 2005;76(1):33–9.
10. Chu CJ, Hussain M, Lok AS. Hepatitis B virus genotype B is associated with earlier HBeAg seroconversion compared with hepatitis B virus genotype C. Gastroenterology. 2002;122(7):1756–62.
11. Livingston SE, Simonetti JP, Bulkow LR, Homan CE, Snowball MM, Cagle HH, et al. Clearance of hepatitis B e antigen in patients with chronic hepatitis B and genotypes a, B, C, D, and F. Gastroenterology. 2007;133(5):1452–7.
12. Westland C, Delaney WT, Yang H, Chen SS, Marcellin P, Hadziyannis S, et al. Hepatitis B virus genotypes and virologic response in 694 patients in phase III studies of adefovir dipivoxil1. Gastroenterology. 2003;125(1):107–16.
13. Yu MW, Yeh SH, Chen PJ, Liaw YF, Lin CL, Liu CJ, et al. Hepatitis B virus genotype and DNA level and hepatocellular carcinoma: a prospective study in men. J Natl Cancer Inst. 2005;97(4):265–72.
14. Kao JH, Chen PJ, Lai MY, Chen DS. Clinical and virological aspects of blood donors infected with hepatitis B virus genotypes B and C. J Clin Microbiol. 2002;40(1):22–5.
15. Yousif M, Mudawi H, Bakhiet S, Glebe D, Kramvis A. Molecular characterization of hepatitis B virus in liver disease patients and asymptomatic carriers of the virus in Sudan. BMC Infect Dis. 2013;13:328.
16. Chu CM, Liaw YF. Genotype C hepatitis B virus infection is associated with a higher risk of reactivation of hepatitis B and progression to cirrhosis than genotype B: a longitudinal study of hepatitis B e antigen-positive patients with normal aminotransferase levels at baseline. J Hepatol. 2005;43(3):411–7.
17. Sanchez-Tapias JM, Costa J, Mas A, Bruguera M, Rodes J. Influence of hepatitis B virus genotype on the long-term outcome of chronic hepatitis B in western patients. Gastroenterology. 2002;123(6):1848–56.
18. Livingston SE, Simonetti JP, McMahon BJ, Bulkow LR, Hurlburt KJ, Homan CE, et al. Hepatitis B virus genotypes in Alaska native people with hepatocellular carcinoma: preponderance of genotype F. J Infect Dis. 2007;195(1):5–11.

19. Yang HI, Yeh SH, Chen PJ, Iloeje UH, Jen CL, Su J, et al. Associations between hepatitis B virus genotype and mutants and the risk of hepatocellular carcinoma. J Natl Cancer Inst. 2008;100(16):1134–43.
20. Kew MC, Kramvis A, Yu MC, Arakawa K, Hodkinson J. Increased hepatocarcinogenic potential of hepatitis B virus genotype a in bantu-speaking sub-saharan Africans. J Med Virol. 2005;75(4):513–21.
21. Lampertico PVM, Soffredini R. Entecavir monotherapy for nuc-na€ıve chronic hepatitis B patients from field practice: high efficacy and favorable 0safety profile over 3 year. Hepatology. 2011;54:A1436.
22. Ono A, Suzuki F, Kawamura Y, Sezaki H, Hosaka T, Akuta N, et al. Long-term continuous entecavir therapy in nucleos(t)ide-naive chronic hepatitis B patients. J Hepatol. 2012;57(3):508–14.
23. Zoutendijk R, Reijnders JG, Zoulim F, Brown A, Mutimer DJ, Deterding K, et al. Virological response to entecavir is associated with a better clinical outcome in chronic hepatitis B patients with cirrhosis. Gut. 2013;62(5):760–5.
24. Kim JH, Jung SW, Byun SS, Shin JW, Park BR, Kim MH, et al. Efficacy and safety of tenofovir in nucleos(t)ide-naive patients with genotype C chronic hepatitis B in real-life practice. Int J Clin Pharm. 2015;37(6):1228–34.
25. Lovett GC, Nguyen T, Iser DM, Holmes JA, Chen R, Demediuk B, et al. Efficacy and safety of tenofovir in chronic hepatitis B: Australian real world experience. World J Hepatol. 2017;9(1):48–56.
26. Malagnino V, Salpini R, Maffongelli G, Battisti A, Fabeni L, Piermatteo L, et al. High rates of chronic HBV genotype E infection in a group of migrants in Italy from West Africa: Virological characteristics associated with poor immune clearance. PLoS One. 2018;13(3):e0195045.
27. Archampong TN, Boyce CL, Lartey M, Sagoe KW, Obo-Akwa A, Kenu E, et al. HBV genotypes and drug resistance mutations in antiretroviral treatment-naive and treatment-experienced HBV-HIV-coinfected patients. Antivir Ther. 2017;22(1):13–20.
28. Boyd A, Maylin S, Moh R, Mahjoub N, Gabillard D, Eholie SP, et al. Hepatitis B surface antigen quantification as a predictor of seroclearance during treatment in HIV-hepatitis B virus coinfected patients from sub-Saharan Africa. J Gastroenterol Hepatol. 2016;31(3):634–44.
29. Boyd A, Moh R, Gabillard D, le Carrou J, Danel C, Anglaret X, et al. Low risk of lamivudine-resistant HBV and hepatic flares in treated HIV-HBV-coinfected patients from cote d'Ivoire. Antivir Ther. 2015;20(6):643–54.
30. Honge BL, Jespersen S, Medina C, Te Dda S, da Silva ZJ, Lewin S, et al. Hepatitis B and Delta virus are prevalent but often subclinical co-infections among HIV infected patients in Guinea-Bissau, West Africa: a cross-sectional study. PLoS One. 2014;9(6):e99971.
31. De Francesco MA, Gargiulo F, Spinetti A, Zaltron S, Giagulli C, Caccuri F, et al. Clinical course of chronic hepatitis B patients receiving nucleos(t)ide analogues after virological breakthrough during monotherapy with lamivudine. The new microbiologica. 2015;38(1):29–37.
32. Boglione L, Cardellino CS, De Nicolo A, Cariti G, Di Perri G, D'Avolio A. Different HBsAg decline after 3 years of therapy with entecavir in patients affected by chronic hepatitis B HBeAg-negative and genotype a, D and E. J Med Virol. 2014;86(11):1845–50.
33. Boglione L, Cariti G, Ghisetti V, Burdino E, Di Perri G. Extended duration of treatment with peginterferon alfa-2a in patients with chronic hepatitis B, HBeAg-negative and E genotype: a retrospective analysis. J Med Virol. 2018; 90(6):1047–52.
34. Boglione L, Cusato J, Cariti G, Di Perri G, D'Avolio A. The E genotype of hepatitis B: clinical and virological characteristics, and response to interferon. The Journal of infection. 2014;69(1):81–7.
35. Erhardt A, Gobel T, Ludwig A, Lau GK, Marcellin P, van Bommel F, et al. Response to antiviral treatment in patients infected with hepatitis B virus genotypes E-H. J Med Virol. 2009;81(10):1716–20.
36. Terrault NA, Lok ASF, McMahon BJ, Chang KM, Hwang JP, Jonas MM, et al. Update on prevention, diagnosis, and treatment of chronic hepatitis B: AASLD 2018 hepatitis B guidance. Hepatology. 2018;67(4):1560–99.
37. Coppola N, Alessio L, Gualdieri L, Pisaturo M, Sagnelli C, Minichini C, et al. Hepatitis B virus infection in undocumented immigrants and refugees in southern Italy: demographic, virological. and clinical features Infectious diseases of poverty. 2017;6(1):33.
38. Ott JJ, Stevens GA, Groeger J, Wiersma ST. Global epidemiology of hepatitis B virus infection: new estimates of age-specific HBsAg seroprevalence and endemicity. Vaccine. 2012;30(12):2212–9.
39. Cuenca-Gomez JA, Salas-Coronas J, Soriano-Perez MJ, Vazquez-Villegas J, Lozano-Serrano AB, Cabezas-Fernandez MT. Viral hepatitis and immigration: a challenge for the healthcare system. Revista clinica espanola. 2016;216(5):248–52.
40. European Association For The Study Of The L. EASL clinical practice guidelines: management of chronic hepatitis B. J Hepatol. 2009;50(2):227–42.
41. European Association For The Study Of The L. EASL clinical practice guidelines: management of chronic hepatitis B virus infection. J Hepatol. 2012;57(1):167–85.
42. Terrault NA, Bzowej NH, Chang KM, Hwang JP, Jonas MM, Murad MH, et al. AASLD guidelines for treatment of chronic hepatitis B. Hepatology. 2016; 63(1):261–83.
43. Bedossa P, Poynard T. An algorithm for the grading of activity in chronic hepatitis C. The METAVIR Cooperative Study Group Hepatology. 1996;24(2): 289–93.
44. Botha JF, Ritchie MJ, Dusheiko GM, Mouton HW, Kew MC. Hepatitis B virus carrier state in black children in Ovamboland: role of perinatal and horizontal infection. Lancet. 1984;1(8388):1210–2.
45. Kew MC. Hepatocellular carcinoma in African blacks: recent progress in etiology and pathogenesis. World J Hepatol. 2010;2(2):65–73.
46. Stasi C, Silvestri C, Voller F, Cipriani F. The epidemiological changes of HCV and HBV infections in the era of new antiviral therapies and the anti-HBV vaccine. Journal of infection and public health. 2016;9(4):389–95.
47. Marcellin P, Zoulim F, Hezode C, Causse X, Roche B, Truchi R, et al. Effectiveness and safety of Tenofovir Disoproxil fumarate in chronic hepatitis B: a 3-year, prospective, real-world study in France. Dig Dis Sci. 2016;61(10):3072–83.
48. Raimondi S, Maisonneuve P, Bruno S, Mondelli MU. Is response to antiviral treatment influenced by hepatitis B virus genotype? J Hepatol. 2010;52(3):441–9.
49. Petersen J, Heyne R, Mauss S, Schlaak J, Schiffelholz W, Eisenbach C, et al. Effectiveness and safety of Tenofovir Disoproxil fumarate in chronic hepatitis B: a 3-year prospective field practice study in Germany. Dig Dis Sci. 2016;61(10):3061–71.
50. Ahn HJ, Song MJ, Jang JW, Bae SH, Choi JY, Yoon SK. Treatment efficacy and safety of Tenofovir-based therapy in chronic hepatitis B: a real life cohort study in Korea. PLoS One. 2017;12(1):e0170362.
51. Pereira CV, Tovo CV, Grossmann TK, Mirenda H, Dal-Pupo BB, Almeida PR, et al. Efficacy of entecavir and tenofovir in chronic hepatitis B under treatment in the public health system in southern Brazil. Memorias do Instituto Oswaldo Cruz. 2016;111(4):252–7.
52. Buti M, Morillas RM, Prieto M, Diago M, Perez J, Sola R, et al. Efficacy and safety of entecavir in clinical practice in treatment-naive Caucasian chronic hepatitis B patients. Eur J Gastroenterol Hepatol. 2012;24(5):535–42.
53. Hou JL, Jia JD, Wei L, Zhao W, Wang YM, Cheng M, et al. Efficacy and safety of entecavir treatment in a heterogeneous CHB population from a 'real-world' clinical practice setting in China. J Viral Hepat. 2013;20(11):811–20.
54. Ridruejo E, Marciano S, Galdame O, Reggiardo MV, Munoz AE, Adrover R, et al. Efficacy and safety of long term entecavir in chronic hepatitis B treatment naive patients in clinical practice. Ann Hepatol. 2014;13(3):327–36.
55. Liu A, Ha NB, Lin B, Yip B, Trinh HN, Nguyen HA, et al. Low hepatitis B envelope antigen seroconversion rate in chronic hepatitis B patients on long-term entecavir 0.5 mg daily in routine clinical practice. Eur J Gastroenterol Hepatol. 2013;25(3):338–43.
56. Luo J, Li X, Wu Y, Lin G, Pang Y, Zhang X, et al. Efficacy of entecavir treatment for up to 5 years in nucleos(t)ide-naive chronic hepatitis B patients in real life. Int J Med Sci. 2013;10(4):427–33.
57. Wang CC, Tseng KC, Peng CY, Hsieh TY, Lin CL, Su TH, et al. Viral load and alanine aminotransferase correlate with serologic response in chronic hepatitis B patients treated with entecavir. J Gastroenterol Hepatol. 2013;28(1):46–50.
58. Yuen MF, Seto WK, Fung J, Wong DK, Yuen JC, Lai CL. Three years of continuous entecavir therapy in treatment-naive chronic hepatitis B patients: VIRAL suppression, viral resistance, and clinical safety. Am J Gastroenterol. 2011;106(7):1264–71.
59. Ahn J, Lee HM, Lim JK, Pan CQ, Nguyen MH, Ray Kim W, et al. Entecavir safety and effectiveness in a national cohort of treatment-naive chronic hepatitis B patients in the US - the ENUMERATE study. Aliment Pharmacol Ther. 2016;43(1):134–44.
60. Pawlowska M, Domagalski K, Smok B, Rajewski P, Wietlicka-Piszcz M, Halota W, et al. Continuous up to 4 years Entecavir treatment of HBV-infected adolescents - a longitudinal study in real life. PLoS One. 2016;11(9):e0163691.
61. Carey INH, Joe D. Denovo antiviral therapy with nucleos(t)ide analogues in 'real-life' patients with chronic hepatitis B infection: comparison of virological response between lamivudine + adefovir, entecavir vs. tenofovir therapy. Hepatology. 2011;54:A1396.

Clinical and genetic factors associated with increased risk of severe liver toxicity in a monocentric cohort of HIV positive patients receiving nevirapine-based antiretroviral therapy

Andrea Giacomelli[1*], Agostino Riva[1], Felicia Stefania Falvella[2], Maria Letizia Oreni[1], Dario Cattaneo[2], Stefania Cheli[2], Giulia Renisi[1], Valentina Di Cristo[1], Angelica Lupo[1], Emilio Clementi[2,3], Stefano Rusconi[1], Massimo Galli[1] and Anna Lisa Ridolfo[1]

Abstract

Background: Nevirapine has been used as antiretroviral agent since early '90. Although nevirapine is not currently recommended in initial anti-HIV regimens, its use remains consistent in a certain number of HIV-1-positive subjects. Thus, our aim was to determine clinical and genetic factors involved in the development of severe nevirapine induced liver toxicity.

Methods: We retrospectively analyzed all HIV positive patients who were followed at the Infectious Diseases Unit, DIBIC Luigi Sacco, University of Milan from May 2011 to December 2015. All patients treated with nevirapine who underwent a genotyping for the functional variants mapping into ABCB1, CYP2B6, CYP3A4 and CYP3A5 genes were included in the analysis. Severe hepatotoxicity was defined as ACTG grade 3–4 AST/ALT increase during the first three months of nevirapine treatment. The causality assessment between NVP exposure and drug-induced liver injury was performed by using the updated Roussel Uclaf Causality Assessment Methods. Hardy Weinberg equilibrium was tested by χ^2 test. A multivariable logistic regression model was constructed using a *backward* elimination method.

Results: Three hundred and sixty-two patients were included in the analysis, of which 8 (2.2%) experienced a severe liver toxicity. We observed no differences between patients with and without liver toxicity as regards gender, ethnicity, age and immune-virological status. A higher prevalence of HCV coinfection (75.0% vs 30.2%; $p = .0013$) and higher baseline AST (58 IU/L vs 26 IU/L; $p = 0.041$) and ALT (82 IU/L vs 27 IU/L; $p = 0.047$) median levels were observed in patients with liver toxicity vs those without toxicity. The genotypes CT/TT at ABCB1 rs1045642 single nucleotide polymorphism (SNP), showed a protective effect for liver toxicity when compared with genotype CC (OR = 0.18, 95%CI 0.04–0.76; $p = 0.020$) in univariate analysis. In the multivariate model, HCV coinfection was independently associated with higher risk of developing liver toxicity (aOR = 8.00, 95%CI 1.27–50.29; $p = 0.027$), whereas ABCB1 rs1045642 CT/TT genotypes (aOR = 0.10, 95%CI 0.02–0.47; $p = 0.004$) was associated with a lower risk.

(Continued on next page)

* Correspondence: andrea.giacomelli@unimi.it; dott.giacomelli@gmail.com
[1]Infectious Diseases Unit, DIBIC Luigi Sacco - University of Milan, Via G.B. Grassi, 74, 20157 Milan, Italy
Full list of author information is available at the end of the article

(Continued from previous page)

Conclusions: According to our findings HCV coinfection and ABCB1 rs1045642 SNP represent independent determinants of severe liver toxicity related to nevirapine. This genetic evaluation could be included as toxicity assessment in HIV-1-positive subjects treated with nevirapine.

Keywords: Nevirapine, Pharmacogenetic, Hepatotoxicity, ABCB1

Background

Nevirapine (NVP) is a potent non-nucleoside reverse transcriptase inhibitor widely prescribed in low-income countries for HIV treatment and prevention of mother-to-child transmission of HIV [1]. In high-resource countries, NVP is no longer included among antiretrovirals recommended for initial antiretroviral treatment (ART), although it still remains a valid component of regimens used as ART simplification strategy due to its high efficacy, good metabolic profile, convenience, and low cost [2–4].

Although generally well tolerated and effective, some individuals exposed to NVP develop in the short-term hypersensitivity reactions which can manifest as hepatotoxicity and/or severe cutaneous adverse reactions [5]. Hepatotoxicity, in particular, has been reported more commonly with NVP than with other antiretroviral drugs [6, 7]. Higher baseline and nadir CD4 cell count have been found to independently influence the risk of NVP-related adverse reactions and the use of NVP in *naive* women (with CD4 > 250 cells/uL) and males (with CD4 > 400 cells/uL) is disallowed [8]. The role of the immune system, i.e. higher CD4 cells count, in the development of NVP induced skin and liver toxicity is corroborated by the higher incidence of these events in HIV negative patients receiving NVP as a component of post exposure prophylaxis [5]. Nevertheless, when NVP is used in ART-*experienced* patients with a controlled viremia the risk of development hepatic or cutaneous adverse events significantly decrease and there is no evident association with CD4 cell count [9–11].

A series of demographic and clinical factors have been found to correlate with an increased risk of NVP-toxicity. In particular, risk factors for ALT and AST elevations during NVP therapy included alteration of liver enzymes before NVP start, co-infection with hepatitis B or hepatitis C viruses, female gender and low body weight [6, 12].

A number of studies have also investigated the possible predictive role of genetic polymorphisms of CYP enzymes or drug-transporters involved in NVP metabolism in predisposing to NVP-related adverse effects. NVP is metabolized by cytochrome P450 enzymes CYP2B6 and CYP3A4 with a minor contribution from CYP3A5 [13]. Single nucleotide polymorphisms (SNPs) have been found to impact NVP pharmacokinetics in ethnic mix populations [14–16]. The genotype TT (c.516/rs3745274) in the CYP2B6 gene, in particular, has been associated with higher plasma concentrations of NVP and its possible role in increasing the risk of hepatotoxicity has been hypothesized [14]. However, there is contrasting evidence of interactions between the presence of variant alleles of CYP2B6 and the development of NVP-induced hepatotoxicity [17–19]. The role of CYP3A4 and CYP3A5 variants in determining NVP plasma concentration and the development of liver toxicity is more controversial, with only one report of association between CYP3A5 variants and transaminase values in African patients exposed to NVP [20]. Moreover, although effects of the efflux transporter P-glycoprotein encoded by the ATP Binding Cassette Subfamily B Member 1 (ABCB1) gene on NVP pharmacokinetics remains controversial, two studies have found a protective effect of ABCB1 c.3435 T allele against NVP-related hepatotoxicity [19, 20].

The majority of the studies that evaluated the correlation between pharmacogenetic profiles and NVP-related hepatotoxicity have been performed mainly on African population. However, genetic variant frequencies can differ markedly between different populations and only few data are available on the mentioned pharmacogenetic profiles in non-African populations.

With this in mind, we assessed clinical and pharmacogenetic factors associated with the risk of severe NVP induced liver toxicity in a population of HIV-positive patients attending a clinical center in Italy.

Methods

This study was conducted on a cohort of adult HIV-positive patients attending the Infectious Diseases Unit, DIBIC Luigi Sacco, University of Milan between May 1 2011 and December 31 2015. Patients who have ever received or were receiving a NVP-containing cART at our clinical center were eligible for the analysis.

Patient's demographic (age, gender, and ethnicity), epidemiological (HIV acquisition risk) and clinical (CDC stage, body mass index, coinfections, previous and current antiretroviral regimens, immune-virological and hemato-biochemical parameters) data registered during medical visits (on average every three months) are routinely collected in a structured database, allowing the use of the database for clinical, epidemiological or therapeutic studies.

Severe hepatotoxicity was defined as ACTG grade 3–4 AST and/or ALT increase (AST or ALT elevation above 5 time the upper reference limit) during the first three months of nevirapine treatment. The causality assessment between NVP exposure and drug-induced liver injury was performed by using the updated Roussel Uclaf Causality Assessment Methods (RUCAM) [21]. According to the RUCAM, patients were firstly assessed for hepatocellular, cholestatic or mixed liver injury. Subsequently, the score was applied and single cases of NVP-induced liver injury were classified accordingly to the RUCAM total score interpretation and causality grading: ≤0, excluded; 1–2, unlikely; 3–5, possible; 6–8, probable and ≥ 9 highly probable [21].

All patients who met the inclusion criteria underwent a genotyping for the functional variants mapping in ABCB1 (c.3435/rs1045642), CYP2B6 (c.516/rs3745274), CYP3A5 (*3/rs776746) and CYP3A4 (*22/rs35599367) genes. Genomic DNA was isolated from peripheral blood cells using an automatic DNA extraction system (Maxwell® 16 System, Promega) according to the manufacturer's instructions. All genotypes were determined by Real-Time PCR, using a panel of LightSNiP from TIB-MolBiol (assays based on SimpleProbe®). At the end of the amplification a melting curve analysis was performed (LightCycler 480, Roche).

Statistical analysis

Baseline clinical characteristics and genotypes of the two groups of interest, i.e. patients who developed severe hepatotoxicity and those who did not, were compared using the $\chi 2$ or Fisher's exact test for categorical variables and the Mann-Whitney test for continuous variables.

Hardy Weinberg equilibrium was tested by χ^2 test.

The association of clinical and genotypic variables with the development of sever liver toxicity was tested by means of a univariate logistic regression model, and all variables were incorporated into a multivariate logistic regression model with a *backward* elimination method. Statistical significance was defined at 2-sided P value < 0.05. The risks were expressed as adjusted odds ratios (aOR) with relative confidence intervals (95% CI). To perform statistical analysis we used the SAS software version 9.3.

The study was reviewed and approved by our ethics committee (Comitato Etico Interaziendale, Milano area 1); all subjects signed a dedicated informed consent.

Results

A total of 362 patients were included in the analysis. Most of them were ART-*experienced* at the time of initiation of NVP-containing regimen, whereas a minority (16.1%) were ART-*naïve*. Overall 8 (2.2%) patients experienced a severe liver toxicity during the first three months from NVP initiation. Table 1 shows the comparison of patients who experienced a severe hepatotoxicity and those who did not. There was no significant difference as regards gender, ethnicity, age and baseline immune-virological status between the two groups although females showed a trend towards a higher frequency of NVP-induced hepatotoxicity (75.0% vs 35.9%; $p = 0.055$). Conversely, patients who developed severe hepatotoxicity were more frequently HCV-coinfected (75.0% vs 30.2%: $p = 0.013$), showed higher baseline AST and ALT median levels (58 IU/L vs 26 IU/L $p = 0.041$, 82 IU/L vs 27 IU/L $p = 0.047$, respectively), and a lower median baseline body mass index value (19.9 kg/m^2 vs 22.6 kg/m^2; $p = 0.017$).

According to RUCAM, the 8 cases of NVP-induced liver toxicity were classified as hepatocellular injury and the likelihood of NVP-induced liver toxicity resulted possible for 3 patients and probable for 5 patients as shown in Table 2. A brief narration for each of the 8 cases is reported in Table 3.

Distribution of different genotypes of ABCB1 rs1045642, CYP2B6 rs3745274 and CYP3A4/A5 combined are shown in Table 4. A statistical significant difference was observed in patient with and without NVP-induced hepatotoxicity according to ABCB1 rs1045642 genotypes ($p = 0.019$).

In univariate analysis (Table 5), male gender (OR = 0.19 95%CI 0.04–0.94; $p = 0.042$), HCV coinfection (OR = 6.93 95%CI 1.38–34.87; $p = 0.019$), AST (OR = 1.02, 95%CI 1.01–1.03; $p = 0.008$) and ALT (OR = 1.01, 95%CI 1.00–1.02; $p = 0.015$) median level at the beginning of NVP have been associated with an increased risk of severe NVP-induced liver toxicity. On the other hand, genotypes CT/TT of ABCB1 rs1045642 (OR = 0.18, 95%CI 0.04–0.76; $p = 0.020$) and greater value of body mass index (OR = 0.7 95%CI 0.51–0.94, p = 0.02) showed a protective effect.

In the multivariate logistic regression model (Table 5), HCV coinfection was confirmed to be independently associated with a higher risk of developing liver toxicity (aOR = 8.00, 95%CI 1.27–50.29; $p = 0.027$), whereas ABCB1 CT/TT genotypes (aOR = 0.10, 95%CI 0.02–0.47; $p = 0.004$) has been associated with a lower risk; a higher body mass index (aOR = 0.72, 95%CI 0.519–1.000; $p = 0.050$) has been barely related to a lower risk (Table 5). On the contrary, the association between gender, baseline AST levels and NVP-induced liver toxicity wasn't confirmed in the final multivariate model.

Discussion

In this study conducted in a monocentric cohort of HIV-1 positive patients exposed to NVP we observed,

Table 1 Baseline characteristics

	Total $n = 362$	Hepatotoxicity $n = 8$	No hepatotoxicity $n = 354$	p*
Age, median (IQR)	38.5 (33.7–45.8)	39.6 (32.7–40.7)	38.5 (33.8–45.9)	0.479
Female, n (%)	133 (36.7)	6 (75.0)	127 (35.9)	0.055
Naïve patients, n (%)	58 (16.0)	1 (12.5)	57 (16.1)	0.783
Risk group, n (%)				
Eterosexual	181 (50.0)	4 (50.0)	177 (50.0)	0.213
MSM	83 (22.9)	0 (0.0)	83 (23.5)	
IVDUs	84 (23.2)	4 (50.0)	80 (22.6)	
Others	14 (3.9)	0 (0.0)	14 (3.9)	
Caucasian, n (%)	330 (91.1)	7 (87.5)	323 (91.2)	0.527
BMI, median (IQR)	22.4 (20.5–24.5)	19.9 (18.3–22.0)	22.6 (20.6–24.5)	*0.017*
AIDS, n (%)	63 (17.4)	1 (12.5)	62 (17.5)	0.999
CD4+/mL, median (IQR)	436 (306–593)	555 (479–611)	433 (300–592)	0.157
HIV-RNA $\log_{10}$ cp/mL,median (IQR)	1.75 (0.00–4.09)	0.00 (0.00–2.16)	1.79 (0.00–4.10)	0.229
HCV coinfection, n (%)	131 (31.2)	6 (75.5)	107 (30.2)	*0.013*
HBV coinfection, n (%)	21 (5.8)	1 (12.5)	20 (5.65)	0.383
AST U/L, median (IQR)	26 (20–38)	58 (29–92)	26 (20–37)	*0.041*
ALT U/L, median (IQR)	28 (18–50)	82 (37–122)	27 (18–49)	*0.047*
ARV backbone, n (%)				
ABC	32 (8.8)	1 (12.5)	31 (8.8)	0.311
AZT/DDI/D4T	223 (61.6)	7 (87.5)	216 (61.0)	
TDF	86 (23.7)	0 (0.0)	86 (24.3)	
Others	21 (5.8)	0 (0.0)	21 (5.9)	

Abbreviations: *n* number, *yrs.* years, *IQR* Inter Quartile Range, *MSM* Man how have sex with man, *IVDUs* Intra venous drug users, *BMI* Body Mass Index, *cps* copies, *ABC* abacavir, *TDF* tenofovir diproxil fumarate. **p*-values are for $\chi 2$ or Fisher's exact test and Mann-Whitney test

during the first three months of treatment, an incidence of severe liver toxicity of 2.2%. This finding is similar to that reported by other cohorts when NVP was used in *experienced* patients [10, 22]. We did not observe a significant association between the development of hepatotoxicity and high CD4 cells count at NVP start, supporting the observation of low frequency of NVP induced liver toxicity in *experienced* patients [10]. The mechanisms involved in the development of severe hepatotoxicity are not well explained and it could be that in patients never exposed to antiretroviral therapy immune-mediated process leading to immune-reconstitution could elicit the development of liver toxicity [23]. On the contrary, in experienced patients with a stable immune-virological situation, hepatotoxicity could be driven by a direct effect of the drug in susceptible patients [24]. We confirm previous findings supporting the importance of HCV coinfection as independent factor associated to the development of NVP-related liver toxicity; HCV infection could play a direct role causing liver injury and also could interfere with the metabolism of the drug [8, 11, 25]. The enhanced risk of development hepatotoxicity in HCV coinfected patients treated with NVP seems to be independent from NVP plasmatic concentrations, since comparable NVP concentration are observed in patients with and without HCV coinfection [26].

A significant correlation between low value of body mass index (< 18.5) such as for increased NVP plasma concentration and increased risk for hepatotoxicity has been previously reported [12, 18], in our study we observed a trend of body weight in predisposing to NVP-hepatotoxicity albeit not confirmed in the multivariate model.

In accordance with previous studies, we did not found a statistically significant association between polymorphisms in CYPs genes (CYP2B6, CYP3A4, CYP3A5) and the development of severe hepatotoxicity. Although these genes are involved in NVP metabolism [27] and their functional variants may significantly affect NVP plasma concentrations [28–30], their role in predisposing NVP induced hepatotoxicity remains unclear [19, 31].

The ABCB1 gene encodes for P-glycoprotein, one of the most important efflux pomp involved in the transport of both NVP and efavirenz and a modification of this protein could determine an alteration in the intracellular concentration of these drugs [32].

Table 2 Updated RUCAM for the nevirapine-induced hepatocellular injury with the total scores for each patient

RUCAM items	Pt 1	Pt 2	Pt 3	Pt 4	Pt 5	Pt 6	Pt 7	Pt 8
1. Time to onset from the beginning of the drug • 5–90 days (rechallenge: 1–15 days) (+ 2) • < 5 or > 90 days (rechallenge: > 15 days) (+ 1) Alternative: Time to onset from cessation of the drug • ≤15 days (except for slowly metabolized chemicals: > 15 days) (+ 1)	+ 2	+ 2	+ 2	+ 2	+ 2	+ 2	+ 2	+ 2
2. Course of ALT after cessation of the drug • Percentage difference between ALT peak and N • Decrease ≥50% within 8 days (+ 3) • Decrease ≥50% within 30 days (+ 2) • No information or continued drug use (0) • Decrease ≥50% after the 30th day (0) • Decrease < 50% after the 30th day or recurrent increase (– 2)	+ 2	+ 2	+ 2	+ 2	+ 2	+ 3	+ 2	0
3. Risk factors • Alcohol use (current drinks/d: > 2 for women, > 3 for men) (+ 1) • Alcohol use (current drinks/d: ≤2 for women, ≤3 for men) (0) • Age ≥ 55 years (+ 1) • Age < 55 years (0)	0	0	+ 1	0	+ 1	+ 0	0	0
4. Concomitant drug(s) • None or no information (0) • Concomitant drug/herb with incompatible time to onset (0) • Concomitant drug/herb with compatible or suggestive time to onset (1) • Concomitant drug/herb known as hepatotoxin and with compatible or suggestive time to onset delete marking right side above (– 2) • Concomitant drug/herb with evidence for its role in this case (positive rechallenge or validated test) (– 3)	0	0	– 2	0	0	0	0	0
5. Search for alternative causes Tick if negative Tick if not done Group I (7 causes) • HAV: Anti-HAV-IgM • Hepatobiliary sonography / colour Doppler • HCV: Anti-HCV, HCV-RNA • HEV: Anti-HEV-IgM, anti-HEV-IgG, HEV-RNA • Hepatobiliary sonography/colour Doppler sonography of liver vessels/endosonography/CT/MRC • Alcoholism (AST/ALT ≥2) • Acute recent hypotension history (particularly if underlying heart disease) Group II (5 causes) • Complications of underlying disease(s) such as sepsis, metastatic malignancy, autoimmune hepatitis, chronic hepatitis B or C, primary biliary cholangitis or sclerosing cholangitis, genetic liverdiseases • Infection suggested by PCR and titer change for - CMV (anti-CMV-IgM, anti-CMV-IgG) - EBV (anti-EBV-IgM, anti-EBV-IgG) - HSV (anti-HSV-IgM, anti-HSV-IgG) - VZV (anti-VZV-IgM, anti-VZV-IgG) Evaluation of groups I and II • All causes-groups I and II—reasonably ruled out (+ 2) • The 7 causes of group I ruled out (+ 1) • 6 or 5 causes of group I ruled out (0) • Less than 5 causes of group I ruled out (– 2) • Alternative cause highly probable (– 3)	0	0	0	0	–2	+ 1	0	0
6. Previous hepatotoxicity of the drug • Reaction labelled in the product characteristics (+ 2) • Reaction published but unlabelled (+ 1) • Reaction unknown (0)	+ 2	+ 2	+ 2	+ 2	+ 2	+ 2	+ 2	+ 2
7. Response to unintentional reexposure • Doubling of ALT with the drug/herb alone, provided ALT below 5 N before reexposure (+3) • Doubling of ALT with the drug(s)/herb(s) already given at the time of first reaction (+ 1) • Increase of ALT but less than N in the same conditions as for the first administration (–2) • Other situations (0)	0	0	0	0	0	0	0	0
Total	+ 6	+ 6	+ 5	+ 6	+ 5	+ 8	+ 6	+ 4

Abbreviations: *pt.* Patient, *ALT* Alanine aminotransferase, *AST* Aspartate aminotransferase, *CMV* Cytomegalovirus, *CT* Computer tomography, *EBV* Epstein Barr virus, *HAV* Hepatitis A virus, *HBc* Hepatitis B core, *HBsAg* Hepatitis B antigen, *HBV* Hepatitis B virus, *HCV* Hepatitis C virus, *HEV* Hepatitis E virus, *HSV* Herpes simplex virus, *MRC* Magnetic resonance cholangiography, *N* upper limit of the normal range, *RUCAM* Roussel Uclaf Causality Assessment Method, *VZV* Varicella zoster virus

Total score and resulting causality grading: ≤0, excluded; 1–2, unlikely; 3–5, possible; 6–8, probable; and ≥ 9, highly probable

Table 3 Clinical characteristics of the 8 cases of NVP-induced liver injury. *HLAB5701 tested absent

	Pt 1	Pt 2	Pt 3	Pt 4	Pt 5	Pt 6	Pt 7	Pt 8
HCV coinfection	no	yes	yes	yes	yes	no	yes	yes
ARV status	Experienced	Experienced	Experienced	Experienced	Naive	Experienced	Experienced	Experienced
Concomitant ARV	d4T + 3TC	d4T + 3TC	ABC* + 3TC	AZT + 3TC	AZT + 3TC	d4T + ddi	AZT + 3TC	d4T + ddi
NVP exposure before treatment interruption (days)	28	61	29	28	58	28	50	38
Concomitant medication	none	none	Vitamin D and folinic acid	none	Phenobarbital and alprazolam	none	None	Folinic acid
Symptoms	Nausea and severe weakness	none	Nausea	none	Weakness	none	Nausea	None
Required hospitalization	yes	no	yes	no	no	no	no	no
Outcome	Recovered without sequelae	Recovered without sequelae	Recovered without sequelae	Recovered without sequelae	Recovered without sequelae	Recovered without sequelae	Recovered without sequelae	Recovered without sequelae
RUCAM	Probable	Probable	Possible	Probable	Possible	Probable	Probable	Possible

Abbreviations: *Pt* Patient, *HCV* Hepatitis C virus, *ARV* Antiretroviral, *d4T* Stavudine, *3TC* Lamivudine, *ABC* Abacavir, *AZT* Zidovudine, *ddi* Didanosine, *RUCAM* Roussel Uclaf Causality Assessment Method

Interestingly, the functional variant c.3435 C > T of ABCB1 gene was associated with an increases risk for severe liver toxicity in a previous study conducted by Hass et al. in South-Africa [19]. Moreover, the variant ABCB1 c.3435 C > T resulted protective for NVP-associated hepatic adverse events in another study conducted in Mozambique [20]. No statistically significant association between ABCB1 c.3435 C > T and NVP adverse events was found in another study conducted by Yuan J et al. in an ethnic mixed population. However, these authors found a significant association between ABCB1 c.3435 C > T variant and hepatic adverse events among Africans but not Asians or Caucasians, despite these latter groups showed increased T-allele frequencies [31].

Overall our study, which was conducted on a prevalently European Caucasian population, disagrees with the study by Yan et al. On the contrary it supports the protective role of T allele of ABCB1 rs1045642 for NVP-hepatotoxicity evidenced by Hass et al. and Ciccacci et al.

The present study has some limitations. In particular, due to the retrospective design we cannot exclude the presence of possible bias related to loss of data. A sub-optimal performance of RUCAM, which is more fitted for a prospective patient evaluation, could be hypothesized because of the

Table 4 Disposition of polymorphisms involved in nevirapine metabolism

	Total	Hepatotoxicity	No hepatotoxicity	*p**
	n = 362	*n* = 8	*n* = 354	
ABCB1 c.3435/rs1045642, n (%)				*0.019*
CC	86 (23.8)	5 (5.8)	81 (94.2)	
CT	178 (49.2)	1 (0.6)	177 (99.4)	
TT	98 (27.0)	2 (2.0)	96 (98.0)	
CYP2B6 c.516/rs3745274, n (%)				0.706
GG	196 (54.1)	6 (3.1)	190 (96.9)	
GT	141 (39.0)	2 (1.4)	139 (98.6)	
TT	25 (6.9)	0 (0.0)	25 (100.0)	
CYP3A4/A5 **, n (%)				0.602
Extensive	58 (16.1)	0 (0.0)	58 (100.0)	
Intermediate	270 (74.5)	8 (3.0)	262 (97.0)	
Poor	25 (6.9)	0 (0.0)	25 (100.0)	
nd	9 (2.5)	0 (0.0)	9 (100.0)	

Abbreviations: *n* number, *nd* not determined, *ABCB* ATP Binding Cassette Subfamily B, *CYP* Cytochrome P450 enzyme
*χ2 test ** CYP3A4*22/rs35599367 and CYP3A5*3/rs776746 combined genotypes for comprehensive functional evaluation [33, 34]

Table 5 Backward logistic regression of factors involved in nevirapine induced liver toxicity

	OR (95%CI)	*p*	aOR (95%CI)	*p*
Male vs Female	0.19 (0.04–0.94)	*0.042*	0.27 (0.06–1.30)	0.102
Age (× 1 year more)	0.96 (0.88–1.04)	0.293	–	
MSM vs HE	0.24 (0.01–4.51)	0.338	–	
IVDUs vs HE	2.20 (0.58–8.41)	0.247	–	
Other vs HE	1.36 (0.06–29.16)	0.844	–	
Caucasian vs Non-Caucasian	0.67 (0.08–5.64)	0.714	–	
BMI (× 1 more)	0.70 (0.51–0.94)	*0.020*	0.72 (0.52–1.00)	0.050
Previous AIDS	0.67 (0.08–5.56)	0.713	–	
Previous therapy duration (× 1 year more)	1.05 (0.90–1.23)	0.518	–	
CD4 200–500 cell/μL vs < 200 cell/μL	1.17 (0.05–25.7)	0.920	1.51 (0.07–32.23)	0.790
CD4 > 500 cell/μL vs < 200 cell/μL	3.97 (0.21–74.51)	0.357	8.12 (0.42–156.90)	0.166
HIV-RNA (× 1 log10 more)	0.80 (0.54–1.18)	0.260	–	
AST (× 1 more)	1.02 (1.01–1.03)	*0.008*	1.01 (0.99–1.03)	0.144
ALT (× 1 more)	1.01 (1.00–1.02)	*0.015*	–	
HCV coinfection	6.93 (1.38–34.87)	*0.019*	8.00 (1.27–50.29)	*0.027*
HBV coinfection	2.39 (0.28–20.36)	0.427	–	
ARV Backbone: AZT/DDI/D4T vs ABC	0.73 (0.12–4.47)	0.731	–	
ARV Backbone: TDF vs ABC	0.12 (0.01–3.141)	0.204	–	
ARV Backbone: Other vs ABC	0.49 (0.02–13.47)	0.672	–	
ABCB1 rs1045642 CT/TT vs CC	0.18 (0.04–0.76)	*0.020*	0.10 (0.02–0.47)	*0.004*

Abbreviations: *OR* Odds Ratio, *aOR* adjusted Odds Ratio, *CI* confidence interval, *HE* Heterosexual, *MSM* Man how have sex with man, *IVDUs* Intra venous drug users, *BMI* Body Mass Index, *cps* copies, *ABC* abacavir, *TDF* tenofovir diproxil fumarate, *BMI* Body Mass Index, *ABCB* ATP Binding Cassette Subfamily B

retrospective nature of the study. Moreover, if on one hand the limited number of NVP induced hepatic adverse events supports the good safety profile of this drug in ART-experienced patients, on the other hand our study could not exclude that the prevalence of the investigated polymorphisms could be driven by chance. Moreover, the prevalence of Caucasian ethnicity limited the comparison of our findings between different ethnic groups.

Conclusion

Beyond to clinical conditions well known to drive the development of hepatotoxicity during NVP treatment, i.e. HCV coinfection and body mass index, pharmacogenomic profiles could also play a role in this phenomenon. Our results suggest the independent role of ABCB1 rs1045642 as a predictive marker of severe liver toxicity related to NVP. Further validation studies, to assess possible clinical application of this marker in countries in which NVP is still widely used and/or in patients with other risk factors for nevirapine related toxicity, are warranted.

Abbreviations

ABCB: ATP Binding Cassette Subfamily B; aOR: Adjusted Odds Ratio; ART: Antiretroviral treatment; CI: Confidence interval; CYP: Cytochrome P450 enzyme; HIV-1: Human immunodeficiency virus type 1; IQR: Inter quartile range; NVP: Nevirapine; OR: Odds Ratio; RUCAM: Roussel Uclaf Causality Assessment Methods; SNPs: Single nucleotide polymorphisms

Acknowledgements

We thank Mrs. Tiziana Formenti for the excellent technical help.

Funding

No financial support to this study.

Authors' contributions

AG, ALR, AR, FSF, MLO, MG, SR designed the study. GR, VDC, AL assessed the patient's documentation and evaluated the inclusion in the study. AG, ALR, GR, VDC, AL, were involved in data collection and interpretation. FSF, EC, DC, SC performed laboratory analyses. AG, MLO were responsible for the statistical analyses. All authors interpreted the data and drafted the manuscript. All authors have critically revised and approved the final version.

Competing interests

S.R. has received consultancy payments and speaking fee from Bristol-Myers Squibb, Gilead, ViiV Healthcare, Merck Sharp Dohme, ABBvie and Janssen. M.G. has received consultancy payments and speaking fee from Bristol-Myers Squibb, Gilead, ViiV Healthcare, Merck Sharp Dohme, ABBvie, Janssen and Roche. Preliminary data of this study were presented as poster presentation (PE10/15) at the 16th European AIDS conference, October 25–27, 2017 Milan, Italy.

Author details

[1]Infectious Diseases Unit, DIBIC Luigi Sacco - University of Milan, Via G.B. Grassi, 74, 20157 Milan, Italy. [2]ASST Fatebenefratelli-Sacco, Clinical Pharmacology Unit, Milan, Italy. [3]E. Medea Scientific Institute, Bosisio Parini, Italy.

References

1. Milinkovic A, Martínez E. Nevirapine in the treatment of HIV. Expert Rev Anti-Infect Ther. 2004;2:367–73.
2. De Boissieu P, Dramé M, Raffi F, et al. Dat'AIDS study group. Long-term efficacy and toxicity of abacavir/lamivudine/nevirapine compared to the most prescribed ARV regimens before 2013 in a French Nationwide cohort study. Medicine (Baltimore). 2016;95(37):e4890.
3. Reliquet V, Allavena C, Morineau-Le Houssine P, Mounoury O, Raffi F. Twelve-year experience of nevirapine use: benefits and convenience for long-term management in a French cohort of HIV-1-infected patients. HIV Clin Trials. 2010;11(2):110–7.
4. Llibre JM, Bravo I, Ornelas A, et al. Effectiveness of a treatment switch to Nevirapine plus Tenofovir and Emtricitabine (or lamivudine) in adults with HIV-1 suppressed viremia. PLoS One. 2015;10(6):e0128131.
5. Patel SM, Johnson S, Belknap SM, et al. Serious adverse cutaneous and hepatic toxicities associated with nevirapine use by non-HIV-infected individuals. J Acquir Immune Defic Syndr. 2004 Feb 1;35(2):120–5.
6. Stern JO, Robinson PA, Love J, et al. A comprehensive hepatic safety analysis of nevirapine in different populations of HIV infected patients. J Acquir Immune Defic Syndr. 2003;34(Suppl. 1):S21–33.
7. Dieterich DT, Robinson PA, Love J, Stern JO. Drug-induced liver injury associated with the use of nonnucleoside reverse-transcriptase inhibitors. Clin Infect Dis. 2004;38(Suppl. 2):S80–9.
8. Wu PY, Cheng CY, Liu CE, et al. Multicenter study of skin rashes and hepatotoxicity in antiretroviral-naïve HIV-positive patients receiving non-nucleoside reverse-transcriptase inhibitor plus nucleoside reverse-transcriptase inhibitors in Taiwan. PLoS One. 2017 Feb 21;12(2):e0171596.
9. Kesselring AM, Wit FW, Sabin CA, Lundgren JD, Gill MJ, Gatell JM, et al. Risk factors for treatment-limiting toxicities in patients starting nevirapine-containing antiretroviral therapy. AIDS. 2009;23:1689–99.
10. Mocroft A, Staszewski S, Weber R, et al. EuroSIDA study group. Risk of discontinuation of nevirapine due to toxicities in antiretroviral-naïve and -experienced HIV-infected patients with high and low CD4+ T-cell counts. Antivir Ther. 2007;12(3):325–33.
11. Van Welzen B, Mudrikova T, Arends J, Hoepelman A. No increased risk of hepatotoxicity in long-term use of nonnucleoside reverse transcriptase inhibitors in HIV-infected patients. HIV Med. 2012;13(7):448–52.
12. Sanne I, Mommeja-Marin H, Hinkle J, et al. Severe hepatotoxicity associated with nevirapine use in HIV-infected subjects. J Infect Dis. 2005;191(6):825–9.
13. Riska P, Lamson M, MacGregor T, Sabo J, Hattox S, Pav J, Keirns J. Disposition and biotransformation of the antiretroviral drug nevirapine in humans. Drug Metab Dispos. 1999;27:895–901.
14. Bertrand J, Chou M, Richardson DM, et al. ANRS 12154 study group. Multiple genetic variants predict steady-state nevirapine clearance in HIV-infected Cambodians. Pharmacogenet Genomics. 2012;22(12):868–76.
15. Penzak SR, Kabuye G, Mugyenyi P, et al. Cytochrome P450 2B6 (CYP2B6) G516T influences nevirapine plasma concentrations in HIV-infected patients in Uganda. HIV Med. 2007;8(2):86–91.
16. Wyen C, Hendra H, Vogel M, et al. Impact of CYP2B6 983T>C polymorphism on non-nucleoside reverse transcriptase inhibitor plasma concentrations in HIV-infected patients. J Antimicrob Chemother. 2008;61:914–8.
17. Rotger M, Colombo S, Furrer H, et al. Influence of CYP2B6 polymorphism on plasma and intracellular concentrations and toxicity of efavirenz and nevirapine in HIV-infected patients. Pharmacogenet Genomics. 2005;15:1–5.
18. Gozalo C, Grard L, Loiseau P, et al. For the ANRS 081 study group pharmacogenetics of toxicity, plasma trough concentration and treatment outcome with Nevirapine-containing regimen in anti-retroviral-nave HIV-infected adults: an exploratory study of the TRIANON ANRS 081 trial. Basic & Clinical Pharmacology & Toxicology. 2011;109:513–20.
19. Haas DW, Bartlett JA, Andersen JW, et al. Pharmacogenetics of nevirapine-associated hepatotoxicity: an adult AIDS Clinical Trials Group collaboration. Clin Infect Dis. 2006;43:783–6.
20. Ciccacci C, Borgiani P, Ceffa S, et al. Nevirapine-induced hepatotoxicity and pharmacogenetics: a retrospective study in a population from Mozambique. Pharmacogenomics. 2010;11:23–31.
21. Danan G, Teschke R. RUCAM in drug and herb induced liver injury: the update. Int J Mol Sci. 2016;17(1):14.
22. Brück S, Witte S, Brust J, et al. Hepatotoxicity in patients prescribed efavirenz or nevirapine. Eur J Med Res. 2008;13:343–8.
23. Bekker Z, Walubo A, du Plessis JB. The role of the immune system in Nevirapine-induced subclinical liver injury of a rat model. ISRN Pharmaceutics. 2012;2012:932542.
24. Núñez M. Hepatotoxicity of antiretrovirals: incidence, mechanisms and management. J Hepatol. 2006;44(1 Suppl):S132–9 Epub 2005 Nov 28.
25. Sulkowski MS, Thomas DL, Chaisson RE, Moore RD. Hepatotoxicity associated with antiretroviral therapy in adults infected with human immunodeficiency virus and the role of hepatitis C or B virus infection. JAMA. 2000;283:74–80.
26. Vogel M, Bertram N, Wasmuth JC, Wyen C, Voigt E, Schwarze-Zander C, Sudhop T, Fätkenheuer G, Rockstroh JK, Reichel C. Nevirapine pharmacokinetics in HIV-infected and HIV/HCV-coinfected individuals. J Antimicrob Chemother. 2009 May;63(5):988–91.
27. Wen B, Chen Y, Fitch WL. Metabolic activation of nevirapine in human liver microsomes: dehydrogenation and inactivation of cytochrome P450 3A4. Drug Metab Dispos. 2009 Jul;37(7):1557–62.
28. Schipani A, Wyen C, Mahungu T, et al. German competence network for HIV/AIDS. Integration of population pharmacokinetics and pharmacogenetics: an aid to optimal nevirapine dose selection in HIV-infected individuals. J Antimicrob Chemother. 2011;66(6):1332–9.
29. Mahungu T, Smith C, Turner F, et al. Cytochrome P450 2B6 516G-->T is associated with plasma concentrations of nevirapine at both 200 mg twice daily and 400 mg once daily in an ethnically diverse population. HIV Med. 2009 May;10(5):310–7.
30. Giacomelli A, Rusconi S, Falvella FS, et al. Clinical and genetic determinants of nevirapine plasma trough concentration. SAGE Open Med. 2018;6: 2050312118780861.
31. Yuan J, Guo S, Hall D, et al. Nevirapine Toxicogenomics study team. Toxicogenomics of nevirapine-associated cutaneous and hepatic adverse events among populations of African, Asian, and European descent. AIDS. 2011;25(10):1271–80.
32. Owen A, Pirmohamed M, Khoo HS, Back DJ. Pharmacogenetics of HIV therapy. Pharmacogenet Genomics. 2006;16:693–703.
33. Zanger UM, Schwab M. Cytochrome P450 enzymes in drug metabolism: regulation of gene expression, enzyme activities, and impact of genetic variation. Pharmacol Ther. 2013 Apr;138(1):103–41.
34. Kitzmiller JP, Sullivan DM, Phelps MA, Wang D, Sadee W. CYP3A4/5 combined genotype analysis for predicting statin dose requirement for optimal lipid control. Drug Metabol Drug Interact. 2013;28(1):59–63.

28

Genetic diversity of drug resistant *Mycobacterium Tuberculosis* in local area of Southwest China

Tao Shi[1*†], Tongxin Li[2†], Jungang Li[2], Jing Wang[2] and Zehua Zhang[3*]

Abstract

Background: By 2014 although tuberculosis (TB) incidence had fallen by an average of 1.5% per year since 2000 and was 18% lower than the level of in 2000, 1.5 million people died for TB in that year. One of reason was that drug resistant *Mycobacterium tuberculosis* (DRTB) spread. This study aims to determine drug resistant characteristics and genotype of DRTB that isolated from patients in a tuberculosis referral hospital of southwest China.

Methods: Five hundred thirty-eight drug resistant tuberculosis samples were collected from July 2013 to March 2015. All the isolates were identified by genomic deletions in region of difference 105 (RD105) and genotyped by mycobacterial interspersed repetitive unit-variable number tandem repeat typing (MIRU-VNTR). Polymorphism and cluster analysis of each locus was carried out using Bionumerics Version 3.0 and phyloviz software.

Results: Five hundred thirty-eight TB strains included 503 *Mycobacterium tuberculosis* (MTB) isolates and 35 non *Mycobacterium tuberculosis* (NMTB) isolates. Of 503 isolates Beijing family type was 447 (88.9%, 447/503) and non-Beijing family type was 56 (11.1%, 56/503). Five hundred three DRTB isolates were divided into 345 genotypes, of which 265 isolates were single genotype and the remaining 238 strains were classified into 80 clusters with cluster rate of 47.3% and cluster ratio of 31.4%. Sixty-nine clusters belonged to Beijing family with cluster rate was 48.3% and clustering ratio was 32.9%. The non - Beijing family had 11 clusters with a cluster rate of 39.3% and the clustering ratio of 19.6%. Beijing genotype had a significant correlation with the age ($P < 0.05$), the retreatment patients ($P < 0.05$) and the city of Chongqing ($P < 0.05$), not with gender ($P > 0.05$). In the 9 Beijing genotype clusters each cluster contained some patients who lived in the same region.

Conclusions: Beijing genotype was the predominant in the patients with DRTB in our hospital. In Chongqing retreatment patients with Beijing genotype MTB may be patient with DRTB. Drug resistance test (DST), regular medication and strict follow-up are very important for patients with Beijing genotype MTB. In Chongqing control and treatment of DRTB should be paid attention. Transmission and relations of patients with DRTB need to be further research.

Keywords: *Mycobacterium tuberculosis*, Drug resistance, Genetic diversity, Transmission

* Correspondence: shitaostone@163.com; shitaostone@163.com; zhangzehuatmmu@163.com
†Tao Shi and Tongxin Li contributed equally to this work.
[1]Department of Orthopedics, The Third Affiliated Hospital of Chongqing Medical University (Gener Hospital), No. 1, Shuanghu Branch Road, Yubei District, Chongqing 401120, China
[3]Department of Orthopedics, Southwest Hospital, Third Military Medical University, No. 30, Gaotanyan Main Street, Shapingba District, Chongqing 400038, China
Full list of author information is available at the end of the article

Background

With the development of tuberculosis diagnosis and treatment methods, the prevention and control of tuberculosis has made great progress. In 2014 tuberculosis (TB) incidence had fallen by an average of 1.5% per year since 2000 and was 18% lower than the level of 2000 according to the "Global Tuberculosis Report 2015" from the World Health Organization (WHO) [1]. Unfortunately about 3.3% of new cases and 20% of previously treated cases were drug resistant *Mycobacterium tuberculosis* (DRTB) [1]. In 2014 about approximately 1.5 million people died of DRTB [1].

China is one of the world's 22 high tuberculosis burden countries and faces the challenge of DRTB, which accounted for 22 to 30% of all cases of tuberculosis [1]. It is unknown whether the spread of DRTB originates from acquire resistance or primary resistance, especially multidrug-resistant tuberculosis (MDR-TB) and extensive drug resistance tuberculosis (XDR-TB). MDR-TB is defined as resistance to at least isoniazid and rifampin, while XDR-TB is defined as having resistance to rifampin and isoniazid as well as any member of the quinolone family and at least one of the remaining second-line anti-TB injectable drugs. The traditional epidemiology investigation lack optimal way to gain answer about this problem.

Early molecular epidemiological tools had provided a reliable way to investigate molecular evolution over shorter and longer periods of time [2–5]. Although IS*6110*-restriction fragment length polymorphism DNA fingerprinting had been the genotyping technique used most widely for MTB and was considered a "gold standard", it is no longer widely used due to time-consuming, technically demanding and requirement of large quantities of high-quality DNA [6]. According to comparison results of different ways, spoligotyping or RD105 was a reliable standard for identifying strains as belonging to the Beijing family because it is simple, highly reproducible and applicable to a digital format and mycobacterial interspersed repetitive unit–variable number tandem repeat typing (MIRU-VNTR) was the most reliable method for the genetic differentiation of MTB isolates because the discriminatory power of this method can be comparable to that of IS*6110* typing [7–9].

Chongqing is the largest municipality located in southwestern China and a city of high incidence of tuberculosis. An epidemiological study demonstrated that the rates of primary and acquired MDR-TB were 3.8 and 26.9%, respectively [10]. Sichuan Province is an adjacent area at the northwest Chongqing and also a high incidence of tuberculosis [8]. Nevertheless; we still have no knowledge of the potential transmission profile of DRTB in these areas. In this study in order to determine drug resistant characteristics, genotype and spread of DRTB, we genotyped the DRTB isolates using RD105 and MIRU-VNTR. The relationship between the molecular characteristics and transmission of DRTB was also analyzed.

Methods

Bacterial strains and culture conditions

From July 2013 to March 2015 a total of 753 samples from The Public Health Medical Center and the 12th People's Hospital of Chongqing were collected. Various *M. tuberculosis* culture and identification systems were used during the study period. The bacterial strains and culture conditions were the same as what Weng described [11]. The first was the BACTEC MGIT 960 system (Becton Dickinson, Sparks, Maryland, USA). Clinical specimens were processed, and the centrifuged sediment was inoculated onto Löwenstein-Jensen (LJ) medium (BBL; Becton Dickinson, Sparks, MD, USA) and Middlebrook 7H9 broth (BBL; Becton Dickinson). The cultures were incubated at 35 °C in 5% carbon dioxide for up to 8 weeks. Identification of *M. tuberculosis* was based on colony morphology and biochemical reactions (nitrate reduction and niacin test). Bacterial cells were isolated from LJ medium.

Drug susceptibility testing

The isolates were determined by conventional proportional drug susceptibility test. The concentrations of drugs in media were as follows: isoniazid (INH) 0.2 μg/ml, rifampicin (RFP) 40 μg/ml, ethambutol (EMB) 2 μg/ml, streptomycin (SM) 4 μg/ml, amikacin (AMK) 30 μg/ml, capreomycin (Cm) 40 μg/ml, levofloxacin (Lofx) 2 μg/ml, protionamide (Pto) 40 μg/ml and dipasic (PAIN) 0.1 μg/ml [10]. A strain was declared resistant to a drug when the growth rate was > 1% compared with the control. MDR-TB strains were defined as those resistant to both isoniazid and rifampicin. In addition, isolates resistant to rifampicin and isoniazid as well as any member of the quinolone family and at least one of the remaining second-line anti-TB injectable drugs were defined as XDR-TB.

Genomic DNA extraction

Genomic DNA was extracted from freshly cultured bacteria. Following centrifugation at 13000 rpm for 2 min, the bacterial cells were transferred to a microcentrifuge tube containing 500 ml Trisethylenediaminetetraacetic acid (TE) buffer. The supernatant was discarded and the pellet was resuspended in 500 ml TE buffer and heated in a 95 °C water bath for 1 h. The cellular debris was isolated by centrifugation at 13000 rpm for 5 min and the DNA in the supernatant was used for PCR amplification reactions.

Genotyping

The identification of genomic deletions in region of difference 105 (RD105) was performed by PCR to distinguish Beijing type from non-Beijing type. Briefly, each PCR mixture was prepared in a volume of 20 μl containing 19 μl RD105 PCR Mix and 1 μl DNA template. The amplification cycle was 10 min at 95 °C followed by 25 cycles of 30 s at 94 °C, 30 s at 68 °C, and 3 min at 72 °C, with a final step for 7 min at 72 °C.

To identify a suitable MIRU-VNTR loci set for genotyping *M. tuberculosis* in this area, the number of tandem repeats was determined in 12 MIRU-VNTR genetic loci: four original MIRU-VNTR loci: MIRU-10, MIRU-26, MIRU-31, MIRU-40; one loci of exact tandem repeats (ETRs): ETR- F; two Mtub loci: Mtub-04, Mtub-21; five Queen's University of Belfast (QUBs) loci: QUB-11b, −18,-26, −4156 and 1895. QUB-11b, QUB-18, QUB-26, QUB-4156, MIRU26, MIRU31, MIRU10, Mtub21 and Mtub04 locus of MTB isolates was amplified separately by PCR using specific primers. Briefly, 1 μl of DNA was added to 19 μl of reagent mix. The amplification parameters consisted of 10 min at 95 °C, followed by 30 cycles of 30 s at 94 °C, 30 s at 58 °C, and 90 s at 72 °C, with a final extension at 72 °C for 7 min. QUB-1895, MIRU40 and ETR-F locus of MTB isolates was amplified separately by PCR using specific primers. Briefly, 1 μl of DNA was added to 19 μl of reagent mix. The amplification parameters consisted of 10 min at 95 °C, followed by 30 cycles of 30 s at 94 °C, 30 s at 64 °C, and 90 s at 72 °C, with a final extension at 72 °C for 7 min. The PCR products were electrophoresed on a 1% agarose gel. The H37Rv strain was assayed in the same manner as a control. The Hunter–Gaston discriminatory index (HGDI) was used to evaluate the discriminatory power of the MIRU-VNTR loci. BioNumerics (version 5.0, Applied Maths, Sint-Martens-Latem, Belgium) was used to construct the Minimal Spanning Trees (MSTs) based on VNTR data. A dendrogram was constructed based on the chi square test and the software package MEGA (version 6.0).

Statistical analysis

All data were presented as mean ± standard deviation (SD) or frequency. Statistical analysis for possible significant association between the different symptoms and different genotype *M. tuberculosis* was performed using Chi-square test. All tests were set as two sides and a P value of < 0.05 was considered statistical significant.

Results

In the 753 samples there were 215 (28.6%) negative culture samples and 538 (71.4%) positive culture samples that included 503 *Mycobacterium tuberculosis (*MTB) isolates and 35 non *Mycobacterium tuberculosis* (NMTB) isolates.

Demography

The mean age of 503 patients including 189 female and 314 male was 38.9 ± 14.9 years old (16–78 years old). There were 201 new patients and 302 previously treated patients. Table 1 displayed distribution of patients in different regions. There are 19 districts and 19 counties in Chongqing and 21 cities in Sichuan Province. Most patients lived in Chongqing regions or near the Chongqing and few patients lived out of Chongqing, but all the patients lived in Chongqing when they suffered from DRTB. Patients from Chongqing accounted for 82.1, 16.1% from Sichuan Province and 1.8% from other regions.

Table 1 Distribution of 503 patients in different regions ($n = 503$)

Chongqing ($n = 413$)						Sichuan Province ($n = 81$)		Other regions ($n = 9$)	
Pengshui	62	Tongliang	10	Dazu	2	Dazhou	44	Tibet	1
Shapingba	33	Yuzhong	10	Fengjie	2	Guangan	23	Jilin Province	1
Banan	29	Wulong	9	Youyang	2	Ziyang	4	Hubei Province	1
Yubei	25	Dadukou	9	Yunyang	2	Yibin	3	Heilongjiang Province	1
Fengdu	21	Yongchuan	6	Wushan	2	Guangyuan	2	Guizhou Dejiang	1
Nanan	20	Jiangjin	6	Tongnan	2	Luzhou	2	Guizhou Fenggang	1
Beibei	20	Nanchuan	6	Rongchang	1	Neijiang	2	Guizhou Qianxi	1
Changshou	19	Bishan	5	Shizhu	1	Chengdu	1	Guizhou Tongren	1
Zhong	16	Kai	5	Wanzhou	1			Guizhou Yinjiang	1
Fuling	15	Qijiang	5	Xiushan	1				
Hechuan	15	Liangping	5	Qiangjiang	1				
Jiulongpo	14	Wansheng	4						
Dianjiang	13	Wuxi	4						

Characteristics of DRTB

All the 503 isolates were MDR-TB. There were 75 (14.9%) XDR-TB in the 503 isolates. Of 503 patients there were some special varieties of resistant drugs. There were 34(6.8%) patients with only resistance to INH and RFP including 27(5.4%) new and 7(1.4%) retreatment patients; 61(12.1%) only resistance to first-line drug including 43(8.5%) new and 18(3.6%) retreatment patients; 54(10.7%) resistance to INH, RFP and any second-line drug including 15(3.0%) new and 39(7.7%) retreatment patients; 17(3.4%) resistance to all test drugs including 5(1.0%) new and 12(2.4%) retreatment patients. The numbers of new and retreatment of patients resistant to Lofx, Pto and PAIN were a significant statistical difference, retreatment patients were more obviously resistant to the above three drugs than new cases (Fig. 1a). Male patients of resistant to AMK and PAIN had a significant statistical difference with female patients; the male was more obviously resistant than the female resistant to AMK and PAIN (Fig. 1b). Resistance to PAIN was more common than the other anti-TB drugs in the retreatment patients and male patients.

The identification of genomic RD105

The collection of 503 DRTB isolates was analyzed by RD105 in this study. 447 (88.9%) isolates belonged to the Beijing genotype, while 56 (11.1%) were from non-Beijing families, demonstrating that Beijing is the predominant genotype.

MIRU-VNTR profiles and genotypes

Five hundred three strains were divided into 345 genotypes that included 265 strains were a single genotype and the remaining 230 strains were classified into 80 clusters (2–24 isolates per cluster). The cluster rate was 47.3% and the cluster ratio was 31.4%. Four hundred forty-seven Beijing genotype isolates were clustered into 69 genotypes and 56 non-Beijing genotype isolates were clustered into 11 genotypes. The cumulative clustering rates of Beijing genotype and non-Beijing genotype strains were 48.3 and 39.3%, respectively. The both clustering ratio were 32.9 and 19.6%, respectively. The non-Beijing genotype isolates came from the newly diagnosed patients.

The details of 80 clusters were displayed in the Table 2 and Fig. 2. Figure 3 displayed the minimum spanning tree of 503 DRTB isolates according to MIRU-VNTR results.

HGDI showed that the 12-site combination had a total resolution index of 0.99. The allelic diversity of each MIRU-VNTR locus was evaluated using the HGDI (Table 3). Overall, the HGDI of four loci (QUB18, Mtub21, QUB26 and QUB11b) exceeded 0.6, classified as highly discriminating loci. The six loci (QUB1895, QUB4156, MIRU26, MIRU31, MIRU40 and Mtub04) showed moderate discrimination (0.3 < HGDI< 0.6). The MIRU10 and ERT-F showed low discrimination loci. A dendrogram was generated based on the genotypes of the 503 isolates using 12 loci.

Comparison between demographic characteristics and DRTB

Clinical factors, including age, gender and treatment history were analyzed between the Beijing and non-Beijing family (Table 4). Beijing genotype had a significant correlation with the age ($P < 0.05$), the retreatment patients ($P < 0.05$) and Chongqing ($P < 0.05$), not with gender ($P > 0.05$). In particular, isolates from patients with retreatment were all Beijing genotype, and there was no statistical result.

Distribution of DRTB

All patients lived in the above regions. The living regions of patients carrying clustering isolates were analyzed. Although all the patients carrying non-Beijing genotype clustering isolates came from different regions of Chongqing, some patients carrying Beijing genotype clustering isolates came from the same regions of Chongqing. Table 5 displayed regional distribution of some patients with Beijing genotype. The patients of the remaining Beijing genotype clusters came from different regions of Chongqing. In each non-Beijing genotype cluster there were no patients who come from the same region. In our study Pengshui, Shapingba and Banan were three regions of high incidence in Chongqing and locate in the southeast Chongqing, while Dazhou and Guangan were two regions of high incidence in Sichuan Province and locate in northeast Sichuan Province (Table 1).

Discussion

The Beijing genotype of *Mycobacterium tuberculosis* was first discovered by Soolingen in 1995 [12]. Since then, several studies have reported that Beijing genotype MTB is the main pathogen type of TB and DRTB patients [13–18]. In our study, a large number of patients with multiple MDR patients in Chongqing were collected. The basic types of DRTB were analyzed systematically. The results showed that DRTB in this region was mainly Beijing family type, accounting for 93.4%, which is similar to most of the current DRTB molecular type of research reports but not exactly the same. The results of the national tuberculosis drug resistance baseline analysis showed that the DR ratio of Beijing genotype strains was 63.97% in China and 59.97% in the southwest China [19], while our study showed the DR ratio of Beijing genotype strains was 88.9% that was significantly higher than the levels of nationwide and southwest

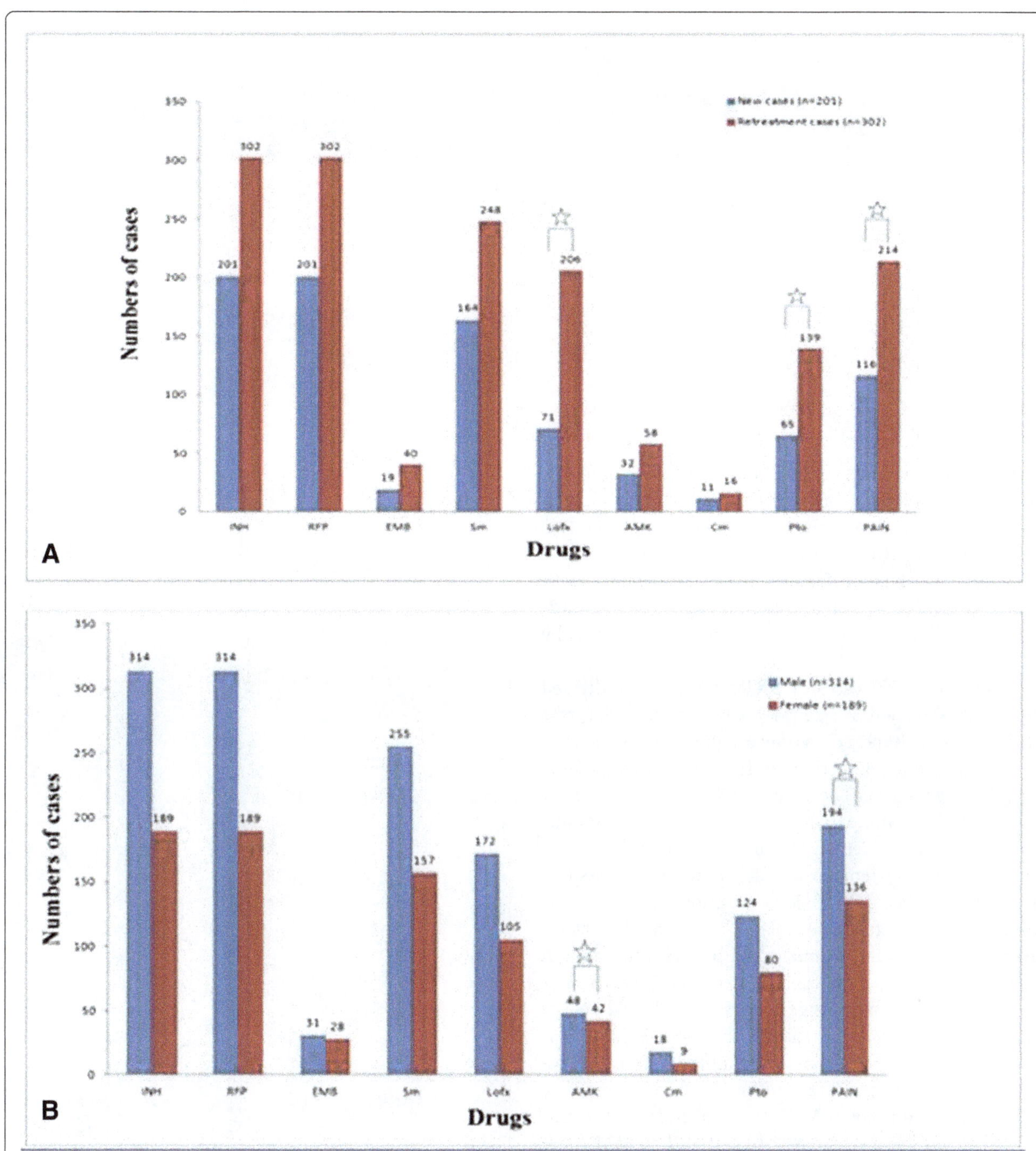

Fig. 1 **a** Distribution of the new cases and retreatment cases in the different anti-TB drugs. **b** Distribution of femal and male patients in the different anti-TB drugs. ☆ Means $P < 0.05$

China. This suggests that the prevalence of the Beijing genotype family in Chongqing may result in the spread of DRTB.

Anti-TB chemotherapy is the cornerstone of treatment of patients with MTB [20]. Unfortunately, evolution of TB leads to be resistant to anti-TB drugs. DRTB is a big challenge to anti-TB treatment. Many researchers studied the DR characteristics of DRTB. Fox example, according to Kapil's research the DR ratio of INH, RFP and SM were 92.7, 81.9 and 69.3%, respectively [21]. Another article showed SM and EMB were most common resistant drugs [10]. In this study INH, RFP and SM were three most common first-line anti-TB resistant drugs and Lofx and PAIN were common second-line

Table 2 Details of 80 clusters

Genotype	No. of cluster	No. of strains in each cluster
Beijing-type		
	1	26
	1	11
	1	10
	1	9
	1	8
	1	7
	4	4
	9	3
	50	2
Non-Beijing-type		
	11	2

anti-TB resistant drugs. In addition DR ratio of Lofx, Pto and PAIN in the retreatment patients was higher than in the new case and resistance to AMK and PAIN was more common in male patients than female. These results may be helpful for treatment of patients with DRTB in southwest China. Different studies have shown the DR ration of different anti-TB drugs varied by regions.

In this study, 503 cases of DRTB strains were divided into 80 clusters and 345 genotypes with a clustering rate of 47.3%. Two hundred sixty-five patients were isolated as a single genotype, accounting for 52.7% of all patients (265/503), which may be considered to be independent isolates and no mutual transmission between patients, but rather independent infection or endogenous recurrent disease. The remaining 238 strains were classified in to 80 clusters, that the largest cluster of which contained 26 Beijing genotype isolates, including 22 isolates from the Chongqing Municipal Public Health Medical Treatment Center and 4 isolates from the Twelfth People's Hospital of Chongqing. By analyzing the redidential regions of patients in the clusters that contained ≥3 isolates, we found some isolates transmitted within one region and had tendency transmitting to an adjacent area. There was a study about MDR transmitting across countries [22]. All these researches suggested the DRTB were transmitting more and more widely. Additional, each cluster of DRTB highly suggested that these isolates belonged to their respective groups and in each group isolates had a certain relationship according to results of MIRU-VNTR. Cross analysis results of MIRU-VNTR and living locations of patients suggested that patients with DRTB were cross-infection, that is, these patients with DRTB are primary resistant, rather than due to withdrawal and relapse. Continue to track these patients to determine the cause of resistance, such as whether patients with the same genotype are relative, contact

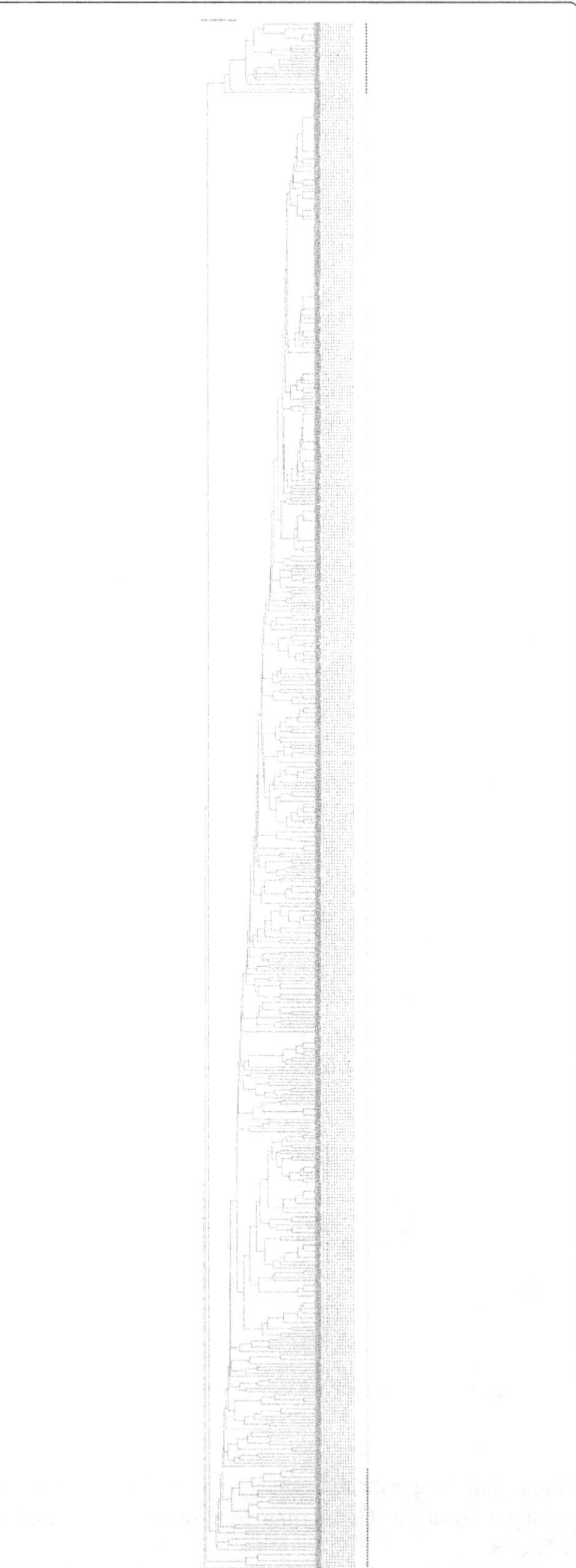

Fig. 2 Dendrogram of 503 DRTB isolates. The phylogenetic tree was generated from the MIRU-VNTR profile

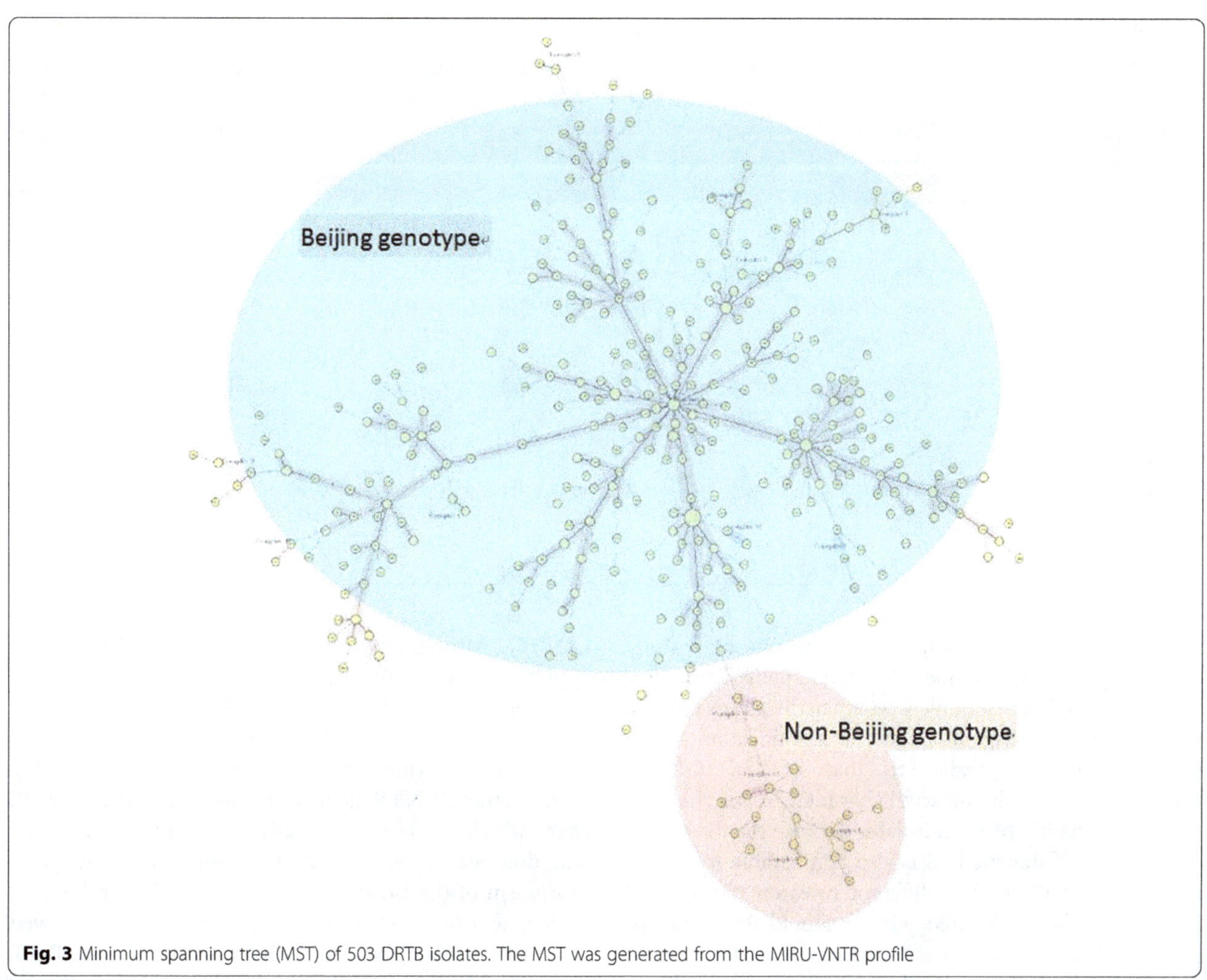

Fig. 3 Minimum spanning tree (MST) of 503 DRTB isolates. The MST was generated from the MIRU-VNTR profile

Table 3 Allelic diversity of 12 different MIRU-VNTR loci among Mycobacterium tuberculosis strains

	Locus	HGDI
1	QUB-11b	0.62
2	QUB-18	0.65
3	QUB-26	0.66
4	QUB-4156	0.37
5	QUB-1895	0.37
6	MIRU26	0.57
7	MIRU31	0.47
8	MIRU10	0.26
9	MIRU40	0.44
10	Mtub21	0.62
11	Mtub04	0.55
12	ETR-F	0.26

history and living in the same community, which is the focus of our follow-up study.

MTB genotyping can explain the epidemiology, infection, pathogenesis and DR of MTB from the molecular level and it is important in TB epidemiological investigation, surveillance and transmission source discovery and transmission pathways. MIRU-VNTR was classified according to the difference of the number of copies between different strains. The method was simple, the result was digitized and the resolution was high, which was convenient for comparison between different laboratories. Compared to IS*6110*-RFLP which used to be the "gold standard" for DNA fingerprints of MTB, MIRU-VNTR has obviously advantages. Using the MIRU-VNTR 191 Beijing family-type MTB were divided into 110 unique genotype and 27 clusters in China [8] and in Sichuan 191 Beijing Mycobacterium tuberculosis has 65 unique genotypes and 8 clusters [23]. In addition, Chinese Center for Disease Control and Prevention analyzed 4017 MTB isolates from 31 different provinces that were divided into 161 clusters and 407 isolates using spoligotyping and

Table 4 Clinical characteristics of the Beijing and non-Beijing family strains

Characteristics	Total	Beijing family	Non-Beijing family	χ^2	*P*-value
Age, years					
≤30	153	150	3	784.00	< 0.05
30–60	306	279	27		
≥60	44	41	3		
Gender					
Male	314	289	25	2.68	> 0.05
Female	189	181	8		
Treatment history					
New cases	201	168	33	214.40	< 0.05
Retreatment	302	302	0		
Regions					
Chongqing	413	402	11	25.40	< 0.05
Sichuan Province	81	78	3		
Other regions	9	6	3		

MIRU-VNTR [24]. According to the results of a study comparing different methods RD105 or spoligotyping is a reliable method for identifying whether the strain belongs to the Beijing cluster, although the identification ability may be not comparable to that of IS*6110*-RFLP. MIRU-VNTR was the most reliable method for the genetic differentiation of MTB isolates because the discriminatory power of this method is also comparable to that of IS*6110* typing [7–9]. The different research purposes of MTB molecular epidemiology study should select the appropriate technological choice ways based on different research purposes, or combined variety of ways in order to improve work efficiency and accuracy of the results.

The discrimination of the MIRU-VNTR depends on the resolution of the site used and the VNTR loci should be selected according to the genetic polymorphism of MTB in different regions. The reports had displayed that QUB18, Mtub21, QUB26, QUB11b, QUB11a, and MIRU26 were highly discriminating loci in Chongqing [25] and Mtub04, Mtub21, Mtub39, QUB26, QUB11b, MIRU10, MIRU26, MIRU39, MIRU40, ETRA and ETRE were highly discriminating loci in Sichuan province [26]. In this study, VNTR genotyping was carried out at 12 sites, which were representative of both international and domestic locations. By analyzing the allelic polymorphism of the isolates, the HGDI of polymorphism of 12 loci was between 0.29 and 0.67. The results showed that the seven loci including QUB-11b, QUB-18, QUB-26, MIRU26, MIRU31, Mtub21 and Mtub04 had high discrimination in MTB in Chongqing area. But the discrimination of MIRU10 in Chongqing is lower than that of Sichuan province. Compared with the typing of Yongchuan in Chongqing the Mtub04 loci selected in this study have a relatively high resolution [10], while

Table 5 Regional Distribution of some patients with Beijing genotype

No. of strains in one cluster	Region	No. of patients	No. of strains in one cluster	Region	No. of patients
26	Pengshui	7	8	Fengjie	2
	Beibei	2		Yubei	2
	Zhong	2		others	4
	others	15	7	Guangan	3
11	Nanan	2		others	4
	Banan	2	4	Zhong	3
	others	7		others	1
10	Pengshui	2	3	Shapingba	2
	others	8		others	1
9	Beibei	3	3	Jiangbei	2
	others	6		others	1

"others" mean "the rest patients came from different regions and only one patient in one region"

MIRU10 and ETR-F are relatively low, which may be related to the size of the selected study sample range. Therefore, in the future the classification work will select high polymorphic combination of sites including QUB-11b, QUB-18, QUB-26, MIRU26, MIRU31, Mtub21 and Mtub04 that is a great help for increasing classification efficiency.

Conclusions

Beijing genotype was the predominant in the patients with DRTB in our hospital. In Chongqing retreatment patients with Beijing genotype MTB may be patient with DRTB. DST, regular medication and strict follow-up are very important for patients with Beijing genotype MTB. In Chongqing control and treatment of DRTB should be paid attention. Transmission and relations of patients with DRTB need to be further research.

Abbreviations

AMK: Amikacin; Cm: Capreomycin; DNA: Deoxyribonucleic acid; DRTB: Drug resistant Mycobacterium tuberculosis; DST: Drug susceptibility testing; EMB: Ethambutol; ETRs: Exact tandem repeats; HGDI: Hunter–Gaston discriminatory index; INH: Isoniazid; Lofx: Levofloxacin; MDR-TB: Multi-drug resistance Tuberculosis; MGIT: Mycobacterium Growth Indicator Tube; MIRU-VNTR: Mycobacterial interspersed repetitive unit-variable number tandem repeat typing; MSTs: Minimal Spanning Trees; NMTB: Non Mycobacterium tuberculosis; PAIN: Dipasic; PCR: Polymerase chain reaction; Pto: Protionamide; QUB: Queen's University of Belfast; RD105: Region of difference 105; RFP: rifampicin; SM: Streptomycin; TB: Tuberculosis; WHO: World Health Organization; XDR-TB: Extensive drug resistance tuberculosis

Acknowledgements

We thank the patients' agreement to participate in this research.

Funding

ZHZ is supported by the Natural Science Foundation of China (grant number: 81772365). The funding sources had no role in the study design, data collection, data analysis, or writing of the report.

Authors' contributions

Conceived and designed the study: TS, TXL. Collected the data: TXL, JGL, JW and ZHZ. Analyzed the data: TXL, JGL, JW. Wrote the paper: TS. Interpreted the results: TXL, JGL, JW. Acquisition of funding: ZHZ. All authors have read and approved the final manuscript.

Competing interests

The authors declare that they have no competing interests.

Author details

[1]Department of Orthopedics, The Third Affiliated Hospital of Chongqing Medical University (Gener Hospital), No. 1, Shuanghu Branch Road, Yubei District, Chongqing 401120, China. [2]Department of Clinical Laboratory, Public Health Medical Center, No. 109, Baoyu Road, Shapingba District, Chongqing 400036, China. [3]Department of Orthopedics, Southwest Hospital, Third Military Medical University, No. 30, Gaotanyan Main Street, Shapingba District, Chongqing 400038, China.

References

1. World Health Organization (WHO). Global tuberculosis report 2015. Geneva: World Health. Organization; 2015.
2. McAdam RA, Hermans PW, van Soolingen D, Zainuddin ZF, Catty D, van Embden JD, et al. Characterization of a Mycobacterium tuberculosis insertion sequence belonging to the IS3 family. Mol Microbiol. 1990;4:1607–13.
3. Supply P, Allix C, Lesjean S, Cardoso-Oelemann M, Rüsch-Gerdes S, Willery E, et al. Proposal for standardization of optimized mycobacterial interspersed repetitive unit–variable-number tandem repeat typing of Mycobacterium tuberculosis. J Clin Microbiol. 2006;44:4498–510.
4. Van Embden JD, Cave MD, Crawford JT, Dale JW, Eisenach KD, Gicquel B, et al. Strain identification of Mycobacterium tuberculosis by DNA fingerprinting: recommendations for a standardized methodology. J Clin Microbiol. 1993;31:406–9.
5. Arnold C. Molecular evolution of Mycobacterium tuberculosis. Clin Microbiol Infect. 2007;13:120–8.
6. Thierry D, Cave MD, Eisenach KD, Crawford JT, Bates JH, Gicquel B, et al. IS6110, an IS-like element of Mycobacterium tuberculosis complex. Nucleic Acids Res. 1990;18:188.
7. Liu Q, Yang D, Xu W, Wang J, LV B, Shao Y, et al. Molecular typing of mycobacterium tuberculosis isolates circulating in Jiangsu Province, China. BMC Infect Dis. 2011;11:288.
8. Guo J-h, Xiang W-l, Zhang G, Luo T, Xie N, Yang ZR, et al. Mycobacterial Interspersed Repetitive Unit typing in Mycobacterium tuberculosis isolates from Sichuan Province in China. Indian J Med Res. 2011;134:362–8.
9. Kam KM, Yip CW, Tse LW, Wong KL, Lam TK, Kremer K, et al. Utility of mycobacterial interspersed repetitive unit typing for differentiating multidrug-resistant Mycobacterium tuberculosis isolates of the Beijing family. J Clin Microbiol. 2005;43(1):306–13.
10. Zhang D, An J, Wang J, Hu C, Wang Z, Zhang R, et al. Molecular typing and drug susceptibility of Mycobacterium tuberculosis isolates from Chongqing municipality, China. Infect Genet Evol. 2013;13:310–6.
11. Weng CY, Ho CM, Dou HY, Ho MW, Lin HS, Chang HL, et al. Molecular typing of Mycobacterium tuberculosis isolated from adult patients with tubercular spondylitis. J Microbiol Immunol Infect. 2013;46(1):19–23.
12. Van Soolingen D, Qian L, de Haas PE, Douglas JT, Traore H, Portaels F, et al. Predominance of a single genotype of Mycobacterium tuberculosis in countries of East Asia. J Clin Microbiol. 1995;33(12):3234–338.
13. Park YK, Shin S, Ryu S, Cho SN, Koh WJ, Kwon OJ, et al. Comparison of drug resistance genotypes between Beijing and non-Beijing family strains of Mycobacterium tuberculosis in Korea. J Microbiol Methods. 2005;63(2):165–72.
14. Ghebremichael S, Groenheit R, Pennhag A, Koivula T, Andersson E, Bruchfeld J, et al. Drug resistant Mycobacterium tuberculosis of the Beijing genotype does not spread in Sweden. PLoS One. 2010;5(5):e10893.
15. Mokrousov I, Jiao WW, Sun GZ, Liu JW, Valcheva V, Li M, et al. Evolution of drug resistance in different sublineages of Mycobacterium tuberculosis Beijing genotype. Antimicrob Agents Chemother. 2006;50(8):2820–3.
16. Liu Y, Tian M, Wang X, Goldbogen J, Southall B. Genotypic diversity analysis of Mycobacterium tuberculosis strains collected from Beijing in 2009, using Spoligotyping and VNTR typing. PLoS One. 2014;9(9):e106787.
17. Chen YY, Chang JR, Kuo SC, Tseng FC, Huang WC, Huang TS, et al. Molecular epidemiology of tuberculosis in Kaohsiung City located at southern Taiwan, 2000–2008. PLoS ONE. 2015;10(1):e0117061.
18. Wang Q, Lau SK, Liu F, Zhao Y, Li HM, Li BX, et al. Molecular epidemiology and clinical characteristics of drug-resistant Mycobacterium tuberculosis in a tuberculosis referral hospital in China. PLoS One. 2014;9(10):e110209.
19. Wang SF, Zhou Y, Pang Y, Zhao YL. Epidemic characteristics of Mycobacterium tuberculosis of Beijing genotype strains and its association with drug resistance—analysis of the data from national drug resistant tuberculosis baseline survey in 2007. Chin J Antitubercul. 2015;37(8):836–42.
20. Tuli SM. Tuberculosis of the spine: a historical review. Clin Orthop Relat Res. 2007;460:29–38.
21. Mohan K, Rawall S, Pawar UM, Sadani M, Nagad P, Nene A, et al. Drug resistance patterns in 111 cases of drug-resistant tuberculosis spine. Eur Spine J. 2013;22(Suppl 4):S647–52.
22. Moonan PK, Teeter LD, Salcedo K, Ghosh S, Ahuja SD, Flood J, et al. Transmission of multidrug-resistant tuberculosis in the USA: a cross-sectional study. Lancet Infect Dis. 2013;13(9):777–84.
23. Guo JH, Xiang WL, Zhang G, Luo T, Xie N, Yang ZR, et al. Mycobacterial interspersed repetitive unit typing in Mycobacterium tuberculosis isolates from Sichuan Province in China. Indian J Med Res. 2011;134:362–8.
24. Pang Y, Zhou Y, Zhao B, Liu G, Jiang G, Xia H, et al. 2012. Spoligotyping and drug resistance analysis of Mycobacterium tuberculosis strains from national survey in China. PLoS One. 2012;7(3):e32976.
25. Zhang D, An J, Wang Y, Pang Y. Genetic diversity of multidrug-resistant tuberculosis in a resource-limited region of China. Int. J Infect Dis. 2014;29: 7–11.

Schistosoma mansoni infection and socio-behavioural predictors of HIV risk

Sergey Yegorov[1,10*], Ronald M. Galiwango[1], Sara V. Good[2,3], Juliet Mpendo[4], Egbert Tannich[5], Andrea K. Boggild[6,7], Noah Kiwanuka[4,8], Bernard S. Bagaya[4,9] and Rupert Kaul[1,6]

Abstract

Background: *Schistosoma mansoni* infection has been associated with increased risk of HIV transmission in African women. This association might be causal or mediated through shared socio-behavioural factors and associated co-infections. We tested the latter hypothesis in a cross-sectional pilot study in a cohort of women from a *S. mansoni* endemic region of Uganda. To validate the immunological effects of *S. mansoni* in this cohort, we additionally assessed known schistosomiasis biomarkers.

Methods: HIV-uninfected non-pregnant adult women using public health services were tested for schistosomiasis using the urine circulating cathodic antigen test, followed by serology and *Schistosoma* spp.-specific PCR. Blood was obtained for herpes simplex virus (HSV)-2 serology, eosinophil counts and cytokine analysis. Samples collected from the genitourinary tract were used to test for classical sexually transmitted infections (STI), for bacterial vaginosis and to assess recent sexual activity via prostate-specific antigen testing. Questionnaires were used to capture a range of socio-economic and behavioral characteristics.

Results: Among 58 participants, 33 (57%) had schistosomiasis, which was associated with elevated levels of interleukin (IL)-10 (0.32 vs. 0.19 pg/ml; $p = 0.038$) and a trend toward increased tumour necrosis factor (TNF) (1.73 vs. 1.42 pg/ml; $p = 0.081$). Eosinophil counts correlated with levels of both cytokines ($r = 0.53$, $p = 0.001$ and $r = 0.38$, $p = 0.019$, for IL-10 and TNF, respectively); the association of eosinophilia with schistosomiasis was not significant (OR = 2.538, $p = 0.282$). Further, schistosomiasis was associated with lower age (per-year OR = 0.910, $p = 0.047$), being unmarried (OR = 0.263, $p = 0.030$), less frequent hormonal contraceptive (HC) use (OR = 0.121, $p = 0.002$, dominated by long acting injectable contraceptives) and a trend to longer time since penile-vaginal sex (OR = 0.350, $p = 0.064$). All women infected by *Chlamydia trachomatis* ($n = 5$), were also positive for schistosomiasis (Fisher's exact $p = 0.064$).

Conclusions: Intestinal schistosomiasis in adult women was associated with systemic immune alterations, suggesting that associations with immunological correlates of HIV susceptibility warrant further investigation. *S. mansoni* associations with socio-behavioral parameters and *C. trachomatis*, which may alter both genital immunity and HIV exposure and/or acquisition risk, means that future studies should carefully control for potential confounders. These findings have implications for the design and interpretation of clinical studies on the effects of schistosomiasis on HIV acquisition.

Keywords: *Schistosoma mansoni*, Intestinal schistosomiasis, HIV susceptibility, HIV risk factors, Injectable hormonal contraceptives, Sexually transmitted infections

* Correspondence: sergey.yegorov@mail.utoronto.ca
[1]Department of Immunology, University of Toronto, Toronto, Canada
[10]Present address: Faculty of Education and Humanities, Suleyman Demirel University, Almaty, Kazakhstan
Full list of author information is available at the end of the article

Background

Schistosomiasis is a neglected tropical disease caused by trematode worms inhabiting the gastrointestinal and/or genitourinary venules. Over 200 million people are infected globally, with a disproportionate burden in Africa, where approximately 90% cases are found alongside significant co-endemicity with HIV-1 (HIV) [1, 2]. Accumulating evidence suggests that schistosomiasis may increase the risk of HIV transmission through complex effects on mucosal immunity and antiviral defenses [2–4]. This association is not only seen for infection by *Schistosoma haematobium*, the cause of genitourinary schistosomiasis, but also for *S. mansoni*, which predominantly affects the gut and causes intestinal/hepatic schistosomiasis [5–10]. Specifically, studies performed in Tanzania reported that *S. mansoni*-infected women were six-fold more likely to be HIV-infected compared to their female peers without schistosomiasis [10]. Subsequently, a prospective study performed in Tanzania found that *S.mansoni*-infected women had a 2.8-fold increased risk of HIV acquisition [11]. Notably, these effects of *S.mansoni* on HIV acquisition in the Tanzanian studies were only seen in women, but not men [9, 11], implying that the effects on HIV susceptibility are mediated by either biological or socio-behavioral factors specific to women.

While various systemic and mucosal immune mechanisms have been hypothesized to explain the latter association [2, 11], the exact underlying cause of increased HIV susceptibility in the context of *S. mansoni* infection remains unclear. Furthermore, studies in this area could be confounded if socio-behavioral factors associated with HIV risk differed between women with and without schistosomiasis.

Active *S. mansoni* infection results in parasite egg-induced granulomatous inflammation in the colon and surrounding internal organs, and subsequent changes in various immunological processes, such as immune cell trafficking [3]. The extent of immune alteration caused by schistosomiasis can be assessed by measuring the levels of specific immune mediators and immune cells in the blood of infected individuals. For example, circulating cytokines interleukin-10 (IL-10) and tumor necrosis factor (TNF) are two biomarkers that have consistently been shown as elevated in human schistosomiasis [12–16]. Eosinophilia (elevated eosinophil counts) is yet another common diagnostic used to assess the severity of helminth infection [17, 18].

As a precursor to studies on the immune impact of schistosomiasis in adults, we performed a cross-sectional observational study, which examined the relationship between schistosomiasis and behavioral HIV risk factors in adult women from Wakiso district, a region endemic for *S. mansoni* [19, 20] (Fig. 1). To this end, we recruited HIV-negative non-pregnant women in Entebbe town and collected from the study participants demographic and diagnostic data, including data on the prevalence of schistosomiasis and classical sexually transmitted infection (STI), as well as measured circulating cytokine levels.

Methods

Study setting and participant recruitment

The study was conducted in Entebbe, a town situated on a peninsula in Lake Victoria (Fig. 1), between September 2015–February 2016. Entebbe has an HIV prevalence of ~ 20% [19] and a schistosomiasis prevalence of ~ 70%, largely due to *S. mansoni* [19] with much lower (< 1%) rates of *S. haematobium* [21]. Consenting women aged 18–45 years ($n = 58$) attending family planning or child vaccination clinics at Entebbe General Hospital or a nearby General Practice clinic were screened for HIV, malaria and pregnancy as previously described [22]; those who tested positive for any of the three conditions were referred for appropriate care according to the Uganda clinical guidelines while those testing negative were eligible for enrolment. This study was designed to provide pilot data for future immune studies, therefore no formal sample size calculations were made.

Sample collection and diagnostic testing

Blood (16 ml) was collected by venipuncture and blood plasma was isolated and stored at -80 °C prior to downstream testing. Eosinophil counts were acquired using an ACT 5diff automated hematology analyzer (Beckman Coulter, USA), and eosinophilia was defined as an eosinophil count > 450 cells per μl of whole blood [17]. Schistosomiasis was diagnosed based on the urine circulating cathodic antigen (CCA), a by-product of adult schistosome metabolism. The CCA test (Rapid Medical Diagnostics, Pretoria, South Africa) is highly sensitive but does not allow schistosome speciation [23]. Therefore, stored plasma was used to extract cell free DNA using QIAamp MinElute extraction kit (Qiagen, Germany) according to the manufacturer's protocol for subsequent species-specific PCR performed as previously described [24–26]. Testing for *Chlamydia trachomatis* (Ct) and *Neisseria gonorrhoeae* (Ng) was performed on urine samples using the Roche Cobas PCR (Roche Diagnostics Corp, Indianapolis, USA). One vaginal swab was tested for *Trichomonas vaginalis* (Tv) using the OSOM rapid test (Sekisui Diagnostics, Framingham, USA), and a second vaginal swab was smeared onto a glass slide, air-dried and Gram's stained to diagnose bacterial vaginosis (BV) using Nugent criteria [27]. A SoftCup (EvoFem, San Diego, USA) was used to collect cervico-vaginal secretions for prostate-specific antigen testing (PSA; Seratec PSA Semiquant kit, Göttingen, Germany) according to the PSA kit manufacturer's instructions. Recent (≤ 3 days) unprotected penile vaginal-sex was defined as a positive PSA test result, since softcup PSA levels increase immediately after unprotected sex and return to baseline levels by approximately 72 h post-exposure. Stored plasma was used to

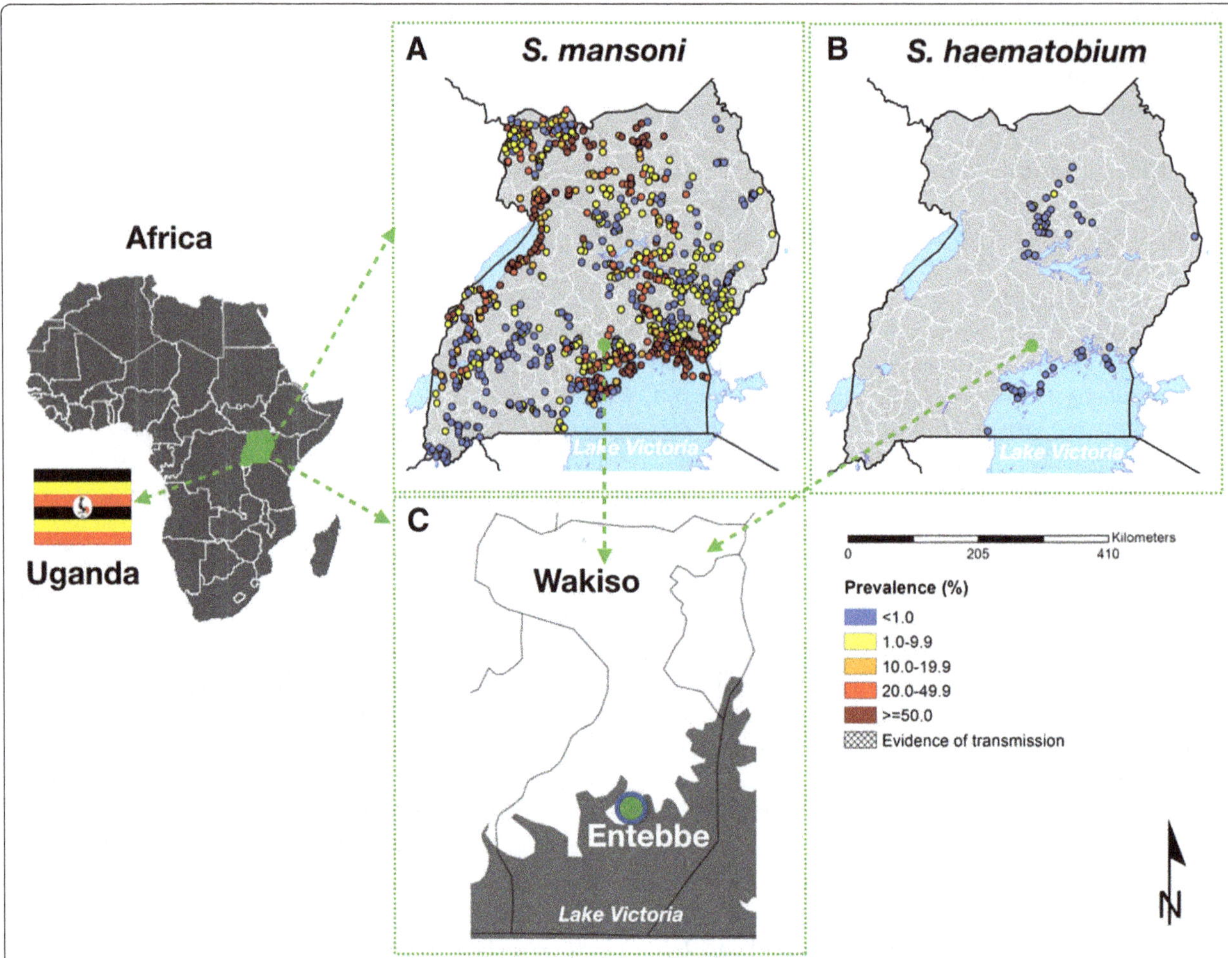

Fig. 1 Distribution of schistosomiasis and the study site location in Uganda. **a**. Prevalence and distribution of *S. mansoni* in Uganda; **b**. Prevalence and distribution of *S. haematobium* in Uganda; **c**. Map of Wakiso district and location of the study site (Entebbe). Note that Entebbe is endemic for *S. mansoni* but not *S. haematobium*. The maps show the location of schistosomiasis surveys and the reported prevalence of schistosomiasis across Uganda. Scale is given for the maps of Uganda. Map source: The Global Atlas of Helminth Infection [21]

perform serology for the presence of antibody specific to *S. mansoni* soluble egg antigen (SmSEA; Scimedx, New Jersey, USA) and optic density (OD) values > 0.2 were considered positive. Herpes simplex virus type 2 (Kalon HSV-2 IgG, Kalon Biological Ltd., UK) testing was performed on stored plasma. Measurements of circulating interleukin-10 (IL-10) and tumor necrosis factor (TNF) were performed on a subset of stored plasma samples using the Meso Scale Discovery electrochemiluminescent ELISA (MD, USA) as done previously [28]. All experimental assays were performed by research personnel blinded to the status of participants. Questionnaires capturing specific socio-economic and behavioral characteristics, such as self-reported sex and contraceptive use (Table 1) were administered.

Statistical analysis

To examine associations between each factor and the presence/absence (+/−) of schistosomiasis, we first performed univariate binomial logistic regression with age as a continuous variable and 10 categorical variables (Table 1) and the schistosomiasis-free (CCA-negative) group ($n = 25$) as the reference category. Then factors found to be significantly associated with schistosomiasis in the binomial regressions (age, marital status, hormonal contraceptive (HC) use (all HC categories combined); recent sex was also included although its association was not significant in the binomial regression) were tested for multicollinearity prior to inclusion in a multivariable binomial regression (Table 2). Cytokine levels between schistosoma +/− groups were compared using a Mann-Whitney U test. Correlations of cytokine levels and eosinophil counts were assessed on log10-transformed values by Pearson's correlation analysis. All statistical analyses were conducted using IBM SPSS V.23 (NY, US). Graphs were plotted using GraphPad Prism V.6.0. (CA, US).

Table 1 Associations of participant characteristics with schistosome infection

Participant characteristic	Entire cohort ($n = 58$)	*Schistosoma* spp. ag -positive ($N = 33$)	*Schistosoma* spp. ag -negative ($N = 25$)	OR for association with schistosomiasis (95% CI)	*P* value ($\alpha = 0.05$)
Median age (IQR)	27.5 (23.8–32.0)	25.0 (22.5–29.5)	30.0 (25.0–34.0)	0.910 (0.830–0.999)	0.047
Married, %	60.7 (34/56)	50.0 (16/32)	79.2 (19/24)	0.263 (0.079–0.878)	0.030
Sexual behaviour					
Hormonal contraceptive use, %	30.4 (17/56)	12.5 (4/32)	54.2 (13/24)	0.121 (0.032–0.452)	0.002
DMPA[a], %	19.6 (11/56)	9.4 (3/32)	33.3 (8/24)		
NetEn[a], %	8.9 (5/56)	3.1 (1/32)	16.7 (4/24)		
Oral pill, %	1.8 (1/56)	0 (0/32)	4.2 (1/24)		
Sex in last 3 days					
PSA+, %	41.8 (23/55)	31.3 (10/32)	56.5 (13/23)	0.350 (0.115–1.064)	0.064[b]
Self-reported, %	29.6 (16/54)	26.7 (8/30)	33.3 (8/24)	0.727 (0.225–2.349)	0.595
Reported condom use in last sex, %	19.2 (10/52)	20.0 (6/30)	18.2 (4/22)	1.125 (0.276–4.585)	1.00
Presence of eosinophilia[a], %	14.3 (8/56)	18.8 (6/32)	8.3 (2/24)	2.538 (0.465–13.868)	0.282
HSV-2 seropositive, %	58.6 (34/58)	63.6 (21/33)	52.0 (13/25)	1.615 (0.561–4.652)	0.374
Genital conditions					
Presence of tested STI, %	12.1 (7/58)	15.2 (5/33)	8.0 (2/25)	2.054 (0.364–11.585)	0.408
T.vaginalis	1.7 (1/58)	0.0 (0/33)	4.0 (1/25)		
C. trachomatis	8.6 (5/58)	**15.2 (5/33)**[b]	0.0 (0/25)		
N. gonorrhoeae	1.7 (1/58)	0.0 (0/33)	4.0 (1/25)		
Self-reporting genital condition in past month, %	30.9 (17/55)	38.7 (12/31)	20.8 (5/24)	2.4 (0.707–8.144)	0.160
Presence of bacterial vaginosis, %	30.6 (11/36)	20.0 (4/20)	43.8 (7/16)	0.321 (0.074–1.405)	0.159

ag antigen, *OR* odds ratio, *DMPA* depot-medroxyprogesterone acetate, *NET-EN* norethisterone enanthate, *PSA* prostate-specific antigen, *STI* sexually transmitted infection; [a]eosinophilia was defined as > 450 eosinophils per ul of blood; [b] trend. Data were assessed using univariate binomial logistic regression with the *Schistosoma* spp. ag-free (CCA-negative) group as the reference category. When OR is above 1, there is a positive association of given factor with schistosomiasis; OR value above 1 represents inverse relationship of given factor with schistosomiasis. OR for age is a per year OR

Results

Participant demographics

A total of 58 women met inclusion criteria and were enrolled; socio-behavioural characteristics are shown in Table 1. The median participant age was 27.5 years, and 56.9% (33/58) of women were diagnosed with schistosomiasis based on urine CCA testing. No participant recalled having received anti-helminthic or anti-schistosomal treatment in the last 10 years.

Table 2 Associations of age, marital status, hormonal contraceptive use and recent sex with schistosome infection as assessed by multivariable logistic regression

Participant characteristic	Entire cohort ($n = 58$)	*Schistosoma* spp. ag -positive ($N = 33$)	*Schistosoma* spp. ag -negative ($N = 25$)	OR for association with schistosomiasis (95% CI)	*P* value ($\alpha = 0.05$)
Median age (IQR)	27.5 (23.8–32.0)	25.0 (22.5–29.5)	30.0 (25.0–34.0)	0.934 (0.838–1.041)	0.216
Married, %	60.7 (34/56)	50.0 (16/32)	79.2 (19/24)	0.590 (0.138–2.527)	0.477
Sexual behaviour					
Hormonal contraceptive use, %	30.4 (17/56)	12.5 (4/32)	54.2 (13/24)	0.151 (0.037–0.611)	0.008
DMPA*, %	19.6 (11/56)	9.4 (3/32)	33.3 (8/24)		
NetEn*, %	8.9 (5/56)	3.1 (1/32)	16.7 (4/24)		
Oral pill, %	1.8 (1/56)	0 (0/32)	4.2 (1/24)		
Sex in last 3 days					
PSA+, %	41.8 (23/55)	31.3 (10/32)	56.5 (13/23)	0.480 (0.130–1.773)	0.271

ag antigen, *OR* odds ratio, *DMPA* depot-medroxyprogesterone acetate, *NET-EN* norethisterone enanthate, *PSA* prostate-specific antigen. Data were assessed using multivariable binomial logistic regression with factors that were found to have significant associations in univariate analysis and the *Schistosoma* spp. ag-free (CCA-negative) group as the reference category. When OR is above 1, there is a positive association of given factor with schistosomiasis; OR value above 1 represents inverse relationship of given factor with schistosomiasis. OR for age is a per year OR

Systemic immune biomarkers of schistosomiasis

First, we examined levels of blood cytokines IL-10 and TNF and eosinophil counts. Participants diagnosed with schistosomiasis based on CCA positivity had increased levels of IL-10 (median of 0.32 pg/ml vs. 0.19 pg/ml in CCA-negative controls, $p = 0.038$, ~ 1.70 fold difference), and tended to have elevated levels of TNF (median of 1.73 pg/ml vs. 1.42 pg/ml, $p = 0.081$, ~ 1.21 fold difference) compared to schistosoma-negative women (Fig. 2a & b). Further, both blood IL-10 and TNF levels were positively correlated with eosinophil counts ($r = 0.53$, $p = 0.001$ and $r = 0.38$, $p = 0.019$, respectively; Fig. 2c & d), although the associations of eosinophilia and eosinophil counts with schistosomiasis were not significant (OR = 2.538, $p = 0.282$ for eosinophilia and $p = 0.866$ for eosinophil counts; Table 1 and Fig. 2e).

Socio-behavioural associations of schistosomiasis

Women with schistosomiasis differed from their infection-free peers in several parameters previously linked to both mucosal immunology and HIV risk. Specifically, CCA-positive participants were younger (median age 25 vs. 30 years; per year OR = 0.910, $p = 0.047$), less likely to be married (50.0% vs. 79.2%; OR = 0.263, $p = 0.030$) and less likely to be using hormonal contraceptives (HC, 12.5% vs. 54.2%; OR = 0.121, $p = 0.002$), mainly consisting of long acting injectable depot-medroxyprogesterone acetate (DMPA, 64.7%) and norethisterone enanthate (NetEn, 29.4%). Recent unprotected penile-vaginal sex, defined as the detection of PSA in cervico-vaginal secretions, tended to be less common in women with schistosomiasis (31.3% vs. 56.5%; OR = 0.350, $p = 0.064$). Although the detection of any classical STI (defined as Ng, Ct or Tv) was not associated with schistosomiasis, all 5 Ct-infected participants were co-infected with schistosomiasis (Fisher's exact $p = 0.064$). No associations were apparent between schistosomiasis and condom use, HSV-2 infection, self-reported genital symptoms or BV (Table 1).

To assess whether the associations with age, marital status, HC use and unprotected sex could be driven by a subset of factors, we assessed the correlation and multicollinearity among factors and performed multivariable regression. Age and marital status were significantly correlated (point-biserial correlation, $p < 0.001$, $r = 0.462$), but multicollinearity was not detected based on a variance inflation factor threshold of three. Thus, we performed multivariable regression with age, marital status, use of hormonal contraceptives and PSA-positivity as independent variables and determined that only the use of long-acting injectable contraceptives remained significantly associated with schistosomiasis status (OR = 0.151, $p = 0.008$; Table 2); inclusion of fewer variables in the model did not significantly change the OR for any of the factors under consideration.

Sub-analysis based on schistosome speciation

The CCA test exhibits high sensitivity for active schistosomiasis, but may give false positive results in the context of urinary tract infections [29]. Therefore, we retrospectively performed PCR and serology testing on stored plasma samples to validate the results derived from CCA alone. When analysis was restricted to CCA+ participants who were positive by either *S. mansoni*-specific PCR and/or serology ($n = 10$), significant associations of schistosomiasis were again seen with marital status (OR = 0.113, $p = 0.011$), long-acting contraceptive use (OR = 0.094, $p = 0.037$) and the presence of blood eosinophilia (OR of 7.33, $p = 0.042$). One CCA-negative woman was found to have a positive PCR result for *S. haematobium* (but not for *S. mansoni*); exclusion of this participant did not have a significant effect on analysis outcomes.

Discussion

In this pilot study, our aim was to examine the relationship between intestinal schistosomiasis and socio-behavioral HIV risk factors in a cohort of adult women from the Wakiso district of Uganda, a region endemic for *S. mansoni*. In addition, we were interested in validating in this cohort the known associations of *S. mansoni* with circulating IL-10, TNF and eosinophilia. To this end, we compared the diagnostic and demographic profiles of adult women with and without schistosomiasis. We observed that *S. mansoni* in this cohort was associated with differences in several socio-behavioral factors, including HC use, and *C. trachomatis* prevalence, which could influence genital immunity and HIV susceptibility. At the same time, schistosomiasis-infected women exhibited previously described systemic immune alterations, emphasizing the relevance of further studies of immunological correlates of HIV susceptibility.

Previously, *S. mansoni* infection has been linked to increased HIV acquisition in women in some [10, 11], but not all [19, 20], epidemiological studies. Since the mucosal immune environment is a key determinant of HIV acquisition risk [30], defining the genital immune impact of schistosomiasis could clarify biological mechanism(s) and lead to novel means of HIV prevention. It is widely recognized that *S. haematobium* infection directly involves the urogenital mucosa, compromising epithelial integrity and causing mucosal inflammation [2, 5]. However, the biologic basis for an association between *S. mansoni* infection and genital HIV susceptibility is less clear, since the parasite primarily infects the gastrointestinal and portal vasculature [2, 11]. While genital immune studies may help to clarify this question, our study demonstrates that schistosomiasis - and *S. mansoni* infection in particular - is associated with differences in

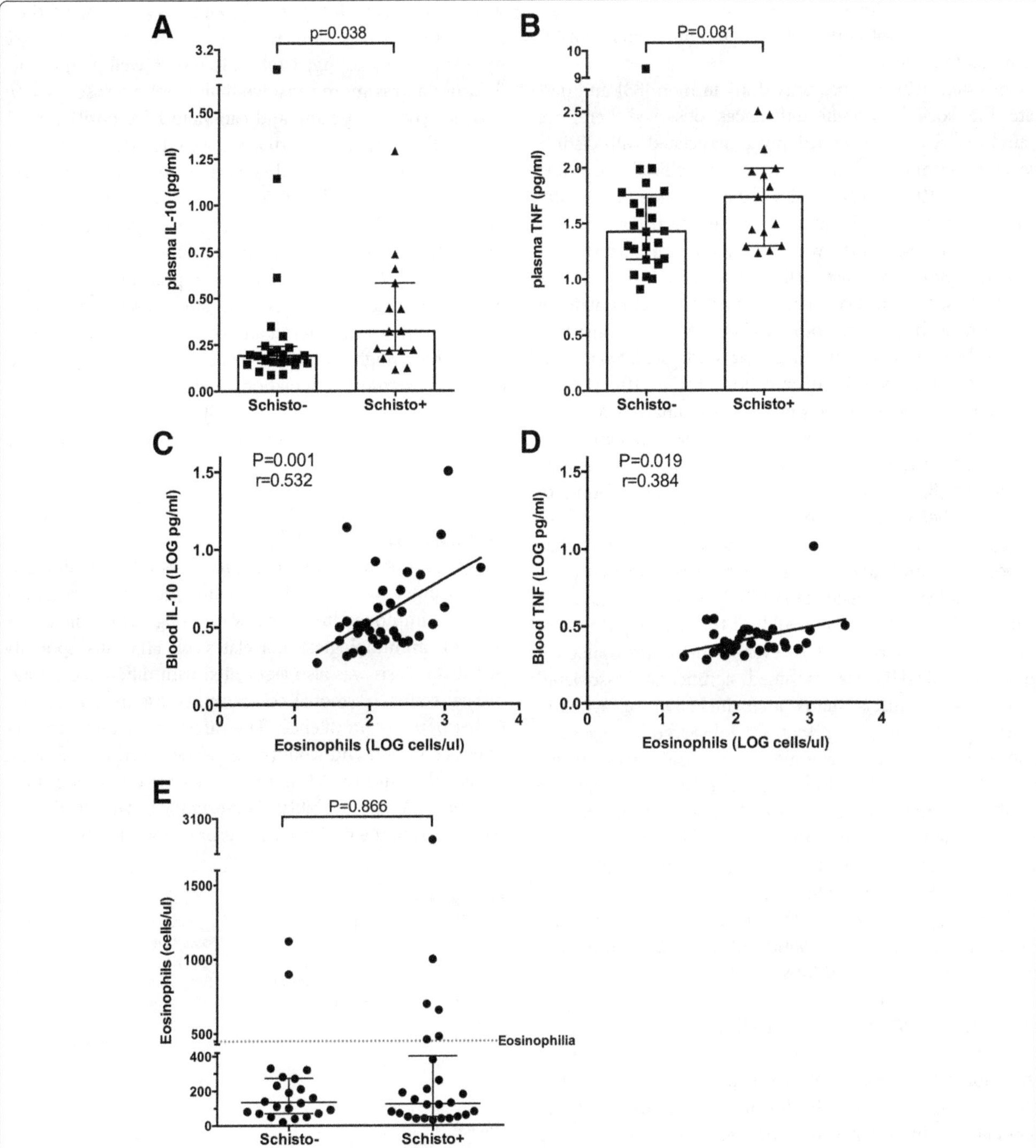

Fig. 2 Systemic immunological differences observed between women with (schisto+) and without schistosomiasis (schisto-). **a.** Plasma IL-10 levels; **b.** Plasma TNF levels; **c** and **d.** Correlations between eosinophil counts and IL-10 (**c**) and TNF (**d**). **e.** Eosinophil counts, where red dotted line depicts the conventional threshold of eosinophilia (450 cells per µl of whole blood). Multiplex ELISA assays were conducted by a technologist blinded to schistosomiasis status on plasma samples available for 39 women (15 positive and 24 negative for schistosomiasis). Cytokine levels and eosinophil counts were compared by Mann-Whitney test ($p = 0.05$); plots depict medians and interquartile ranges. Correlations were assessed on LOG-transformed values by Spearman test ($p = 0.05$)

women's age, marital status, hormonal contraceptive use, sexual behavior and *C. trachomatis* prevalence. Since all of these parameters can both modulate HIV risk and alter genital immunology [30–32], they may confound clinical studies of the impact of schistosomiasis on mucosal HIV susceptibility. Potential study designs to overcome this barrier would include a large enough sample size to permit robust multivariable analysis, or longitudinal studies that control for inter-individual confounders by assessing changes in mucosal immunology before and after schistosomiasis treatment.

Consistent with our previous study in men [33] and despite the socio-behavioral differences observed here, we found that *S. mansoni* infection was associated with distinct systemic immunological signatures. Specifically, elevated levels of IL-10 and TNF indicate the presence of parasite-driven inflammation in schistosoma-infected women, suggesting that associations with immunological correlates of HIV susceptibility warrant further investigation.

Our observation that schistosomiasis-infected women are younger than schistosomiasis-free women is consistent with other reports indicating that both schistosomiasis prevalence and intensity of infection peak at 10–20 years and then decline with age due to a combination of changing behavioural patterns of exposure to schistosome-contaminated water and build-up of anti-schistosomal immunity [8, 34]. Younger women were also found to have a higher prevalence of *C. trachomatis* [35] and, not surprisingly, were less likely to be married. The latter has important implications for hormonal contraceptive choices and the frequency of sex [32], so that the age association of schistosomiasis could be the primary driver of the observed differences. However, in the multivariable regression, only HC use remained significantly associated with schistosomiasis status after inclusion of age and marital status, implying that the observed associations may not be driven by age alone, and could also involve other latent socio-behavioral characteristics. Notably, no significant multi-collinearity was detected among the factors included in the multivariable model, suggesting that each factor contributes independently to the overall interaction with *S. mansoni* infection.

To our best knowledge, the current study is the first to report the inverse association of injectable contraceptive use with *S. mansoni* infection in African women. To date, several studies have assessed the epidemiological association of *S. mansoni* with HIV, with conflicting results. Tanzanian women (but not men) with *S. mansoni* infection were more likely to acquire HIV [9–11], but studies in Uganda [19, 20] did not find similar HIV risk associations in either women or men. Interestingly, none of these studies assessed injectable contraceptive use, known to considerably vary across East African countries [36, 37], to be linked with both HIV acquisition [38] and altered genital immunology [31], and was less common in women with schistosomiasis in this study.

Our findings should be interpreted in the light of several limitations. First, the study was designed as a pilot with a small sample size, precluding a more detailed assessment of parameters such as HSV-2 infection, the prevalence of which tended to be increased in schistosomiasis-infected women despite their lower age. Therefore, larger studies will be necessary for a more robust assessment of these parameters. In addition, we screened for schistosomiasis by urine CCA testing; while this test is well adapted for field use and is more sensitive than stool microscopy [39], it is not species-specific and can yield false positive readouts in the presence of urinary tract infections [29]. However, our results remained consistent in participants, who were demonstrated by PCR/serology to have *S. mansoni* infection ($n = 10$); this subset would be expected to have a relatively high worm burden (as confirmed by a significant association with eosinophilia), and represent a minority of infected individuals. Lastly, our study recruitment took place at clinics that offered and/or monitored family planning, which might amplify the observed hormonal contraceptive-*S.mansoni* association. Nevertheless, the overall rate of HC use in our study (~ 30%) was similar to that observed in broader communities from the Lake Victoria region [40].

Conclusions

This study demonstrated that *S. mansoni* infection in Ugandan women was associated with previously described systemic immune alterations, warranting further investigation of immunological correlates of HIV susceptibility. Schistosomiasis was also associated with differences in age, marital status, hormonal contraceptive use, recent sex and *C. trachomatis* prevalence. The direction of these associations is complex and would be expected to confound future studies that aim to define the impact of *S. mansoni* infection on HIV susceptibility. These findings will need to be considered in the design and interpretation of such studies.

Acknowledgements

We thank the participants and members of all research teams involved in the study. We are especially grateful to Dr. Moses Muwanga, Irene Wesonga and Shardiah Namusisi (Entebbe General Hospital), Dr. George Miiro, Obenyu P. Akiteng and David A. Drajole (UVRI clinic), Sanja Huibner (University of Toronto), Rachel Lau (Public Health Ontario Laboratories) and to the staff of the UVRI-IAVI and UVRI-MRC Clinical Laboratories. We thank Dr. Dominic Wichmann (University Hospital Hamburg-Eppendorf) for his expert advice on *Schistosoma* spp.-specific PCR.

Funding

This study was supported by the Canadian Institutes of Health Research (CIHR) to RK (TMI-138656), CIHR Vanier Canada Graduate Scholarship to SY and the Fogarty HIV Research Training Program of the National Institutes of Health to RMG (4D43TW009578–04).

Authors' contributions

SY, RK: conceived, designed and implemented the study, drafted the manuscript. SY, RMG, SVG: data collection and analysis. JM: contributed to study design and supervision at clinical sites. ET, AB: oversaw schistosomiasis PCR/serology testing. NK, BSB, RK: overall study conception, design, implementation and supervision. All authors critically reviewed the draft of the paper and approved the final version of the manuscript.

Competing interests

The authors declare that they have no competing interests.

Author details

[1]Department of Immunology, University of Toronto, Toronto, Canada. [2]Genetics and Genome Biology Program, The Hospital for Sick Children, Toronto, Canada. [3]Community Health Sciences, University of Manitoba, Winnipeg, Canada. [4]Uganda Virus Research Institute –International AIDS Vaccine Initiative HIV Vaccine Program, Entebbe, Uganda. [5]Bernhard Nocht Institute for Tropical Medicine, Hamburg, Germany. [6]Department of Medicine, University of Toronto, Toronto, Canada. [7]Public Health Ontario Laboratories, Toronto, Canada. [8]Department of Epidemiology and Biostatistics, School of Public Health, College of Health Sciences, Makerere University, Kampala, Uganda. [9]Department of Immunology and Molecular Biology, School of Biomedical Sciences, College of Health Sciences, Makerere University, Kampala, Uganda. [10]Present address: Faculty of Education and Humanities, Suleyman Demirel University, Almaty, Kazakhstan.

References

1. World Health Organization. Schistosomiasis Fact Sheet [Internet]. 2017. Available from: http://www.who.int/en/news-room/fact-sheets/detail/schistosomiasis. Accessed 22 Feb 2018.
2. Secor WE. The effects of schistosomiasis on HIV/AIDS infection, progression and transmission. Curr Opin HIV AIDS. 2012;7(3):254–9.
3. Mouser EE, Pollakis G, Paxton WA. Effects of helminths and Mycobacterium tuberculosis infection on HIV-1: a cellular immunological perspective. Curr Opin HIV AIDS. 2012;7(3):260–7.
4. Hotez PJ, Fenwick A, Kjetland EF. Africa's 32 cents solution for HIV/AIDS. PLoS Negl Trop Dis. 2009;3(5):e430.
5. Mbabazi PS, Andan O, Fitzgerald DW, Chitsulo L, Engels D, Downs JA. Examining the relationship between urogenital schistosomiasis and HIV infection. PLoS Negl Trop Dis. 2011;5(12):e1396.
6. Kjetland EF, Ndhlovu PD, Gomo E, Mduluza T, Midzi N, Gwanzura L, et al. Association between genital schistosomiasis and HIV in rural Zimbabwean women. AIDS. 2006;20(4):593–600.
7. Mbah MLN, Poolman EM, Drain PK, Coffee MP, van der Werf MJ, Galvani AP. HIV and Schistosoma haematobium prevalences correlate in sub-Saharan Africa. Tropical Med Int Health. 2013;18(10):1174–9.
8. Downs JA, Mguta C, Kaatano GM, Mitchell KB, Bang H, Simplice H, et al. Urogenital schistosomiasis in women of reproductive age in Tanzania's Lake Victoria region. Am J Trop Med Hyg. 2011;84(3):364–9.
9. Downs JA, de Dood CJ, Dee HE, McGeehan M, Khan H, Marenga A, et al. Schistosomiasis and human immunodeficiency virus in men in Tanzania. Am J Trop Med Hyg. 2017;96(4):856–62.
10. Downs JA, van Dam GJ, Changalucha JM, Corstjens PL, Peck RN, de Dood CJ, et al. Association of Schistosomiasis and HIV infection in Tanzania. Am J Trop Med Hyg. 2012;87(5):868–73.
11. Downs JA, Dupnik KM, van Dam GJ, Urassa M, Lutonja P, Kornelis D, et al. Effects of schistosomiasis on susceptibility to HIV-1 infection and HIV-1 viral load at HIV-1 seroconversion: a nested case-control study. PLoS Negl Trop Dis. 2017;11(9):e0005968.
12. de Jesus AR, Silva A, Santana LB, Magalhaes A, de Jesus AA, de Almeida RP, et al. Clinical and immunologic evaluation of 31 patients with acute schistosomiasis mansoni. J Infect Dis. 2002;185(1):98–105.
13. Zwingenberger K, Irschick E, Vergetti Siqueira JG, Correia Dacal AR, Feldmeier H. Tumour necrosis factor in hepatosplenic schistosomiasis. Scand J Immunol. 1990;31(2):205–11.
14. Mwatha JK, Kimani G, Kamau T, Mbugua GG, Ouma JH, Mumo J, et al. High levels of TNF, soluble TNF receptors, soluble ICAM-1, and IFN-gamma, but low levels of IL-5, are associated with hepatosplenic disease in human schistosomiasis mansoni. J Immunol. 1998;160(4):1992–9.
15. Secor WE. Immunology of human schistosomiasis: off the beaten path. Parasite Immunol. 2005;27(7–8):309–16.
16. Elfaki TE, Arndts K, Wiszniewsky A, Ritter M, Goreish IA, Atti El Mekki Mel Y, et al. Multivariable regression analysis in Schistosoma mansoni-infected individuals in the Sudan reveals unique Immunoepidemiological profiles in uninfected, egg+ and non-egg+ infected individuals. PLoS Negl Trop Dis. 2016;10(5):e0004629.
17. Fulkerson PC, Rothenberg ME. Targeting eosinophils in allergy, inflammation and beyond. Nat Rev Drug Discov. 2013;12(2):117 29.
18. Pardo J, Carranza C, Muro A, Angel-Moreno A, Martin AM, Martin T, et al. Helminth-related eosinophilia in African immigrants, gran Canaria. Emerg Infect Dis. 2006;12(10):1587–9.
19. Sanya RE, Muhangi L, Nampijja M, Nannozi V, Nakawungu PK, Abayo E, et al. Schistosoma mansoni and HIV infection in a Ugandan population with high HIV and helminth prevalence. Tropical Med Int Health. 2015;20(9):1201–8.
20. Ssetaala A, Nakiyingi-Miiro J, Asiki G, Kyakuwa N, Mpendo J, Van Dam GJ, et al. Schistosoma mansoni and HIV acquisition in fishing communities of Lake Victoria, Uganda: a nested case-control study. Tropical Med Int Health. 2015; 20(9):1190–5.
21. London Applied & Spatial Epidemiology Reseach Group The Global Atlas of Helminth Infection [Internet]. 2017 [Accessed 26 July 2018]. Available from: http://www.thiswormyworld.org/maps/distribution-of-schistosomiasis-survey-data-in-uganda.
22. Yegorov S, Galiwango RM, Ssemaganda A, Muwanga M, Wesonga I, Miiro G, et al. Low prevalence of laboratory-confirmed malaria in clinically diagnosed adult women from the Wakiso district of Uganda. Malar J. 2016;15(1):555.
23. Kildemoes AO, Vennervald BJ, Tukahebwa EM, Kabatereine NB, Magnussen P, de Dood CJ, et al. Rapid clearance of Schistosoma mansoni circulating cathodic antigen after treatment shown by urine strip tests in a Ugandan fishing community - relevance for monitoring treatment efficacy and re-infection. PLoS Negl Trop Dis. 2017;11(11):e0006054.
24. Cnops L, Soentjens P, Clerinx J, Van Esbroeck M. A Schistosoma haematobium-specific real-time PCR for diagnosis of urogenital schistosomiasis in serum samples of international travelers and migrants. PLoS Negl Trop Dis. 2013;7(8):e2413.
25. Wichmann D, Poppert S, Von Thien H, Clerinx J, Dieckmann S, Jensenius M, et al. Prospective European-wide multicentre study on a blood based real-time PCR for the diagnosis of acute schistosomiasis. BMC Infect Dis. 2013;13:55.
26. Wichmann D, Panning M, Quack T, Kramme S, Burchard GD, Grevelding C, et al. Diagnosing schistosomiasis by detection of cell-free parasite DNA in human plasma. PLoS Negl Trop Dis. 2009;3(4):e422.
27. Nugent RP, Krohn MA, Hillier SL. Reliability of diagnosing bacterial vaginosis is improved by a standardized method of gram stain interpretation. J Clin Microbiol. 1991;29(2):297–301.
28. Shannon B, Yi TJ, Perusini S, Gajer P, Ma B, Humphrys MS, et al. Association of HPV infection and clearance with cervicovaginal immunology and the vaginal microbiota. Mucosal Immunol. 2017;10:1310–9.
29. Technical brochure for "Schisto POC-CCA cassette based test". Rapid Medical Diagnostics 2017. http://www.rapid-diagnostics.com/products.html. Accessed 26 July 2018.
30. Yi TJ, Shannon B, Prodger J, McKinnon L, Kaul R. Genital immunology and HIV susceptibility in young women. Am J Reprod Immunol. 2013;69 Suppl 1:74–9.
31. Hall OJ, Klein SL. Progesterone-based compounds affect immune responses and susceptibility to infections at diverse mucosal sites. Mucosal Immunol. 2017;10(5):1097–107.
32. Ramjee G, Daniels B. Women and HIV in sub-Saharan Africa. AIDS Res Ther. 2013;10(1):30.
33. Prodger JL, Ssemaganda A, Ssetaala A, Kitandwe PK, Muyanja E, Mpendo J, et al. Schistosoma mansoni infection in Ugandan men is associated with increased abundance and function of HIV target cells in blood, but not the foreskin: a cross-sectional study. PLoS Negl Trop Dis. 2015;9(9):e0004067.
34. Kabatereine NB, Brooker S, Tukahebwa EM, Kazibwe F, Onapa AW. Epidemiology and geography of Schistosoma mansoni in Uganda: implications for planning control. Tropical Med Int Health. 2004;9(3):372–80.
35. Masese L, Baeten JM, Richardson BA, Deya R, Kabare E, Bukusi E, et al. Incidence and correlates of chlamydia trachomatis infection in a high-risk cohort of Kenyan women. Sex Transm Dis. 2013;40(3):221–5.
36. United Nations Department of Economic and Social Affairs, Population Division. World Contraceptive Use 2017; 2017 [Accessed 22 Feb 2018]. Available from: http://www.un.org/en/development/desa/population/publications/dataset/contraception/wcu2017.shtml.
37. Dennis ML, Radovich E, Wong KLM, Owolabi O, Cavallaro FL, Mbizvo MT, et al. Pathways to increased coverage: an analysis of time trends in contraceptive need and use among adolescents and young women in Kenya, Rwanda, Tanzania, and Uganda. Reprod Health. 2017;14(1):130.

Permissions

All chapters in this book were first published in ID, by BioMed Central; hereby published with permission under the Creative Commons Attribution License or equivalent. Every chapter published in this book has been scrutinized by our experts. Their significance has been extensively debated. The topics covered herein carry significant findings which will fuel the growth of the discipline. They may even be implemented as practical applications or may be referred to as a beginning point for another development.

The contributors of this book come from diverse backgrounds, making this book a truly international effort. This book will bring forth new frontiers with its revolutionizing research information and detailed analysis of the nascent developments around the world.

We would like to thank all the contributing authors for lending their expertise to make the book truly unique. They have played a crucial role in the development of this book. Without their invaluable contributions this book wouldn't have been possible. They have made vital efforts to compile up to date information on the varied aspects of this subject to make this book a valuable addition to the collection of many professionals and students.

This book was conceptualized with the vision of imparting up-to-date information and advanced data in this field. To ensure the same, a matchless editorial board was set up. Every individual on the board went through rigorous rounds of assessment to prove their worth. After which they invested a large part of their time researching and compiling the most relevant data for our readers.

The editorial board has been involved in producing this book since its inception. They have spent rigorous hours researching and exploring the diverse topics which have resulted in the successful publishing of this book. They have passed on their knowledge of decades through this book. To expedite this challenging task, the publisher supported the team at every step. A small team of assistant editors was also appointed to further simplify the editing procedure and attain best results for the readers.

Apart from the editorial board, the designing team has also invested a significant amount of their time in understanding the subject and creating the most relevant covers. They scrutinized every image to scout for the most suitable representation of the subject and create an appropriate cover for the book.

The publishing team has been an ardent support to the editorial, designing and production team. Their endless efforts to recruit the best for this project, has resulted in the accomplishment of this book. They are a veteran in the field of academics and their pool of knowledge is as vast as their experience in printing. Their expertise and guidance has proved useful at every step. Their uncompromising quality standards have made this book an exceptional effort. Their encouragement from time to time has been an inspiration for everyone.

The publisher and the editorial board hope that this book will prove to be a valuable piece of knowledge for researchers, students, practitioners and scholars across the globe.

List of Contributors

Jill Morse, Dora Luhanga, Helene J Smith, Stable Besa, Nzali Kancheya and Monde Muyoyeta
Centre for Infectious Disease Research in Zambia (CIDRZ), Lusaka, Zambia

Michael E Herce
Centre for Infectious Disease Research in Zambia (CIDRZ), Lusaka, Zambia
Division of Infectious Diseases, Department of Medicine, University of North Carolina School of Medicine, Chapel Hill, North Carolina, USA

Jennifer Harris and Stewart E Reid
Centre for Infectious Disease Research in Zambia (CIDRZ), Lusaka, Zambia
Division of Infectious Diseases, Department of Medicine, University of Alabama at
Birmingham School of Medicine, Birmingham, AL, USA

Graham Samungole
Lusaka District Health Office, Ministry of Health, Government of the Republic of Zambia, Lusaka, Zambia

George Kiwanuka and Juliet Nabirye
Department of Health Policy Planning and Management, Makerere University School of Public Health, Kampala, Uganda

Noah Kiwanuka, Fiston Muneza and Magdalene A. Odikro
Department of Epidemiology and Biostatistics, School of Public Health, Makerere University College of Health Sciences, Kampala, Uganda

Frederick Oporia and Rhoda K. Wanyenze
Department of Disease Control and Environmental Health, Makerere University School of Public Health, Kampala, Uganda

Barbara Castelnuovo
Department of Research, Infectious Diseases Institute, Makerere University College of Health Sciences, Kampala, Uganda

Alexander J Stockdale and Melita A Gordon
Malawi Liverpool Wellcome Trust Clinical Research Programme, Chichiri 3, Blantyre, Malawi
Institute of Infection and Global Health, University of Liverpool, Ronald Ross Building, 8 West Derby Street, Liverpool L69 7BE, UK

Dean Everett
Malawi Liverpool Wellcome Trust Clinical Research Programme, Chichiri 3, Blantyre, Malawi
MRC Centre for Inflammation Research, The Queen's Medical Research Institute, University of Edinburgh, 47 Little France Crescent, Edinburgh EH16 4TJ, UK

Anna Maria Geretti
Institute of Infection and Global Health, University of Liverpool, Ronald Ross Building, 8 West Derby Street, Liverpool L69 7BE, UK

Collins Mitambo
HIV and AIDS Department, Malawi Ministry of Health, Lilongwe, Malawi

Che-Liang Chung
Department of Internal Medicine, Yuanlin Christian Hospital, Changhua, Taiwan

Yen-Fu Chen
Department of Internal Medicine, National Taiwan University Hospital Yunlin Branch, Douliu, Yunlin, Taiwan

Yen-Ting Lin and Jann-Yuan Wang
Department of Internal Medicine, National Taiwan University Hospital, #7, Chung-Shan South Road, Zhongzheng District, Taipei 10002, Taiwan

Shuenn-Wen Kuo and Jin-Shing Chen
Division of Thoracic Surgery, Department of Surgery, National Taiwan University Hospital and National Taiwan University College of Medicine, Taipei, Taiwan

Avital Hirsch, Ilan Gofer, Maya Leventer-Roberts and Ran Balicer
Chief Physician's Office, Clalit Health Services, Clalit Research Institute, Tel Aviv, Israel

Mark A. Katz
Chief Physician's Office, Clalit Health Services, Clalit Research Institute, Tel Aviv, Israel

School of Public Health, Medical School for International Health, Faculty of Health Sciences, Ben Gurion University of the Negev, Beer Sheva, Israel
Department of Epidemiology, University of Michigan School of Public Health, Ann Arbor, MI, USA

Arnold S. Monto, Emily Toth Martin and Ryan E. Malosh
Department of Epidemiology, University of Michigan School of Public Health, Ann Arbor, MI, USA

Alon Laufer Peretz
Rabin Medical Center, Occupational Medicine Department, Petah Tikva, Israel

David Greenberg
Pediatric Infectious Disease Unit, Soroka University Medical Center, Beer Sheva, Israel

Rachael Wendlandt, Gabriella Newes-Adeyi and William Campbell
Abt Associates, Inc, Atlanta, GA, USA

Yonat Shemer Avni
Clinical Virology, Soroka University Medical Center, Ben Gurion University of the Negev, Beer Sheva, Israel

Nadav Davidovitch, Anat Rosenthal and Rachel Gur-Arie
Department of Health Systems Management, School of Public Health, Faculty of Health Sciences, Ben Gurion University of the Negev, Beer Sheva, Israel

Tomer Hertz
Department of Microbiology Immunology and Genetics, Faculty of Health Sciences, Ben Gurion University of the Negev, Beer Sheva, Israel
Vaccine and Infectious Disease Division, Fred Hutch Cancer Research Center, Seattle, WA, USA

Aharona Glatman-Freedman
Israel Center for Disease Control, Ministry of Health, Tel Hashomer, Ramat Gan, Israel
Department of Epidemiology and Preventive Medicine, School of Public Health, Sackler Faculty of Medicine, Tel Aviv University, Tel Aviv, Israel

Eduardo Azziz-Baumgartner, Jill Morris Ferdinands, Min Levine and Mark G. Thompson
Influenza Division, Centers for Disease Control and Prevention (CDC), Atlanta, GA, USA

Joan Manuel Neyra Quijandría
U.S. Naval Medical Research Unit N° 6 - Lima, Lima, Peru

Qingyu Li and Fei Wang
Department of Clinical Pharmacy, Affiliated Hangzhou First People's Hospital, Zhejiang University School of Medicine, Hangzhou, China

Changcheng Shi
Department of Clinical Pharmacy, Affiliated Hangzhou First People's Hospital, Zhejiang University School of Medicine, Hangzhou, China
Department of Clinical Pharmacy, Hangzhou First People's Hospital, Nanjing Medical University, Hangzhou, China

Nengming Lin
Department of Clinical Pharmacy, Affiliated Hangzhou First People's Hospital, Zhejiang University School of Medicine, Hangzhou, China
Department of Clinical Pharmacy, Hangzhou First People's Hospital, Nanjing Medical University, Hangzhou, China
Department of Clinical Pharmacology, Translational Medicine Research Center, Affiliated Hangzhou First People's Hospital, Zhejiang University School of Medicine, Hangzhou, China

Qi Zhang
Department of Clinical Pharmacy, Hangzhou First People's Hospital, Nanjing Medical University, Hangzhou, China

Yubo Xiao
Department of Pharmacometrics, Mosim Co., Ltd, Shanghai, China

Jing Wu
Department of Pharmacy, Hangzhou Obstetrics and Gynecology Hospital, Hangzhou, China

Dezi Kouhounina Batsimba, Alida Malonga-Massanga, Reyna Ibara Ottia, Ghyslain Kimbassa Ngoma, Brice Pembet Singana, Gabriel Ahombo and Simon Charles Kobawila
Faculté des Sciences et Techniques, Université Marien Ngouabi, BP 69, Brazzaville, République du Congo

Pembe Issamou Mayengue and Roch Fabien Niama
Faculté des Sciences et Techniques, Université Marien Ngouabi, BP 69, Brazzaville, République du Congo

Laboratoire National de Santé Publique, BP 120, Brazzaville, République du Congo

Igor Louzolo, Nadia Claricelle Loukabou Bongolo, Lucette Macosso and Henri Joseph Parra
Laboratoire National de Santé Publique, BP 120, Brazzaville, République du Congo

Louis Régis Dossou-Yovo
Laboratoire National de Santé Publique, BP 120, Brazzaville, République du Congo
Ecole Normale Supérieure, Université Marien Ngouabi, BP 69, Brazzaville, République du Congo

Géril Sekangue Obili
Centre Hospitalier Universitaire de Brazzaville, BP 1846, Brazzaville, République du Congo

Naomi Kemunto and Eric Osoro
Paul G. Allen School for Global Animal Health, Washington State University, Pullman, USA
Washington State University Global Health Program Kenya, Nairobi, Kenya

M. Kariuki Njenga and S. M. Thumbi
Paul G. Allen School for Global Animal Health, Washington State University, Pullman, USA
Washington State University Global Health Program Kenya, Nairobi, Kenya
Center for Global Health Research, Kenya Medical Research Institute, Nairobi, Kenya

Eddy Mogoa
Faculty of Veterinary Medicine, University of Nairobi, Nairobi, Kenya

Austin Bitek
Food and Agriculture Organization of the United Nations, Nairobi, Kenya

Peizhen Zhao, Ye Zhang, Cheng Wang and Bin Yang
Dermatology Hospital, Southern Medical University, Guangzhou, China

Weiming Tang
Dermatology Hospital, Southern Medical University, Guangzhou, China
SESH study group of University of North Carolina at Chapel Hill, Guangzhou, China
University of North Carolina at Chapel Hill Project-China, Guangzhou 510095, China
School of Medicine of University of North Carolina at Chapel Hill, Chapel Hill, USA

Li Liu
Nanjing Municipal Center for Disease Control and Prevention, Jiangsu, China

Huanhuan Cheng
The Third Affiliated Hospital, Sun Yat-Sen University, Guangzhou, China

Chuncheng Liu
SESH study group of University of North Carolina at Chapel Hill, Guangzhou, China

Bolin Cao
SESH study group of University of North Carolina at Chapel Hill, Guangzhou, China
University of North Carolina at Chapel Hill Project-China, Guangzhou 510095, China

Joseph D. Tucker
SESH study group of University of North Carolina at Chapel Hill, Guangzhou, China
University of North Carolina at Chapel Hill Project-China, Guangzhou 510095, China
School of Medicine of University of North Carolina at Chapel Hill, Chapel Hill, USA

Chongyi Wei
Social and Behavioral Health Sciences, School of Public Health, Rutgers University, Piscataway, NJ, USA

Mark Anthony Stevenson and Rebecca Justine Traub
Faculty of Veterinary and Agricultural Sciences, University of Melbourne, Parkville, VIC 3052, Australia

Dinh Ng-Nguyen
Faculty of Veterinary and Agricultural Sciences, University of Melbourne, Parkville, VIC 3052, Australia
Faculty of Animal Sciences and Veterinary Medicine, Tay Nguyen University, Dak Lak, Vietnam

Van-Anh Thi Nguyen
Faculty of Animal Sciences and Veterinary Medicine, Tay Nguyen University, Dak Lak, Vietnam

Kathleen Breen
Department of Livestock, Montana Veterinary Diagnostic Lab, Bozeman, MT, USA

Trong Van Phan
Faculty of Medicine and Pharmacy, Tay Nguyen University, Dak Lak, Vietnam

Tinh Van Vo
Department of Physiology, Pathology and Immunology, Pham Ngoc Thach University of Medicine, Ho Chi Minh, Vietnam

Ploenpit Hanond
Department of Microbiology, Faculty of Medicine, Khon Kaen University, Khon Kaen, Thailand

Jureeporn Chuerduangphui, Kanisara Proyrungroj, Chamsai Pientong, Saowarop Hinkan and Tipaya Ekalaksananan
Department of Microbiology, Faculty of Medicine, Khon Kaen University, Khon Kaen, Thailand
HPV and EBV and Carcinogenesis Research Group, Khon Kaen University, Khon Kaen, Thailand

Jiratha Budkaew
Department of Social Medicine, Khon Kaen Center Hospital, Khon Kaen, Thailand

Charinya Pimson
Department of Animal Health Science, Faculty of Agro-Industrial Technology, Kalasin University, Kalasin, Thailand
HPV and EBV and Carcinogenesis Research Group, Khon Kaen University, Khon Kaen, Thailand

Bandit Chumworathayi
Department of Obstetrics and Gynecology, Faculty of Medicine, Khon Kaen University, Khon Kaen, Thailand
HPV and EBV and Carcinogenesis Research Group, Khon Kaen University, Khon Kaen, Thailand

Yun Qian
Department of Orthopedics, Shanghai Jiao Tong University Affiliated Sixth People's Hospital, 600 Yishan Road, Shanghai 200233, People's Republic of China

Cunyi Fan
Department of Orthopedics, Shanghai Jiao Tong University Affiliated Sixth People's Hospital, 600 Yishan Road, Shanghai 200233, People's Republic of China
Department of Orthopedics, Shanghai Sixth People's Hospital East Affiliated to Shanghai University of Medicine and Health Sciences, Shanghai 201306, China

Qixin Han
Center for Reproductive Medicine, Renji Hospital, School of Medicine, Shanghai Jiao Tong University, Shanghai 200135, China
Shanghai Key Laboratory for Assisted Reproduction and Reproductive Genetics, Shanghai 200135, China

Wenjun Liu
Department of Orthopedics, Shanghai Sixth People's Hospital East Affiliated to Shanghai University of Medicine and Health Sciences, Shanghai 201306, China
Taishan Medical University, Taian 271016, China

Wei-En Yuan
Engineering Research Center of Cell and Therapeutic Antibody, Ministry of Education, and School of Pharmacy, Shanghai Jiao Tong University, Shanghai 200240, China

Sören Schubert and Gabriele Liegl
Chair of Medical Microbiology and Hospital Epidemiology, Max von Pettenkofer Institute, Faculty of Medicine, LMU Munich, Marchioninistr. 17, 81377 Munich, Germany

Ahmed Zeynudin
Chair of Medical Microbiology and Hospital Epidemiology, Max von Pettenkofer Institute, Faculty of Medicine, LMU Munich, Marchioninistr. 17, 81377 Munich, Germany
Institute of Health Sciences, Jimma University, Jimma, Ethiopia
Center for International Health (CIH), University of Munich (LMU), 80802 Munich, Germany

Michael Pritsch
Chair of Medical Microbiology and Hospital Epidemiology, Max von Pettenkofer Institute, Faculty of Medicine, LMU Munich, Marchioninistr. 17, 81377 Munich, Germany
Division of Infectious Diseases and Tropical Medicine, Medical Center of the University of Munich (LMU), 80802 Munich, Germany
German Center for Infection Research (DZIF), Partner Site Munich, 80802 Munich, Germany

Andreas Wieser
Chair of Medical Microbiology and Hospital Epidemiology, Max von Pettenkofer Institute, Faculty of Medicine, LMU Munich, Marchioninistr. 17, 81377 Munich, Germany
Institute of Health Sciences, Jimma University, Jimma, Ethiopia
Division of Infectious Diseases and Tropical Medicine, Medical Center of the University of Munich (LMU), 80802 Munich, Germany

German Center for Infection Research (DZIF), Partner Site Munich, 80802 Munich, Germany

Tefara Belachew
Institute of Health Sciences, Jimma University, Jimma, Ethiopia

Michael Hoelscher
Center for International Health (CIH), University of Munich (LMU), 80802 Munich, Germany
Division of Infectious Diseases and Tropical Medicine, Medical Center of the University of Munich (LMU), 80802 Munich, Germany
German Center for Infection Research (DZIF), Partner Site Munich, 80802 Munich, Germany

Maxim Messerer
Plant Genome and Systems Biology, Helmholtz Center Munich, German Research Center for Environmental Health, 85764 Neuherberg, Germany

Kaidi Telling and Irja Lutsar
Department of Microbiology, Institute of Biomedicine and Translational Medicine, University of Tartu, Ravila 19, 50411 Tartu, Estonia

Mailis Laht, Veljo Kisand and Tanel Tenson
Institute of Technology, University of Tartu, Tartu, Estonia

Age Brauer and Maido Remm
Institute of Molecular and Cell Biology, University of Tartu, Tartu, Estonia

Matti Maimets
Department of Infection Control, Tartu University Hospital, Tartu, Estonia

Nguyen Thanh Long and Nguyen Dinh Hong Phuc
Department of Infectious Diseases, Hanoi Medical University, no 1 Ton That Tung street, Dong Da district, Hanoi, Vietnam

Vu Quoc Dat
Department of Infectious Diseases, Hanoi Medical University, no 1 Ton That Tung street, Dong Da district, Hanoi, Vietnam
Wellcome Trust Major Overseas Programme, Oxford University Clinical Research Unit, Hanoi, 78 Giai Phong street, Dong Da district, Hanoi, Vietnam
National Hospital for Tropical Diseases, 78 Giai Phong street, Dong Da district, Hanoi, Vietnam

Ana Bonell
Wellcome Trust Major Overseas Programme, Oxford University Clinical Research Unit, Hanoi, 78 Giai Phong street, Dong Da district, Hanoi, Vietnam

H. Rogier van Doorn and Behzad Nadjm
Wellcome Trust Major Overseas Programme, Oxford University Clinical Research Unit, Hanoi, 78 Giai Phong street, Dong Da district, Hanoi, Vietnam
Nuffield Department of Clinical Medicine, Centre for Tropical Medicine, University of Oxford, Oxford, UK

Nguyen Van Kinh
National Hospital for Tropical Diseases, 78 Giai Phong street, Dong Da district, Hanoi, Vietnam

Nguyen Vu Trung
National Hospital for Tropical Diseases, 78 Giai Phong street, Dong Da district, Hanoi, Vietnam
Department of Microbiology, Hanoi Medical University, no 1 Ton That Tung street, Dong Da district, Hanoi, Vietnam

Vu Ngoc Hieu
Department of Microbiology, Hanoi Medical University, no 1 Ton That Tung street, Dong Da district, Hanoi, Vietnam

Liping Yan, Heping Xiao and Qing Zhang
Department of Tuberculosis, Shanghai Pulmonary Hospital, Tongji University School of Medicine, 507 Zhengmin Road, Shanghai 200433, People's Republic of China

Ons Haddad, Aida Elargoubi, Hajer Rhim, Yosr Kadri and Maha Mastouri
Laboratoire de Microbiologie, CHU Fatouma Bourguiba de Monastir, Monastir, Tunisie
Laboratoire des Maladies Transmissible et Substances Biologiquement Actives, LR99ES27, Faculté de Pharmacie de Monastir, Université de Monastir, Monastir, Tunisie

Abderrahmen Merghni
Laboratoire des Maladies Transmissible et Substances Biologiquement Actives, LR99ES27, Faculté de Pharmacie de Monastir, Université de Monastir, Monastir, Tunisie

Tomas Reischig, Martin Kacer and Mirko Bouda
Department of Internal Medicine I, Faculty of Medicine in Pilsen, Charles University, Czech Republic and Teaching Hospital, 30460 Pilsen, Czech Republic
Biomedical Centre, Faculty of Medicine in Pilsen, Charles University, 32300 Pilsen, Czech Republic

Petra Hruba
Biomedical Centre, Faculty of Medicine in Pilsen, Charles University, 32300 Pilsen, Czech Republic
Transplant Laboratory, Institute for Clinical and Experimental Medicine, 14021 Prague, Czech Republic

Daniel Lysak
Biomedical Centre, Faculty of Medicine in Pilsen, Charles University, 32300 Pilsen, Czech Republic
Department of Hemato-oncology, Teaching Hospital, 30460 Pilsen, Czech Republic

Ondrej Hes
Biomedical Centre, Faculty of Medicine in Pilsen, Charles University, 32300 Pilsen, Czech Republic
Department of Pathology, Faculty of Medicine in Pilsen, Charles University, Czech Republic and Teaching Hospital, 30460 Pilsen, Czech Republic

Stanislav Kormunda
Biomedical Centre, Faculty of Medicine in Pilsen, Charles University, 32300 Pilsen, Czech Republic
Division of Information Technologies and Statistics, Faculty of Medicine in Pilsen, Charles University, 32300 Pilsen, Czech Republic

Hana Hermanova
Department of Hemato-oncology, Teaching Hospital, 30460 Pilsen, Czech Republic

Evanson Z. Sambala and Anelisa Jaca
Cochrane South Africa, South African Medical Research Council, Box 19070, Cape Town, PO 7505, South Africa

Chinwe Juliana Iwu
Cochrane South Africa, South African Medical Research Council, Box 19070, Cape Town, PO 7505, South Africa
Division of Health Systems and Public Health, Department of Global Health, Faculty of Medicine and Health Sciences, Stellenbosch University, Cape Town, South Africa

Charles S. Wiysonge
Cochrane South Africa, South African Medical Research Council, Box 19070, Cape Town, PO 7505, South Africa
Division of Epidemiology and Biostatistics, School of Public Health and Family Medicine, University of Cape Town, Cape Town, South Africa
Centre for Evidence-Based Health Care, Division of Epidemiology and Biostatistics, Department of Global Health, Faculty of Medicine and Health Sciences, Stellenbosch University, Cape Town, South Africa

Tiwonge Kanyenda
Vaccines for Africa Initiative, Division of Medical Microbiology and Institute of Infectious Disease and Molecular Medicine, University of Cape Town, Cape Town, South Africa

Chidozie Declan Iwu
Department of Biochemistry and Microbiology, University of Fort Hare, Alice, South Africa

Karla T. Tafur, Cynthia Pinedo, Carmen Contreras, Roger Calderon and Milagros J. Mendoza
Socios En Salud Sucursal Perú, Av. Túpac Amaru 4480, Comas, Lima, Peru

Leonid Lecca
Socios En Salud Sucursal Perú, Av. Túpac Amaru 4480, Comas, Lima, Peru
Department of Global Health and Social Medicine, Harvard Medical School,
Boston, MA, USA

Julia Coit, Segundo R. Leon and Molly F. Franke
Department of Global Health and Social Medicine, Harvard Medical School,
Boston, MA, USA

Silvia S. Chiang
Department of Pediatrics, Alpert Medical School of Brown University, Providence, RI, USA
Center for International Health Research. Rhode Island Hospital, Providence, RI, USA

Talita Rantin Belucci
Hospital Israelita Albert Einstein, São Paulo, Brazil
Division of Medical Practice, Hospital Israelita Albert Einstein, Avenida Albert Einstein, 627 - bloco A1, 1° andar, Morumbi, São Paulo 05651-901, Brazil

Paula Kiyomi Onaga Yokota and Oscar Fernando Pavão dos Santos
Division of Medical Practice, Hospital Israelita Albert Einstein, Avenida Albert Einstein, 627 -bloco A1, 1° andar, Morumbi, São Paulo 05651-901, Brazil

Alexandre R. Marra
Division of Medical Practice, Hospital Israelita Albert Einstein, Avenida Albert Einstein, 627 -bloco A1, 1° andar, Morumbi, São Paulo 05651-901, Brazil
Office of Clinical Quality, Safety and Performance Improvement, University of Iowa Hospitals and Clinics, Iowa City, IA, USA

Michael B. Edmond
Office of Clinical Quality, Safety and Performance Improvement, University of Iowa Hospitals and Clinics, Iowa City, IA, USA
Division of Infectious Diseases, Department of Internal Medicine, University of Iowa Carver College of Medicine, Iowa City, IA, USA

João Renato Rebello Pinho
Clinical Laboratory, Hospital Israelita Albert Einstein, São Paulo, Brazil
LIM 03/07, Faculdade de Medicina da USP, São Paulo, Brazil

Ana Carolina Cintra Nunes Mafra
Statistics Department, Instituto Israelita de Ensino e Pesquisa Albert Einstein, Hospital Israelita Albert Einstein, São Paulo, Brazil
Núcleo de Indicadores e Sistemas de Informações, Hospital Israelita Albert Einstein, São Paulo, Brazil

Ewa Janczewska and Brygida Adamek
Department of Basic Medical Sciences, School of Public Health in Bytom, Medical University of Silesia, ID Clinic, Janowska 19, 41-400 Mysłowice, Bytom, Poland

Dorota Zarębska-Michaluk
Department of Infectious Diseases, Wojewódzki Szpital Zespolony, Kielce, Poland

Hanna Berak
Hospital of Infectious Diseases, Warszawa, Poland

Anna Piekarska
Department of Infectious Diseases and Hepatology, Medical University of Łódź, Łódź, Poland

Andrzej Gietka
Department of Internal Medicine and Hepatology, Central Clinical Hospital of the MSWiA, Warszawa, Poland

Dorota Dybowska and Waldemar Halota
Department of Infectious Diseases and Hepatology, Faculty of Medicine, Collegium Medicum Bydgoszcz, Nicolaus Copernicus University Toruń, Bydgoszcz, Poland

Włodzimierz Mazur
Department of Infectious Diseases, Infectious Hepatology and Acquired Immunodeficiency, Medical University of Silesia in Katowice, Chorzów, Poland

Teresa Belica-Wdowik and Barbara Baka-Ćwierz
Regional Center for Diagnosis and Treatment of Viral Hepatitis and Hepatology, John Paul II Hospital, Kraków, Poland

Witold Dobracki
MED-FIX Medical Center, Wrocław, Poland

Magdalena Tudrujek-Zdunek and Krzysztof Tomasiewicz
Department of Infectious Diseases, Medical University of Lublin, Lublin, Poland

Zbigniew Deroń
Ward of Infectious Diseases and Hepatology, Biegański Regional Specialist Hospital, Łódź, Poland

Iwona Buczyńska and Krzysztof Simon
Department of Infectious Diseases and Hepatology, Wrocław Medical University, Wrocław, Poland

Marek Sitko and Aleksander Garlicki
Department of Infectious and Tropical Diseases, Collegium Medicum, Jagiellonian University, Kraków, Poland

Agnieszka Czauż-Andrzejuk and Robert Flisiak
Department of Infectious Diseases and Hepatology, Medical University of Białystok, Białystok, Poland

Beata Lorenc
Pomeranian Center of Infectious Diseases, Department of Infectious Diseases, Medical University of Gdansk, Gdansk, Poland

Jolanta Białkowska-Warzecha
Department of Infectious and Liver Diseases, Medical University of Łódź, Łódź, Poland

Jolanta Citko
Medical Practice of Infections, Regional Hospital, Olsztyn, Poland

Łukasz Laurans, Łukasz Socha and Marta Wawrzynowicz-Syczewska
Department of Infectious Diseases, Hepatology and Liver Transplantation, Pomeranian Medical University, Szczecin, Poland

Jerzy Jaroszewicz
Department of Infectious Diseases and Hepatology, Medical University of Silesia in Katowice, Bytom, Poland

Olga Tronina
Department of Transplantation Medicine, Nephrology, and Internal Diseases, Medical University of Warsaw, Warszawa, Poland

Andrzej Horban
Warsaw Medical University and Hospital of Infectious Diseases Warszawa, Warszawa, Poland

Lianxin Liu
Department of Hepatobiliary Surgery, the First Affiliated Hospital of Harbin Medical University. Key Laboratory of Hepatosplenic Surgery, Ministry of Education, No. 23 Youzheng Street, Harbin 150001, China

Yuxing Ni
Department of Hospital Infection Control, Rui Jin Hospital, Shanghai Jiao Tong University School of Medicine, No. 197 Rui-Jin 2nd Road, Shanghai 200025, China

M. Bahena-Román and V. Madrid-Marina
Chronic Infectious Diseases and Cancer Division, Center for Research on Infectious Diseases, Instituto Nacional de Salud Pública (INSP), Cuernavaca, Morelos, Mexico

K. Torres-Poveda
Chronic Infectious Diseases and Cancer Division, Center for Research on Infectious Diseases, Instituto Nacional de Salud Pública (INSP), Cuernavaca, Morelos, Mexico
CONACYT-INSP, Cuernavaca, Morelos, Mexico

K. Delgado-Romero
Centro de Atención para la Salud de la Mujer (CAPASAM) (Center for Women's Health), Health Services of the State of Morelos, Cuernavaca, Mexico

Daphne A. van Wees and Janneke C. M. Heijne
Centre for Infectious Disease Control, National Institute for Public Health and the Environment, Bilthoven, The Netherlands

Mirjam E. E. Kretzschmar
Centre for Infectious Disease Control, National Institute for Public Health and the Environment, Bilthoven, The Netherlands
Julius Centre for Health Sciences and Primary Care, University Medical Centre Utrecht, Utrecht, The Netherlands

Chantal den Daas
Centre for Infectious Disease Control, National Institute for Public Health and the Environment, Bilthoven, The Netherlands
Department of Interdisciplinary Social Science, Faculty of Social and Behavioural Sciences, Utrecht University, Utrecht, The Netherlands

Titia Heijman
Public Health Service Amsterdam, Amsterdam, The Netherlands

Karlijn C. J. G. Kampman
Public Health Service Twente, Enschede, The Netherlands

Karin Westra
Public Health Service Hollands Noorden, Alkmaar, The Netherlands

Anne de Vries
Public Health Service Kennemerland, Haarlem, The Netherlands

José Ángel Cuenca-Gómez, Ana Belén Lozano-Serrano, María Teresa Cabezas-Fernández, Manuel Jesús Soriano-Pérez, Isabel Cabeza-Barrera and Joaquín Salas-Coronas
Tropical Medicine Unit, Hospital de Poniente, Carretera de Almerimar s/n, PD: 07400 Almería, El Ejido, Spain

José Vázquez-Villegas
Tropical Medicine Unit, Distrito Poniente, Almería, Spain

Matías Estévez-Escobar
Digestive Service, Hospital de Poniente, Almería, El Ejido, Spain.

Andrea Giacomelli, Agostino Riva, Maria Letizia Oreni, Giulia Renisi, Valentina Di Cristo, Angelica Lupo, Stefano Rusconi, Massimo Galli and Anna Lisa Ridolfo
Infectious Diseases Unit, DIBIC Luigi Sacco - University of Milan, Via G.B. Grassi, 74, 20157 Milan, Italy

Felicia Stefania Falvella, Dario Cattaneo and Stefania Cheli
ASST Fatebenefratelli-Sacco, Clinical Pharmacology Unit, Milan, Italy

Emilio Clementi
ASST Fatebenefratelli-Sacco, Clinical Pharmacology Unit, Milan, Italy
E. Medea Scientific Institute, Bosisio Parini, Italy

Tao Shi
Department of Orthopedics, The Third Affiliated Hospital of Chongqing Medical University (Gener Hospital), No. 1, Shuanghu Branch Road, Yubei District, Chongqing 401120, China

Tongxin Li, Jungang Li and Jing Wang
Department of Clinical Laboratory, Public Health Medical Center, No. 109, Baoyu Road, Shapingba District, Chongqing 400036, China

Zehua Zhang
Department of Orthopedics, Southwest Hospital, Third Military Medical University, No. 30, Gaotanyan Main Street, Shapingba District, Chongqing 400038, China

Ronald M. Galiwango
Department of Immunology, University of Toronto, Toronto, Canada

Rupert Kaul
Department of Immunology, University of Toronto, Toronto, Canada
Department of Medicine, University of Toronto, Toronto, Canada

Sergey Yegorov
Department of Immunology, University of Toronto, Toronto, Canada
Present address: Faculty of Education and Humanities, Suleyman Demirel University, Almaty, Kazakhstan

Sara V. Good
Genetics and Genome Biology Program, The Hospital for Sick Children, Toronto, Canada
Community Health Sciences, University of Manitoba, Winnipeg, Canada

Juliet Mpendo
Uganda Virus Research Institute -International AIDS Vaccine Initiative HIV Vaccine Program, Entebbe, Uganda

Noah Kiwanuka
Uganda Virus Research Institute -International AIDS Vaccine Initiative HIV Vaccine Program, Entebbe, Uganda
Department of Epidemiology and Biostatistics, School of Public Health, College of Health Sciences, Makerere University, Kampala, Uganda

Bernard S. Bagaya
Uganda Virus Research Institute -International AIDS Vaccine Initiative HIV Vaccine Program, Entebbe, Uganda
Department of Immunology and Molecular Biology, School of Biomedical Sciences, College of Health Sciences, Makerere University, Kampala, Uganda

Egbert Tannich
Bernhard Nocht Institute for Tropical Medicine, Hamburg, Germany

Andrea K. Boggild
Department of Medicine, University of Toronto, Toronto, Canada
Public Health Ontario Laboratories, Toronto, Canada

Index

www.ingramcontent.com/pod-product-compliance
Lightning Source LLC
Chambersburg PA
CBHW061313190326
41458CB00011B/3794
* 9 7 8 1 6 3 2 4 1 6 5 0 6 *